Hip & Pelvis Injuries in Sports Medicine

Hip & Pelvis Injuries in Sports Medicine

Carlos A. Guanche, MD

Southern California Orthopaedic Institute
Van Nuys, CA

Wolters Kluwer | Lippincott Williams & Wilkins
Health

Philadelphia • Baltimore • New York • London
Buenos Aires • Hong Kong • Sydney • Tokyo

Acquisitions Editor: Robert Hurley
Product Manager: Dave Murphy
Production Manager: Bridgett Dougherty
Senior Manufacturing Manager: Benjamin Rivera
Marketing Manager: Lisa Parry
Design Coordinator: Doug Smock
Production Service: SPi Technologies

Printed in China

Library of Congress Cataloging-in-Publication Data
978-0-7817-7771-1
0-7817-7771-2

Library of Congress Cataloging-in-Publication Data
Hip and pelvis injuries in sports medicine/[edited by] Carlos A. Guanche. — 1st ed.
p. ; cm.
Includes bibliographical references and index.
ISBN 978-0-7817-7771-1 (alk. paper)
1. Hip joint—Wounds and injuries. 2. Pelvis—Wounds and injuries. 3. Sports injuries.
I. Guanche, Carlos A.
[DNLM: 1. Hip Injuries—diagnosis. 2. Hip Injuries—therapy. 3. Athletic Injuries.
4. Pelvis—injuries. WE 855 H66725 2010]

RD549.H497 2010
617.5' 81044—dc22

2009022056

Care has been taken to confirm the accuracy of the information presented and to describe generally accepted practices. However, the authors, editors, and publisher are not responsible for errors or omissions or for any consequences from application of the information in this book and make no warranty, expressed or implied, with respect to the currency, completeness, or accuracy of the contents of the publication. Application of the information in a particular situation remains the professional responsibility of the practitioner.

The authors, editors, and publisher have exerted every effort to ensure that drug selection and dosage set forth in this text are in accordance with current recommendations and practice at the time of publication. However, in view of ongoing research, changes in government regulations, and the constant flow of information relating to drug therapy and drug reactions, the reader is urged to check the package insert for each drug for any change in indications and dosage and for added warnings and precautions. This is particularly important when the recommended agent is a new or infrequently employed drug.

Some drugs and medical devices presented in the publication have Food and Drug Administration (FDA) clearance for limited use in restricted research settings. It is the responsibility of the health care provider to ascertain the FDA status of each drug or device planned for use in their clinical practice.

To purchase additional copies of this book, call our customer service department at (800) 638-3030 or fax orders to (301) 223-2320. International customers should call (301) 223-2300.

Visit Lippincott Williams & Wilkins on the Internet: at LWW.com. Lippincott Williams & Wilkins customer service representatives are available from 8:30 am to 6 pm, EST.

10 9 8 7 6 5 4 3 2 1

CCS1009

To my wife, Anna
My inspiration

Contributing Authors

Michael B. Banffy, MD
Resident in Orthopaedic Surgery
Department of Orthopaedic Surgery
Harvard Combined Orthopaedic Residency Program
Boston, MA

Aaron A. Bare, MD
OAD Orthopaedics
Warrenville, IL

James Bond, MD
Oklahoma Sports and Orthopaedics Institute
Oklahoma University Health Sciences Center
Department of Orthopaedics and Rehabilitation
Oklahoma City, OK

Karen K. Briggs, MPH
Steadman Hawkins Clinic
Steadman Hawkins Research Foundation
Vail, CO

Adam G. Brooks, BA
Keck School of Medicine
University of Southern California
Los Angeles, CA

Javier Camacho-Galindo, MD
Assistant Professor of Hip and Knee Surgery
Universidad Nacional Autónoma de México
Service of Adult Hip and Knee Reconstruction
National Rehabilitation Institute of Mexico
Mexico City, Mexico

Kevin S. Caperton, MD
Oklahoma University Health Sciences Center
Department of Orthopaedics and Rehabilitation
Oklahoma City, OK

C. Chambliss Harrod
Resident in Orthopaedic Surgery
Department of Orthopaedic Surgery
Harvard Combined Orthopaedic Residency Program
Boston, MA

Benjamin G. Domb, MD
Orthopaedic Sports Medicine and Hip Injuries
Loyola University Chicago
Hinsdale Orthopaedic Associates

Andrew Ebert, MD
Oklahoma University Health Sciences Center
Department of Orthopaedics and Rehabilitation
Oklahoma City, OK

Gary B. Fetzer, MD
TRIA Orthopaedic Center
Minneapolis, MN

David A. Fischer, MD
TRIA Orthopaedic Center
Minneapolis, MN

Hollis M. Fritts, MD
Center for Diagnostic Imaging
St Louis Park, MN

Reinhold Ganz, MD
Professor emeritus
Department of Orthopaedic Surgery
Inselspital
University of Berne
Berne, Switzerland

Michael W. Geary, MD
Sports Medicine Fellowship
Southern California Orthopaedic Institute
Van Nuys, CA

Pau Golanó, MD
Laboratory of Arthroscopic and Surgical Anatomy
Department of Pathology and Experimental Therapeutics
(Human Anatomy Unit)
University of Barcelona
Barcelona, Spain

Carlos A. Guanche, MD
Southern California Orthopaedic Institute
Van Nuys, CA

Mitchel B. Harris, MD, FACS
Associate Professor
Department of Orthopaedic Surgery
Harvard Medical School
Brigham & Women's Hospital
Boston, MA

Connor J. Hay, BA
Steadman Hawkins Clinic
Steadman Hawkins Research Foundation
Vail, CO

Benton E. Heyworth, MD
Orthopaedic Surgery Resident
Department of Orthopaedic Surgery
Hospital for Special Surgery
New York, NY

George P. Hobbs, MD
Assistant Professor of Radiology
Musculoskeletal Staff
Methodist Hospital Division
Thomas Jefferson University Hospital
Philadelphia, PA

Devyani Hunt, MD
Assistant Professor
Section of Physical Medicine and Rehabilitation
Department of Orthopaedic Surgery
Washington University School of Medicine
St. Louis, MO

Victor M. Ilizaliturri Jr, MD
Professor of Hip and Knee Surgery
Universidad Nacional Autónoma de México
Chief of Adult Hip and Knee Reconstruction
National Rehabilitation Institute of Mexico
Mexico City, Mexico

Bryan T. Kelly, MD
Assistant Attending
Orthopaedic Surgeon
Department of Orthopaedic Surgery
Hospital for Special Surgery
Assistant Professor
Department of Orthopaedic Surgery
New York-Presbyterian Hospital
Weill Medical College
New York, NY

David A. Kuppersmith, BS
Steadman Hawkins Clinic
Steadman Hawkins Research Foundation
Vail, CO

Jason Kurian, MD
Orthopedic & Fracture Clinic
Portland, OR

Christopher M. Larson, MD
Director of Education
Minnesota Sports Medicine Fellowship Program
Minnesota Orthopaedic Sports Medicine Institute
Eden Prairie, MN

Martin L. Lazarus, MD
Vice Chairman
Academic Affairs
Associate Professor of Radiology
Chief, Section of Musculoskeletal Radiology and Sports Medicine Imaging
Evanston Hospital
NorthShore University Health System
University of Chicago Pritzker School of Medicine
Department of Radiology
Evanston, IL

Michael Leunig, MD
Department of Orthopaedics
Hip Service
Schulthess Clinic
Zürich, Switzerland
Associate Professor
University of Bern
Switzerland

Greg Lovell, MBBS, Dip DHM, FACSP
Sports Physician
Department of Sports Medicine
Australian Institute of Sport
Bruce ACT, Australia

Travis G. Maak, MD
Hospital for Special Surgery
New York, NY

Benjamin A. MacArthur, BS
Medical Student
Baylor College of Medicine
Houston, TX

Luis Pérez-Carro, MD, PhD
Department of Orthopedic and Trauma Surgery
Centro Médico Lealtad and Hospital Universitario Marqués de Valdecilla
Santander, Spain

Marc J. Philippon, MD
Steadman Hawkins Clinic
Steadman Hawkins Research Foundation
Vail, CO

Heidi Prather, DO
Associate Professor
Chief, Section of Physical Medicine and Rehabilitation
Department of Orthopaedic Surgery
Washington University School of Medicine
St. Louis, MO

Anil S. Ranawat, MD
Assistant Attending
Hospital for Special Surgery
Instructor
Weill Medical College of Cornell University
New York, NY

Andrew J. Schoenfeld, MD
Orthopaedic Spine Fellow
Department of Orthopaedic Surgery
Harvard Medical School
Brigham & Women's Hospital
Boston, MA

Jon K. Sekiya, MD
Associate Professor
University of Michigan
MedSport—Department of Orthopaedic Surgery
Ann Arbor, MI

J. W. Thomas Byrd, MD
Nashville Sports Medicine Foundation
Nashville, TN

Alexander Tomic-Loftkjaer, MD
Clinical and Research Fellow of Hip and Knee Surgery
Service of Adult and Knee Reconstruction
National Rehabilitation Institute of Mexico
Mexico City, Mexico

Jeffrey R. Vargo, PT
CEO
Vargo Physical Therapy, Inc
Westlake Village, CA

Jordi Vega, MD
Department of Orthopedic and Trauma Surgery
Hospital Asepeyo Sant Cugat
Sant Cugat del Vallès
Barcelona, Spain

James E. Voos, MD
Hospital for Special Surgery
New York, NY

Mark R. Williams, MD
Visiting Fellow
Department of Orthopaedics
Hip Service
Schulthess Clinic
Zürich, Switzerland

Erik J. Wolpert, PT
Partner and Regional Director
Vargo Physical Therapy
Valencia, CA

Brett Wolters, MD
Orthopaedic Surgeon and Sports Medicine
Department of Orthopaedics
Springfield Clinic
Springfield, IL

Adam C. Zoga, MD
Associate Professor of Radiology
Director of Musculoskeletal MRI and Ambulatory Imaging Services
Program Director
Musculoskeletal and Combined MRI Fellowships
Thomas Jefferson University Hospital
Philadelphia, PA

Introduction

It is safe to say that over the last 10 years an explosion in the knowledge of the hip joint has occurred. The treatment of many entities that were previously unrecognized is now commonplace around the world. In the past, many patients with significant hip pathologies were told to simply modify their lifestyles and seek nonoperative avenues of treatment (including chronic pain management) since a firm diagnosis for many of their problems was not obvious.

This book is a response to the need for education in the diagnosis and management of a variety of hip conditions that were previously unknown or unrecognized. It is the first comprehensive attempt to catalog much hip pathology that we are just now beginning to understand. While there are a plethora of books dealing with the surgical reconstruction of the hip joint with the use of implants, this book is different. It covers many of the other problems that do not require a hip replacement. Many team physicians are not familiar with a lot of these diagnoses and their specific treatment algorithms, but certainly need to understand them to provide comprehensive care to their athletes. In putting together this book, I hope to stimulate further knowledge and research in the area so that the hip joint can be looked at comprehensively, much like the knee, shoulder and other joints with which we are so familiar.

Contents

CHAPTER

1

Pau Golanó
Jordi Vega
Luis Pérez-Carro
James Bond
Andrew Ebert
Kevin S. Caperton

Hip Anatomy for the Arthroscopist: Gross Anatomy

An intimate knowledge of the anatomy of the hip is a prerequisite for any orthopaedic surgeon interested in performing arthroscopy of this joint. Nonetheless, in this chapter we will not attempt to describe hip anatomy in meticulous detail—the classic anatomy texts accomplish this task to perfection—but instead to provide anatomic information that is useful and applicable to performing arthroscopic procedures in this region.

The hip joint is a highly constrained diarthrodial articulation with a configuration most analogous to a ball and socket. It possesses several anatomic characteristics that make it more complex than other regions or articulations for undertaking arthroscopic techniques. The acetabulum has a fibrocartilaginous rim that grips the femoral head. This configuration, together with a strong surrounding fibrous capsule and ligament complex, makes arthroscopic access to the joint difficult. In addition, the large muscle groups around the hip relegate the joint to a deep plane, further complicating the arthroscopic approach. Finally, the hip region is crossed by numerous vessels and nerves, which are essential for proper functioning of the limb and are susceptible to injury during arthroscopic access. Because of these factors, arthroscopic surgery of the hip is complicated by the requirement for longer instruments and more difficult triangulation with greater depth from the working surface. Thus, before contemplating hip arthroscopy, it is important for the surgeon to have not only a detailed anatomic knowledge of the region but also considerable experience in the arthroscopic techniques used in other joints.

TOPOGRAPHIC ANATOMY OF THE HIP

Topography is the first challenge the orthopaedic surgeon will encounter in the evaluation and management of hip disease; therefore, it must be mastered. Because the hip is a deep articulation, a proper understanding of the surface anatomy is essential for surgical tasks in and around the joint. The surface features of the region will orient us to the location of key anatomic structures relevant to arthroscopic procedures. The value of the surface references is made clear by the difficulty encountered when attempting to perform a routine procedure in a joint with distorted or absent topography.

In the surface anatomy of the hip region, it is possible to palpate the greater trochanter, anterior superior iliac spine (ASIS), iliac crest, posterior superior iliac spine, anterior inferior iliac spine (AIIS), pubic symphysis, and ischial tuberosity (Fig. 1.1). As related to arthroscopy, the main surface references to be aware of are the greater trochanter and ASIS. The iliac crest and the ASIS are easily palpable in the majority of patients. The AIIS lies inferior and slightly medial to the ASIS. Laterally, on the outer proximal portion of the thigh, the greater trochanter can be seen and palpated as a flattened, depressed area. A line extending horizontally from the tip of the greater trochanter will intersect the center of the acetabulum (Fig. 1.1). The reference provided by the greater trochanter can vary depending on the position of the leg; hence, it must be repeatedly localized by palpation when the position changes.

THE HIP JOINT

The hip is a diarthrotic joint formed by the surface of the acetabulum and the head of the femur (Fig. 1.2A–C). These two highly congruent juxtaposed articular surfaces are lubricated by fluid from the synovial lining and are surrounded by a strong capsule and ligament complex. The architecture of the joint provides a nearly exact match between the cuplike acetabulum and femoral head and makes the freely mobile articulation perfectly suited for weight-bearing locomotion. In addition, the configuration of the bony architecture provides inherent stability and limits overall range of motion, while allowing multiaxial articulation and minimizing the need for soft tissue constraint. Because of these characteristics, the hip joint plays a pivotal role in lower extremity gait advancement and can bear up to four times the body weight during walking.[1]

The acetabulum is a confluence of the ilium, superiorly; the ischium, laterally and inferiorly; and the pubis, medially. These

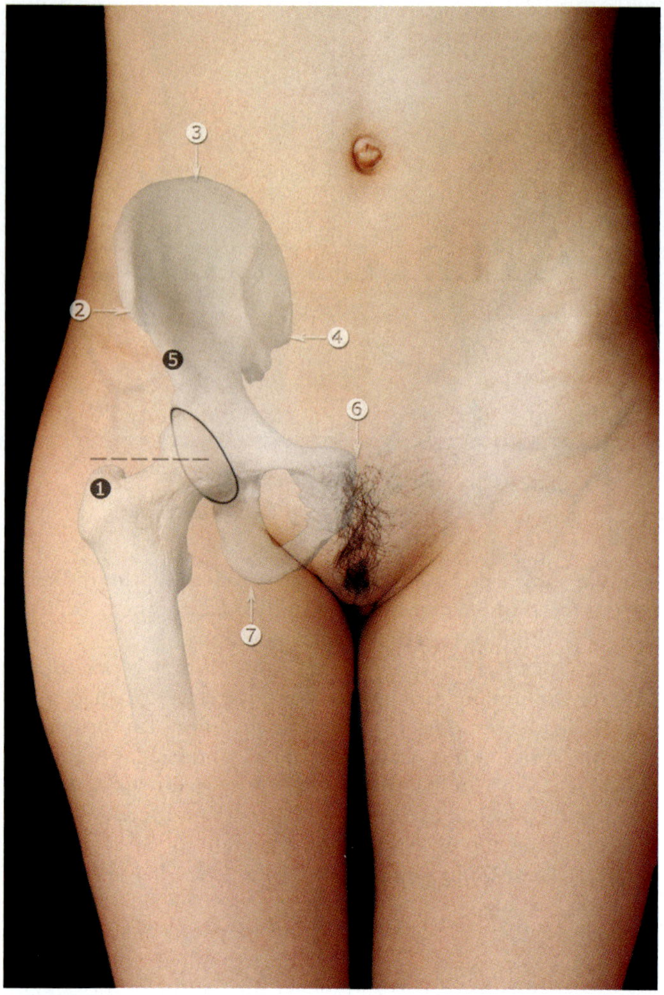

Figure 1.1. Surface anatomy of the hip region. **1.** Greater trochanter. **2.** Anterior superior iliac spine. **3.** Iliac crest. **4.** Posterior superior iliac spine. **5.** Anterior inferior iliac spine. **6.** Pubic symphysis. **7.** Ischial tuberosity. The discontinued line extending horizontally from the tip of the greater trochanter goes to the center of the acetabulum. (Figure copyright © Pau Golano)

three bones fuse at the triradiate cartilage during growth and development to form the coxal bone or innominate bone (Fig. 1.3). The acetabulum is hemispheric in shape and is partially covered at the weight-bearing surface by articular cartilage, creating a lunate-shaped cartilage configuration, the lunate articular surface, with a nonarticular portion in the center and inferior regions. This lunate-shaped cartilage is the thickest at its most superior portion owing to the load it bears during ambulation. At the anteroinferior region of the acetabulum, there is a focal bone indentation, the acetabular notch, which is spanned by the transverse ligament. The central, nonarticular cavity or acetabular fossa, often referred to as the cotyloid fossa, contains the pulvinar and ligamentum teres (Figs. 1.4 & 1.5). The bony acetabulum has a fibrocartilaginous rim, the labrum, that increases the depth and extension of the cotyloid fossa. The acetabular labrum the ligamentum teres and pulvinar are important structures to recognize during hip arthroscopy; thus, they will be explained in detail in the chapter on arthroscopic anatomy (Fig. 1.5).

The ball portion of the hip joint is comprised of the femoral head, which is reciprocally shaped to the acetabular socket, but is not perfectly congruent. The head is conceptualized as two-thirds of a sphere, but during development becomes more ovoid than spherical. The head is attached at its base to the femoral neck, and the neck is attached distally to the femoral shaft. The femoral head is fully encased in articular cartilage, except the fovea capitis. Similar to the acetabulum, the thickest portion of cartilage lies in the position of greatest load bearing. This anterolateral area corresponds to the region of the head opposed to the superior dome of the acetabulum. In the area posterior and slightly inferior to the true center of the femoral head, there is a small depression corresponding to the femoral insertion site of the ligamentum teres. This small depression, the only area of the femoral head that is not covered by articular cartilage, is the fovea capitis (Figs. 1.6 & 1.7).[2]

When performing the arthroscopic portals, it is important to be aware of the spatial orientation of the two components of the hip joint to avert injury to the joint cartilage. Anatomically, the coxal bone is described from an anteroposterior and lateromedial view. Nevertheless, this bone has an oblique orientation that is demonstrated radiographically in the outlet view in which the X-ray beam is aimed in a caudal to cephalad direction to obtain a true anteroposterior view of the pelvis. Because the acetabulum has 30° to 40° of inferior and lateral inclination, it overhangs the femoral head, forming a partial roof that comprises the weight-bearing dome.[3] In addition, the acetabulum is usually oriented in approximately 20° of anteversion compared to the sagittal plane, but this position can vary considerably, even to the point of retroversion. As is the case of the acetabulum, the femoral portion of the hip joint has several important angular relationships. Distally, the angle subtended by the axis of the femoral shaft and neck averages 125° in adulthood. Together with acetabular anteversion, there is femoral anteversion. This is produced as the transverse axis of the neck averaging 15° anterior to the epicondylar axis of the femur.

THE CAPSULOLIGAMENTOUS COMPLEX OF THE HIP JOINT

The capsule of the hip joint is in intimate relationship with the extra-articular ligamentous structures of the hip (intrinsic ligaments), and these elements form a strong capsuloligamentous complex. This complex, which reaches a thickness of 0.5 cm in some parts, is the most important stabilizer of the joint (Fig. 1.8).

The capsule encases the hip joint from the acetabulum to the base of the femoral neck. Anatomically, the posterior capsular insertion on the femur is more proximal than the anterior insertion, and the posterior wall of the acetabular fossa together with the strong labrum occupies a great part of this area, reducing the volume of the posterior region of the peripheral compartment. The joint capsule has several reinforcing elements. The most important of these is the zona orbicularis or annular ligament, a thick bundle of fibers circularly arranged in the medial, deep region of the capsule that forms a reinforcing ring around the femoral neck. This structure

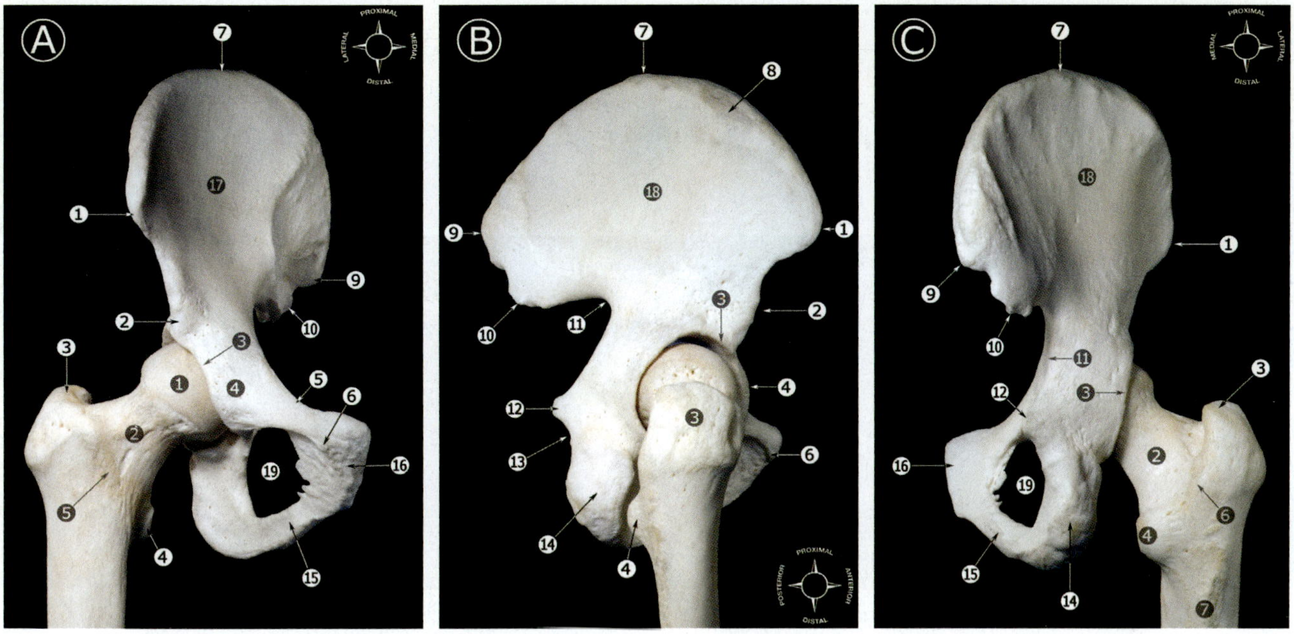

Figure 1.2. Bones of the hip joint. **A:** Anterior view. **B:** Lateral view. **C:** Posterior view. Hip bone or coxal. Anterior border: **1.** Anterior superior iliac spine. **2.** Anterior inferior iliac spine. **3.** Rim of the acetabulum. **4.** Iliopubic eminence. **5.** Pectineal line or pecten of pubis. **6.** Pubic tubercle. Superior border: **7.** Iliac crest. **8.** Tubercle of the iliac crest. Posterior border: **9.** Posterior superior iliac spine. **10.** Posterior inferior iliac spine. **11.** Greater sciatic notch. **12.** Ischial spine. **13.** Lesser sciatic notch. Inferior border: **14.** Ischial tuberosity. **15.** Ramus of ischium. **16.** Body of pubis. **17.** Iliac fossa. **18.** Gluteal surface. **19.** Obturator foramen. **Femur. 1.** Head. **2.** Neck. **3.** Greater trochanter. **4.** Lesser trochanter. **5.** Intertrochanteric line. **6.** Intertrochanteric crest. **7.** Gluteal tuberosity. (Figure copyright © Pau Golano)

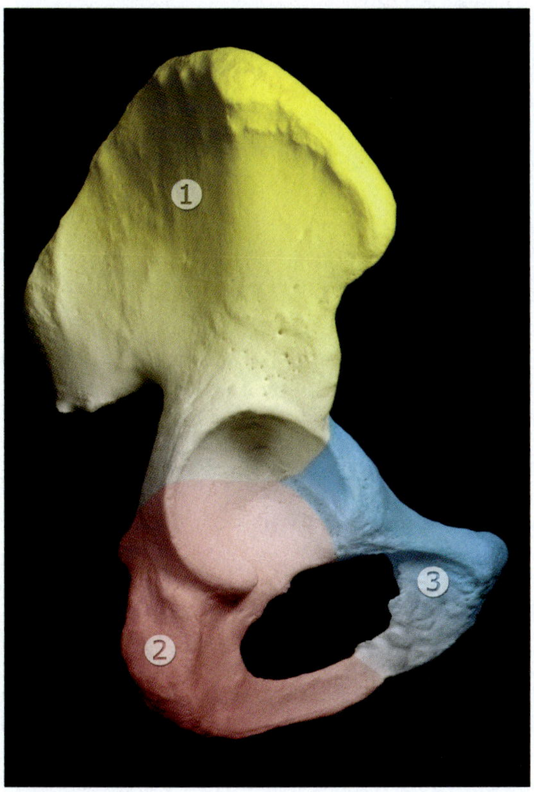

Figure 1.3. The ilium (**1**), the ischium (**2**), and the pubis (**3**) fuse at the triradiate cartilage during the development of the coxal. (Figure copyright © Pau Golano)

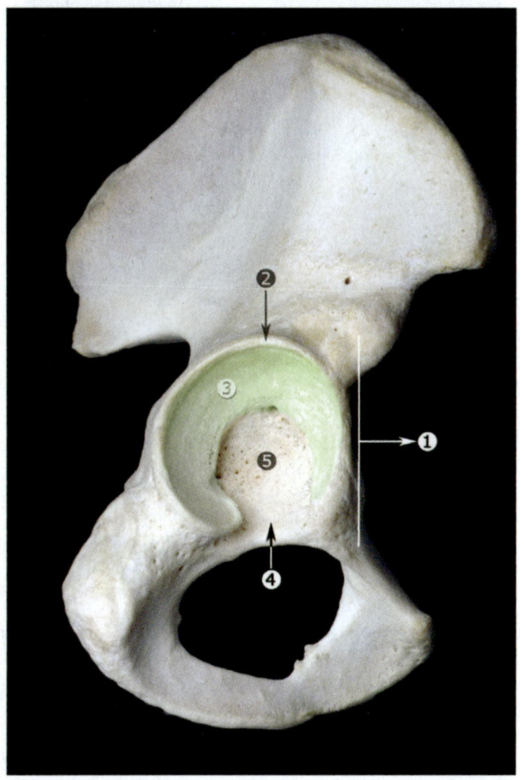

Figure 1.4. Lateral view of hip bone or coxal. **1.** Acetabulum. **2.** Rim of acetabulum. **3.** Lunate articular surface (*painted in green*). **4.** Acetabular notch. **5.** Acetabular fossa or cotyloid fossa. (Figure copyright © Pau Golano)

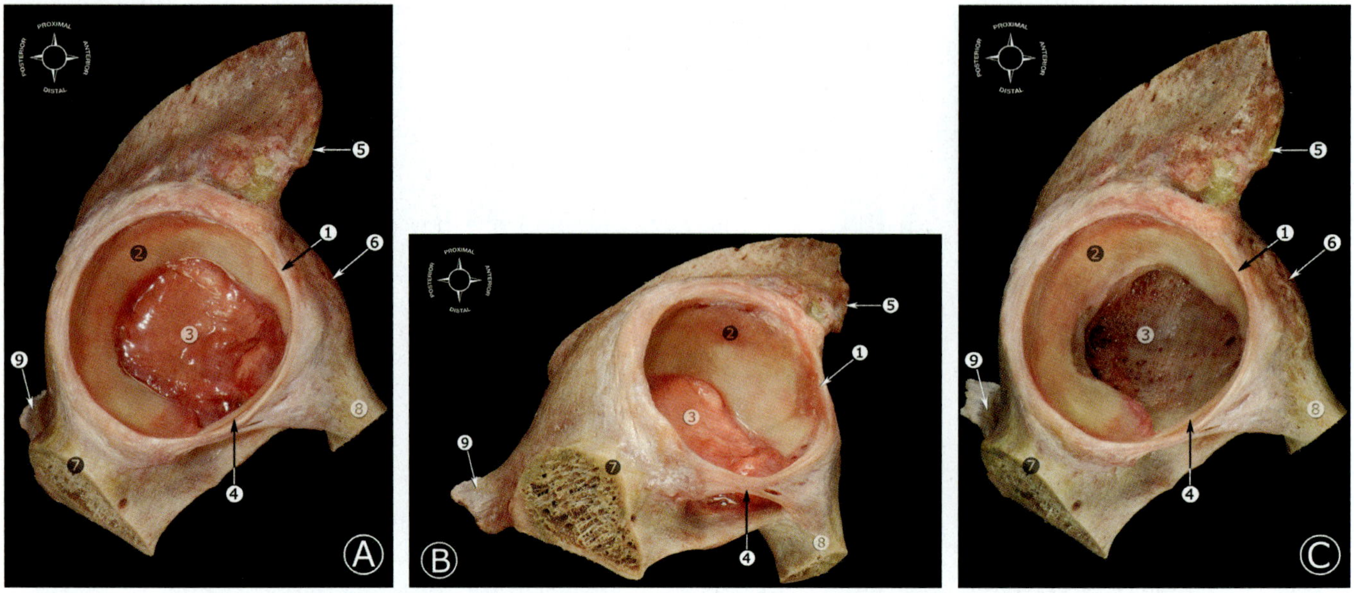

Figure 1.5. Detail of acetabulum in an osteoarticular dissection. Lateral view **(A & C)**, inferior view **(B)**. **1.** Acetabular labrum. **2.** Lunate articular surface. **3.** Acetabular fossa or cotyloid fossa, with the pulvinar (the ligamentum teres is removed). **4.** Acetabular notch and the transverse ligament. **5.** Anterior inferior iliac spine. **6.** Iliopubic eminence **7.** Body of ischium. **8.** Superior pubic ramus. **9.** Ischial spine. In **(C)**, the pulvinar is removed from the acetabular fossa (**3**). (Figure copyright © Pau Golano)

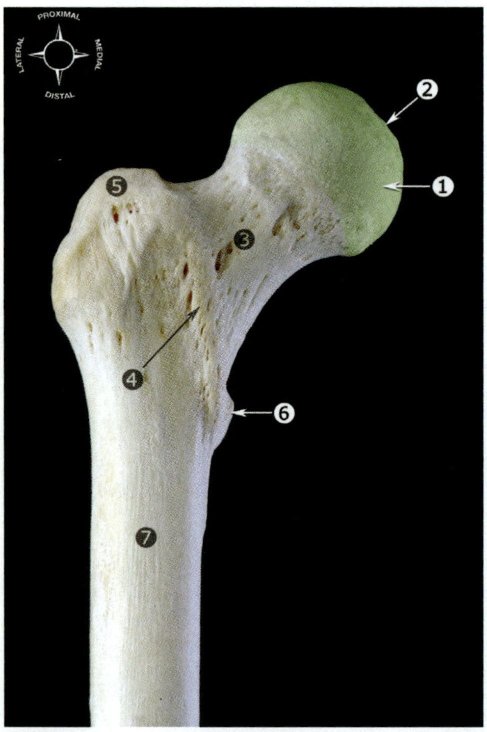

Figure 1.6. Anterior view of the proximal femur. **1.** Head and articular surface (*painted in green*). **2.** Fovea for ligamentum teres. **3.** Neck. **4.** Intertrochanteric line. 5. Greater trochanter. **6.** Lesser trochanter. **7.** Shaft of femur. (Figure copyright © Pau Golano)

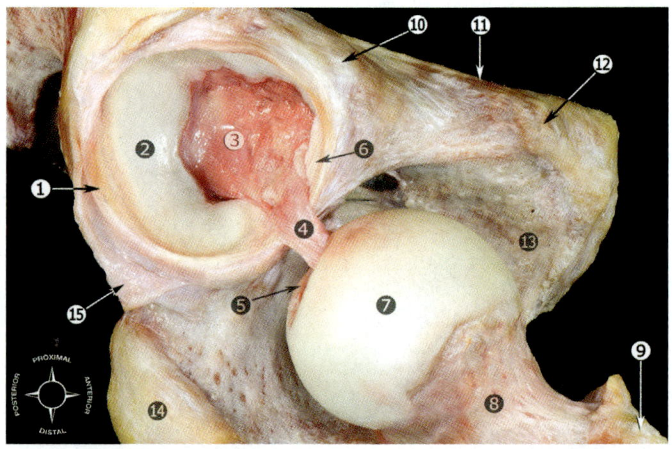

Figure 1.7. Anatomical dissection of the hip joint (lateral view). **1.** Acetabular labrum. **2.** Lunate articular surface. **3.** Acetabular fossa or cotyloid fossa, with the pulvinar. **4.** Ligamentum teres. **5.** Fovea capitis. **6.** Transverse ligament. **7.** Head of femur. **8.** Neck of femur. **9.** Greater trochanter. **10.** Iliopubic eminence. **11.** Pectineal line or pecten of pubis. **12.** Pubic tubercle. **13.** Body of pubis. **14.** Ischial tuberosity and insertions of posterior muscles of the thigh. **15.** Capsule of the hip joint (resected). (Figure copyright © Pau Golano)

is thought to act as another checkrein to aid in maintaining the head in a reduced position within the acetabulum. A portion of the orbicular fibers is derived from deep tendons of the gluteal region and the reflected head of the rectus femoris muscle. The zona orbicularis of the anterior capsule is easily seen in the arthroscopic view of the peripheral compartment of the hip joint and should not be confused with the acetabular labrum.[4] The inner surface of the capsule and the intra-articular femoral neck are covered by the synovium. This synovial tissue forms a series of folds that descend along the neck of the femur. The medial synovial fold passes below the zona orbicularis, and both these structures are a good reference for arthroscopic orientation.

Surrounding and reinforcing the capsule are three ligaments, the intrinsic ligaments of the hip. All three are external to the joint capsule and connect the iliac, pubic, and ischial

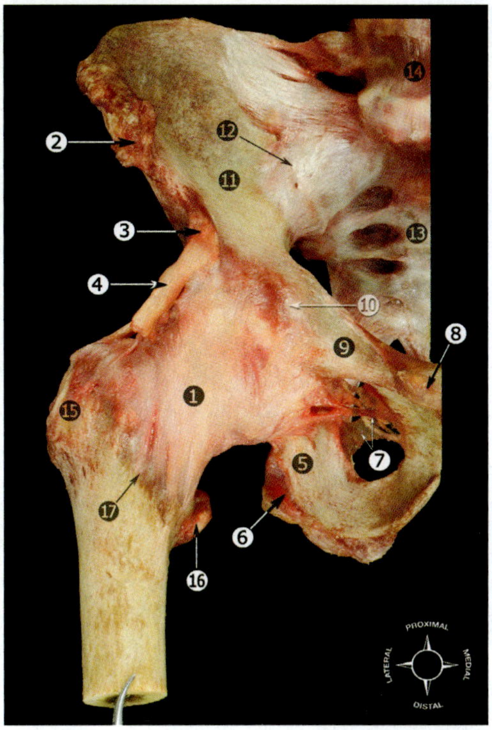

Figure 1.8. Osteoarticular dissection showing capsuloligamentous complex of the hip joint (anterior view). **1.** Capsuloligamentous complex. **2.** Anterior superior iliac spine. **3.** Anterior inferior iliac spine. **4.** Straight head tendon of the rectus femoris muscle. **5.** Body of ischium. **6.** Ischial tuberosity with insertion of posterior muscles of the thigh. **7.** Obturator foramen and obturator membrane. **8.** Pubic tubercle. **9.** Superior pubic ramus. **10.** Iliopubic eminence. **11.** Iliac fossa. **12.** Sacroiliac joint. **13.** Sacrum. **14.** Body of lumbar (L5). **15.** Greater trochanter. **16.** Lesser trochanter. **17.** Intertrochanteric line. (Figure copyright © Pau Golano)

portions of the pelvis and acetabulum to the femur. There is one ligament for each component of the coxal bone. The iliofemoral and pubofemoral ligaments are found in the anterior region of the hip joint, whereas the ischiofemoral ligament is located in the posterior region.

The iliofemoral ligament (Y ligament or ligament of Bigelow), the largest of the three capsular ligaments, is exceedingly thick and one of the strongest ligaments in the human body. The iliofemoral ligament is comprised of two bands of fibers, one medial and one lateral (Fig. 1.9A & B). In a detailed anatomic study, Fuss and Bacher[5] reported a third band, which has not been observed by other authors in more recent studies[6]; nor have we encountered this band in our anatomic dissections. The medial band originates between the AIIS and the iliac portion of the acetabular rim. It runs distally in a nearly vertical course and inserts in a protuberance in the distal intertrochanteric line of the femur. The lateral band originates proximal to the AIIS. This band has a more horizontal course than the medial band, and inserts in the anterior region of the crest of the greater trochanter. The configuration of these two bands is classically described as an inverted Y. The medial band tightens in external rotation and extension, whereas the lateral band tightens in external rotation and flexion or in internal and external rotation during extension of the hip (Fig. 1.10A & B).[6] Because the iliofemoral is the thickest and most powerful of the three ligaments that surround the joint, its position in relaxation (internal rotation and flexion) facilitates intra-articular access during arthroscopy of the central and peripheral compartments of the hip joint by allowing greater anterior capsular distension (Fig. 1.11).

The pubofemoral ligament is comprised of a single fiber band that is thinner than the two bands of the iliofemoral ligament. The pubofemoral ligament originates from the superior pubic ramus and inserts on the distal region of the intertrochanteric line of the femur, blending with the medial band of the iliofemoral ligament. Although the pubofemoral tightens in external rotation and extension of the hip, it has a less important limiting role in the joint and acts more as a reinforcing element of the anteroinferior joint capsule (Fig. 1.12).[6]

The ischiofemoral ligament is located at the posterior part of the hip joint capsule and consists of an upper and lower band. These bands have a common origin at the ischial part of the acetabular rim. The upper band inserts at a site medial to the anterosuperior base of the greater trochanter. The lower band inserts at a posteromedial site at the base of the greater trochanter, at the posterior intertrochanteric crest. Internal rotation of the hip in flexion and extension tightens both bands of the ischiofemoral ligament (Fig. 1.13).[6]

EXTRA-ARTICULAR HIP ANATOMY

This section includes a description of the anatomy of the various muscle groups and neurovascular structures found in the hip region.

MUSCULATURE

The hip joint is enclosed by 18 different muscles. This not only contributes to the inherent stability of the joint, but also complicates surgical exposure of the hip because of the depth required to adequately visualize the acetabulum and femoral head and neck. The arrangement of muscles relative to the center of the hip, specifically the origins and insertions, creates long lever arms that increase the range of excursion and power of the individual muscles.[7]

The anatomy of the muscles around the hip can be described in several ways. A simple system for understanding the hip musculature is by classifying the muscles according to their main function in the joint.

The anterior muscles of the hip mainly have a flexor function. The iliopsoas muscle, which is found in a proximal position, has an external rotator function in addition to the flexor function. The sartorius and rectus femoris muscles are located distally and additionally act as extensors of the leg.

The extensor muscles of the hip are found in the posterior region. The gluteus maximus muscle and tensor of the fasciae lata are located in a proximal position. The gluteus maximus has the added function of external rotation. Distally, one encounters the semitendinosus muscle, the biceps femoris, and the semimembranosus muscle. These last three muscles also function as flexors of the leg.

The abductor muscles of the hip, which include the gluteus medius and gluteus minimus, are also located in the posterior region. The gluteus minimus muscle additionally has an internal rotator function owing to the action of its anterior fibers and an external rotator function owing to its posterior fibers.[8]

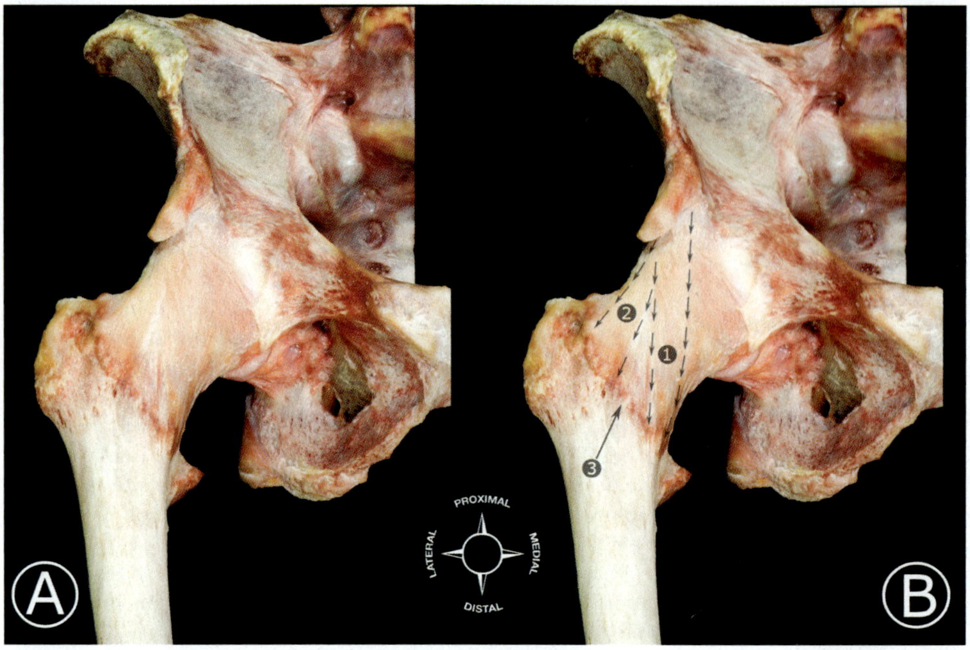

Figure 1.9. **A:** Anterior view of capsuloligamentous complex of the hip. **B:** Bands of fibers of the iliofemoral ligament (between *arrows*) that originates at the anterior inferior iliac spine. **1.** Medial band. **2.** Lateral band. **3.** Intertrochanteric line. (Figure copyright © Pau Golano)

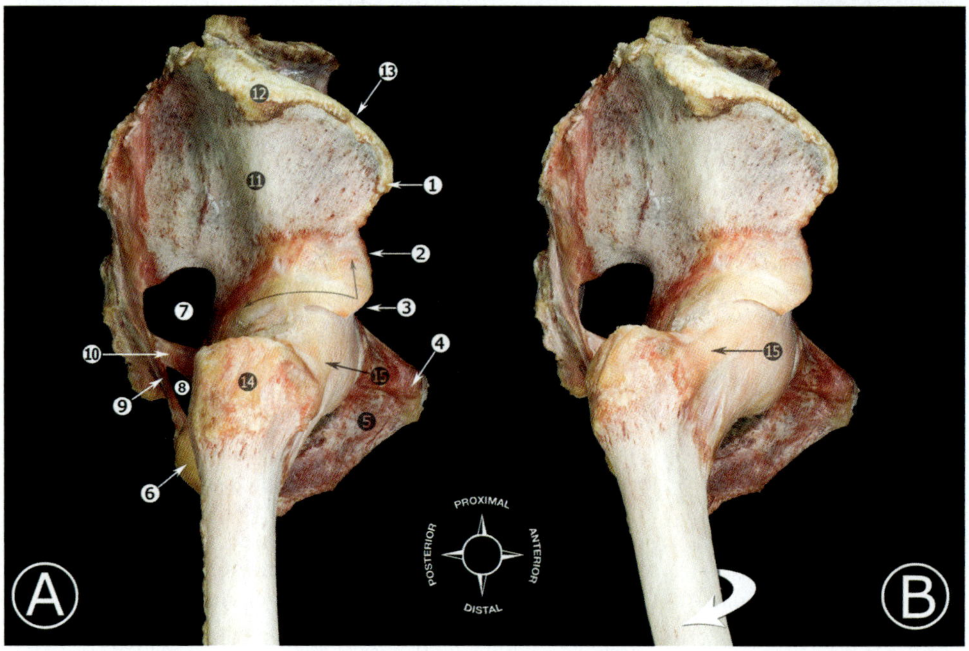

Figure 1.10. Lateral view of the hip in neutral **(A)** and external rotation **(B)** of the femur. **1.** Anterior superior iliac spine. **2.** Anterior inferior iliac spine. **3.** Rectus femoris tendon cut (reflected and straight heads of the rectus femoris tendon with *arrows*). **4.** Pubic tubercle. **5.** Body of pubis. **6.** Ischial tuberosity with insertion of posterior muscles of the thigh. **7.** Greater sciatic foramen. **8.** Lesser sciatic foramen. **9.** Sacrotuberous ligament. **10.** Sacrospinous ligament. **11.** Gluteal surface. **12.** Gluteal tuberosity. **13.** Iliac crest. **14.** Greater trochanter. **15.** Lateral band fiber of the iliofemoral ligament. The lateral band is relaxed in neutral position **(A)** and tightened in external rotation of the hip **(B)**. (Figure copyright © Pau Golano)

Anterior to gluteus minimus an accessory muscle is occasionally observed, which has been named gluteus quartus or gluteus scansorius.[9] Although its function remains uncertain, it seems to collaborate with the anterior fibers of gluteus minimus in internal rotation.[8]

The adductor hip muscles are located in a medial position. At the proximal level are found the gracilis and pectineus, and distally the adductor longus in the superficial plane, adductor brevis in the middle plane, and the adductor magnus in the deep plane.

Most of the muscles that rotate the leg are located in a deep plane. In the posterior region and from proximal to distal are found the gluteus minimus (which additionally has an abductor function), piriformis (also an abductor), superior gemellus, obturator internus, inferior gemellus, obturator externus, and quadratus femoris (also an adductor). Located in the anterior region, the iliopsoas can also perform external rotation of the hip. The gluteus maximus muscle, found at a more superficial and posterior plane, has the secondary function of external hip rotation.

The piriformis muscle is an important reference structure in open hip surgery. The superior gluteal neurovascular bundle emerges between the superior border of the piriformis muscle and the greater sciatic notch. The internal pudendal neurovascular bundle, ischial vessels, and sciatic nerve course between the inferior border of the piriformis muscle and the sciatic spine.[10] The superior border of the piriformis muscle corresponds to the line of the femoral neck.

As related to arthroscopy, the muscles of the hip are less crucial than other anatomic structures. Because the hip is a deep

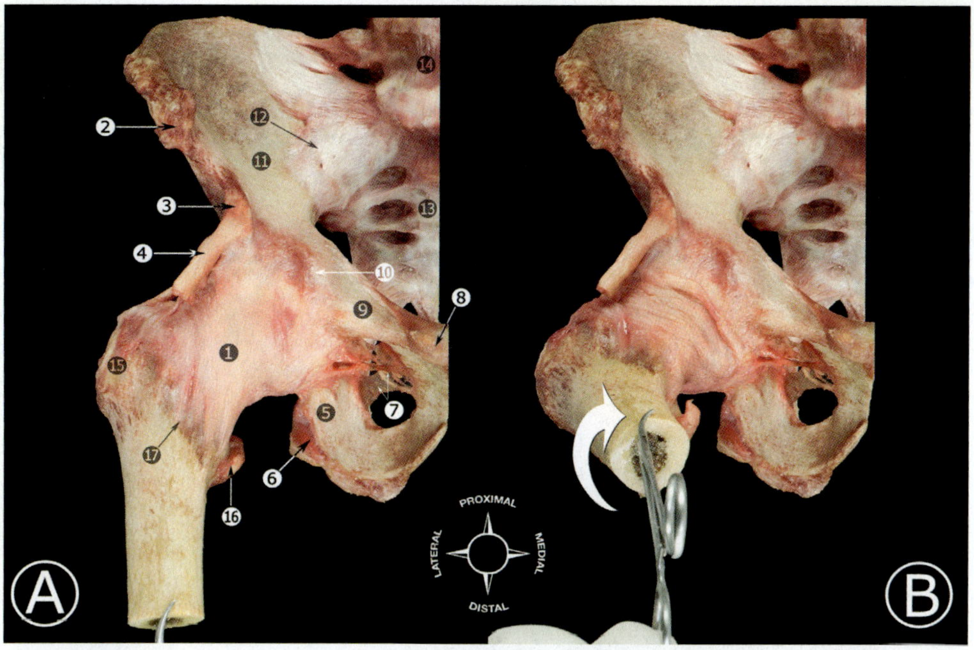

Figure 1.11. Anterior view of the hip. **A: 1.** Capsuloligamentous complex. **2.** Anterior superior iliac spine. **3.** Anterior inferior iliac spine. **4.** Straight head tendon. **5.** Body of ischium. **6.** Ischial tuberosity with insertion of posterior muscles of the thigh. **7.** Obturator foramen and obturator membrane. **8.** Pubic tubercle. **9.** Superior pubic ramus. **10.** Iliopubic eminence. **11.** Iliac fossa. **12.** Sacroiliac joint. **13.** Sacrum. **14.** Body of lumbar (L5). **15.** Greater trochanter. **16.** Lesser trochanter. **17.** Intertrochanteric line. **B:** The iliofemoral ligament is relaxed in internal rotation and flexion of the femur, facilitating intra-articular access during arthroscopy. (Figure copyright © Pau Golano)

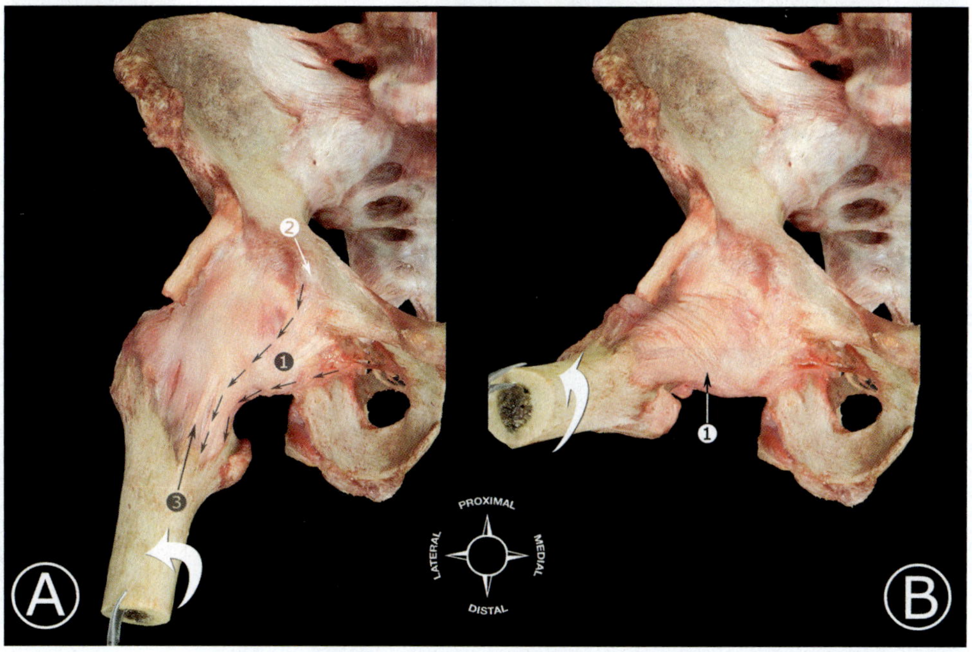

Figure 1.12. Anterior view of the hip. The Pubofemoral ligament is tightened in external rotation and extension **(A)**, and relaxed in flexion of the hip **(B)**. **1.** Pubofemoral ligament (between *arrows*). **2.** Iliopubic eminence. **3.** Medial band fibers of the iliofemoral ligament. (Figure copyright © Pau Golano)

joint, many muscles can be crossed by the arthroscopic portals without any repercussions.

Nevertheless, some of these muscles deserve mention because of their implication in pathological processes. This is the case of the insertions of the gluteus medius and minimus muscles at the level of the greater trochanter of the femur and their relationship with the iliotibial tract and trochanteric bursa in what has been termed greater trochanter pain syndrome (Figs. 1.14–1.16). This relationship is similar to that of the supraspinatus muscle tendon and the acromion and subacromial bursa in subacromial syndrome of the shoulder. Because of this similarity, the combined insertion of the gluteus medius and gluteus minimus has been termed the rotator cuff of the hip[11,12] even though the main function of the muscles is abduction. As occurs with the shoulder, it is possible to treat lesions to the rotator cuff of the hip and the related processes encompassed in greater trochanter pain syndrome with arthroscopic-endoscopic techniques (Fig. 1.17).[13–16]

The common insertion site of the gluteus medius and gluteus minimus muscles in the greater trochanter is comprised of a broad musculotendinous anchor. The insertion site may show slight variations and there is an evident insertion impression in the greater trochanter. The greater trochanter has four facets: the anterior, lateral, posterior, and superoposterior.[8,17–20] The posterior facet does not possess a muscle insertion, being occupied by the trochanter bursa. The other three facets form the footprint of the rotator cuff of the hip. The insertional anatomy of this area has been studied in detail (Fig. 1.18).[8,19,21,22]

The gluteus medius insertion site is divided into two parts, a superoposterior and a lateral component. The thicker and

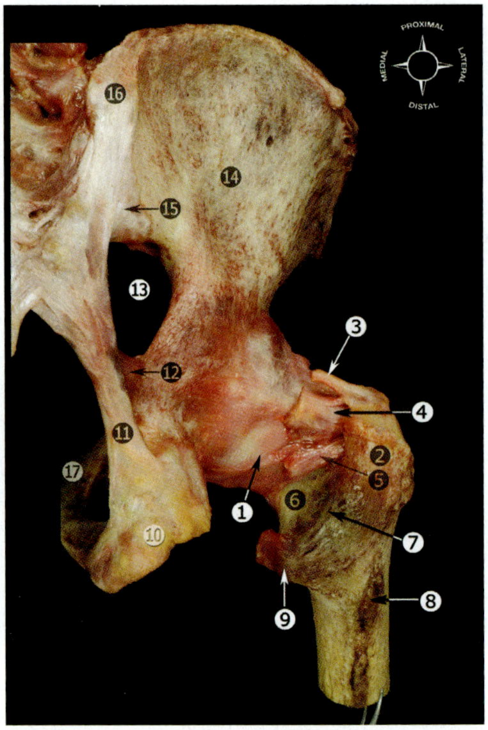

Figure 1.13. Posterior view of the hip. **1.** Ischiofemoral ligament. **2.** Greater trochanter. **3.** Piriformis muscle tendon. **4.** Obturator internus and, gemellus superior and inferior muscles. **5.** Obturator externus. **6.** Extra-articular neck of the femur. **7.** Intertrochanteric crest. **8.** Gluteal tuberosity. **9.** Lesser trochanter with iliopsoas muscle tendon insertion. **10.** Ischial tuberosity and insertions of posterior muscles of the thigh. **11.** Sacrotuberous ligament. **12.** Sacrospinous ligament. **13.** Greater sciatic foramen. **14.** Gluteal surface. **15.** Sacroiliac joint. **16.** Posterior superior iliac spine. **17.** Body of pubis. (Figure copyright © Pau Golano)

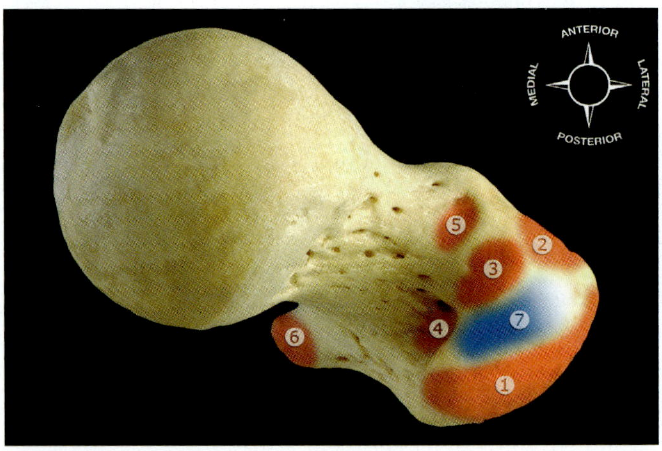

Figure 1.14. Superior view of the proximal femur with areas of muscular insertion painted in red. **1.** Gluteus medius. **2.** Gluteus minimus. **3.** Piriformis. **4.** Obturator externus. **5.** Obturator internus with superior and inferior gemellus. **6.** Iliopsoas. **7.** Bald area (*painted in blue*). (Figure copyright © Pau Golano)

more important posterior component inserts at the superoposterior surface of the greater trochanter. The smaller component is located central and anterior to the muscle and inserts at the lateral surface of the trochanter. These two insertion sites are located in different planes; hence, the action of the muscle on each of these insertion areas results in a different function.[22]

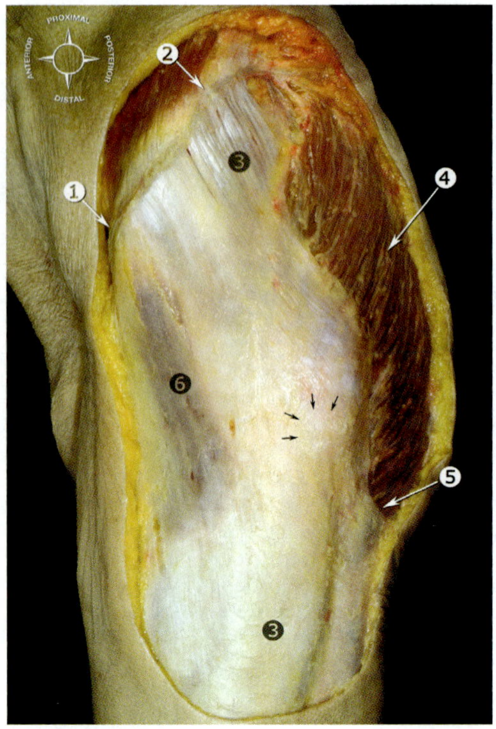

Figure 1.15. Lateral view of the iliotibial tract and lateral trochanteric area. Trochanteric area delimited with arrows (left hip). **1.** Anterior superior iliac spine. **2.** Iliac crest. **3.** Iliotibial tract. **4.** Gluteus maximus. **5.** Insertion of gluteus maximus. **6.** Tensor of the fasciae lata muscle. (Figure copyright © Pau Golano)

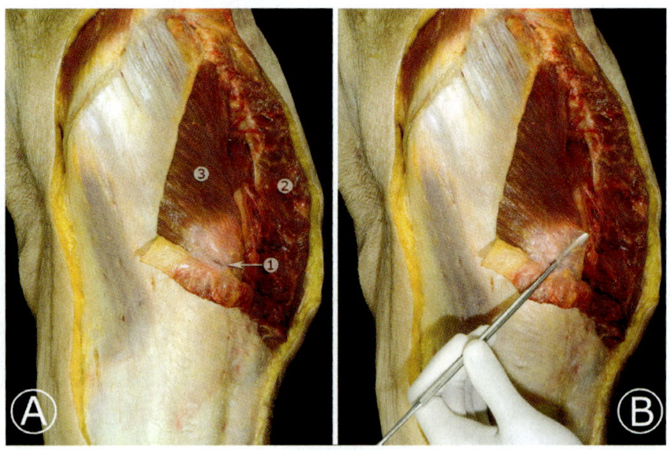

Figure 1.16. Lateral view of the hip joint with iliotibial tract cut and gluteus maximus removed (left hip). **A: 1.** Trochanteric bursa. **2.** Gluteus maximus. **3.** Gluteus medius. **B:** Dissector inside the trochanteric bursa. (Figure copyright © Pau Golano)

The posterior component of the muscle has an abductor action, whereas the central, anterior component exerts external rotation of the hip.[21,22] Most injuries to the gluteus medius occur in the more anterior portion of the muscle, where it inserts on the lateral surface of the greater trochanter.[12,23,24] The insertion of the anterior component of gluteus medius can be mistaken for the gluteus minimus insertion on the anterior surface of the greater trochanter.[19]

Gluteus minimus also has two distinct insertion sites on the greater trochanter. The larger component inserts on the anterior surface of the trochanter in its inferior area, and the smaller component, which has a myotendinous nature, inserts on the anterior surface of the trochanter in its superior area and on the anterosuperior capsule of the hip joint.

Between the lateral insertion of gluteus medius (central and anterior components of the muscle) and the anterior insertion of gluteus minimus in the superior area (myotendinous component), there is a bald area with no muscle insertions[22] that should not be mistaken for an insertional injury of the rotator cuff of the hip (Figs. 1.14 & 1.18).

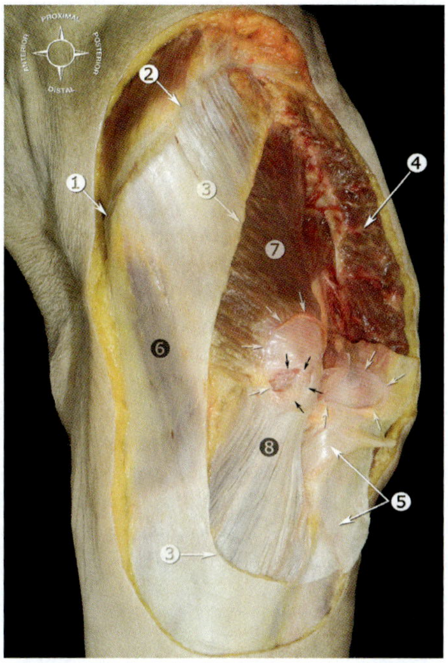

Figure 1.17. Lateral view of the hip joint with iliotibial tract removed. Limits of the trochanteric bursa with white arrows, and tear of the rotator cuff of the hip delimited with black arrows (left hip). **1.** Anterior superior iliac spine. **2.** Iliac crest. **3.** Iliotibial tract. **4.** Gluteus maximus. **5.** Insertion of gluteus maximus. **6.** Tensor of the fasciae lata muscle. **7.** Gluteus medius. **8.** Vastus lateralis muscle. (Figure copyright © Pau Golano)

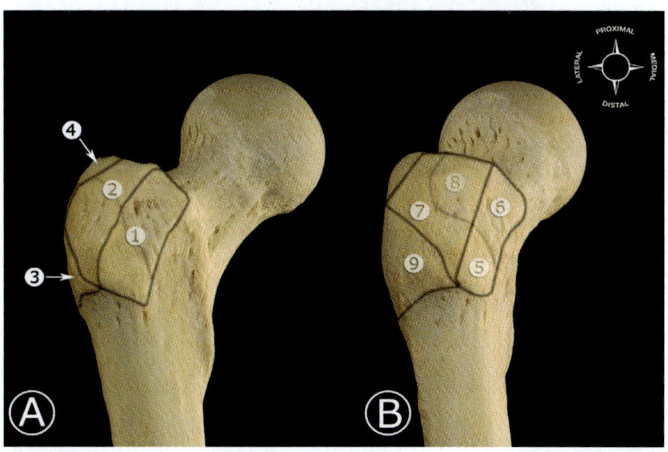

Figure 1.18. Anatomy facets of the greater trochanter **(A)** and their relationship with muscle insertions **(B)**. **1.** Anterior facet. **2.** Lateral facet. **3.** Posterior facet. **4.** Superoposterior facet. **5.** Gluteus minimus insertion. **6.** Subgluteus minimus bursa. **7.** Gluteus medius insertion. **8.** Subgluteus medius bursa. **9.** Trochanteric bursa. (Figure copyright © Pau Golano)

NEUROVASCULAR ANATOMY

The hip region contains numerous important neurological and vascular structures. We will focus on those that are susceptible to injury during arthroscopic procedures because of their proximity to the portals or the trajectory of the instruments toward the joint. These include the femoral neurovascular bundle, the lateral femoral cutaneous nerve (LFC), and the sciatic nerve. Nonetheless, the arthroscopist should also be aware of the multiple neurologic structures that innervate the muscles and cutaneous areas in the hip region, or simply cross the hip in a distal direction.

THE FEMORAL NEUROVASCULAR BUNDLE

The femoral neurovascular bundle is located in an anteromedial position in the thigh and can be palpated at the most proximal portion, in the area of the inguinal fold. In a lateral to medial direction, the bundle is comprised of the femoral nerve, the femoral artery and vein, and the corresponding lymphatic system (Fig. 1.19).

A line descending from the ASIS is the reference boundary that delimits the safe work area; the femoral neurovascular bundle is located medial to this line. Palpation of the femoral artery

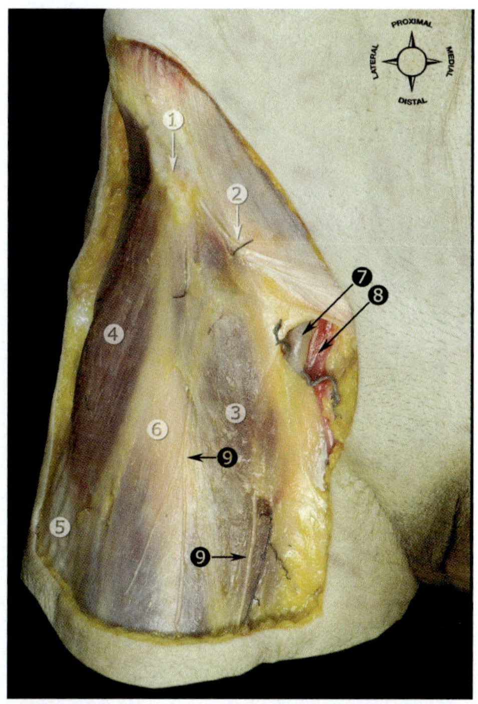

Figure 1.19. Anatomic dissection showing superficial area of the inguinal and proximal thigh region. **1.** Anterior superior iliac spine. **2.** Inguinal ligament. **3.** Sartorious muscle. **4.** Tensor of the fasciae lata muscle. **5.** Iliotibial tract. **6.** Rectus femoris muscle. **7.** Femoral artery. **8.** Femoral vein. **9.** Cutaneous branches of the femoral nerve. (Figure copyright © Pau Golano)

pulse is the reference to localize the femoral nerve, which lies lateral to the artery.

The femoral nerve begins as the L2–L4 nerve roots leave the lumbar plexus. The nerve pierces the psoas muscle and runs in the groove between the psoas and iliacus, passing under the inguinal ligament and continuing distally just lateral to the femoral artery, vein, and lymphatics. The location of the femoral nerve in the groin can be estimated as halfway between the ASIS and the pubic tubercle, both of which are topographic landmarks.

The iliopsoas muscle separates the femoral nerve from the hip joint. Approximately 2 cm below the inguinal ligament, the femoral nerve divides, innervating muscular, articular, and cutaneous structures throughout the thigh, hip, and knee. Finally the femoral nerve terminates as the saphenous nerve, traveling with the superficial femoral artery in the subsartorial adductor canal (canal of Hunter). The femoral nerve innervates the sartorius, quadriceps, and pectineus muscles and sends branches via the rectus femoris to the hip joint and via the vastus lateralis to the knee (Fig. 1.20).[3]

The femoral artery, vein, and lymphatics are contained within the femoral sheath, which is located medial to the femoral nerve as it courses in the anterior region of the hip. The femoral artery is a continuation of the external iliac artery. As the femoral artery courses distally, it divides into the superficial and deep femoral arteries. The deep femoral or profunda femoris artery originates from the femoral artery approximately 3.5 cm below the inguinal ligament.[3] Several branches of the deep femoral are relevant to any description of the vascular anatomy of the hip joint. The lateral and medial circumflex femoral branches leave the deep femoral artery to supply the head, neck, and proximal portions of the femur (Fig. 1.21).

The lateral circumflex femoral leaves the deep femoral and divides into the ascending, transverse, and descending branches. The ascending branch courses in a superior and oblique direction toward the intertrochanteric line to provide a small portion of the blood supply to the femoral head and neck. The transverse branch travels toward the quadratus femoris, and the descending branch runs inferiorly to form part of the anastomotic blood supply around the knee.

The medial circumflex femoral artery is typically a branch of the deep femoral artery. Nonetheless, in 17% of individuals it arises directly from the common femoral artery.[25] The medial circumflex femoral provides a substantial part of the blood supply to the adult femoral head[26,27] and its importance cannot be overstated. The medial circumflex femoral artery runs behind the hip joint, toward the intertrochanteric crest between the iliopsoas and pectineus muscles, and continues posterolaterally through the quadratus muscle. At this point the medial circumflex femoral artery divides. At least one of the divisions, the trochanteric branch, runs behind the tendon of the obturator externus muscle and anterior to the tendons of the superior gemellus, obturator internus, and inferior gemellus. The trochanteric branch perforates the joint capsule just above the insertion site of the tendon of the superior gemellus muscle, and then divides into two to four terminal branches.[28] These vessels pass along a synovial fold in the posterosuperior region of the femoral neck and perforate the cartilage-bone junction of the femoral head some 2 to 4 mm in the lateral area. Approximately 80% of the perforating vessels are located in the anterosuperior and posterosuperior

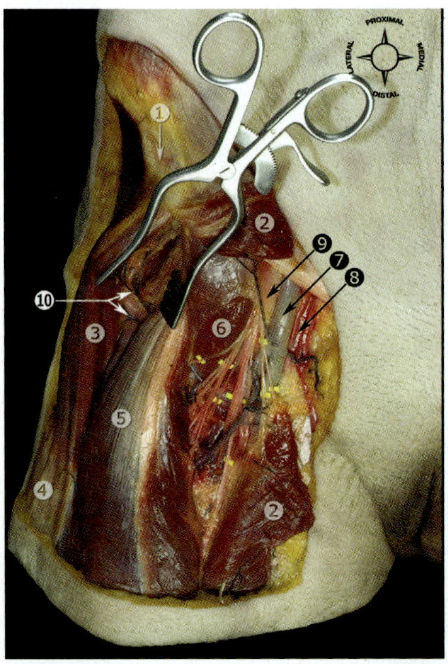

Figure 1.20. Anatomic dissection showing neurovascular structures in the inguinal area (vascular structures filled up with black latex). Sartorious muscle cut and rejected. **1.** Anterior superior iliac spine. **2.** Sartorious muscle. **3.** Tensor of the fasciae lata muscle. **4.** Iliotibial tract. **5.** Rectus femoris muscle. **6.** Iliopsoas muscle. **7.** Femoral artery. **8.** Femoral vein. **9.** Femoral nerve and branches. **10.** Retractor between tensor of the fasciae lata and rectus femoris muscle showing the lateral circumflex femoral artery and their branches. (Figure copyright © Pau Golano)

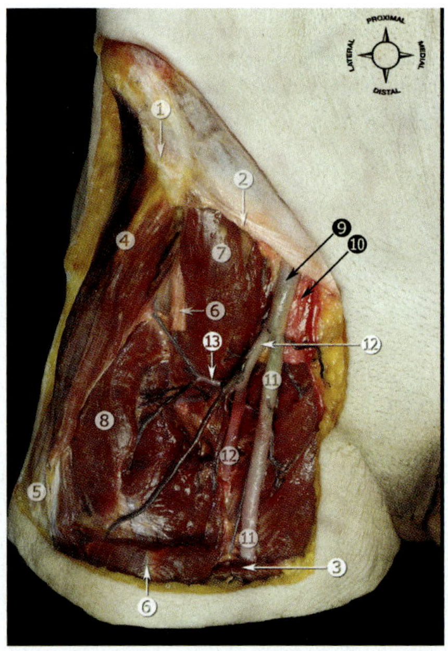

Figure 1.21. Anatomic dissection showing femoral artery and their branches. Femoral nerve and their branches removed. **1.** Anterior superior iliac spine. **2.** Inguinal ligament. **3.** Sartorious muscle cut. **4.** Tensor of the fasciae lata muscle. **5.** Iliotibial tract. **6.** Rectus femoris muscle cut. **7.** Iliopsoas muscle. **8.** Vastus lateralis muscle. **9.** Femoral artery. **10.** Femoral vein cut. **11.** Superficial femoral artery. **12.** Deep femoral artery. **13.** Lateral circumflex femoral artery and their branches. (Figure copyright © Pau Golano)

quadrant of the femoral neck.[28] It is important to keep in mind the anatomic relationships of the femoral head vascularization. Injury to the medial circumflex femoral artery or its perforating vessels at the junction of the femoral neck and head during treatment of conditions such as femoroacetabular impingement, can compromise vascularization of the head.

The contribution of the ligamentum teres artery to the femoral head blood supply is small in adulthood, although it plays a larger role during growth and development. The artery of the ligamentum teres is a branch of the obturator artery within the pelvis, resulting from a division of the internal iliac artery, and is absent in approximately 20% of the population (Fig. 1.8).[29] Because the ligamentum teres artery is not an essential structure for femoral head vascularization, surgical dislocation of the hip joint can be safely performed; there have been no reported cases of osteonecrosis in studies involving conservative surgery of the hip joint.[30–32]

THE LATERAL FEMORAL CUTANEOUS NERVE

The LFC, although smaller and seemingly less significant than the other nerves of the hip region, has considerable clinical importance, particularly in relation to surgery of the hip, iliac crest, and acetabulum. The LFC originates from the L2–L4 nerve roots of the lumbar plexus and courses under the inguinal ligament near the ASIS in 58.5% of specimens.[33] Its location and variability in relation to the ASIS place it at risk for compression or iatrogenic injury during anterior approaches to the hip, pelvis, or acetabulum, as well as during iliac crest bone harvesting.[33–35] Compression or iatrogenic injury to the LFC causes a painful condition known as meralgia paresthetica.[36] Due to its variability and vulnerability, the location of the LFC has been studied at length to establish a safe zone during surgical approaches. Cadaveric studies have shown its wide variability: the relationship to the ASIS is up to 2 cm posterior along the iliac crest and up to 7.3 cm medial along the inguinal ligament (Fig. 1.22).[35,37] Four types of nerve positions have been described in relation to the ASIS.[33] In 27.6% of individuals, the nerve divides before crossing the inguinal ligament.[35] The nerve or its branches acquire a course lateral to the sartorius after crossing the inguinal ligament, from 2.2 to 11.3 cm distal to the ASIS.[35] Placement of the anterior arthroscopic portal of the hip, which is useful for examining the central compartment, can result in injury to the LFC or its anterolateral branch.[38,39] Although the nerve has been localized at some 0.3 cm from the standard anterior arthroscopic portal,[40] our experience has shown that this distance can vary considerably. Thus, it is essential to perform this portal according to a protocoled technique similar to that used in arthroscopic surgery of other joints (skin incision and blunt dissection with a mosquito forceps to the deep plane), or alternatively, to perform a small incision to visualize and avert injury to this nerve.[41]

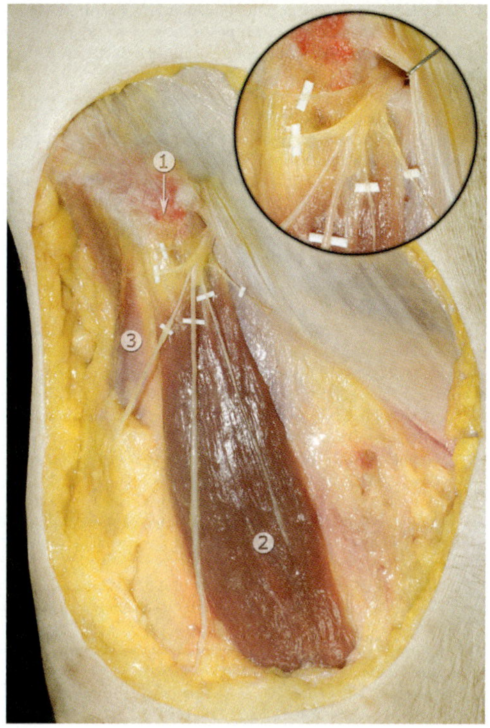

Figure 1.22. Anatomic dissection showing lateral femoral cutaneous nerve **1.** Anterior superior iliac spine. **2.** Sartorius muscle. **3.** Tensor of the fasciae lata muscle. (Figure copyright © Pau Golano)

THE SCIATIC NERVE

The sciatic nerve is the largest nerve structure around the hip and the longest in the human body. The course of the sciatic in relation to the piriformis muscle is somewhat variable. If the nerve divides into its tibial and peroneal divisions within the pelvis, the peroneal portion usually pierces the piriformis muscle. This is an important consideration in surgical exposures involving retraction of the piriformis; it is believed that this configuration may predispose patients to piriformis syndrome. This aberrant course occurs in approximately 10% of the population.[3]

From the viewpoint of arthroscopy, the importance of the sciatic nerve lies in its anatomical relationship with the lesser trochanter and the insertion of the iliopsoas muscle tendon, particularly when treating internal snapping hip.[42,43] When the patient is in the supine decubitus position with the leg in neutral position, the sciatic nerve at the level of the lesser trochanter is posterior and medial to the femur. This relationship can vary, however, with distances of 4 mm lateral to the medial margin of the trochanter and up to 7.7 mm medial to the trochanter being observed.[44] At the deep level of the lesser trochanter, the sciatic nerve is found at a distance similar to the distance between the femur and the skin, between 3 and 4 cm.[45] Rotation of the limb can result in variations in this relationship, such that in internal rotation the nerve is located medial to the femur, whereas in external rotation it is lateral to the femur.[46,47]

Although injury to the sciatic nerve as a consequence of establishing the various arthroscopic portals has not been reported, neuropraxia because of excessive traction during arthroscopy of the central compartment has been observed.[48,49]

REFERENCES

1. Hughes PE, Hsu JC, Matava MJ. Hip anatomy and biomechanics in the athlete. *Sports Med Arthrosc.* 2002;10:103–114.
2. Keene GS, Villa RN. Arthroscopic anatomy of the hip: An in vivo study. *Arthroscopy.* 1994;10:392–399.
3. O'Brien M, Delaney M. The anatomy of the hip and groin. *Sports Med Arthrosc.* 1997;5:252–267.
4. Stoller DW. *Magnetic Resonance Imaging in Orthopaedics and Sports Medicine.* Philadelphia, PA: Lippincott-Raven; 1997.
5. Fuss FK, Bacher A. New aspects of the morphology and function of the human hip joint ligaments. *Am J Anat.* 1991;192:1–13.
6. Martin HD, Savage A, Braly BA, et al. The function of the hip capsular ligaments: A quantitative report. *Arthroscopy.* 2008;24:188–195.

7. Iannotti J, Godstein S, Kuhn J, et al. The formation and growth of skeletal tissues. In: Buckwalter J, Einhorn T, Simon S, eds. *Orthopaedic Basic Science: Biology and Biomechanics of the Musculoskeletal System.* 2nd Ed. Rosemont, IL: American Academy of Orthopaedic Surgeons; 2000, pp. 77–109.
8. Beck M, Sledge JB, Gautier E, et al. The anatomy and function of the gluteus minimus muscle. *J Bone Joint Surg Br.* 2000;82B:358–363.
9. Testut L, Latarjet A. *Traité d'anatomie humaine.* 9ème Ed. *G Doin & Cie*, 1948, pp. 1112–1114.
10. Testut L, Jacob O. *Tratado de anatomía topográfica.* 8ª Ed. *Salvat Editores*; 1979, pp. 873–874.
11. Bunker TD, Esler CNA, Leach WJ. Rotator-cuff tear of the hip. *J Bone Joint Surg Br.* 1997;79B:618–620.
12. Kagan A II. Rotator cuff tears of the hip. *Clin Orthop.* 1999;368:135–140.
13. Fox JL. The role of arthroscopic bursectomy in the treatment of trochanteric bursitis. *Arthroscopy.* 2002;18:E34.
14. Kandemir U, Bharam S, Philippon MJ, et al. Endoscopic treatment of calcific tendinitis of gluteus medius and minimus. *Arthroscopy.* 2003;19:E4.
15. Ilizaliturri VM Jr, Martinez-Escalante FA, Chaidez PA, et al. Endoscopic iliotibial band release for external snapping hip syndrome. *Arthroscopy.* 2006;22:505–510.
16. Voos JE, Rudzki JR, Shindle MK, et al. Arthroscopic anatomy and surgical techniques for peritrochanteric space disorders in the hip. *Arthroscopy.* 2007; 23:1246.e1–1246.e5.
17. Armbuster TG, Guerra J Jr, Resnick D, et al. The adult hip: An anatomic study. Part I: The bony landmarks. *Radiology.* 1978;128(1):1–10.
18. Nazarian S, Tisserand P, Brunet C, et al. Anatomic basis of the transgluteal approach to the hip. *Surg Radiol Anat.* 1987;9(1):27–35.
19. Pfirrmann CWA, Chung CB, Theumann NH, et al. Greater trochanter of the hip: Attachment of the abductor mechanism and a complex of three bursae – MR imaging an MR bursography in cadavers and MR imaging in asymptomatic volunteers. *Radiology.* 2001;221(2):469–477.
20. Dwek J, Pfirrmann C, Stanley A, et al. MR imaging of the hip abductors: Normal anatomy and commonly encountered pathology at the greater trochanter. *Mag Reson Imaging Clin N Am.* 2005;13:691–704.
21. Gottschalk F, Kourosh S, Leveau B. The functional anatomy of tensor fasciae latae and gluteus medius and minimus. *J Anat.* 1989;166:179–189.
22. Robertson WJ, Gardner MJ, Barker JU, et al. Anatomy and dimensions of the gluteus medius tendon insertion. *Arthroscopy.* 2008;24:130–136.
23. Chung CB, Robertson JE, Cho GJ, et al. Gluteus medius tendon tears and avulsive injuries in elderly women: Imaging findings in six patients. *Am J Roentgenol.* 1999;173:351–353.
24. Bird PA, Oakley SP, Shnier R, et al. Prospective evaluation of magnetic resonance imaging and physical examination findings in patients with greater trochanteric pain syndrome. *Arthritis Rheum.* 2001;44:2138–2145.
25. Gautier E, Ganz K, Krugel N, et al. Anatomy of the medial femoral circumflex artery and its surgical implications. *J Bone Joint Surg Br.* 2000;82B:679–683.
26. Beaulé P, Campbell P, Hoke R, et al. Notching of the femoral neck during resurfacing arthroplasty of the hip: A vascular study. *J Bone Joint Surg Br.* 2006;88B:35–39.
27. Beaulé P, Campbell P, Shim P. Femoral head blood flow during hip resurfacing. *Clin Orthop.* 2006;456:148–152.
28. Beaulé P, Campbell P, Lu Z, et al. Vascularity of the arthritic femoral head and hip resurfacing. *J Bone Joint Surg Am.* 2006;88A:85–96.
29. Byrd JW. Gross anatomy. In: Byrd JW, ed. *Operative Hip Arthroscopy.* 2nd Ed. New York: Springer; 2005, pp. 100–109.
30. Ganz R, Gill TJ, Gautier E, et al. Surgical dislocation of the adult hip: A technique with full access to the femoral head and acetabulum without the risk of avascular necrosis. *J Bone Joint Surg Br.* 2001;83B:1119–1124.
31. Murphy S, Tannast M, KimY, et al. Debridement of the adult hip for femoroacetabular impingement: Indications and preliminary clinical results. *Clin Orthop.* 2004;429: 178–181.
32. Beaulé P. A soft tissue sparing approach to surface arthroplasty of the hip. *Oper Tech Orthop.* 2004;429:178–181.
33. Murata Y, Takahashi K, Yamagata M, et al. The anatomy of the lateral femoral cutaneous nerve, with special reference to the harvesting of iliac bone graft. *J Bone Joint Surg Am.* 2000;82A:746–747.
34. De Ridder VA, De Lange S, Popta JV. Anatomical variations of the lateral femoral cutaneous nerve and the consequences for surgery. *J Orthop Trauma.* 1999;13:207–211.
35. Grothaus MC, Holt M, Mekhail AO, et al. Lateral femoral cutaneous nerve: An anatomic study. *Clin Orthop.* 2005;437:164–168.
36. Sunderland S. Lateral femoral cutaneous nerve: Meralgia paraesthetica. In: Sunderland S, ed. *Nerves and Nerve Injuries.* 2nd Ed. New York: Churchill Livingstone; 1978, pp. 1007–1010.
37. Murata Y, Takahashi K, Yamagata M, et al. Injury to the lateral femoral cutaneous nerve during harvest iliac bone graft, with reference to the size of the graft. *J Bone J Surg Br.* 2002;84B:798–801.
38. Eriksson E, Arvidsson I, Arvidsson H. Diagnostic and operative arthroscopy of the hip. *Orthopedics.* 1986;9:169–176.
39. Frich LH, Lauritzen J, Juhl M. Arthroscopy in diagnosis and treatment of hip disorders. *Orthopedics.* 1989;12:389–392.
40. Byrd JWT, Pappas JB, Pedley MJ. Hip Arthroscopy: An anatomic study of portal placement and relationship to the extra-articular structures. *Arthroscopy.* 1995;11:418–423.
41. Sekiya JK, Wojtys EM, Loder RT, et al. Hip arthroscopy using a limited anterior exposure: An alternative approach for arthroscopic access. *Arthroscopy.* 2000;16:16–20.
42. Ilizaliturri VM, Villalobos FE, Chaidez PA, et al. Internal snapping hip syndrome: Treatment by endoscopic release of the iliopsoas tendon. *Arthroscopy.* 2005;21:1375–1380.
43. Wettstein M, Jung J, Dienst M. Arthroscopic psoas tenotomy. *Arthroscopy.* 2006;22:907.e1–907.e4.
44. Ericksen ML, Swenson JD, Pace NL. The anatomic relationship of the sciatic nerve to the lesser trochanter: Implications for anterior sciatic nerve block. *Anesth Analg.* 2002;95:1071–1074.
45. Chelly JE, Delaunay L. A new anterior approach to the sciatic nerve block. *Anesthesiology.* 1999;91:1655–1660.
46. Hadzic A, Reiss W, Dilberovic F, et al. Rotation of the leg influences ability to approach the sciatic nerve through the anterior approach. *Reg Anesth Pain Med.* 1998;23:38.
47. Vloka JD, Hadzic A, April E, et al. Anterior approach to the sciatic nerve block: The effects of leg rotation. *Anesth Analg.* 2001;92:460–462.
48. Funke EL, Munzinger U. Complications in hip arthroscopy. *Arthroscopy.* 1996;12:156–159.
49. Clarke MT, Arora A, Villar RN. Hip arthroscopy: Complications in 1054 cases. *Clin Orthop Relat Res.* 2003;406:84–88.

CHAPTER

2

Martin L. Lazarus

Imaging the Hip

INTRODUCTION

Imaging of the hip has undergone dramatic changes over the last decade. Previously, plain radiography, radionuclide scintigraphy (bone scanning), and computed tomography (CT) provided the bulk of the imaging armamentarium. This has subsequently evolved to include predominantly plain radiography and magnetic resonance imaging (MRI). While the prior focus of imaging was placed on the extra-articular structures of the hip and surrounding pelvis, the current focus is directed to the intra-articular structures. MRI and, more specifically, MR arthrography (MRA) have assumed an important and leading role in the assessment of these structures. Imaging, to a great degree, has simply followed the lead of clinical sports medicine as greater emphasis has been placed on the intra-articular structures and the concept of femoroacetabular impingement (FAI).

Only recently, with the advent of MRA, has the radiologic assessment of the hip been able to approach that of other major joints such as the shoulder and knee. Improved visualization of intra-articular structures such as the acetabular labrum, articular cartilage, and ligamentum teres has allowed for improved diagnosis and treatment of athletes with hip pain. This chapter will discuss the general utility of multiple imaging modalities, followed by detailed descriptions of different hip and pelvis injuries in athletes and the current concepts regarding their radiologic imaging.

RADIOLOGIC MODALITY: GENERAL REVIEW

PLAIN FILM RADIOGRAPHY

There are several invasive and noninvasive imaging modalities available for the evaluation of hip pain, both acute and chronic, in the athlete. Plain film radiography has been and remains the primary screening means in the evaluation of this patient population. Plain films are inexpensive and readily available. In general, plain radiography detects gross fractures, tumors, advanced arthrosis and hip dysplasias as well. In addition, pathology involving other joints within the pelvis, such as the symphysis pubis and sacroiliac joints, can also be detected. Unfortunately, plain radiographs do not detect the early changes of joint space narrowing, as well as many subtle stress or insufficiency fractures. Many disorders of the hip and pelvis in young athletes manifest bone marrow edema (such as early avascular necrosis [AVN] or transient bone marrow edema syndrome). Plain radiography is unable to detect these changes as well. Even so, the role of plain radiography is preserved.

At our institution, AP, frog leg lateral, and standing AP pelvis views are routinely obtained. If FAI is suspected, a true cross-table lateral film is added.

MAGNETIC RESONANCE IMAGING

After screening plain films have been obtained, MRI is the next (and often final) imaging modality to be employed in the evaluation of the injured athlete. It is, currently, the diagnostic imaging modality of choice. The importance of various factors on the ultimate quality of MRI images cannot be overstated. In general, the higher the field strength of the magnet, the greater the quality of the examination; 1.5 T or above is considered high field strength. Additionally, type of coil, placement of coil, plane of imaging, use of contrast, and imaging parameters all play a major role in the final product. However, possibly the most important factor regarding MRI is the image interpretation and relationship with and confidence in the interpreter. This should encompass the entire imaging facility including the technologists.

From a technical standpoint, each MRI exam should be tailored to answer the specific question pertaining to the individual patient. Certain entities require imaging of a single hip only, while others require imaging of the entire pelvis and both hips. Most extra-articular causes of pathology do not need intravenous contrast. However, some (such as soft tissue or osseous tumors) do necessitate IV contrast. Currently, direct MRA is used to evaluate most causes of intra-articular pathology of the hip. T1-weighted and fluid sensitive sequences (such as T2-weighted and short tau inversion recovery [STIR]) are needed in all exams. T1 images are essential for anatomic detail and marrow imaging, while fluid sensitive sequences are essential for the evaluation of soft tissue edema, joint effusions, and marrow abnormalities. It is critical, particularly, when dealing with athletes who tend to develop overuse injuries within the musculature and in particular, the bone marrow that fat-suppression techniques are employed with the fluid sensitive sequences. This increases conspicuity of both subcutaneous fat and bone marrow edema.

COMPUTED TOMOGRAPHY

CT is most commonly used for the assessment of cortical fractures. This includes simple and complex acetabular fractures and pubic rami fractures. In athletes, CT scanning may detect stress type fractures, particularly if there is an associated periosteal reaction. However, MRI is currently the modality of choice in the assessment of stress injury based on its superior ability to image the bone marrow. CT is able to demonstrate avulsion fractures in the hip and pelvis adequately because of its excellent delineation of the cortical bone. In addition, CT is used for assessing many bone lesions (often times in conjunction with plain radiography and MRI) and can detect cortical bone destruction associated with these lesions, as well as matrix mineralization. Osteoid osteoma is typically imaged with CT and the central nidus is well seen. There is excellent ability to image developmental disorders of the hip in children and adolescents. Helical single CT and multidetector row CT (MDCT) with three-dimensional volume rendering have been successful in evaluating slipped capital femoral epiphysis as well as developmental dysplasia of the hip (DDH) in these patients.[1]

Overall, although CT scanning can be very useful in specific circumstances, its use in imaging the injured athlete remains limited.

RADIONUCLIDE SCANNING

Radionuclide (bone) scanning, or scintigraphy, has, for the most part, been supplanted by MRI in the evaluation of hip injuries in the athlete. This is predominantly due to the increased sensitivity and specificity of MRI for the detection of bone and soft tissue abnormalities. Radionuclide scanning is most often reserved for screening the entire skeleton to assess for systemic involvement of osseous and joint pathology.

ULTRASONOGRAPHY

In the athlete, ultrasound is reserved for specific indications and, overall, has a limited role in imaging the hip. It may be used to assess for iliopsoas tendon involvement in the internal snapping hip syndrome.[2–5] Sonography may also be used to image soft tissue fluid collections about the hip and thigh and is especially useful in postoperative patients who have metallic hardware (such as ORIF of femoral shaft fractures). Because ultrasound does not reliably evaluate intra-articular structures, other imaging modalities such as MRI with direct arthrography are generally used for assessing patients with suspected intra-articular etiology of their hip pain.[5]

OCCULT AND STRESS FRACTURES

Breithrupt gave the first clinical description of stress fractures in soldiers with painful and edematous feet two years after the discovery of the X-ray in 1897. This was revealed as fracture of the metatarsal shaft and was termed "March Fracture."[6,7]

Occult fracture is a term used to describe a fracture not initially visible on plain radiography. This includes fractures detected by other imaging modalities or eventually on radiographs. MRI may or may not reveal a fracture line. MRI will display patchy areas of increased T2 or STIR signal intensity and decreased T1 signal intensity[8–10] (Fig. 2.1).

Stress fractures may be divided into fatigue and insufficiency fractures. Fatigue fractures are seen in a healthy bone subjected to repetitive microtrauma, while insufficiency fractures occur when a normal physiologic load is applied to weak, deficiently mineralized bone, as is seen in osteoporosis and osteomalacia.[11] If the bone is subjected to excessive muscular action or abnormal torque, fatigue fractures occur (assuming it contains sufficient mineral content and elasticity). Stress response may

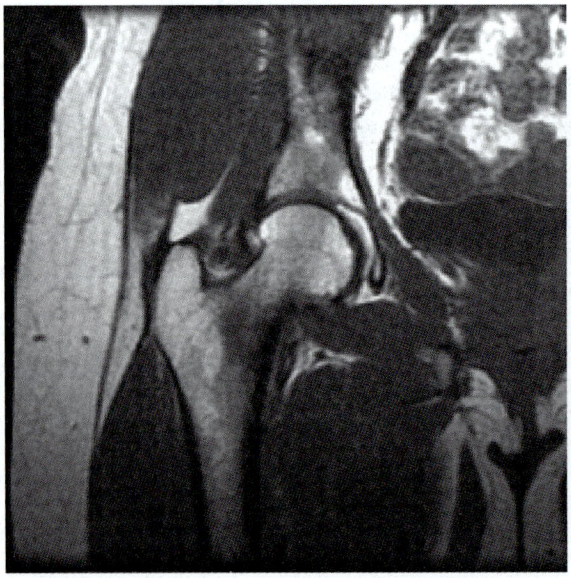
A

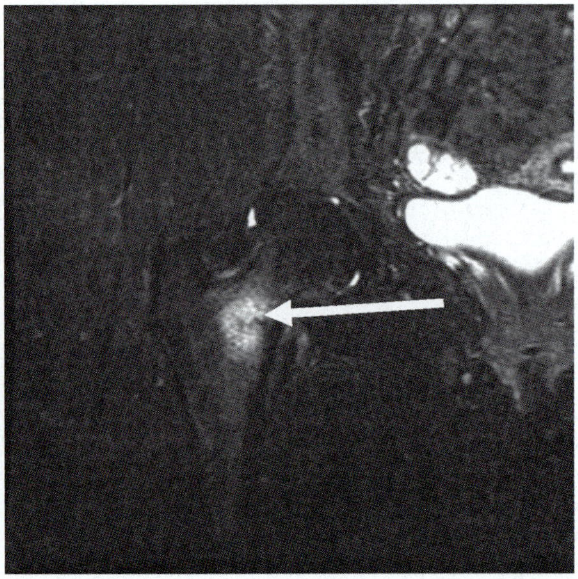
B

Figure 2.1. Coronal T1-weighted (**A**) and inversion recovery (**B**) MR images of the hip show decreased T1 signal and increased IR signal within the medial aspect of the femoral neck with a subtle linear focus of low IR signal representing incomplete fracture line (*arrow*).

be considered a subclinical stress fracture.[8] A fracture line is not visible, either radiographically or by MRI. For the purposes of this chapter, fatigue fracture and stress fracture will be used interchangeably.

Imaging is important in the evaluation of stress injuries to bones, as clinical assessment is often times difficult. As stress injury is a continuum from mild stress change to fracture, imaging findings are variable and somewhat unpredictable. Factors such as type of bone involved, athletic activity, and timing of the imaging procedure all have an effect on the imaging characteristics.[6]

Running is responsible for the highest number of stress fractures, and in many series, running caused more stress fractures than all other sports combined.[12]

Plain radiography should be the first study obtained. Two distinct types of femoral neck stress fractures have been described based on their causative mechanisms. A "compressive" variety is seen along the lower medial border and is usually nondisplaced and sclerotic on plain films. A "distraction" type is seen along the superior portion of the femoral neck.[7,13] The sensitivity of early radiographs is as low as 15% while follow-up radiographs will be positive in only 50% of cases.[7,14,15]

Sacral stress fractures have been described in athletes such as marathon runners. These appear to be more common in women[16] and typically parallel to the sacroiliac joint. Oblique coronal MR images through the sacrum with STIR or fat-suppressed T2-weighted fast spin echo (FSE) sequences are useful for examining the young athlete with buttock pain[8,11] (Fig. 2.2).

MR will reveal decreased T1-weighted and increased T2-weighted fat-suppressed or STIR signal. Shin et al. demonstrated that MRI was 100% accurate in correctly differentiating femoral neck stress fractures from other causes of hip pain.[17,18] Slocum et al. showed that 90% of patients with femoral neck stress fractures showed normalization of their signal intensity changes on STIR imaging within 6 months of initial diagnosis. Thus, when diffuse signal abnormality is seen on STIR greater than 6 months after initial diagnosis, this most likely represents a new injury.[19] Stress fractures may also be seen in the pubic rami and acetabulum in athletes.

MUSCLE AND TENDON INJURIES OF THE HIP

Although ultrasound has been found to be cost-effective and sensitive in the early detection and grading of muscle-tendon injuries, and conventional radiography and CT may be useful in specific types of injuries, such as osseous avulsions, the superior soft tissue contrast resolution of MRI has proven most effective in the evaluation of most posttraumatic musculotendinous disorders about the hip and thigh.[20]

MRI is able to visualize injury to all major components of the musculotendinous unit. This encompasses the tendinous origin and insertion sites, myotendinous junction (which, in the hamstring musculature, may run the entire length of the muscle), as well as the muscle belly.[20–24] MRI is also able to quantify the extent and degree of injury using axial, sagittal, and coronal imaging planes parallel to the long and short axes of the involved muscle-tendon unit.[23]

Fluctuations in water content in damaged musculotendinous tissue are seen in virtually all acute traumatic injuries.[21,23,24] T1-weighted imaging is relatively insensitive to these types of changes. Fat-suppressed T2-weighted or STIR sequences are highly sensitive in detecting subtle or overt edema in these tissues and are the workhorse in diagnosing these injuries.[21,24] T1-weighted imaging (in conjunction with T2) becomes useful in the detection of soft tissue hematoma, as in its subacute state methemoglobin is increased in signal intensity on T1-weighted pulse sequences (Fig. 2.3). Intramuscular hemorrhage can also

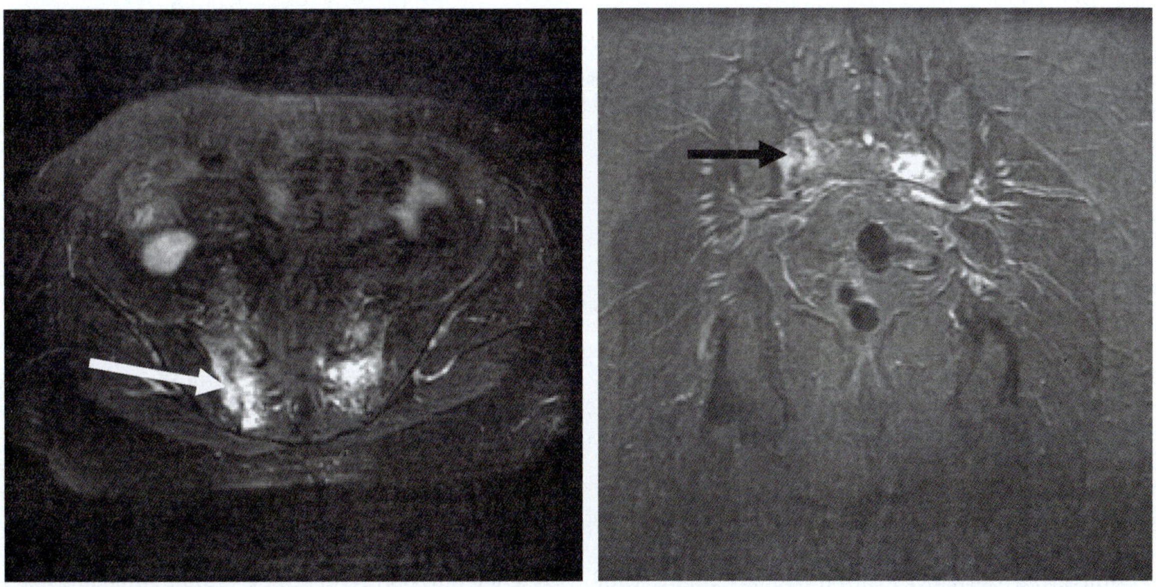

A B

Figure 2.2. Sacral stress fracture. Axial T2-weighted (**A**) and coronal inversion recovery (**B**) MR images of the pelvis demonstrate abnormal increased signal within both sacral ala with an irregular vertical fracture line in the right sacral wing (*arrow*).

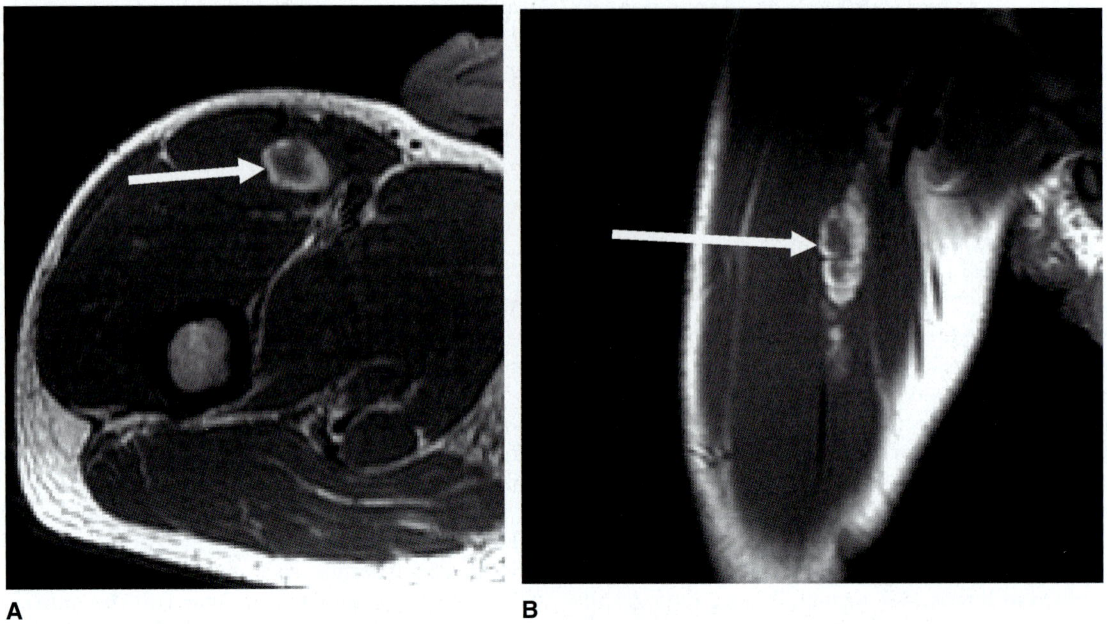

Figure 2.3. Intramuscular hematoma. (**A**) Axial and (**B**) coronal T1-weighted MR images demonstrate ovoid area of low signal intensity surrounded by hyperintensity within the rectus femoris muscle (*arrow*).

be imaged utilizing gradient echo T2-weighted pulse sequences due to the presence of blooming artifact related to the presence of blood products within the muscle. In addition, gadolinium-enhanced MRI has been suggested as a means to detect subtle musculotendinous injuries.[25]

PROXIMAL DISORDERS

AVULSION INJURIES

These types of injuries typically occur from forceful eccentric muscle contraction or from passive lengthening.[26,27] This may manifest as an avulsion fracture (Fig. 2.4) or avulsion injury of the proximal tendon (Fig. 2.5). Hamstring avulsion fractures off of the ischial tuberosity are fairly uncommon and are typically seen in adolescent athletes prior to closure of the apophysis.[28] These are usually diagnosed by plain radiography.[29,30] Acutely, the fracture appears as a crescentic, sharply marginated osseous fragment adjacent to the tuberosity. In chronic cases, marked periosteal reaction, callus, and oftentimes osteolysis at the fracture site may mimic a more aggressive lesion, often necessitating further workup. If there is a lack of marrow within the fragment, MR may miss small cortical fragments. Hematoma and periosteal stripping at the tendinous insertion with waviness and retraction of the tendon may be seen.

Hamstring tendon avulsion injuries at the ischial tuberosity are seen in adult athletes occasionally. Although the semimembranosus and conjoint tendon of the biceps femoris and semitendinosus are usually involved, some patients will preserve their semimembranosus. MRI adequately assesses tendon retraction and morphology of tendon edges and has been found to be highly sensitive and specific compared with ultrasound[30] (Fig. 2.6).

TENDINOPATHY

Tendinosis and tendinopathy are seen in athletes of all ages and are felt to be secondary to repetitive microtrauma and intrasubstance degeneration. MRI demonstrates increased cross-sectional area of the tendon with inhomogeneous intrasubstance increased T2 signal intensity (Fig. 2.7). Reactive marrow edema may be seen in the subjacent tendon insertion site, with the conjoint biceps femoris–semitendinosis tendon being affected in the majority of cases, relatively sparing the semimembranosus.[30]

MUSCLE STRAINS

Muscle strains occur most frequently at the myotendinous junction because of forceful muscle contraction.[21,26,31,32] Strains can be classified on MRI depending on the amount of disruption present.[21,33,34] First-degree strains produce a feathery appearance on T2-weighted or STIR images. This is a result of minor fiber disruption and associated mild interstitial edema and hemorrhage at the musculotendinous junction. Small areas of intramuscular and extramuscular laminar fluid may be seen (Fig. 2.8). Second-degree strains are characterized by partial-thickness tears without retraction, with a hematoma usually present. Third-degree strains represent complete rupture of the musculotendinous unit. MRI will demonstrate high T2 and STIR signal fluid within a gap (Fig. 2.9).

De Smet et al. reported the geographic distribution of hamstring injury within all segments of the musculotendinous unit. All strains in their study occurred at the musculotendinous junction, proximal (60%) slightly more common than distal.[35]

Pomeranz and Heidt[36] looked at multiple imaging parameters and found longer convalescence in athletes who had complete muscle transection, ganglionlike fluid collections, hemorrhage signal intensity, distal musculotendinous injury, and greater than 50% cross-sectional involvement. Another study found a significant

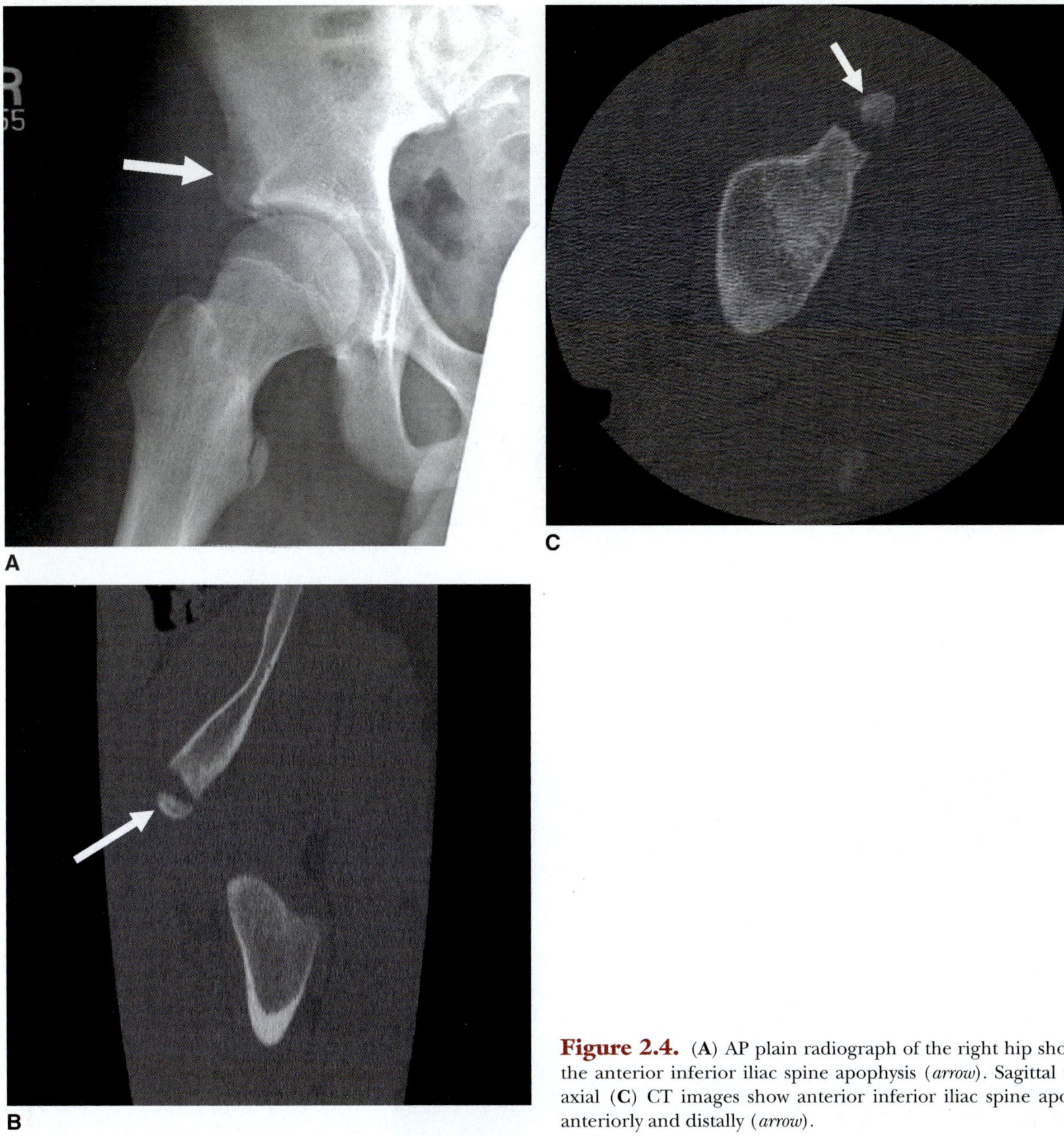

Figure 2.4. (**A**) AP plain radiograph of the right hip shows subtle avulsion of the anterior inferior iliac spine apophysis (*arrow*). Sagittal reformatted (**B**) and axial (**C**) CT images show anterior inferior iliac spine apophysis displacement anteriorly and distally (*arrow*).

association of pain with cross-sectional area and volume of abnormal muscle, but only a cross-sectional area of greater than or equal to 50% involvement was associated with longer rehabilitation times.[37] Connell et al.[38] found that multiple parameters were associated with a longer convalescent time including injury specific to the biceps femoris, percentage of cross-sectional area, length of injury, and injury outside the musculotendinous junction. Persistent MRI abnormalities were seen in up to 30% of players at a 6-week follow-up, although all but one were symptom-free.

MUSCLE CONTUSION

Muscle contusions are usually seen in contact sports such as football and rugby. These are secondary to direct blunt impaction and ensuing blood vessel disruption, interstitial edema and hemorrhage, and muscle inflammation. MRI reveals increased signal on T2 and STIR images with a feathery, infiltrative appearance and lack of architectural distortion[32] (Fig. 2.10). If a hematoma is present, MRI may show a focal mass with variable signal characteristics, depending on maturity and age of the hematoma.

A common complication of muscle contusion is myositis ossificans. This represents focal calcification or ossification at the site of injury. Radiographs and CT commonly demonstrate the typical rim of calcification or ossification. On MRI, however, signal intensity is often nonspecific and the peripheral, mineralized rim is often difficult to detect.[20]

Myofascial Herniation

Myofascial herniation represents a focal protrusion of muscle through a fascial defect. This is most frequently seen in the leg,

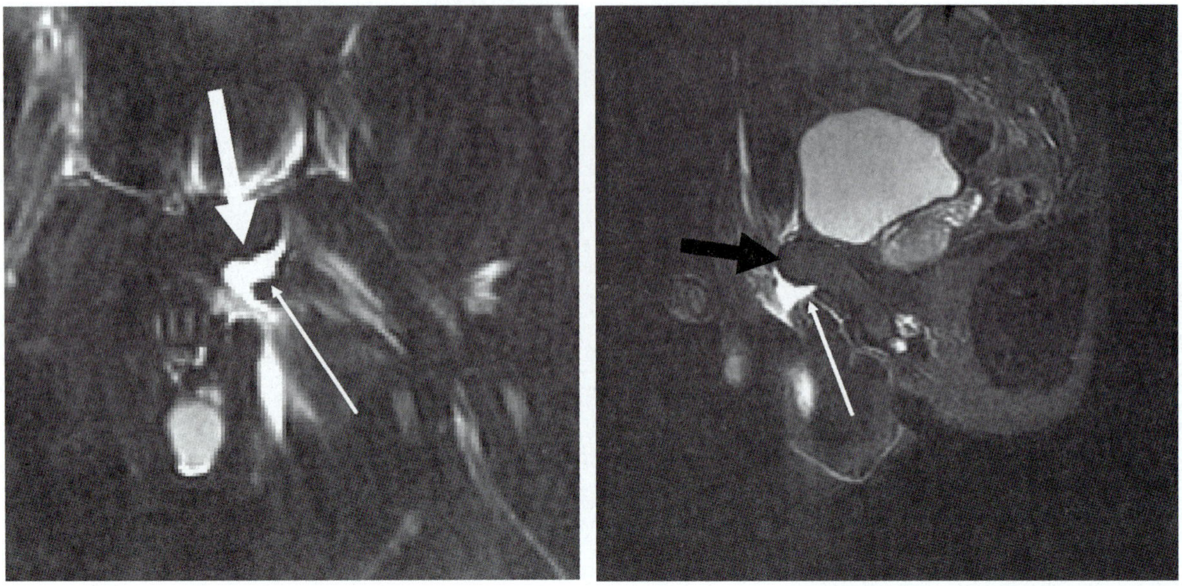

A B

Figure 2.5. Coronal inversion recovery (**A**) and sagittal T2-weighted fat-suppressed (**B**) images through the parasymphyseal region of the pelvis. High signal fluid (*thin arrow*) outlines complete avulsion of the adductor tendons from the pubic body (*arrow*) in this professional football player.

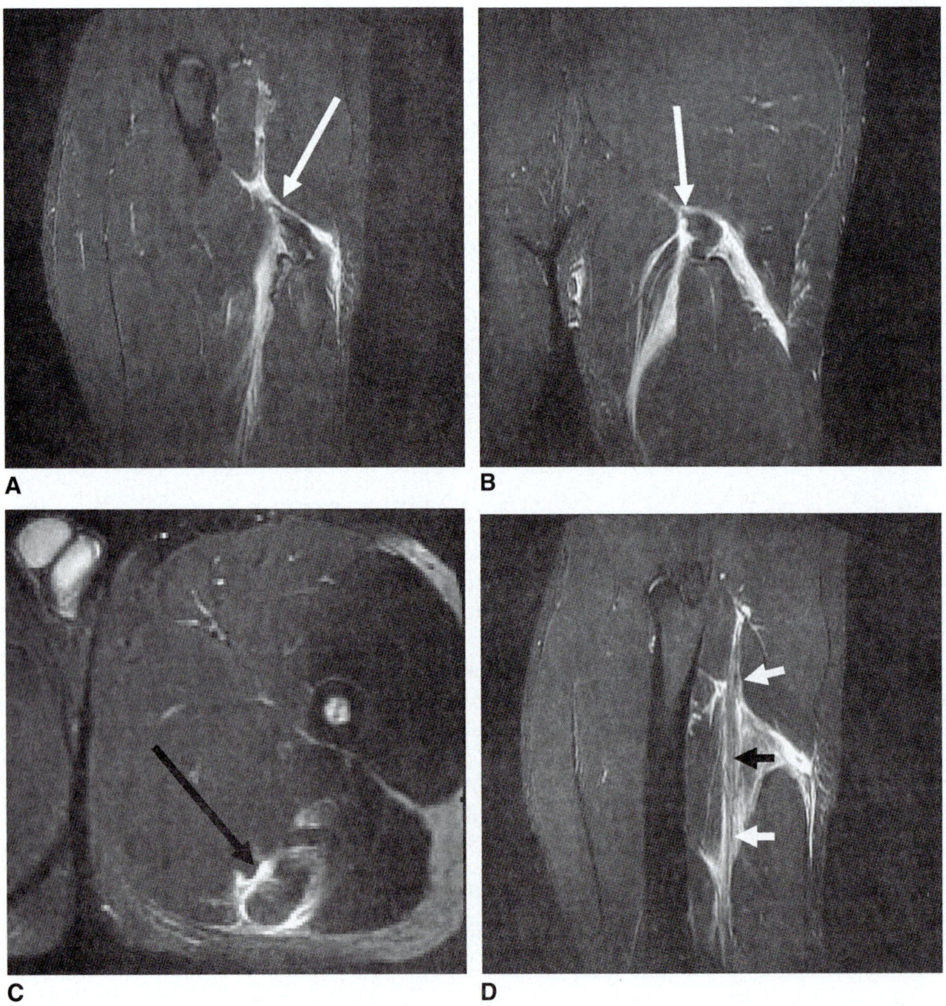

Figure 2.6. Complete hamstring avulsion in a professional football player. Sagittal T2-weighted fat-suppressed (**A**) and coronal inversion recovery (**B**) MR images demonstrate retracted, redundant ruptured tendon margin located within the mid-to-upper thigh (*arrows*). Axial (**C**) and sagittal (**D**) T2-weighted fat-suppressed MR images demonstrate thickened tendon with surrounding high signal hematoma (*long arrow*) as well as thickening and increased signal within the adjacent sciatic nerve (*short arrows*) representing neuritis.

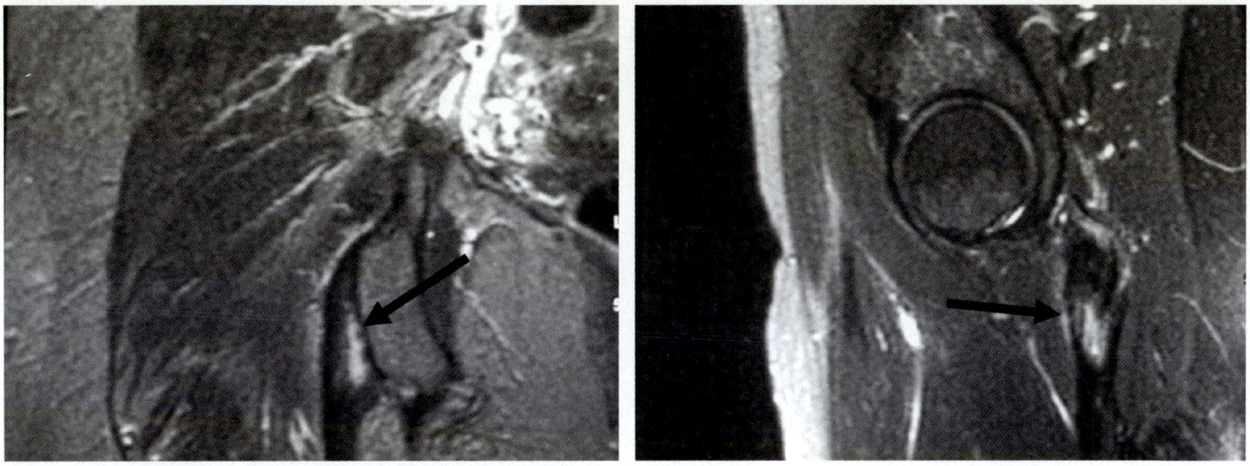

A B

Figure 2.7. Hamstring tendon strain. (**A**) Coronal inversion recovery and (**B**) sagittal T2-weighted images of the right ischial tuberosity reveal increased signal within the origin of the conjoined tendon of the biceps femoris and semitendinosis (*arrows*).

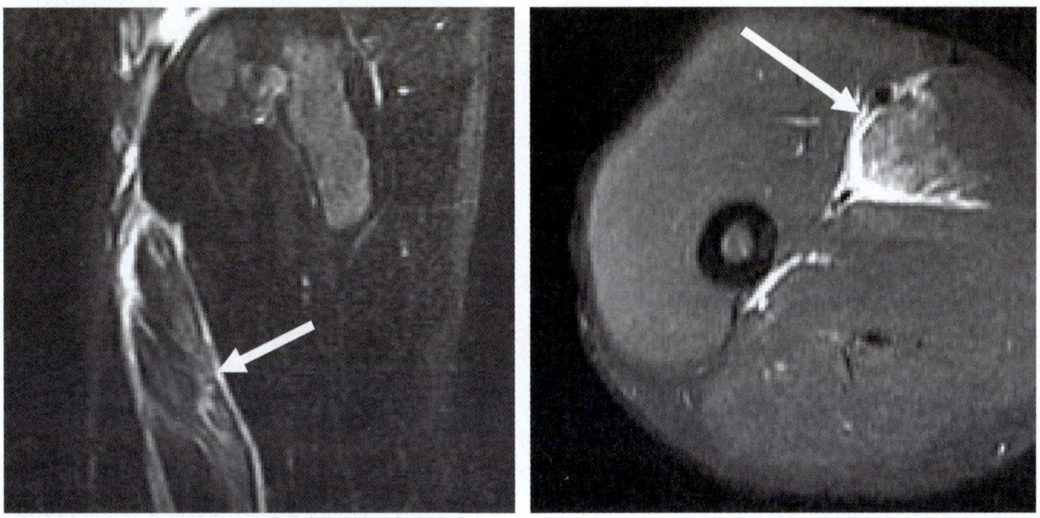

A B

Figure 2.8. Type I (first degree) strain. (**A**) Sagittal and (**B**) axial T2-weighted fat-suppressed images of the proximal thigh demonstrates increased signal within the adductor longus with a feathery appearance (*arrows*).

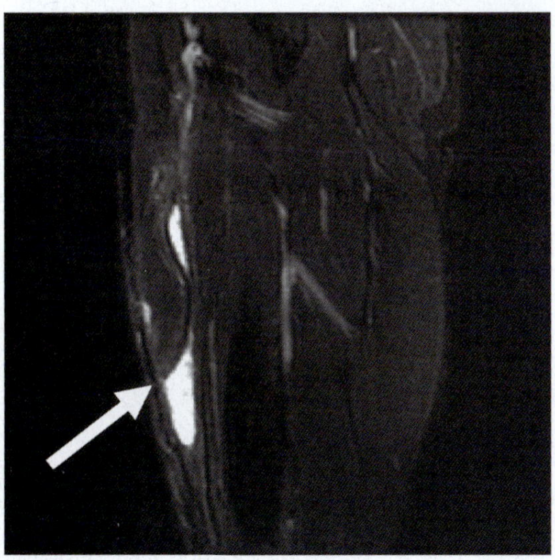

Figure 2.9. Type III (third degree) strain of the rectus femoris. Sagittal T2-weighted fat-suppressed image shows fluid within a gap with a smooth, retracted tendon margin, indicating a chronic injury (*arrow*).

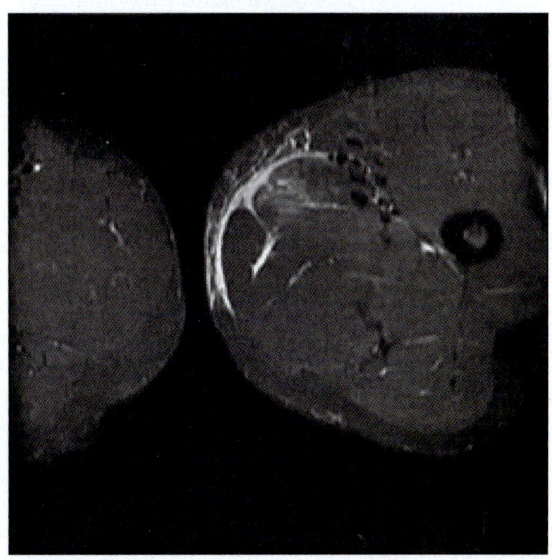

Figure 2.10. Axial T2-weighted fat-suppressed image. Abnormal increased signal within the adductor longus muscle with a feathery appearance and surrounding thin layer of fluid representing a muscle contusion. Note the lack of architectural distortion.

especially the middle and lower thirds. This is less common in the thigh. Hernias usually present in athletes or soldiers. MRI may be helpful to clarify the diagnosis when herniation is suspected, as well as to exclude other soft tissue masses.[20] A subtle bulge of the muscle belly may be seen. Fast, dynamic, and kinematic MRI during active contraction may reveal the abnormality.[20] Alternatively, MRI after rigorous exercise, particularly activity reported to reproduce the bulge, may help visualize the myofascial herniation.

DELAYED ONSET MUSCLE SORENESS

Delayed onset muscle soreness may be present several hours to days following rigorous exercise, usually in a new activity or increased activity level. Abnormal increased signal intensity on T2-weighted or STIR pulse sequences will be present, in a pattern mimicking a grade I muscle strain. Maximum changes are seen 48 to 72 h postexercise, and symptoms usually resolve within a week. Abnormal increased T2 or STIR signal intensity may persist up to 80 days postexercise.[39]

INTRA-ARTICULAR PATHOLOGY AND FEMOROACETABULAR IMPINGEMENT

A great deal of attention has been focused recently on the acetabular labrum, articular cartilage, and mechanisms by which they are injured.[40,41] A relationship between FAI, acetabular labral, and adjacent chondral lesions, and, thus, the development of subsequent osteoarthritis have been proposed.[42] Subtle anatomical findings and the concept of FAI have underscored the importance of the increasing role of imaging in the evaluation of intra-articular abnormalities in athletes with a painful hip. The mainstays of this imaging are plain radiography and MRA.[43–46] These athletes are prone to develop osteoarthritis of the hip as young and middle-aged adults.

FAI is defined as an abnormal contact between the anterior femoral head–neck junction and the anterior acetabular rim and labrum. FAI may be divided into two distinct types: "cam" and "pincer." Although most individuals have predominantly one or the other, combinations of the two may be seen. In cam FAI, a nonspherical shape of the femoral head at the head–neck junction as well as reduced depth of the femoral neck causes abnormal contact with the acetabular rim.[40,43,47] This nonspherical shape usually manifests itself as a "bump" along the lateral femoral neck (Fig. 2.11). Contact of the abnormal femur with the acetabulum is believed to lead to subsequent tearing of the adjacent labrum.[39,41,47]

In pincer FAI, acetabular overcoverage leads to decreased range of motion and abutment between the femur and acetabulum.[48] This process may be local, as is seen in acetabular retroversion or of a more general cause, such as coxa profunda and acetabuli protrusio. This type of FAI leads to labral tears with osseous proliferation at the acetabular rim. In addition, a "contre-coup" injury to the cartilage of the posteroinferior acetabulum may be seen.[43,47]

RADIOGRAPHIC ASSESSMENT OF THE HIP

Weight bearing AP views of the pelvis, as well as AP views of the hip, allow for measurement of acetabular coverage and orientation.[48,49] The lateral center edge angle (of Wiberg) is used to assess for acetabular dysplasia. This is obtained by creating a line from the center of the femoral head to the lateral aspect of the acetabulum and a perpendicular dropped through the femoral head (Fig. 2.12). This angle is considered abnormal if less than 20° to 25°.[50] The false profile view (anterior lateral edge) angle has also been used (Fig. 2.13). The horizontal toit externe (HTE) angle (acetabular index) of the weight bearing surface is obtained by drawing a line parallel to the weight

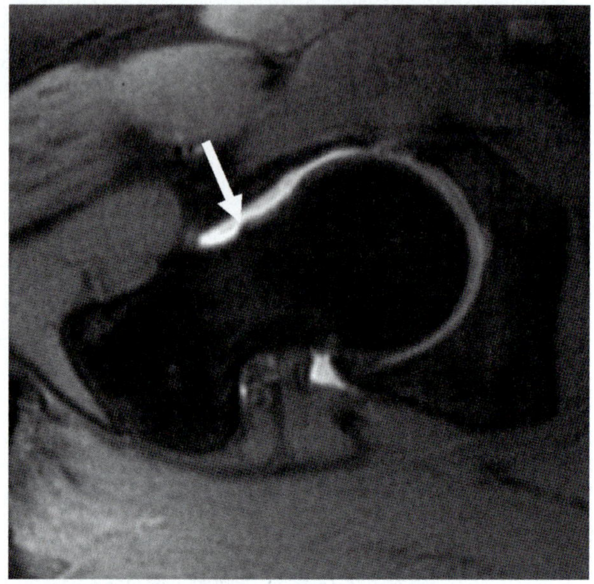

Figure 2.11. Axial proton density fat-suppressed image from an MR arthrogram reveals a "bump" at the anterior aspect of the femoral head-neck junction (*arrow*).

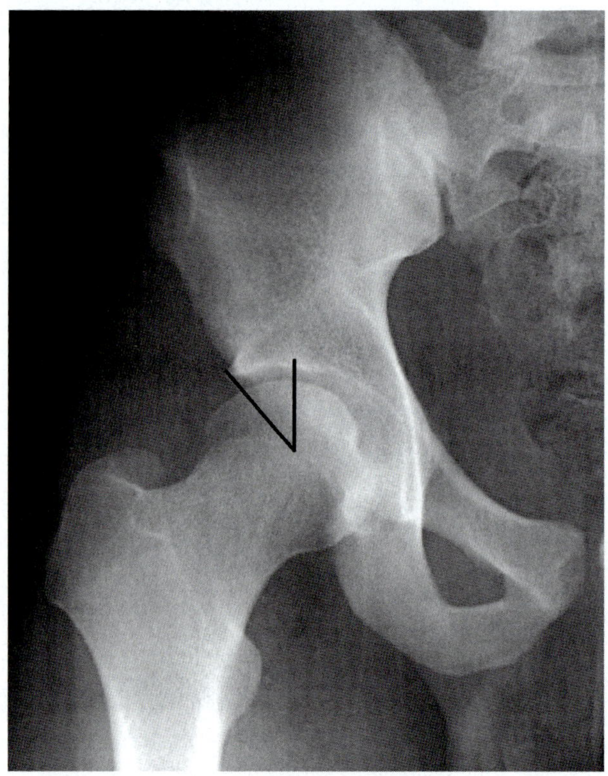

Figure 2.12. AP radiograph of the right hip. Normal lateral center edge angle.

bearing surface of the acetabulum referenced to a horizontal line (Fig. 2.14). Greater than 10° is considered abnormal.

Although the AP view of the hip is the most common, other lateral views are also obtained. These include the frog lateral (flexion and external rotation) as well as a Dunn view (90° flexion and 20° abduction) and cross-table lateral.[43,51,52] The cross-table lateral is obtained by placing the film cassette adjacent to the involved hip with the patient supine, with the opposite knee bent to allow the X-ray beam to pass. Head–neck offset is measured by drawing a line through the longitudinal axis of the femoral head and two parallel lines: one through the anterior femoral neck cortex and the other through the most anterior aspect of the femoral head. Distance between the two most anterior lines should be less than 7.2 mm (SD 2.6) in abnormal cases and 11.5 mm (SD 2.2) in normal patients. In cam FAI, the "bump" should be visible on all the lateral views. Another means to measure an abnormal femoral head–neck offset is the alpha angle. It is measured most frequently on a lateral radiograph, sagittal oblique, or radial MR image. The angle is formed by starting with a perpendicular line through the femoral neck at its narrowest point. Bisect the femoral neck perpendicular to this line. Create a best-fit circle onto the femoral head. The alpha angle is formed between the line through the femoral neck, and a line drawn from the center of the head to the point where the neck intersects the circular head[43] (Fig. 2.15). The angle should be less than 55°.

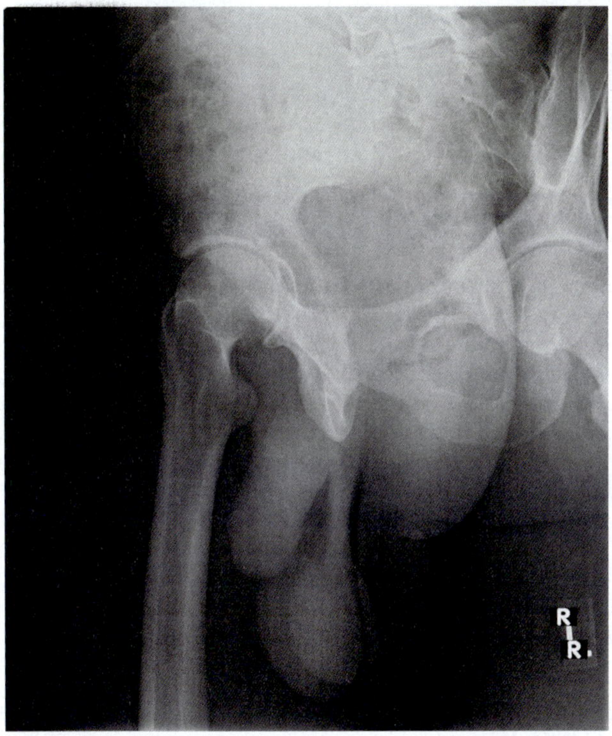

Figure 2.13. False profile view. (Reprinted from Beigler D, Chicago, Ils, with permission.)

Pincer FAI is generally associated with acetabular retroversion. This can be seen when the anterior acetabular rim projects more laterally than the posterior rim, usually superiorly. This is termed the "crossover" or "figure-8" sign on plain films (Fig. 2.16). The posterior acetabular rim should lie medial to the center of the femoral head as well (posterior wall sign). These abnormalities should be assessed on a well-centered view of the pelvis with the distance between the sacrococcygeal joint and pubic symphysis measuring 3 to 5 cm (3.2 cm in male, 4.7 cm in female)[53] or when the coccyx is about 1 cm from the pubic symphysis[54] (Fig. 2.17).

ADDITIONAL PLAIN RADIOGRAPHIC FINDINGS OF FEMOROACETABULAR IMPINGEMENT

A periacetabular ossicle (os acetabuli) is suggestive of FAI. Kassarjian et al.[49] looked at 42 hips with cam FAI and found an abnormal alpha angle in 93% and an os acetabulum in 40%. Rim ossification has also been associated with FAI (double-rim sign).[43]

Synovial herniation pits have been considered a normal variant, seen in 5% of the normal population. These were felt to be considered secondary to anterior pressure of the iliofemoral ligament on the joint capsule during hip extension (Fig. 2.18).[55] More recent reports raise the possibility of a pathologic component, with soft tissue impingement, enlargement, and association with pain.[50,56,57] Leunig et al.[57] studied 117

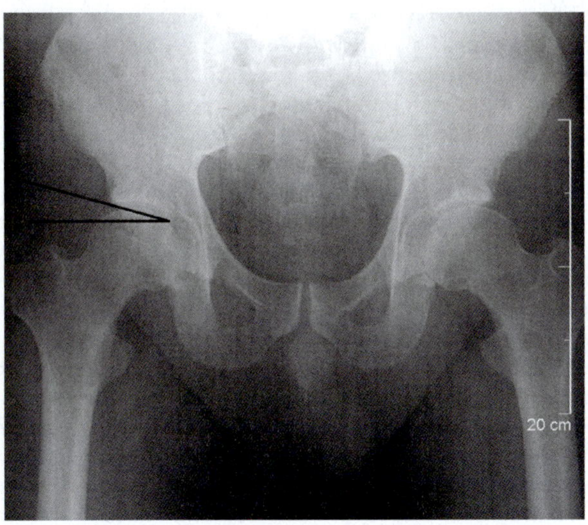

Figure 2.14. Acetabular index.

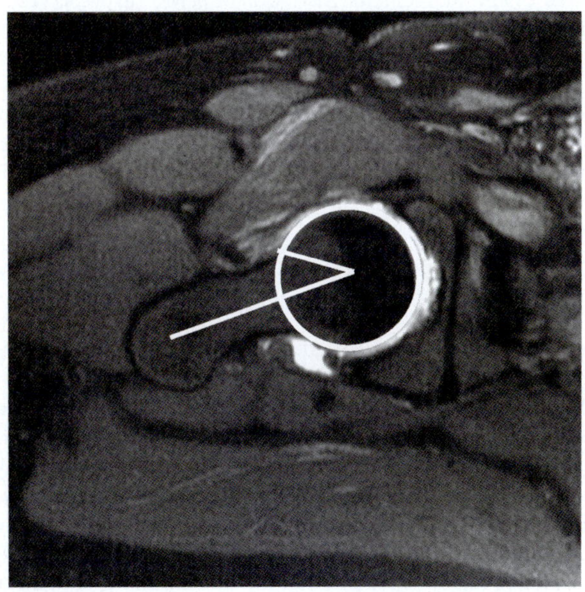

Figure 2.15. Normal alpha angle.

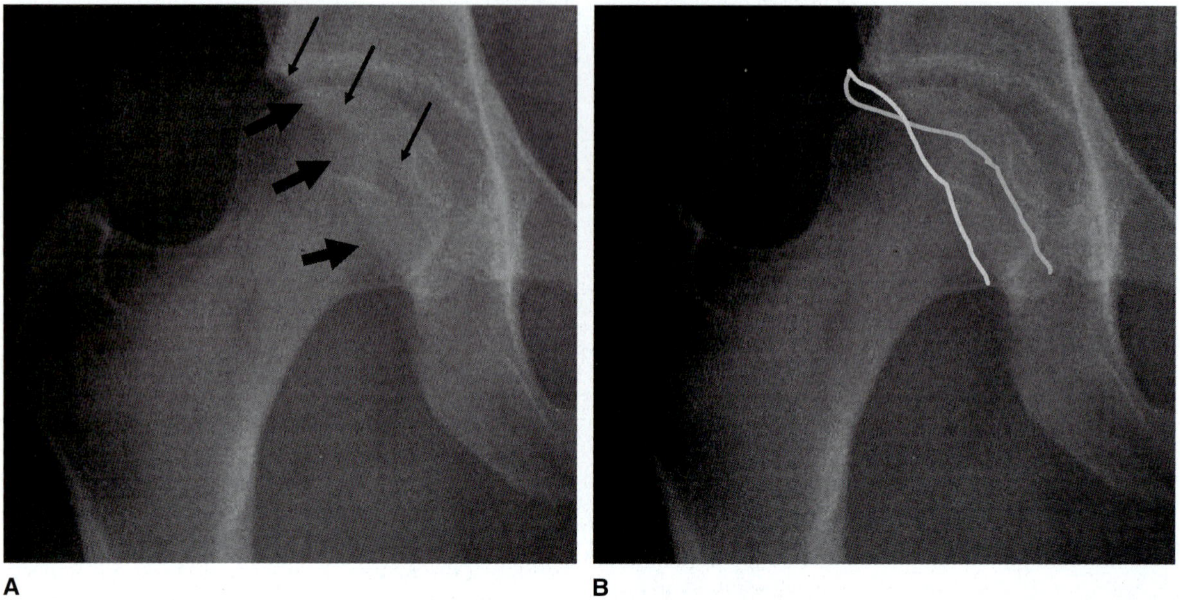

Figure 2.16. AP radiographs. **A**: Anterior acetabulum (*thin arrows*) and posterior acetabulum (*thick arrows*). **B**: *Crossover sign.*

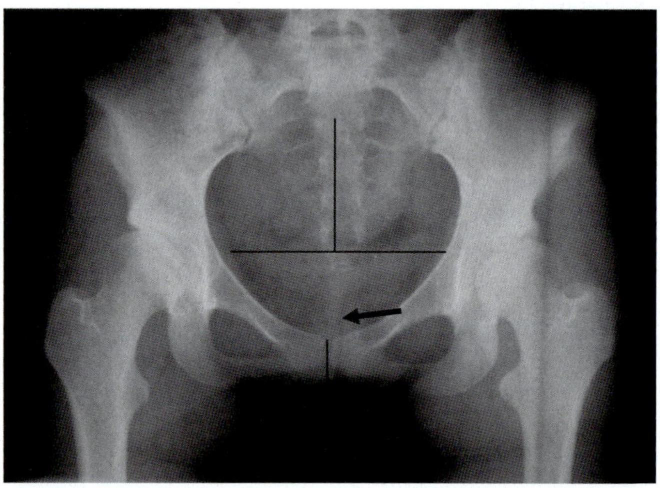

Figure 2.17. Well-centered AP view of the pelvis. Tip of coccyx within 1 cm of pubic symphysis (*arrow*). Sacroccygeal junction (*inverted* "*T*").

hips with FAI and found that 33% showed these herniation (fibrocystic) pits. Another recent study found 15% of patients with findings suggestive of FAI on frog leg lateral views had herniation pits and 30% had periacetabular ossicles.[58]

MAGNETIC RESONANCE IMAGING OF INTRA-ARTICULAR PATHOLOGY

Direct MRA of the hip is used for assessment of intra-articular pathology. Multiple studies have shown increased accuracy for direct MRA compared with noncontrast MRI. Czerny et al.[45] found that sensitivity increased from 30% to 90% and accuracy increased from 36% to 91% in going from noncontrast MRI to contrast MRI in a study of 57 hips in 56 patients. Hodler's group found increased conspicuity of the acetabular labral complex with administration of intra-articular contrast material utilizing 12 cadaveric hips.[59] Byrd assessed the labrum in 40 patients and compared noncontrast MR with MRA. A 42% false negative rate was obtained for labral tears with plain MRI as opposed to an 8% false negative rate for MRA.[60] Chen et al. more recently evaluated the sensitivity and accuracy of MRA with true sagittal scout images and radial reformation in detecting and localizing labral tears. They looked at 30 patients and compared their findings with hip arthroscopy. The sensitivity and accuracy for the diagnosis of hip labral tears were 100% and 96%, respectively.[61] Another study, however, obtained less encouraging results: 71% sensitivity, 44% specificity, and a positive predictive value of 93% and accuracy of 69%.[62] Toomayan et al.[63] compared MRA with a small field of view to noncontrast MRI with a large or small field of view and found MRA to be more sensitive than either type of noncontrast MRI.

MAGNETIC RESONANCE ARTHROGRAPHIC TECHNIQUE

Direct MRA is typically performed under fluoroscopic guidance. At our institution, an anterior or anterolateral approach is used and the proximal or mid femoral neck is localized. The foot is in slight internal rotation with the knee slightly flexed and supported, to create a lax anterior capsule. Two milliliters of iodine-based contrast to ensure positioning are instilled, followed by a mixture of dilute gadolinium (1:250 dilution), 8 mL of saline, and 0.25 mL of epinephrine (to allow retention of fluid within the joint via vasoconstriction). We also instill 2 to 4 mL of lidocaine and a steroid such as solumedrol. Preinjection and postinjection provocative log roll and flexion internal and external rotation maneuvers are performed to help determine an intra-articular or extra-articular cause of symptomatology. About 8 to 12 mL of total fluid is injected which allows for distension of the joint capsule and improved visualization of the labrum and cartilage. Overdistension of the joint may have deleterious effects such as decreased blood flow to the femoral head with increased intra-capsular pressure.[64] A recent study looked at the two common locations for injection (lateral femoral head and femoral neck) and found that the femoral neck injection caused less discomfort but was associated with more contrast extravasation.[65]

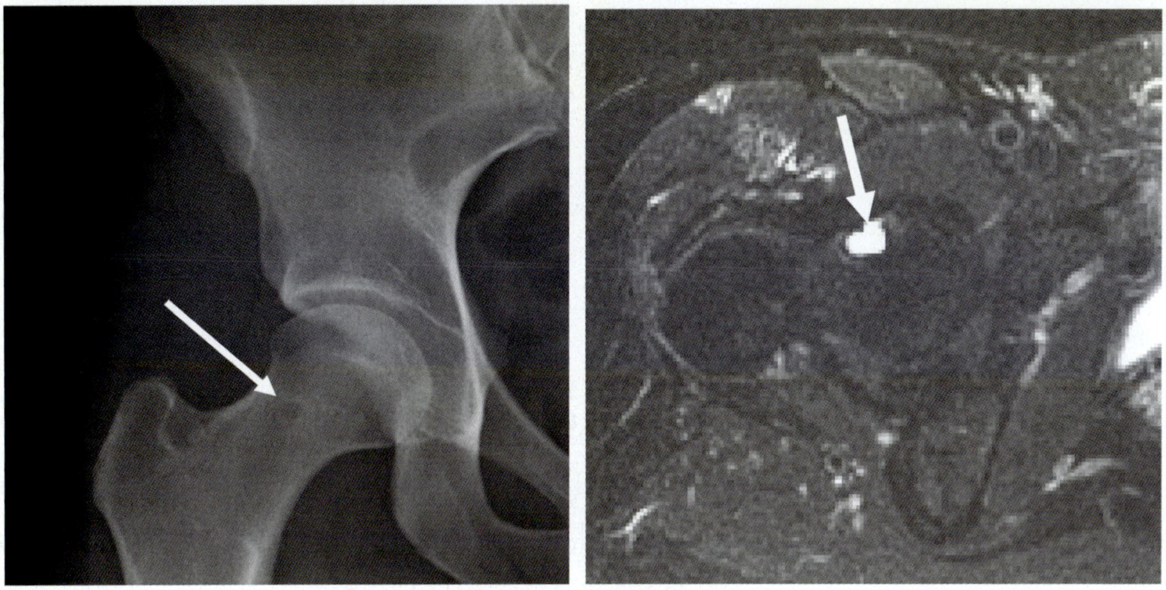

A B

Figure 2.18. **A:** AP radiograph. **B:** Axial T2-weighted fat-suppressed MR image. Rounded lucency within the femoral neck representing herniation pit (impingement fibrocyst) (*arrow*).

Unilateral, direct MRA of the hip should be performed with a phased-array surface coil in a high field strength scanner (≥1.5 T). A smaller field of view (14 to 16 cm) is used to increase resolution and enhance labral lesion conspicuity. Four imaging planes are obtained: axial, sagittal, coronal, and oblique sagittal. This last pulse sequence is obtained by imaging parallel to a line drawn through the long axis of the femoral neck (Fig. 2.19).

The specific protocols used at our institution include: true sagittal T1, fat saturation (repetition time [TR] 500, echo time (TE)[77], echo train length 2, 16 to 20 cm field of view, number of excitations [nex] = 2, frequency and phase matrix 256 × 192, slice thickness 4 mm with 0.5 mm interslice gap), true axial T1, fat saturation (TR 500, TE[77], echo train length 2, 16 to 20 nex = 2, matrix 256 × 192, slice thickness 4 mm with 0.5 mm interslice gap), true coronal inversion recovery (TR 4100 TE 42 inversion time 100, echo train length 8, matrix 265 × 160, 20 cm FOV, slice thickness 4 mm with interslice gap 0.5 mm), sagittal T2 fat sat (TR 2500 TE 68, echo train length 17, nex = 2, matrix 256 × 224, slice thickness 4 mm with interslice gap 0.5 mm), axial T2 FSE fat sat (TR 2500, TE 68, echo train length 17, 20 cm FOV, nex = 2, slice thickness 4 mm with interslice gap 0.5 mm, matrix 256 × 224), and oblique sagittal proton density fat sat (TR 1500 TE 11, echo train length 4, 20 cm FOV, 320×160 matrix, slice thickness 4 mm with interslice gap 0.5 mm). Radial imaging has also been

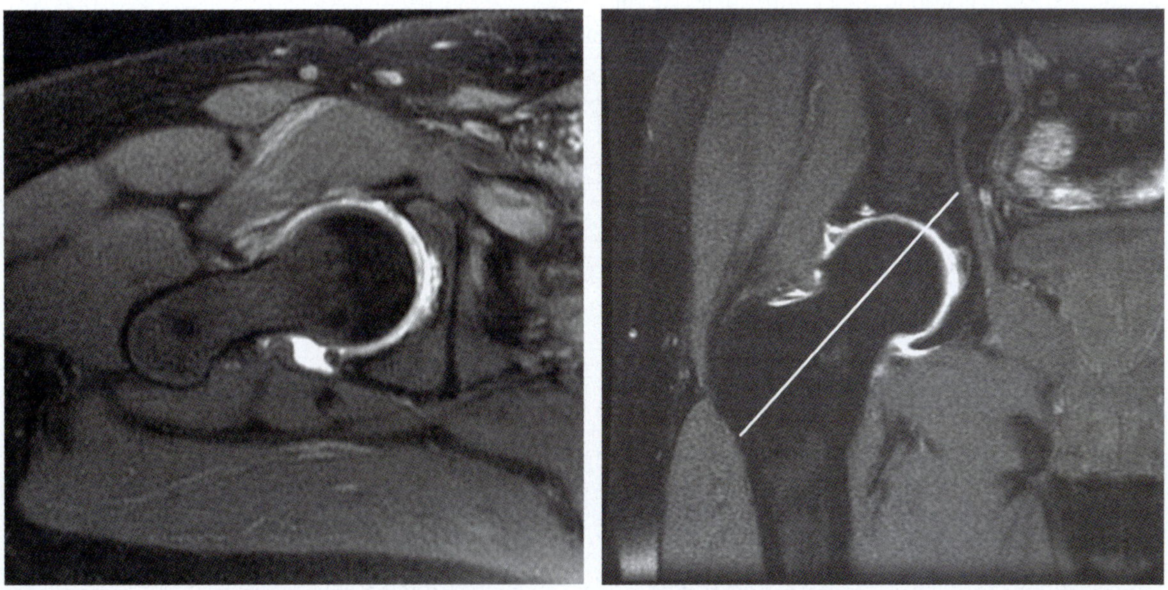

A B

Figure 2.19. Oblique sagittal proton density image (**A**) prescribed off of coronal image (**B**) through the long axis of the femoral neck.

employed in the evaluation of the labrum.[44,66] These are usually performed at 10° or 15° intervals from the geometrical center of the acetabulum in a double oblique fashion. T2-weighted pulse sequences remain essential for two reasons: (a) gadolinum does not usually penetrate paralabral cysts and (b) T1-weighted sequences do not adequately image the bone marrow.

THE LABRUM

The acetabular labrum has increasingly been recognized as a source of hip pain in the young, athletic population.[67] Anatomically, the labrum is triangular in shape. The base of this fibrocartilaginous structure is attached to the acetabular rim with the apex extending laterally along the capsular side. When the labrum is torn, forces are transmitted to the subjacent cartilage at the labral–chondral junction. This suggests a causal relationship between labral tears and subsequent osteoarthritis.[68] The majority of the athletic and traumatic tears of the labrum occur in the anterior, anterosuperior or superior portion, with some variations as a result of the different types of impingement.[47]

Because of a preponderance of organized collagen, as well as a relative lack of water, the labrum appears low in signal on all MR pulse sequences. The apex (free margin) may appear flattened, rounded, or mildly irregular, as well as sharp, in normal individuals (Fig. 2.20). However, rounding, enlargement, and increased intrasubstance signal intensity may be seen with aging.[50,69–71] This latter appearance, however, should not be seen in the young athlete.

There are several pitfalls in the interpretation of labral tears. One is the presence of a normal paralabral recess (labral recessus) between the capsule at its superior insertion and the capsular side of the labrum and adjacent acetabulum. This is often seen after capsular distention during MRA and is often absent in patients with acetabular dysplasia.[72] A second pitfall is the presence of a sublabral sulcus under the labrum. This has been, and remains, a controversial issue. Byrd,[73,74] in 1996, referred to an anterosuperior sulcus and stated that sublabral sulci were common in a follow-up review. One study employing second look arthroscopies in 100 patients showed a single posteroinferior sulcus, while another found several examples of posterinferior sulci.[75,76] Another study comparing MRI with arthroscopy showed that 22% of patients had sublabral sulci, and these were found at all anatomic positions (anterosuperior, anteroinferior, posterosuperior, and posterinferior) about the hip.[77] At our institution, we currently state the presence of a sublabral sulcus in all locations if the contrast outlines a smooth defect seen on multiple images at the base of the labrum at the labral–chondral junction (Fig. 2.21). A third pitfall is the occasional presence of mild, increased signal on all pulse sequences at the labral–chondral junction which should not be confused with a tear. Finally, the junction of the anterior labrum and transverse ligament can frequently demonstrate an irregular appearance which should not be confused with a tear (Fig. 2.22).

Lage et al.[78] described an arthroscopic classification for acetabular labral tears. Type 1 is a radial flap tear with disruption of the free margin (Fig. 2.23) and accounts for 57% of all tears. Type 2 is a chronic degenerative tear and appears as radial fibrillation (22%). Type 3 is a longitudinal peripheral (16%) tear at the junction of the labrum and acetabulum (Fig. 2.24),

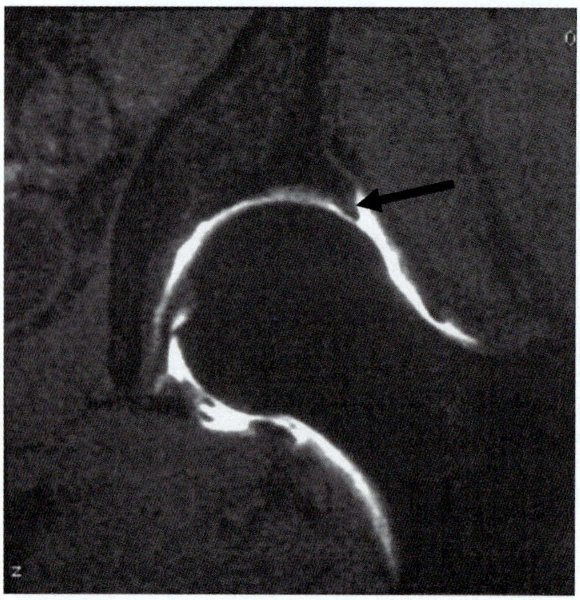

Figure 2.20. Normal triangular-shaped acetabular labrum (*arrow*).

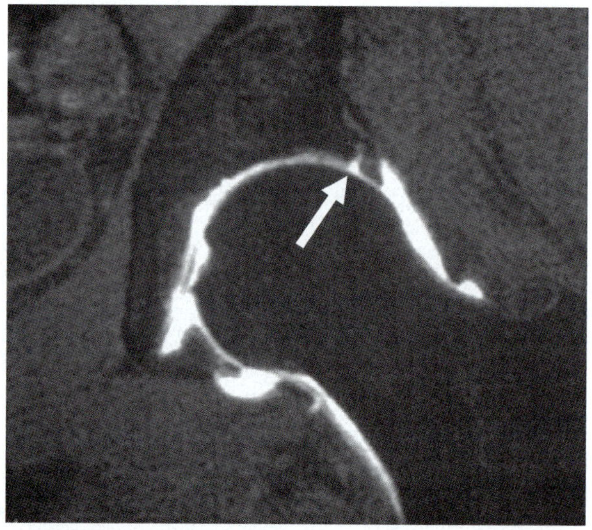

Figure 2.21. Normal sublabral sulcus (*arrow*).

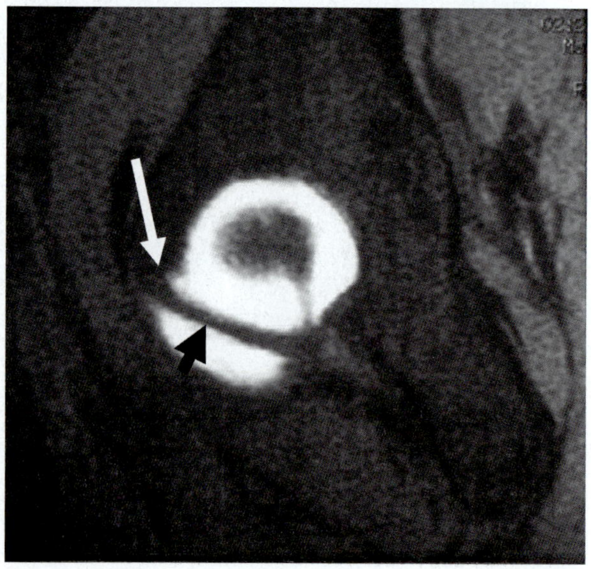

Figure 2.22. Sagittal postcontrast image demonstrates normal irregularity (*long arrow*) at the junction of the transverse ligament (*short arrow*) and anterior acetabulum.

and type 4 is an abnormally mobile, unstable tear. Although MR classifications of labral tears have been presented, the usefulness of these systems has been questioned. However, newer arthroscopic techniques that aim to repair the labrum and salvage tissue have been developed and for this reason MR description of labral tears should be as descriptive and specific as possible.[79] Much as in the glenoid labrum, tears may be described as partially or completely detached. Linear contrast or fluid will be seen extending partially or completely through the base of the labrum, near its attachment to the acetabulum. The labrum may be displaced or nondisplaced. The orientation of the tear is also included, such as radial or flap, as well as the length. Intrasubstance tears may be seen, in which the contrast extends into the midsubstance of the labrum, usually along the articular side. A degenerated labrum demonstrates abnormal contour with either thinned or diffusely enlarged morphology and abnormal fluid or contrast signal within the substance (Fig. 2.25).[50] When the degenerated labrum extends longitudinally from anterior to posterior, this may reveal a linear high signal focus on true coronal images, surrounded above and below by linear low signal, what we term the "oreo cookie" sign (Fig. 2.26). MR may detect paralabral cystic fluid collections seen best on T2-weighted sequences and is a reliable sign of an associated acetabular labral tear (Fig. 2.27).[80,81]

HYALINE CARTILAGE INJURY

There is a strong association between FAI, labral tears, and cartilage abnormalities.[47,82] So, clearly, close inspection of all portions of articular cartilage is essential for the complete

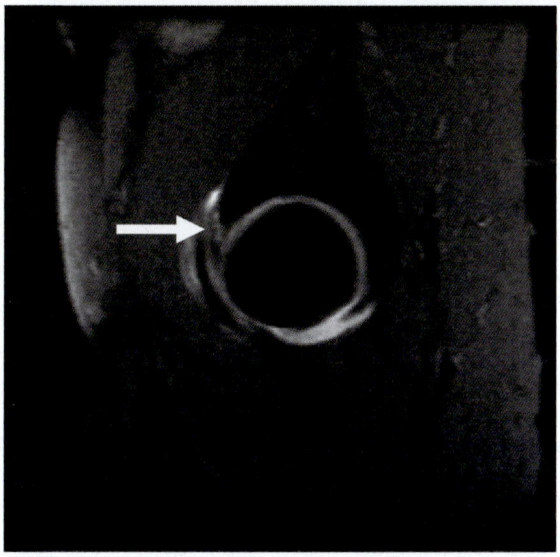

Figure 2.23. Sagittal T1-weighted MR arthrographic image. Linear high signal within the base of the anterior labrum (*arrow*) representing type I tear.

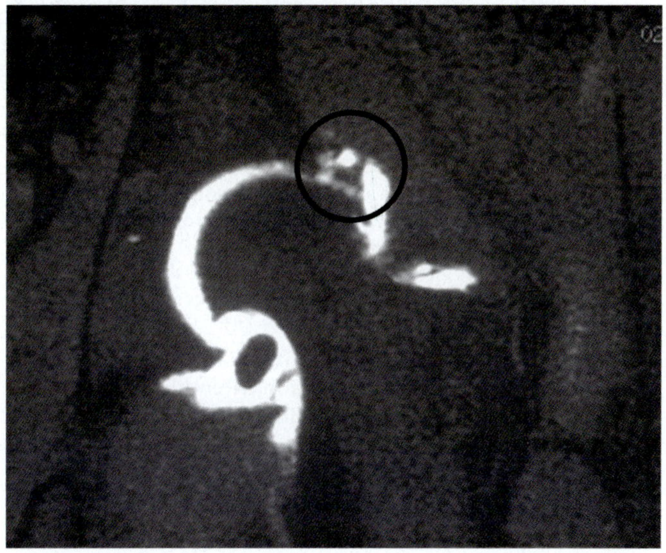

Figure 2.25. Coronal T1-weighted postcontrast image demonstrates abnormal morphology, intrasubstance contrast, and detachment of a degenerated labrum (*circle*).

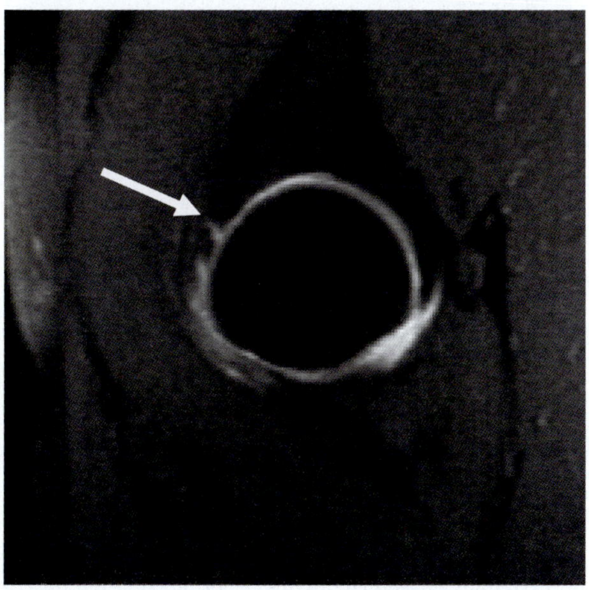

Figure 2.24. Sagittal T1-weighted MR arthrographic image demonstrates linear high signal at the base of the anterior labrum representing detached, nondisplaced type III tear (*arrow*).

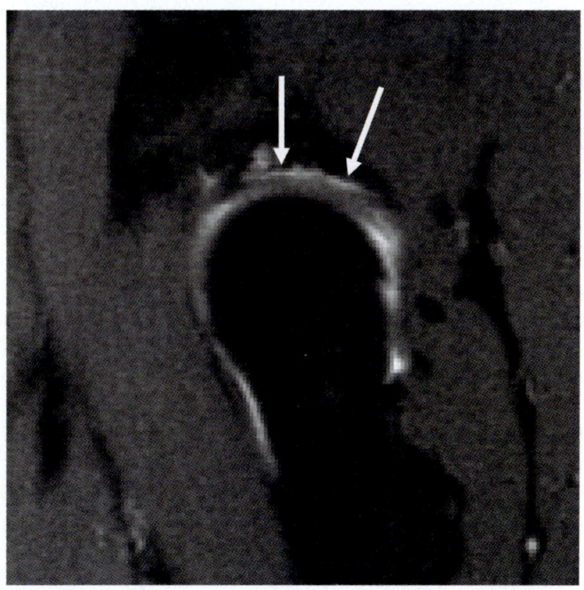

Figure 2.26. Sagittal T1-weighted MR arthrographic image through the superolateral labrum. Linear high signal extending from anterior to posterior representing an intrasubstance longitudinal tear (*arrows*).

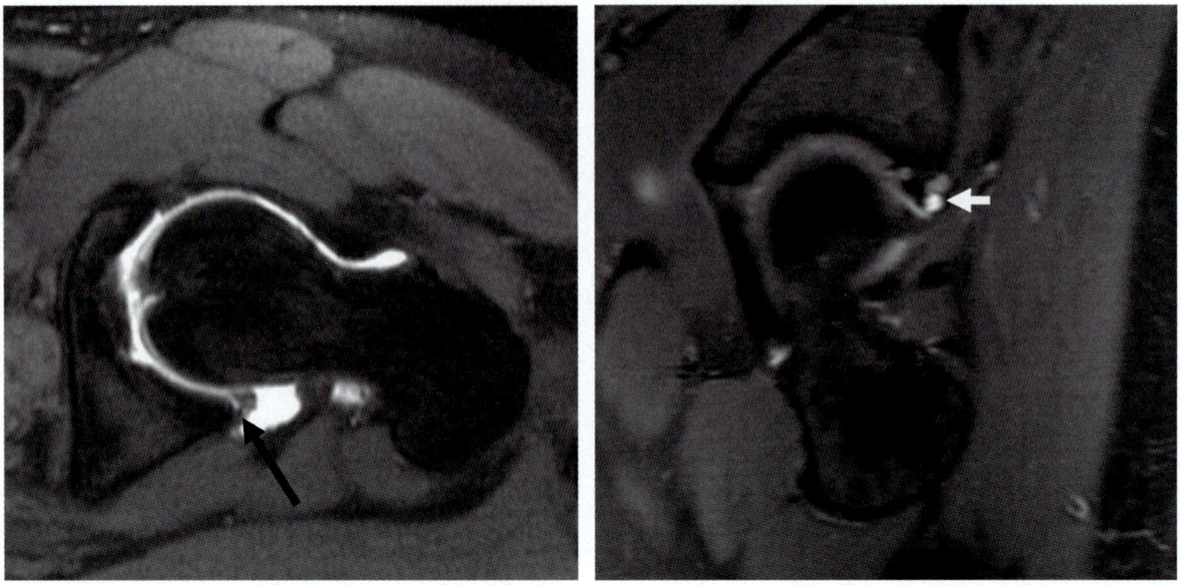

Figure 2.27. Posterior labral tear and paralabral cyst. (**A**) Oblique sagittal and (**B**) true sagittal T1-weighted MR arthrographic images. Abnormal signal within the base of the posterior labrum (arrow) representing tear. There is a small rounded focus of high signal at the posterior margin of the posterior labrum indicative of a paralabral cyst (*short arrow*).

evaluation of intra-articular structures. Unfortunately, only moderate sensitivity for the detection of chondral lesions has been reported. A range of sensitivities from 47% to 79% and specificities from 77% to 89% has been reported for articular pathologies.[62,83]

Cartilage damage is felt to be the primary etiology of early osteoarthritis and one study has found significant lesions in 63% of hips, predominantly in an associated anterior location (Fig. 2.28).[84] In this study, 73% of labral lesions had accompanying chondral lesions, while only 6% of chondral lesions did not have labral lesions. It is difficult to assess the articular cartilage of the hip by imaging for several reasons. This includes inadequate filling of defects in the acetabular hyaline cartilage, relatively thin cartilage, particularly when compared with cartilage in the knee, and the hip's curved structure and inherent problems of volume averaging. Beck et al. described different patterns of cartilage loss with different types of FAI. They found that pincer type FAI resulted in diffuse, circumferential chondral injury, while cam type FAI resulted in primarily anterosuperior chondral injury.[85] The MR classification for osteochondral lesions of the hip is as follows: Grade 1 shows intact cartilage with subchondral bone signal changes, grade 2 shows a partial detachment of cartilage with subchondral signal changes, grade 3 shows complete detachment of a nondisplaced fragment, and grade 4 shows a detached and displaced fragment (Fig. 2.29).[31] Grades 1 and 2 are more accurately depicted by MRA than grades 3 and 4 at this time, and much of the research is currently geared toward detection of these earlier chondral lesions.

Delayed gadolinium-enhanced MRI of cartilage (dGEMRIC) is a promising means of possibly assessing these early stages of cartilage degradation. This technique has been applied to the articular cartilage of the knee previously,[86–88] and more recently has been applied to the hip, particularly in patients with hip dysplasia, by Kim et al.[87] The dGEMRIC acts under the premise that loss of glycosaminoglycan (GAG) is a prelude to early osteoarthritis.[89] The dGEMRIC is a molecular imaging technique that estimates GAG distribution in articular cartilage by T1 mapping in the presence of Gd-DTPA2- (T1, Gd).[86,90] The "delay" refers to the time necessary for the contrast to diffuse into the cartilage after IV injection. A color-coded mapping of the cartilage is obtained that displays regions of early GAG degradation (Fig. 2.30). Tiderius et al. have looked at optimal timing protocols for this type of study[91] and

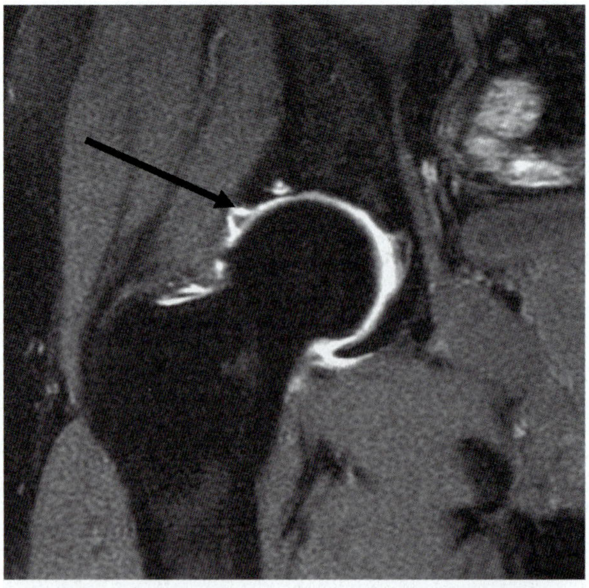

Figure 2.28. Osteoarthritis and labral tear. Coronal T1-weighted MR arthrographic image demonstrates high signal at the base of the labrum (*arrow*). There is prominent chondromalacia involving the superior acetabulum with subchondral cyst formation.

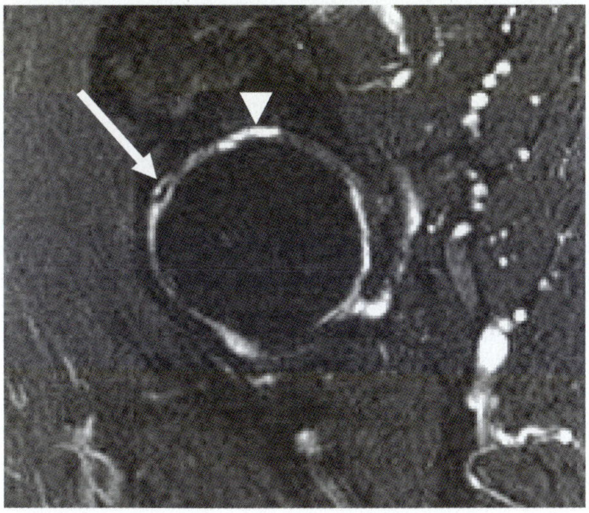

Figure 2.29. Sagittal T2-weighted image of the hip reveals chondral flap anteriorly (grade II lesion) at the chondral–labral junction (*arrow*) with a chondral defect (grade IV lesion) at the superior aspect of the acetabulum (*arrowhead*).

found higher sensitivity to the disease 30 to 65 min after contrast injection, but more reproducibility closer to 100 min after injection. At all times, the dGEMRIC index was 20% to 30% lower in osteoarthritic patients than healthy volunteers. This indicates that dGEMRIC is a sensitive measure of early cartilage degradation in the hip joint.[91,87] Using the dGEMRIC technique, Boesen et al.[92] found that intra-articular gadolinium provided better delineation of hip joint cartilage than intravenous injection.

LIGAMENTUM TERES

Increasingly, ligamentum teres abnormalities have become an indication for MRA of the hip, since they represent the third most common cause of intra-articular pathology.[93,94] Anatomically, the ligamentum teres courses from the fovea of the femoral head proximally to the transverse ligament and posteroinferior portion of the cotyloid fossa of the acetabulum.[95,96] The shape changes from round or oval proximally to trapezoidal at the transverse ligament (Fig. 2.31).[93] On MR, the normal ligament appears homogeneous with low signal intensity on T1- and T2-sequences. Oblique sagittal images may help alleviate partial volume averaging seen on some true sagittal and coronal images.[50] Ligamentous intrasubstance signal change, discontinuity, or fraying all indicate injury (Fig. 2.32). A hypertrophied ligamentum teres may also be identified. This is present when the ligament extends more than 2 mm beyond its foveal insertion on oblique axial images. The exact significance of a hypertrophied ligamentum teres is unclear. Guanche and Sikka[97] looked at elite runners and found hypertrophic changes in the ligamentum teres during arthroscopy and postulated a relationship with chronic instability.

LOOSE OSTEOCHONDRAL BODIES

MRA is excellent for the detection of loose osteochondral bodies within the joint. Hip joint distention with contrast (or joint fluid) will increase conspicuity of loose bodies that otherwise may be concealed by a contracted joint capsule (Fig. 2.33).

DEVELOPMENTAL DYSPLASIA OF THE HIP

While DDH and FAI have many clinical similarities, such as presentation of groin pain, symptoms of acetabular overload, and early onset of osteoarthritis, the imaging findings may differ significantly. Evaluation for the presence of DDH begins with measuring the acetabular coverage of the femoral head including the center-edge angle of Wiberg.[41,98] The hip should also be evaluated for sphericity and concentricity of the femoral head and acetabulum. In addition, focal retroversion of the anterosuperior acetabulum is a common finding in these patients.[49] The abnormal acetabular coverage leads to microinstability and subsequent shear stresses resulting in enlargement of the labrum with degeneration, fraying, and tearing.[99] Associated chondral injury ensues, usually at the anterosuperior aspect of the joint.[100]

TRANSIENT OSTEOPOROSIS OF THE HIP

Transient osteoporosis of the hip (TOH) has also been recently termed "bone marrow edema syndrome" and "transient bone marrow edema."[101] This entity was first described in 1959 and has been the focus of much debate. There is no consensus regarding its etiology or pathophysiology. Some believe TOH to be a distinct

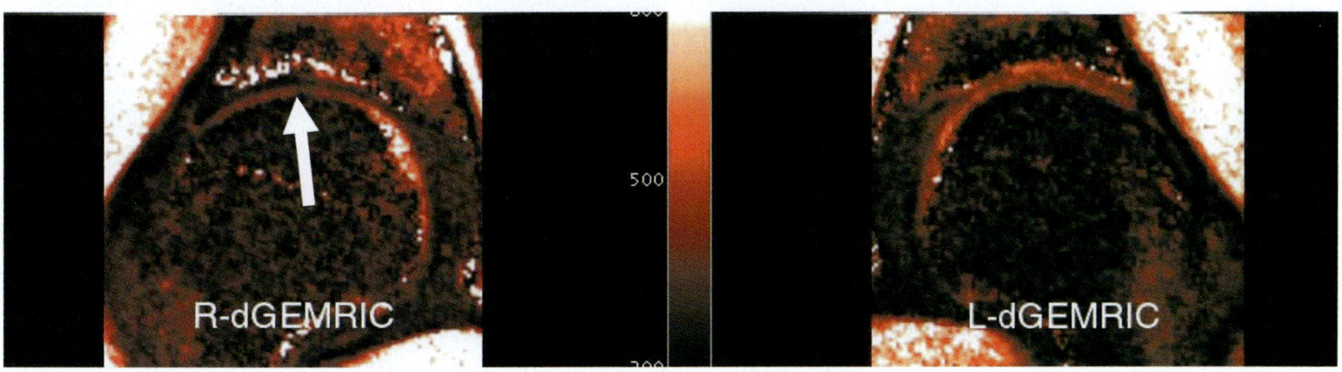

Figure 2.30. Decreased dGEMRIC index (*darker shading*) within the articular cartilage of the right hip (*arrow*) relative to the left hip indicative of cartilage degradation. (Reprinted from Kim YJ, Boston, MA, with permission.)

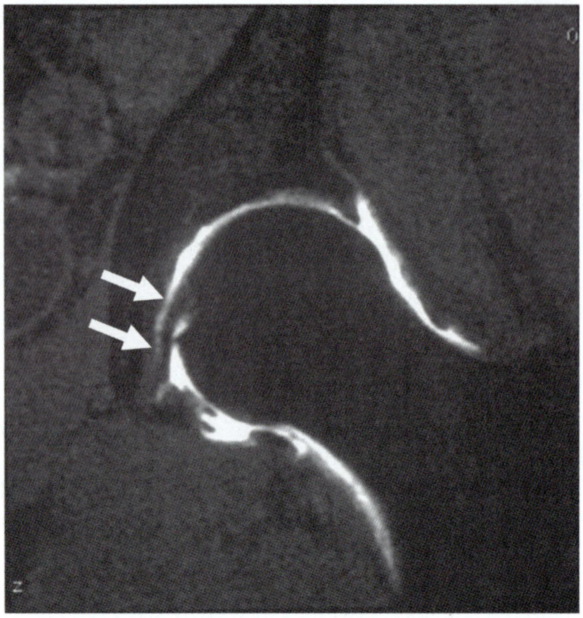

Figure 2.31. Normal ligamentum teres. Coronal T1-weighted postcontrast image reveals normal course and appearance of the ligamentum teres.

entity attributed to a process similar to reflex sympathetic dystrophy, while others believe it represents an early form of AVN.[101,103,104]

This entity was originally described in pregnant women in their third trimester but is now most commonly seen in young and middle-aged men, and is seen in more and more athletes in these age groups. Clinically, patients experience sudden onset of hip pain which may significantly restrict mobility. Plain radiographs may be normal or demonstrate osteoporosis of the femoral head and neck.[105] In the past, bone scintigraphy has been the imaging modality of choice after plain films. MR demonstrates a nonspecific bone marrow edema pattern consisting of diffuse decreased T1-weighted and increased T2-weighted signals within the femoral head, usually extending into the femoral neck and intertrochanteric region (Fig. 2.34). Occasionally, subchondral marrow changes are seen as small fractures (0% to 5%).[102,106] In an attempt to differentiate irreversible lesions from transient bone marrow edema lesions within the femoral head, Vande Berg et al. reviewed 72 lesions in 42 men and 25 women. The presence of a subchondral focus of low T2 signal intensity, at least 4 mm thick or 12.5 mm long, had positive predictive values of 85% and 75%, respectively, for irreversible lesions. Lack of subchondral change on T2-weighted images had a 100% positive predictive value for transient lesions.[107] TOH is considered a self-limited disease with much controversy of what is the most effective treatment.[108,109]

OSTEONECROSIS

Osteonecrosis is a dynamic process which is characterized by bone marrow ischemia progressing to cell death and subsequent attempted repair.[110] Pathophysiologic studies of the femoral head have shown that AVN develops as a result of insufficient blood flow to the bone. The etiology is multifactorial in most situations.[111–115] With disruption of femoral head blood flow, local PO_2 is reduced, and with as little as 2 to 3 h of ischemia, osteocyte necrosis ensues. After necrosis, a reparative phase takes place. MRI can be used to evaluate this process and has been determined to be the most sensitive imaging modality for the evaluation of osteonecrosis.[116,117]

MRI findings of osteonecrosis include a geographic area of variable signal intensity surround ed by a peripheral rim of T1 and T2 hypointensity. The peripheral hypointense rim represents sclerosis and demarcates viable from nonviable bone.[116] In up to 80% of cases, a "double-line" sign is present, a band of high signal intensity within the hypointense rim which is virtually

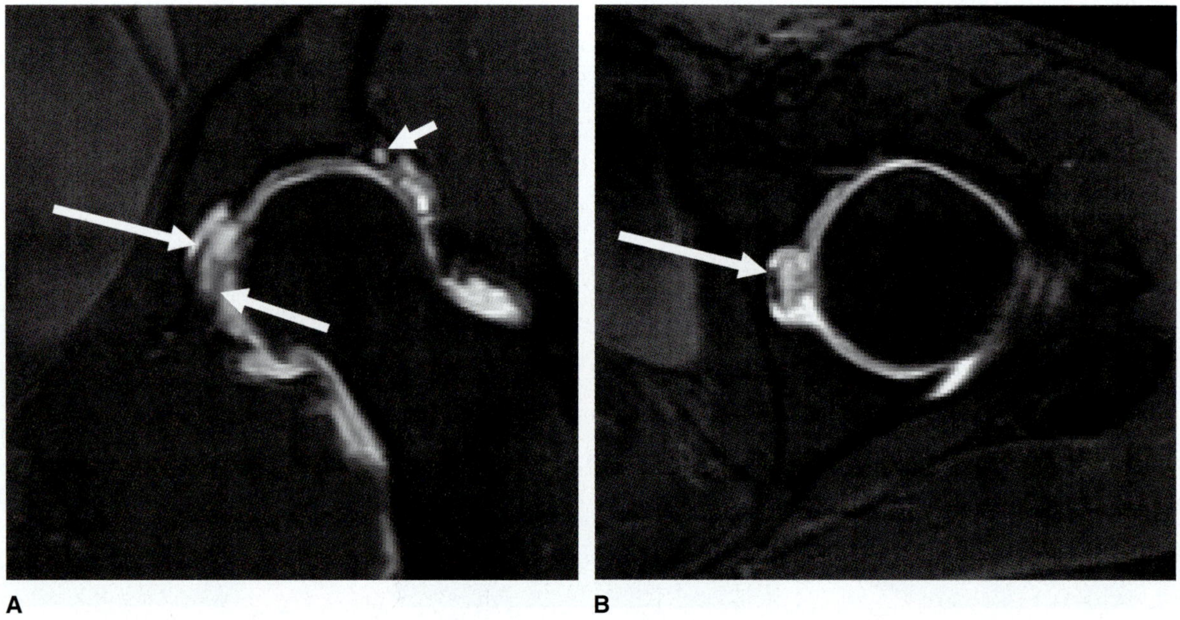

Figure 2.32. Ligamentum teres tear. Coronal (**A**) and axial (**B**) T1-weighted MR arthrographic images demonstrate abnormal contrast within a thickened but grossly intact ligamentum teres (*arrows*) representing partial thickness tear. Note degenerated, fluid-filled labrum (*short arrow*).

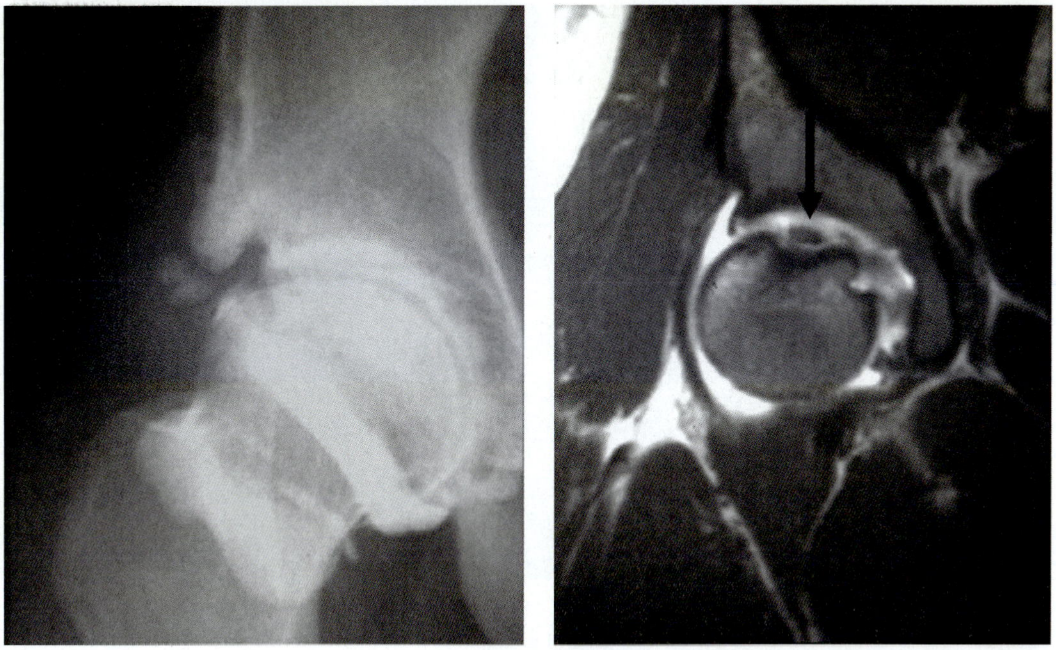

A B

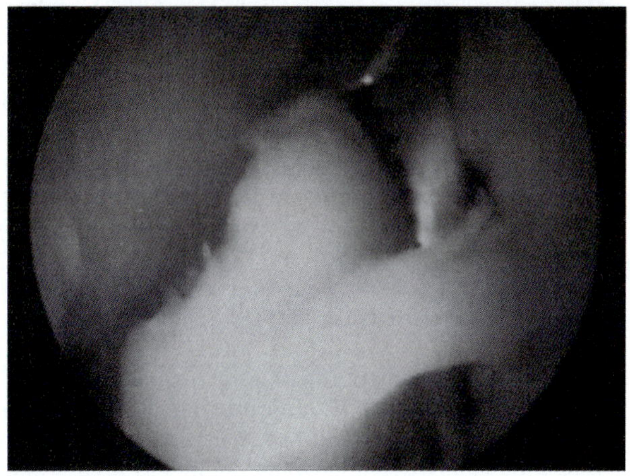

C

Figure 2.33. AP view of the right hip (**A**) and coronal T1-weighted MR arthrographic view (**B**) in a 15-year-old elite distance runner with sudden onset of locking and a history of DDH. Postoperative changes on the plain film with uncovering of the femoral head and acetabular dysplasia. The MR reveals an ovoid loose body in the superior aspect of the femoral head lying within its crater (*arrow*) (grade III chondral lesion). (**C**). Arthroscopic image shows loose body sitting within the superior aspect of the femoral head. DDH, developmental dysplasia of the hip.

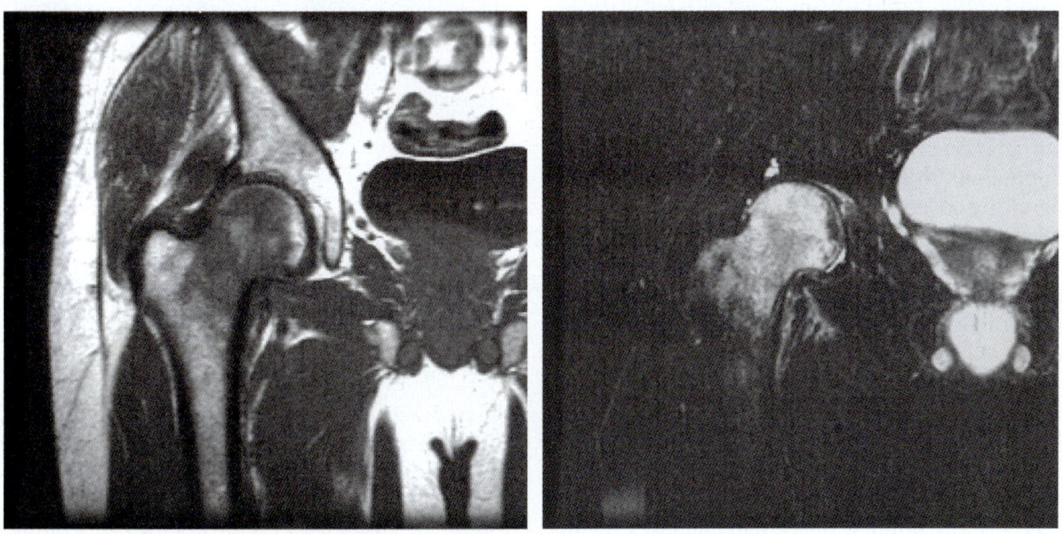

A B

Figure 2.34. Transient osteoporosis of the hip. Coronal T1-weighted (**A**) and inversion recovery (**B**) images reveal diffuse, homogeneous low T1, high T2 signal within the femoral head and neck.

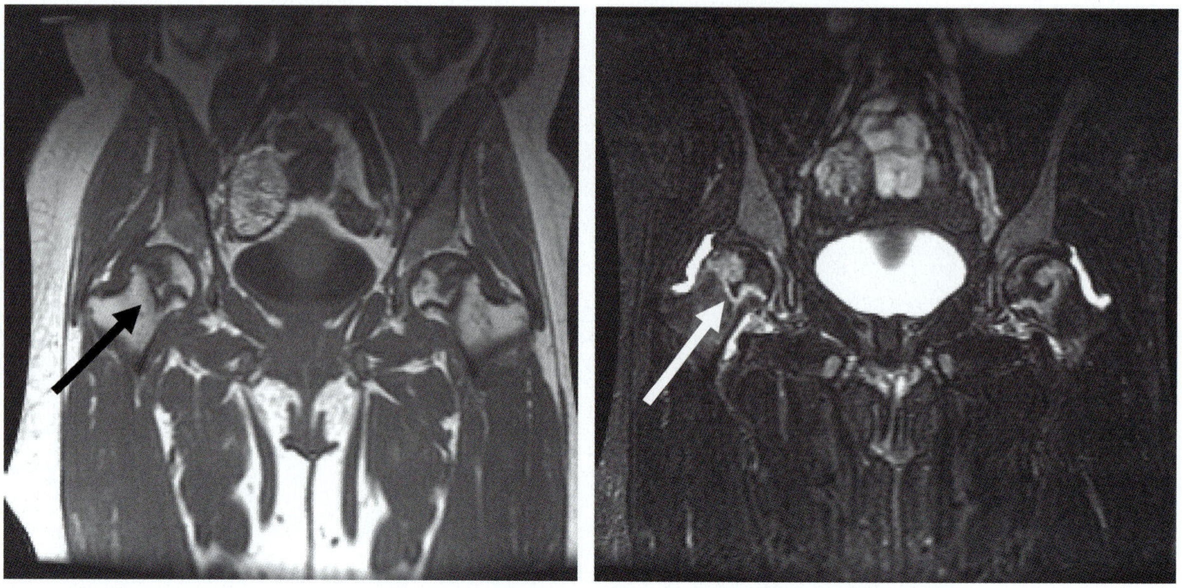

A **B**

Figure 2.35. Coronal T1 (**A**) and inversion recovery (**B**) MR images reveal bilateral serpiginous foci of high surrounded by low signal within the femoral heads representing AVN (*arrows*).

pathognomonic for osteonecrosis (Fig. 2.35). Some studies attribute the inner hyperintense band to hyperemic granulation tissue, while others attribute it to chemical shift misregistration (artifact).[118]

Plain radiographic findings of AVN are best described by the Ficat classification system.[119] In stage I disease, the radiographic appearance of the hip is normal. In stage II, subtle sclerosis, cyst formation, and/or osteopenia are present, indicative of osseous reaction and repair adjacent to the region of bone necrosis. Stage III disease demonstrated subchondral collapse with flattening of the femoral head. The crescent sign, linear subchondral lucency, represents early subchondral osseous collapse. In stage IV disease, secondary osteoarthritis develops with joint space narrowing. Steinberg et al.[120] modified this classification, describing stages III as subchondral collapse (crescent sign), stage IV as flattening of the femoral head, and stage V as joint narrowing, with or without acetabular involvement. With the advent of MRI, the system was further modified to include a stage O, representing asymptomatic patients with normal radiographs and a positive MRI examination.

Mitchell et al.[121] proposed a classification system to describe the signal characteristics of the marrow space proximal to the "double-line" within the femoral head. Infarcted marrow with signal intensity similar to fat is class A; class B marrow parallels the signal intensity of blood with high signal intensity on T1- and T2-weighted pulse sequences, while class C marrow signal parallels fluid, with low T1- and high T2-weighted signals. Finally, class D marrow is similar to fibrous tissue, with low signal intensity on both T1- and T2-weighted images.

Unfortunately, the MR classification is not clinically predictive. Rather, location and percentage of femoral head weight-bearing surface involved by AVN have proven important.[122,123] One study has evaluated 50 patients over 44 months and found that 74% of the femoral heads had collapsed when AVN affected more than two thirds of the weight-bearing surface area.[124]

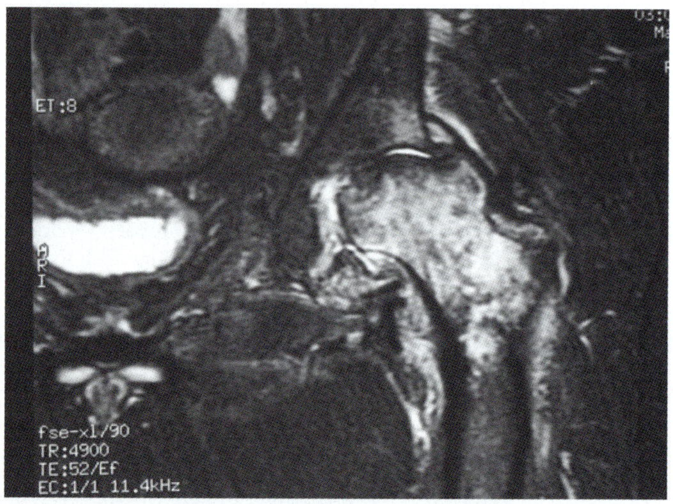

Figure 2.36. Advanced AVN. Coronal inversion recovery image demonstrates abnormal increased signal within the femoral head and neck with collapse of the articular surface and degenerative joint disease (DJD).

If early AVN is not recognized and treated, osteoarthritis and joint replacement are the ultimate endpoint (Fig. 2.36). Diagnosis needs to be made prior to subchondral fractures and articular cartilage damage.

Pelvic Fractures

Pelvic fractures in the athlete can range from simple, nondisplaced avulsion fractures to complex fractures involving the acetablum and pelvic ring. Diagnosis of these fractures may be made on plain radiographs. However, most often, supplemental imaging with CT or MRI is required to adequately assess for displacement of fragments, amount of comminution, and exact locations of fragments (Fig. 2.37). In addition, cross-sectional imaging with CT or MRI often detects occult fractures not seen with plain radiography. MRI detects a large number of pelvic fractures not seen on plain radiographs.[125] Fractures appear as poorly defined or well-defined linear regions of T1 hypointensity (Fig. 2.38). These zones are of increased signal intensity on T2-weighted and STIR pulse sequences. Other groups have described radiographically occult fractures as presenting with low T2-weighted signal intensity.[126]

Proximal femoral fractures, although uncommon in the athlete, are usually detected radiographically. Once again, several studies have shown that MRI is extremely helpful in diagnosing radiographically occult or indeterminant fractures.[127,128]

Bursae

Inflammation within a bursa is termed bursitis and is usually a result of excessive rubbing and associated friction. Hematoma formation from a direct blow may also lead to bursitis.[31] The most commonly inflamed bursae within the pelvis are the trochanteric, ischial, and iliopsoas.[129]

Trochanteric bursitis (greater trochanteric pain syndrome) is a common cause of pain about the hip in the athlete and nonathlete alike.[130] The iliopsoas bursa is a synovial outpouching anteriorly from the hip joint which originates between the iliofemoral and pubofemoral ligamentous bands of capsular thickening. It is the largest bursa about the hip

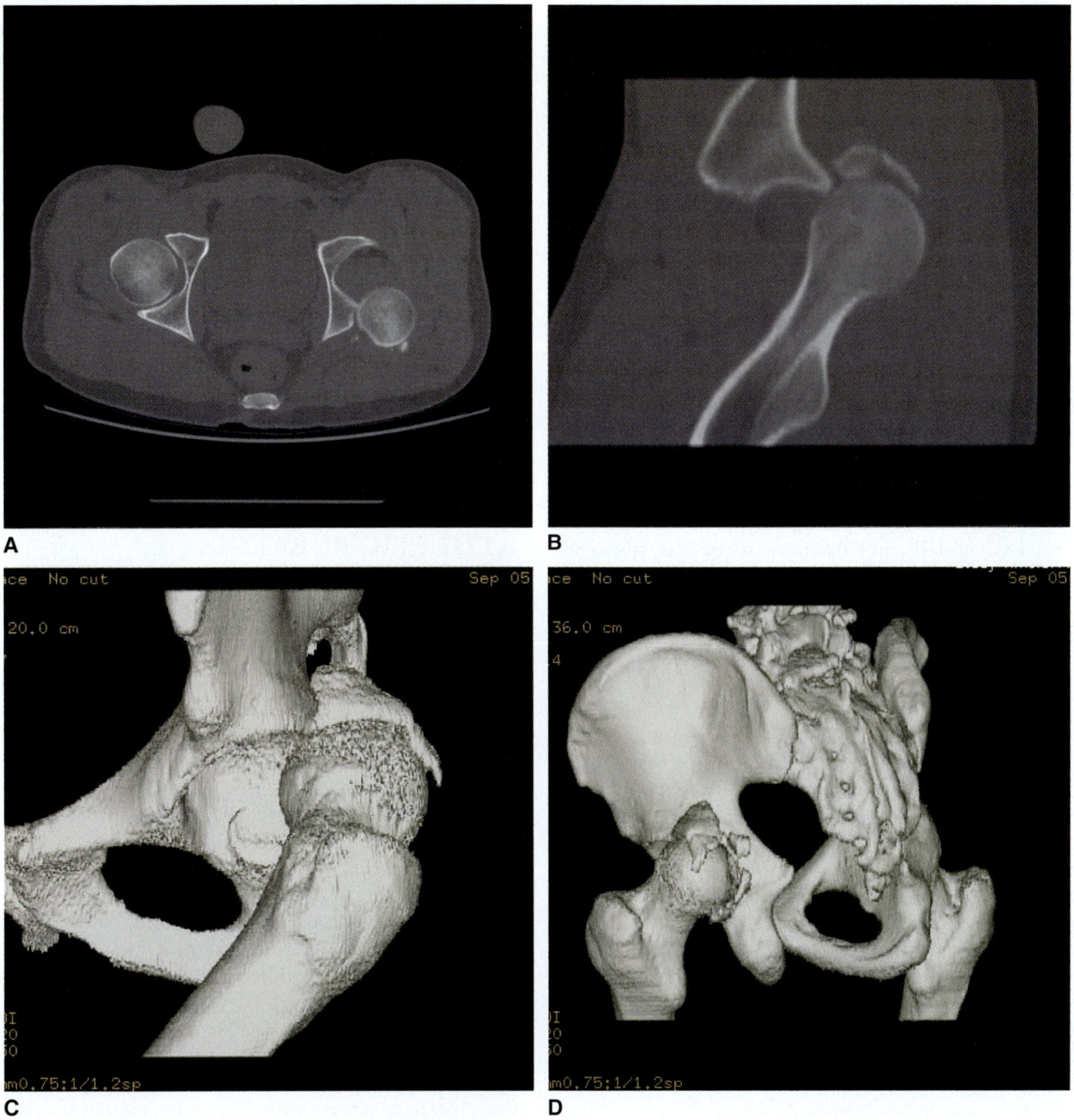

Figure 2.37. Direct axial (**A**) and sagittal (**B**) reformatted images of the left hip show posterior fracture-dislocation of the femoral head. Multiple posterior acetabular rim fragments have been displaced posteriorly. Three-dimensional reconstructed images in the same patient reveal a relationship between femoral head, acetabulum, and rim fragments.

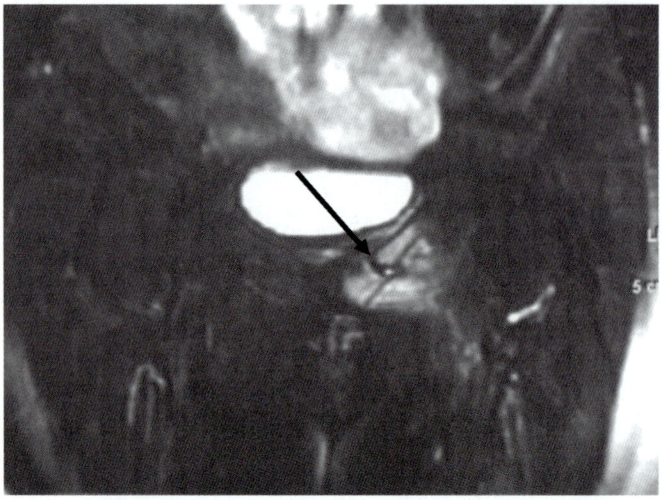

Figure 2.38. Coronal inversion recovery MR image of the pelvis demonstrates a transverse fracture through the left superior pubic ramus (*arrow*) with surrounding increased signal within the musculature.

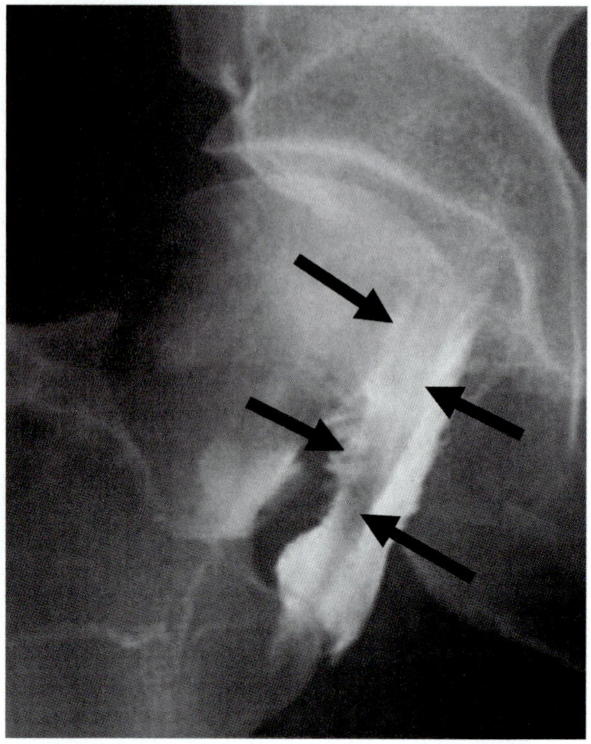

Figure 2.39. Snapping hip syndrome. Direct fluoroscopic injection into the tendon sheath outlines the tendon margins (*arrows*) prior to assessment for abnormal excursion.

joint and communicates with the joint in approximately 15% of cases. It may extend, when distended, into the anterolateral pelvis along the sheath of the iliopsoas.[131] Finally, the obturator externus bursa communicates with and extends from the posteroinferior aspect of the hip joint deep into the obturator externus tendon. Obturnator externus bursitis will often be associated with a joint effusion, as will iliopsoas bursitis.[132]

Plain radiographs may demonstrate calcification in the region of a chronically inflamed bursa, particularly about the greater trochanter. MR may demonstrate a high signal in the region of the bursa on T2-weighted and STIR pulse sequences. It should be remembered that some bursal distention with fluid may be related to associated adjacent joint pathology via the previously described anatomic communication.

Snapping Hip Syndrome

The snapping hip syndrome is comprised of symptoms characterized by an audible snapping or popping sensation, as well as hip pain with particular, and usually reproducible, hip movements. The syndrome can be classified as intra-articular and extra-articular.[133] Dynamic sonography of the iliopsoas tendon is considered the most useful imaging modality to detect abnormal excursion of the tendon over the iliopectineal eminence during extension of the flexed, abducted, and externally rotated hip.[134] Direct injection of the iliopsoas tendon sheath with iodinated contrast material under fluoroscopy is another means of assessment (Fig. 2.39). The patient's movements, as well as the excursion of the iliopsoas tendon, may be recorded and reviewed after the procedure. The drawback of this second technique to evaluate the snapping hip is (a) it is invasive, (b) it is technically somewhat difficult, and (c) it is often difficult for the patient to reproduce symptoms under the constraints of the fluoroscopy table and while in discomfort from the injection. A steroid injection into the tendon sheath may be performed for symptomatic relief.

ATHLETIC PUBALGIA

"Pubalgia" refers to activity-related groin or pubic pain without conclusive physical examination findings.[131,135,136] There is a high incidence in sports such as soccer, track, rugby, American and Australian rules football and ice hockey that involve kicking, sprinting, and change in direction.[131] The ventral abdominal wall, inguinal canal, pubis, perineum, and femoral triangle converge at the groin to form a complex intersection.[138,139] The pubic symphysis is a secondary, synovial amphiarthrodial joint lined by hyaline cartilage. Between the hyaline cartilages lies a thick fibrocartilaginous disc, similar to an intervertebral disc.[140,141] Secondary ossification centers appear at the anterior margins of the symphysis at puberty and fuse with the pubis in late adolescence or early adulthood. Thus, in adolescents the symphysis appears as an anterior opening "V" in axial images (Fig. 2.40).[141] In adults, the symphyseal margins become parallel.

Superiorly, the symphysis is stabilized by the superior pubic ligament, while inferiorly, the symphysis is strengthened by the arcuate pubic ligament, as well as a broad insertion of the superficial fibers of the linea alba, medial heads of the rectus abdominus, and the pyramidalis muscle.[138,142] The inguinal canal extends obliquely parallel to the inguinal ligament with the posterior wall comprised of the transversalis fascia and the

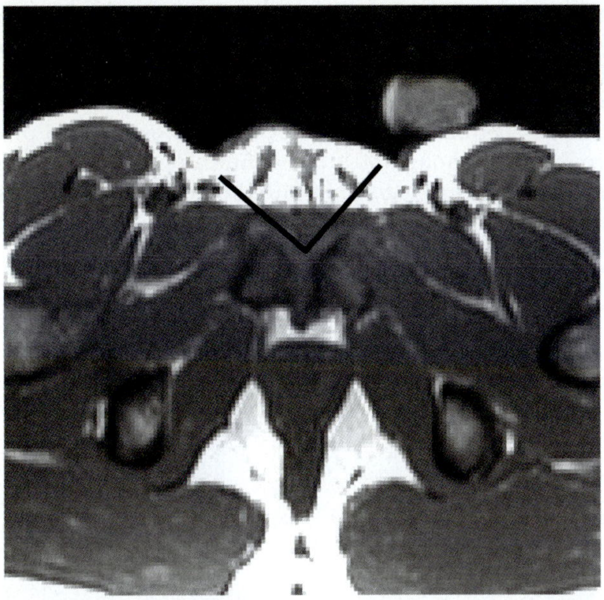

Figure 2.40. "V"-shaped configuration to the anterior symphysis in an adolescent on an axial T1-weighted MR image.

conjoined tendon. The lack of striated muscle within the posterior wall, and the passage of the spermatic cord, predispose to weakness.[143] The external (superficial) inguinal ring is found anterior to the distal conjoined tendon.[144]

IMAGING TECHNIQUES

Conventional radiography remains the initial imaging modality of choice in the assessment of the athlete with groin pain. Standard anteroposterior views of the pelvis and anteroposterior and frog-lateral views of the symptomatic hip are obtained. Alternating bilateral flamingo views are useful to stress the symphysis (anteroposterior weight-bearing views). Periarticular soft tissues are well seen on a properly exposed conventional radiograph, and digital radiography can enhance the soft tissues by adjusting the window and level settings. In addition, juxta-articular fat pads and their associated displacement can be well seen on plain radiography.

MRI is complimentary to conventional radiography for examining athletes with groin/pubic pain. The entire pelvis is usually imaged to start the examination utilizing a torso array coil. At our institution, axial T2-weighted fat-suppressed, axial T1-weighted, coronal inversion recovery (STIR), and coronal T1-weighted pulse sequences are obtained. Dedicated imaging of the hip or symphysis pubis may be performed. However, imaging of the entire pelvis, with particular attention to the SI joints, should be obtained at some point in the study, as many patients with anterior (symphyseal) pathology will also demonstrate sacroiliac instability and pathology.

HERNIOGRAPHY

Previously, herniography was the only imaging modality that was able to detect a hernia sac. In this exam, contrast is injected directly into the peritoneal cavity, and fluoroscopic spot images and radiographs are obtained. Although easy to perform, the procedure is invasive and lacks the ability to determine the relationship of the hernia sac with adjacent soft tissue structures.[145] However, since the advent of CT (Fig. 2.41) and MRI, herniography has been, for the most part, replaced.

COMPUTED TOMOGRAPHY

CT is useful in the detection and characterization of radiographically occult fractures or osseous lesions. Muliplanar and three-dimensional reconstruction can also assist in the morphologic assessment of fracture fragments. Subtle soft tissue calcification or cortical erosion, particularly about the symphysis pubis, is also well seen with CT.

SCINTIGRAPHY

Bone scintigraphy is a highly sensitive means to detect metabolically active bone pathology within the pelvis. As mentioned previously, however, it lacks the specificity and ability to provide anatomic detail of MRI and CT. At our institution, bone scintigraphy has largely been replaced by MRI in the evaluation of athletes with pubalgia.

OSTEITIS PUBIS

Osteitis pubis is diagnosed clinically by the presence of increasing groin, pubic, or lower abdominal pain and the presence of tenderness to palpation over the symphysis pubis, the superior pubic ramus, or the proximal adductor muscles.[138,146] There are multiple radiographic findings associated with osteitis pubis. Variable amounts of diastasis of the symphysis pubis may be present, as well as periarticular cortical irregularity and erosions. Subchondral sclerosis and subchondral cyst formation

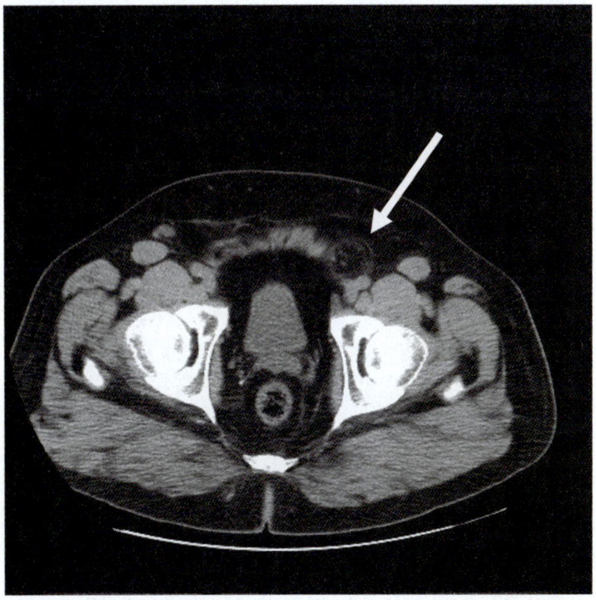

Figure 2.41. Axial CT image through the femoral heads. Rounded focus of low density (*arrow*) within the left inguinal region representing a fat-filled inguinal hernia.

are often present. CT may show these same subchondral changes as well as "stamp erosions" and periarticular calcification or ossification. There is frequent deformity of the superior margin of the symphysis with "beaking," which may impress upon the inferior aspect of the bladder.[147]

Extrusion of the symphysis disc is common in athletes, particularly soccer players, and usually occurs in a posterior or superior direction and the MRI may show this discal extrusion. MRI will also reveal bone marrow edema on one or both sides of the joint on T2-weighted or STIR images (Fig. 2.42). Stress or insufficiency fractures in the parasymphyseal region may also be noted (Fig. 2.43).[141] A secondary cleft sign, seen on STIR or T2-weighted pulse sequences as an oblique inferior extension of the primary cleft, may be present (Fig. 2.44). Increased T2-weighted or STIR signal intensity often continues into the ipsilateral adductor and gracilis entheses, lending credence to the theory that chronic adductor enthesopathy and osteitis pubis are related phenomena.[148] Sacral stress fractures or sacroiliac joint degenerative change or instability should be considered in any athlete with osteitis pubis and low back or sciatic pain.[149]

MUSCULOFASCIAL PATHOLOGY AND "THE SPORTSMAN'S HERNIA"

Abdominal wall abnormalities, anterior abdominal wall hernias, and groin hernias are increasingly diagnosed in the athletic population.[138,150–152] Athletes typically present with chronic groin pain localized to the pubic tubercle that increases with valsalva or other provocative activity. A precise anatomic abnormality is elusive and controversial.[153] Gilmore originally attributed a torn external oblique aponeurosis as a cause of dilation of the external (superficial) inguinal ring.[154–156]

Rectus abdominus muscle abnormalities seem to be the primary cause of groin pain in one group of athletes studied. MRI in these athletes with "pubalgia caused by abdominal musculofascial abnormalities" demonstrated attenuation or focal convexities of the abdominal wall musculature and macroscopic defects or thinning of the associated fascial layers. Preoperative imaging is helpful in planning a unilateral or bilateral procedure.[135,136,138] Although MRI can define and visualize inguinal hernias and their relationship with the inguinal rings and surrounding soft tissues and vessels, the "sportsman's hernia" has

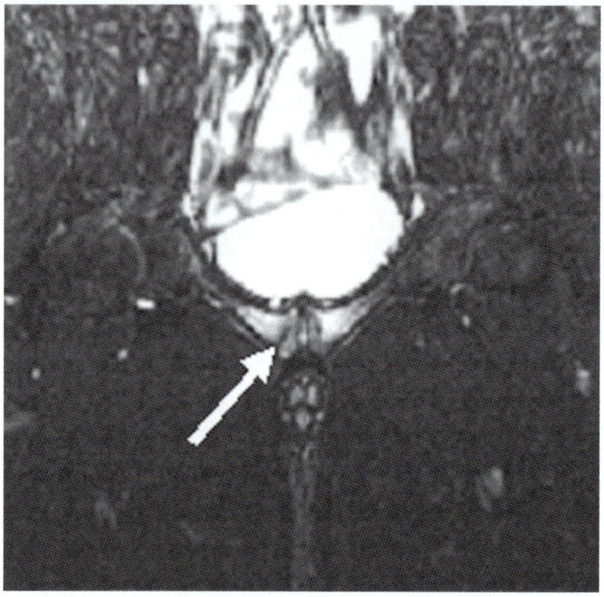

Figure 2.43. Coronal inversion recovery image of the pelvis. Marrow edema within the pubic body bilaterally with a linear low signal fracture line within the right pubic body (*arrow*).

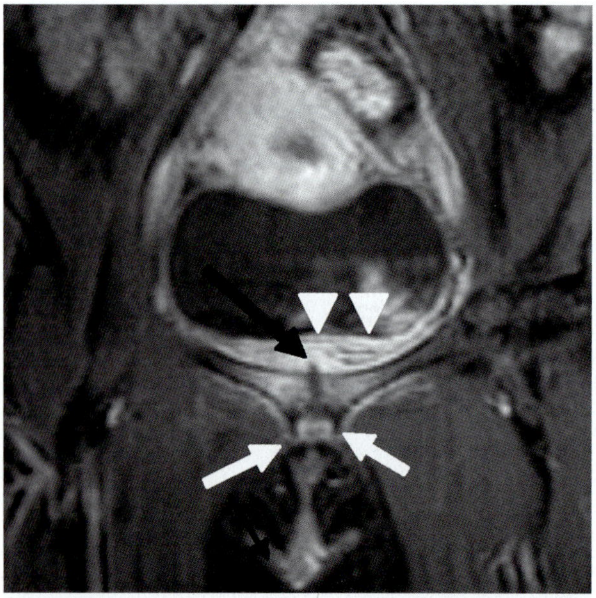

Figure 2.42. Coronal inversion recovery MR image of the symphysis pubis reveals superior protrusion of the disc (*arrow*) with surrounding swelling and impression upon the bladder base (*arrowheads*). There is marrow edema within the pubic body bilaterally. Note tendinous insertion of the adductors (*short arrows*).

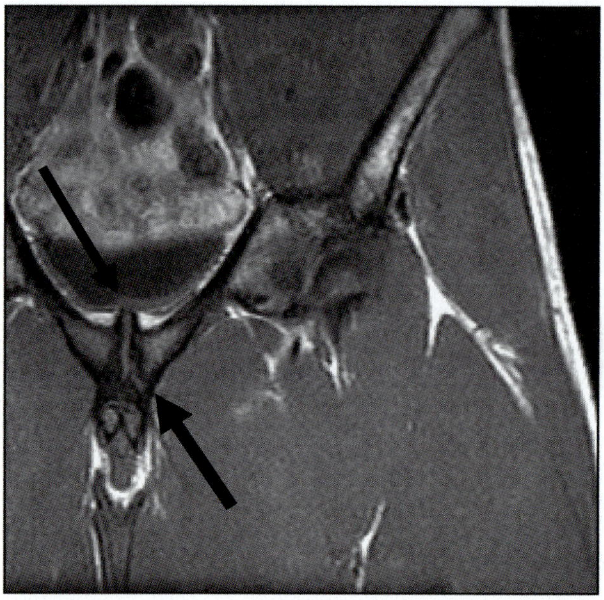

Figure 2.44. Secondary cleft. Coronal T1-weighted image shows an obliquely oriented linear focus of increased signal (*arrow*) extending from the primary cleft of the symphysis inferiorly toward the adductor origin. Also note superior discal protrusion and spurring impressing upon the base of the bladder (*thin arrow*).

less reliable imaging findings (Fig. 2.45). Cross-sectional imaging with CT or MRI is still critical to exclude all other causes of athletic pubalgia in these athletes, aside from hernias, that may be responsible for the patient's symptoms.[143]

SYNOVIAL PROLIFERATIVE DISORDERS

Pigmented villonodular synovitis (PVNS) and synovial osteochondromatosis are two proliferative processes which affect younger individuals and demonstrate rather unique appearances on imaging studies. The hip is the second most commonly affected joint after the knee (80% of cases).[157–162] Plain radiographs may demonstrate multiple, juxta-articular erosions, often about the femoral neck with osteoarthritic-like changes.[158,162,163] There is typically no mineralization associated with this condition, making early radiographic diagnosis difficult. MRI is the modality of choice. Synovial-based nodules and thickening are commonly identified, with characteristic low T1- and T2-weighted signal intensity (Fig. 2.46). Scattered foci of increased T1 signal may be seen due to the presence of lipid-laden macrophages.[158,164]

Synovial osteochondromatosis can be divided into primary and secondary forms. The primary form is an uncommon, benign, idiopathic disorder which typically demonstrates synovial metaplasia and transformation. Large joints such as the hip and knee are frequently involved.[165]

Secondary osteochondromatosis is seen in association with trauma, osteoarthritis, osteonecrosis, and neuropathic arthropathy. In this form, the loose intra-articular bodies tend to be

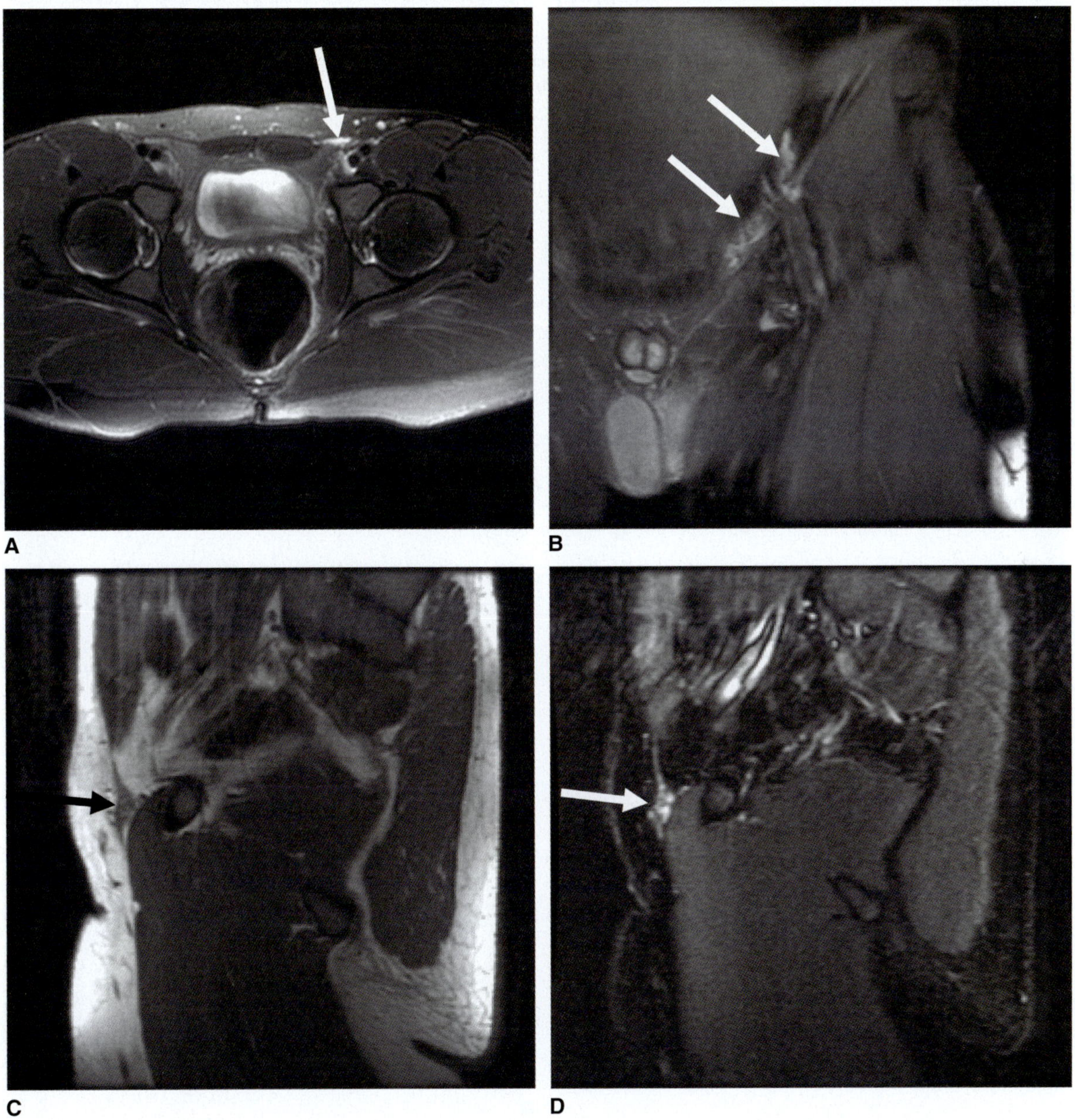

Figure 2.45. Sportsman's hernia. (**A**) axial and (**B**) coronal T2-weighted images of the inguinal region reveal asymmetric focus of hyperintensity on the left in the inguinal canal (*arrows*). Sagittal T1 (**C**) and T2-weighted (D) images through the pelvis show subtle focus of low T1 and high T2 signal in the inguinal region (*arrows*).

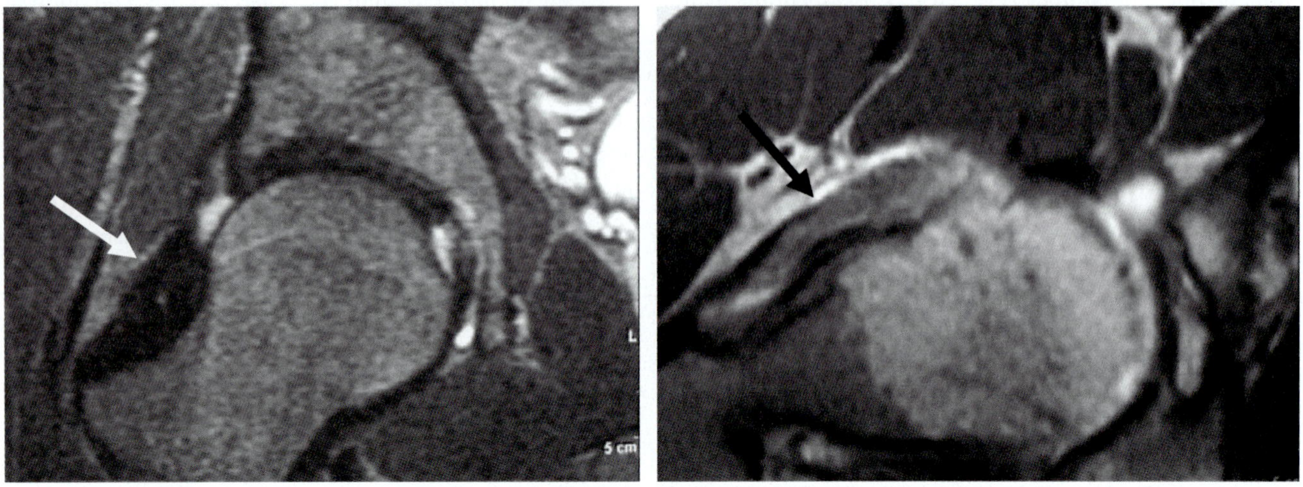

A B

Figure 2.46. Pigmented villonodular synovitis. Coronal T2 (**A**) and axial T1-weighted MR arthrographic image (**B**) show markedly thickened capsule anterolaterally with low signal on all pulse sequences (*arrows*).

larger, fewer, and less uniform than in the primary form and is usually associated with severe osteoarthritis.[157,158] MR reveals synovial thickening, intra-articular loose bodies, bone erosions, and synovial herniation (Fig. 2.47).[166] Ossified loose bodies may be hypointense or hyperintense on T1-weighted pulse sequences depending on the absence or presence of fatty marrow.[158]

BONE LESIONS

Common tumors of the proximal femur include osteoid osteoma, osteoblastoma, chondroblastoma, chondrosarcoma, and, in the older population, metastases and multiple myeloma.[167] While plain radiography remains the primary modality of choice in the evaluation of bone tumors, CT is optimal in anatomically complex regions such as the hip.[158] MRI is useful to determine the extent of tumor, as well as determine the intramedullary and extraosseous involvement of bone lesions. Lesion detectability (sensitivity) is high with MRI, but specificity is low. Tumors typically exhibit intermediate to low signal intensity on T1-weighted images and high signal intensity on T2-weighted pulse sequences (Fig. 2.48). It must be stressed that MRI cannot reliably differentiate benign from malignant neoplasms in most cases.[168]

Osteoid osteoma is a fairly common lesion which is frequently seen in the young, athletic age group. About half of the patients are between the ages of 10 and 20 years. Intra-articular lesions are most commonly seen in the hip.[169] Radiographically, the osteoid osteoma is often referred to as the "nidus" because

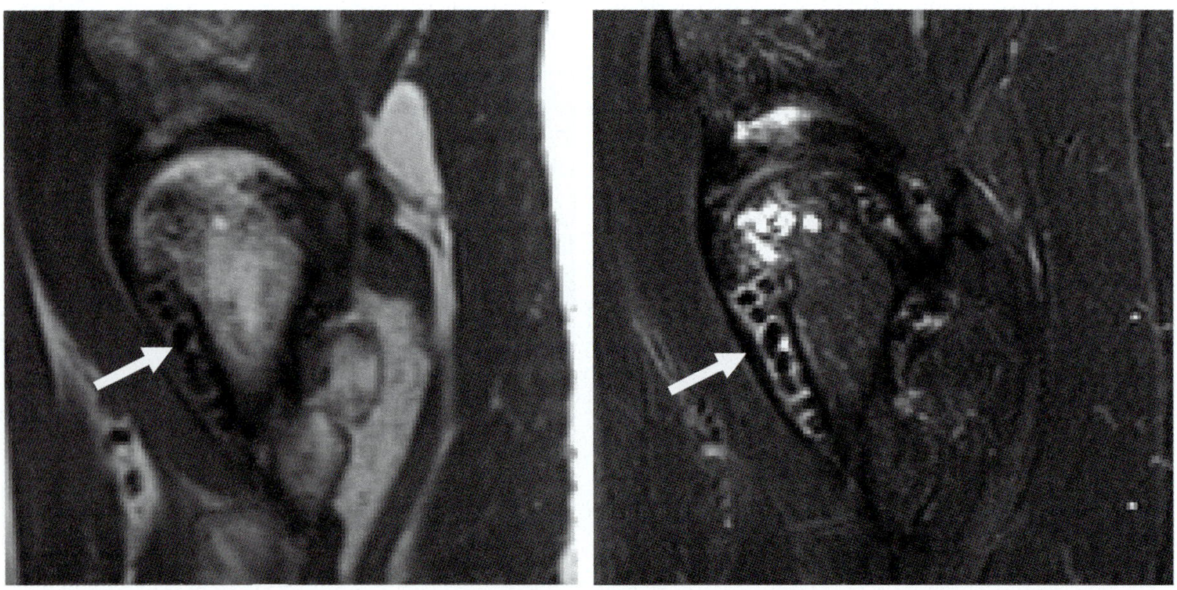

A B

Figure 2.47. Secondary osteochondromatosis. Sagittal T2-weighted (**A**) and T1-weighted (**B**) images of the hip demonstrate multiple loose bodies of varying sizes and shapes (*arrows*). There is associated joint space narrowing, subchondral cyst formation and spurring.

it is the focus of underlying pathology and is centrally located within an area of dense reactive sclerosis. This nidus is usually lucent and may contain matrix mineralization.[169] When the osteoid osteoma is intra-articular (as in the hip), sclerosis may be absent (in contrast to cortical lesions), and initial radiographs may be normal. CT demonstrates the nidus and associated mineralization as well as periosteal reaction and sclerosis.[170] Lui et al.[171] looked at 11 patients with osteoid osteoma, comparing CT with dynamic, enhanced MRI and nonenhanced MRI (Fig. 2.49), and found osteoid osteomas can be imaged with greater lesion conspicuity by using dynamic gadolinium-enhanced MRI, and with conspicuity equal to or better than thin-section CT.

MOREL-LAVALLÉE LESIONS

Morel-Lavallée[172] (ML) first described posttraumatic fluid collections dissecting the subcutaneous fatty tissues in 1863. Although these posttraumatic fluid collections may be found in the subcutaneous soft tissues of the abdominal wall, buttock, lower lumbar spine, scapular region, and calf, they are particularly common

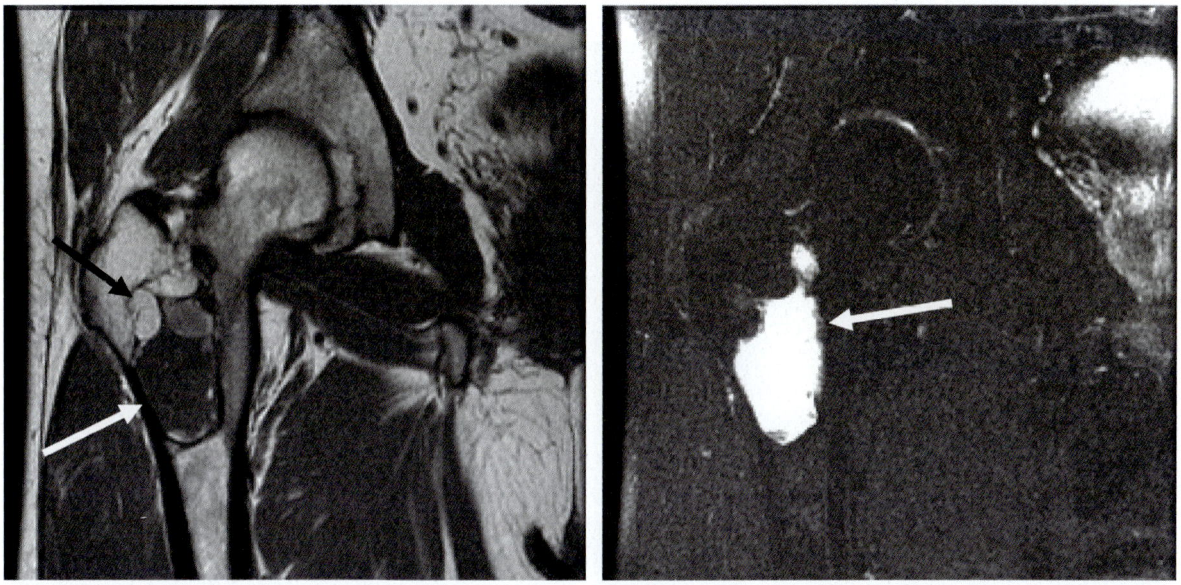

A B

Figure 2.48. **A:** Coronal T1-weighted MR image through the proximal femur demonstrates an inhomogeneous lesion with both fat (*black arrow*) and fluid (*white arrow*) signal intensity within the intertrochanteric and subtrochanteric regions of the femur. **B:** Coronal inversion recovery MR image of the proximal femur demonstrates the cystic component (*white arrow*) to the lesion. Lesion diagnosed as benign intra-osseous lipoma.

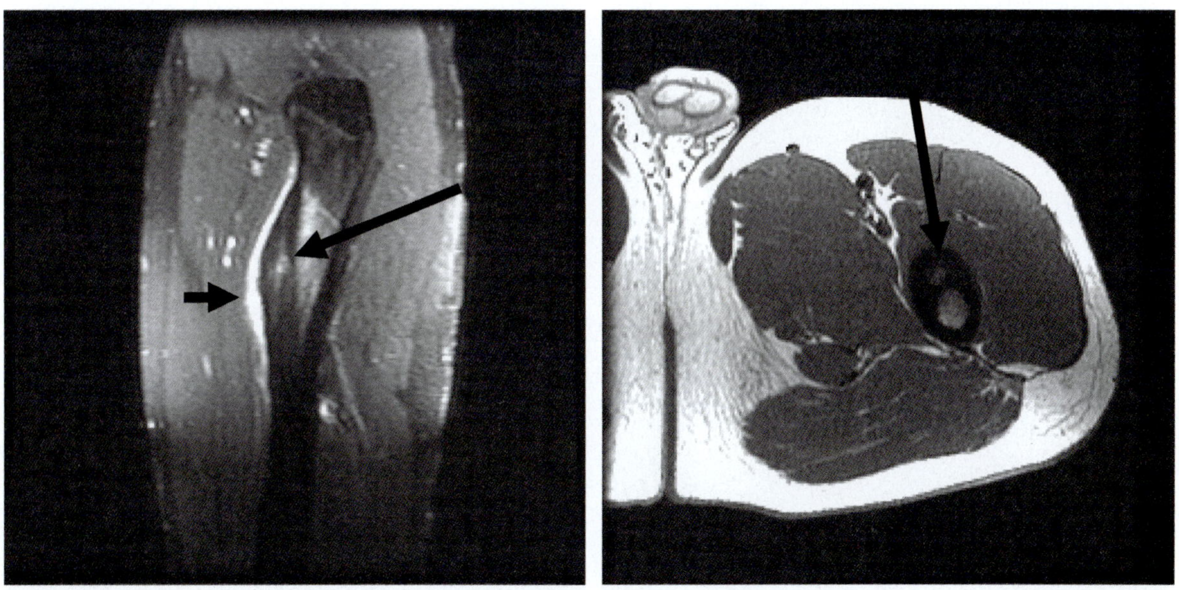

A B

Figure 2.49. Osteoid osteoma of the proximal femur. Sagittal T1-weighted (**A**) and axial T1-weighted (**B**) MR images of the proximal thigh reveal marked cortical thickening with marrow edema, a cortically based nidus (*long arrow*) and periosteal reaction (*short arrow*).

in the trochanteric region and proximal thigh.[173] ML lesions of the trochanteric and upper thigh region typically dissect perifascial planes adjacent to the fascia lata and iliotibial band.[173–179] The presence of ML lesions may initially be missed in up to one third of cases and may be detected months or years after trauma, when acute lesions have long resolved.[173,175,177,178]

On ultrasound, the ML lesion has the appearance of a complex, cystic mass, either anechoic or mildly hyperechoic.[180,181] CT will demonstrate a well-defined, encapsulated fluid collection with occasional fluid–fluid levels.[180,181] Because of its unparalleled soft tissue contrast, MR is utilized most frequently for assessment.[174] MRI reveals unilateral or bilateral, well-defined oval fusiform-shaped lesions with tapering margins within the subcutaneous perifascial planes. The lesions may demonstrate variable internal signal intensity, septations, and fluid–fluid levels and are often surrounded, at least partially, by a peripheral hypointense fibrous rim (Fig. 2.50). An MRI classification for staging these lesions has been proposed and includes Type I lesions exhibiting fluidlike signal (low on T1-weighted, high on T2-weighted sequences) most likely representing serous or hemorrhagic effusion (Fig. 2.51). Type II ML lesions demonstrate hyperintensity on T1- and

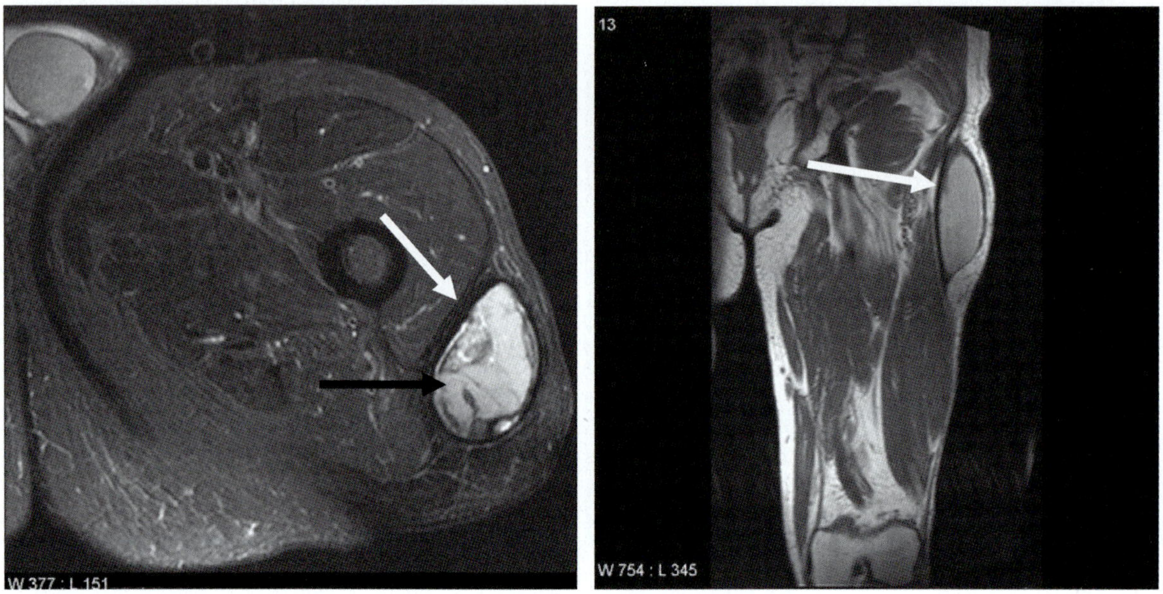

A B

Figure 2.50. ML lesion. Axial T2 (**A**) and coronal T1 (**B**) weighted images demonstrate ovoid fluid collection within the superficial fascia (*black arrow*) which contains septations and a hypointense fibrous capsule (*white arrows*).

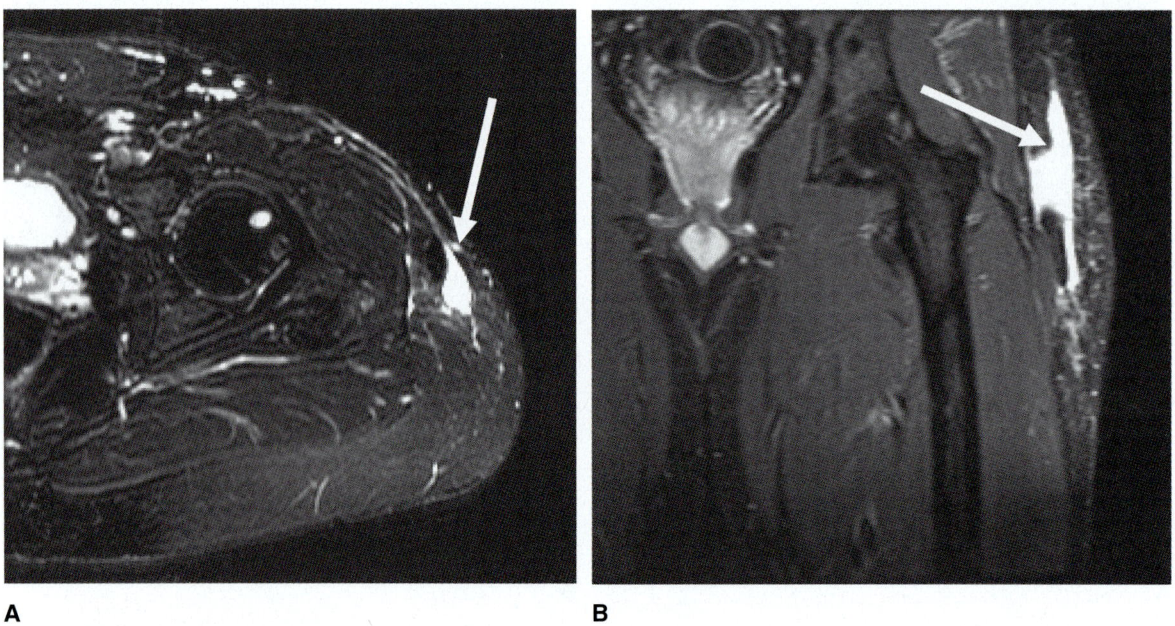

A B

Figure 2.51. Type I ML lesion. Axial (**A**) and coronal (**B**) T2 and inversion recovery images of the thigh demonstrate focal high signal fluid within the deep subcutaneous soft tissues lateral to the greater trochanter (*arrows*).

T2-weighted sequences, most likely representing subacute hematoma. Type III ML lesions demonstrate intermediate T1-weighted, heterogeneous hyperintensity on T2-weighted sequences (most likely representing chronic blood products). Type IV lesions show a combined perifascial dissection and closed fat laceration with or without fluid. Type V lesions display a pseudonodular appearance, while type VI ML lesions represent an infected lesion, which may present with a thick, enhancing peripheral capsule, internal septations, inflammatory reaction, peripheral fluid leakage, and sinus tract formation.[174]

REFERENCES

1. Lawler LP, Sponsellar P, Fishman EK. Helical single and multi detector row CT with three-dimensional volume rendering of the young hip. *Crit Rev Comput Tomogr.* 2004;45:111–145.
2. Blankenbaker DG, Tuite MJ. The painful hip: New concepts. *Skeletal Radiol.* 2006;34:352–370.
3. Janzen DL, Patridge E, Logan M, et al. The snapping hip: Clinical and imaging findings in transient subluxation of the ilippsoas tendon. *Can Assoc Radio J.* 1996;47:202–208.
4. Pelsser V, Cardinal E, Hobden R, et al. Extraarticular snapping hip: Sonographic findings. *Am J Roentgenol.* 2001;176:67–73.
5. Cardinal E, Kenneth B, Capello W, et al. US of the snapping ilippsoas tendon. *Radiology.* 1996;198:521–522.
6. Pentecost RL, Murray RA, Brindley HH. Fatigue, insufficiency, and pathologic fractures. *J Am Med Assoc.* 1964;187:1001–1004.
7. Anderson MW, Greenspan A. Stress fractures. *Radiology.* 1996;199:1–12.
8. Edelman RR, Hesselink JR, Crues JV, et al. *Clinical MRI.* Philadelphia, PA: W.B. Saunders, 2006;108: pp. 3545–3575.
9. Wishaupt D, Schweitzer ME. MR imaging of the foot and ankle: Patterns of bone marrow signal abnormalities. *Eur Radiol.* 2002;12:416–426.
10. Schweitzer ME, Karasick D. MR of the ankle and Hindfoot, Semin Ultrasound, CT, MRI. 1994;15:410–422.
11. Hassankhani A, Bencardino JT. MRI of sports injuries of the spine. *Top Magn Reson Imaging.* 2003;14(1):87–102.
12. Jones BH, Harris JM, Vin TN, et al. Exercise induced stress fractures and stress reactions of bone: Epidemiology, etiology, and classification. *Exerc Sport Sci Rev.* 1989;17:379–422.
13. Devas M. *Stress Fractures.* Edinburgh, Scotland: Churchill Livingstone; 1975.
14. Greaney RB, Gerber FN, Laughlin RL, et al. Distribution and natural history of stress fractures in U.S. marine recruits. *Radiology.* 1983;146:339–346.
15. Nielsen MB, Hansen K, Holmes P, et al. Tibial periosteal reactions in soldiers: A scintigraphic study of 29 cases of lower leg pain. *Acta Orthop Scand.* 1991;62:531–534.
16. Bottomley MB. Sacral stress fractures in a runner. *Br J Sports Med.* 1990;24:243–244.
17. Shin AY, Morin WK, Gorman JD, et al. The superiority of magnetic resonance imaging in differentiating the cause of pain in endurance athletes. *Am J Sports Med.* 1996;24:168–176.
18. Bencardino JT, Kassarjian A, Palmer WE. Magnetic resonance imaging of the hip: Sports related injuries. *Top Magn Reson Imaging.* 2003;14(2):145–160.
19. Slocum KA, Gorman JD, Puckett ML, et al. Resolution of abnormal MR signal intensity in patients with stress fractures of the femoral neck. *Am J Roentgenol.* 1997;168:1295–1299.
20. Bencardino JT, Mellado JM. Hamstring injuries of the hip. *Magn Reson Imaging Clin N Am.* 2005 Nov.;13(4):677–690.
21. Palmer WE, Kuong SJ, Elmadbouh HM. MR imaging of myotendinous strain. *Am J Roentgenol.* 1999;173:703–709.
22. De Smet A. Magnetic resonance findings in skeletal muscle tears. *Skeletal Radiol.* 1993;22:479–484.
23. Shellock FG, Mink J, Deutsch AL. MR imaging of muscle injuries. *Appl Radiol.* 1994;(February):11–18.
24. Steinbach LS, Fleckenstein JL, Mink JH. Magnetic resonance imaging of muscle injuries. *Orthopedics.* 1994;17:991–999.
25. EL-Noueam KI, Schweitzer ME, Bhatia M, et al. The utility of contrast enhance MRI in diagnosis of muscle injuries occult to conventional MRI. *J Comput Assist Tomogr.* 1997;21:965–968.
26. Stevens MA, EL Khoury GY, Kathol MH, et al. Imaging features of avulsion injuries. *Radiographics.* 1999;19:655–682.
27. Bordalo-Rodrigues M, Rosenberg ZS. MR imaging of the proximal rectus femoris musculoteninous unit. *Magn Reson Imaging Clin N Am.* 2005 Nov.;13(4):717–725.
28. Paletta GA, Andrish JT. Injuries about the hip and pelvis in the young athlete. *Clin Sports Med.* 1995;14:591–628.
29. Manaster BJ. Adult chronic hip pain: Radiographic evaluation. *Radiographics* 2000:20:S3–S25.
30. Kolouris G, Connell D. Evaluation of the hamstring muscle complex following acute injury. *Skeletal Radiol.* 2003;32:582–589.
31. Overdeck KH, Palmer WE. Imaging of hip and groin injuries in athletes. *Semin Musculoskelet Radiol.* 2004;8(1):41–53.
32. May DA, Disler DG, Jones EA, et al. Abnormal signal intensity in skeletal muscle at MR imaging: Patterns, pearls and pitfall. *Radiographics.* 2000;20:5295–5315.
33. Temple HT, Kuklo TR, Sweet DE, et al. Rectus femoris muscle tear appearing as a pseudotumor. *Am J Sports Med.* 1998;26:544–548.
34. Blankenbaker DG, De Smet AA. MR imaging of muscle injuries. *Appl Radiol.* 2004;33:14–26.
35. De Smet AA, Best TM. MRI of the distribution and location of acute hamstring injuries in athletes. *Am J Roentgenol.* 2000;174:393–399.
36. Pomeranz SJ, Heidt RS. MRI in the prognostication of hamstring injury. *Radiology.* 1993;189:897–900.
37. Slavotinek JP, Verral GM, Fon GT. Hamstring injury in athletes: Using MRI measurements to compare extent of muscle injury with amount of time lost from competition. *Am J Roentgenol.* 2002;179:1621–1628.
38. Connell DA, Schneider-Kolsky ME, Hoving JL, et al. Longitudinal study comparing sonographic and MRI assessments of acute and healing hamstring injuries. *Am J Roentgenol.* 2004;183:975–984.
39. Fleckenstein JL, Weatherall PT, Parkey RW, et al. Sports-related muscle injuries: Evaluation with MRI imaging. *Radiology.* 1989;172:793–798.
40. Ito K, Leunig M, Ganz R. Histopathologic features of the acetabular labrum in femoroacetabular impingement. *Clin Orthop.* 2004;429:262–271.
41. Beall DP, Sweet CF, Martin HD, et al. Imaging findings of femoroacetabular impingement syndrome. *Skeletal Radiol.* 2005;34:691–701.
42. Newberg AH, Newman JS. Imaging the painful hip. *Clin Orthop.* 2003;406:17–28.
43. Manaster BJ, Zakel S. Imaging of femoral acetabular impingement syndrome. *Clin Sports Med.* 2006;25:635–657.
44. Petersilge CA, Hague MA, Petersilge WJ, et al. Acetabular labral tears: Evaluation with MR arthrography. *Radiology.* 1986;200:231–235.
45. Czerny C, Hofmann S, Neuhold A, et al. Lesions of the acetabular labrum: Accuracy of MR imaging and MR arthrography in detection and staging. *Radiology.* 1996;200:225–230.
46. Kassarjian A. Hip MR arthrography and femoroacetabular impingement. *Semin Musculoskelet Radiol.* 2006;10:208–219.
47. Pfirmann CW, Mengiardi B, Dora C. Cam and pincer femoroacetabular impingement: Characteristic MR arthrographic findings in 50 patients. *Radiology.* 2006;240(3):778–785.
48. Li PL, Ganz R. Morphologic features of congenital acetabular dysplasia: One in six is retroverted. *Clin Orthop Relat Res.* 2003;416:245–253.
49. Mast JW, Brunner RL, Zebrack J. Recognizing acetabular version in the radiographic presentation of hip dysplasia. *Clin Orthop Relat Res.* 2004;428:48–53.
50. Armfield DR, Towers JD, Robertson DD. Radiographic and MR imaging of the athletic hip. *Clin Sports Med.* 2006;25:211–239.
51. Siebenrock KA, Wahab KH, Werlen S, et al. Abnormal extension of the femoral head epiphysis as a cause of Cam impingement. *Clin Orthop Relat Res.* 2004;418:54–60.
52. Eijer H, Leunig M, Mahomed N, et al. Cross-table lateral radiographs for screening of anterior femoral head-neck offset in patients with FAI. *Hip Int.* 2001;11:37–41.
53. Siebenrock KA, Kalbermatten DF, Ganz R. Effect of pelvic tilt on acetabular retroversion: A study of pelves from cadavers. *Clin Orthop Relat Res.* 2003;407:241–248.
54. Giori NJ, Trousdale RT. Acetabular retroversion is associated with osteoarthritis of the hip. *Clin Orthop Relat Res.* 2003;417:263–269.
55. Pitt MJ, Graham AR, Shipman JH, et al. Herniation pit of the femoral neck. *AJR.* 1982;138:1115–1121.
56. Thomason CB, Silverman ED, Walter RD, et al. Focal bone tracer uptake associated with a herniation pit of the femoral neck. *Clin Nucl Med.* 1983;8:304–305.
57. Leunig M, Beck M, Kalhor M, et al. Fibrocystic changes at anterosuperior femoral neck: Prevalence in hips with FAI. *Radiology.* 2005;236:237–246.
58. Gerguis S, Motamedi K, Seeger L. Review of the secondary signs of FAI and correlation with the head-neck angle measured on the frog-leg lateral view. *Soc Skeletal Radiol,* 2005;35–39.
59. Hodler J, YU JS, Goodwin D, et al. MR arthrography of the hip: Improved imaging of the acetabular labrum with histologic correlation in cadavers. *Am J Roentgenol.* 1995;165:887–891.
60. Byrd JWT, Jones KS. Diagnostic accuracy of clinical assessment, MRI, MR arthrography, and intra-articular injection in hip arthroscopy patients. *Am J Sports Med.* 2004;32:(7):1668–1674.
61. Chan YS, Lien LC, Hsu HL, et al. Evaluating hip labral tears using MR arthrography: A prospective study comparing hip arthroscopy and magnetic resonance arthrography diagnosis. *Arthroscopy.* 2005;21(10):1250–1256.
62. Keeney JA, Peelle MW, Jackson J, et al. Magnetic resonance arthrography versus arthroscopy in the evaluation of articular hip pathology. *Clin Orthop.* 2004;429:163–169.
63. Toomayan GA, Holman WR, Major NM, et al. Sensitivity of MR arthrography in the evaluation of acetabular labral tears. *Am J Roentgenol.* 2006;186:449–453.
64. Beck M, Siebenrock KA, Affolter B, et al. Increased intraarticular pressure reduces blood flow to the femoral head. *Clin Orthop Relat Res.* 2004;424:149–152.
65. Duc SR, Hodler J, Schmid MR, et al. Prospective evaluation of two different injection techniques for MR arthrography of the hip. *Eur Radiol.* 2006;16:473–478.
66. Kubo T, Horii M, Yamaguchi J, et al. Acetabular labrum in hip dysplasia evaluated by radial MRI. *J Rheumatol.* 2000;27:1955–1960.
67. Phillipon M, Hip Biomechanics. AANA hip arthrography course, Masters Series, Rosemont, IL, March 2006.
68. Ferguson SJ, Bryant JT, Ganz R, et al. The influence of the acetabular labrum on hip joint consolidation: A poroelastic finite element model. *J Biomech.* 2000;33:953–960.
69. Cotton A, Boutry N, Demondion X, et al. acetabular labrum: MRI in asymptomatic volunteers. *J Comput Assist Tomogr.* 1998;22:1–7.
70. Lecouvet FE, Vande Berg BC, Malghem J, et al. MR imaging of the acetabular labrum: Variations in 200 asymptomatic hips. *Am J Roentgenol.* 1996;167:1025–1028.
71. Abe I, Haraday Y, Oinuma K, et al. Acetabular labrum: Abnormal findings at MR imaging in asymptomatic hips. *Radiology.* 2000;216:576–582.
72. Klaue K, Durnin CW, Ganz R. The acetabular rim syndrome. A clinical presentation of dysplasia of the hip. *J Bone Joint Surg BR.* 1991;73:423–429.
73. Byrd JWT. Labral lesions: An elusive source of hip pain-case reports and literature review. *Arthroscopy.* 1996;12:603–612.
74. Byrd JWT. Hip arthroscopy the supine position. *Clin Sports Med.* 2001;20:703–731.
75. Keene GS, Villar RN. Arthroscopic anatomy of the hip: An in vitro study. *Arthroscopy.* 1994;10:392–399.
76. Dinauer PA, Murphy KP, Carroll JF. Sublabral sulcus at the postero inferior acetabulum: A potential pitfall in MR arthrography diagnosis of acetabular tear. *Am J Roentgenol.* 2004;183:1745–1753.

77. Saddik D, Troupis J, Tirman P, et al. Prevalence and location of acetabular sublabral sulci at hip Arthroscopy with retrospective MRI review. *Am J Roentgenol.* 2006;187:W507–W511.
78. Lage LA, Patel JV, Villar RN. The acetabular labral tear: An Arthroscopic classification. *Arthroscopy.* 1996;12(3):269–272.
79. Kelly BT, Williams III RJ, Philippon MJ. Hip arthroscopy current indications, treatment options, and management issues. *Am J Sports Med.* 2003;31:1020–1037.
80. Magee T, Hinson G. Association of paralabral cysts with acetabular disorders. *Am J Roentgenol.* 2000;174:1381–1384.
81. Petersilge CA. Chronic adult hip pain: MR arthrography of the hip. *Radiographics.* 2000;20:543–52.
82. Kassarjian A, Yoon LS, Belzile E, et al. Triad of MR arthrographic findings in patients with cam-type FAI. *Radiology.* 2005;236:588–592.
83. Scmid MR, Motzli HP, Zanetti M, et al. Cartilage lesions in the hip: Diagnostic effectiveness of MR arthrography. *Radiology.* 2003;226:382–386.
84. McCarthy JC, Noble PC, Schuch MR, et al. The role of labral lesions to the development of early degenerative hip disease. *Clin Orthop Relat Res.* 2001;393:25–37.
85. Beck M, Kalhor M, Leunig M, et al. Hip morphology influences the pattern of damage to the acetabular cartilage: FAI as a cause of early osteoarthritis of the hip. *J Bone Joint Surg BR.* 2005;87:1012–1018.
86. Bashir A, Gray ML, Burstein D. Gd-DTPA[2-] as a measure of cartilage degradation. *Magn Reson Med.* 1996;36:665–675.
87. Kim YJ, Jaramillo D, Millis MB, et al. Assessment of early osteoarthritis in hip dysplasia with delayed gadolinium enhanced MRI of cartilage. *J Bone Joint Surg AM.* 2003;85-A:1987–1992.
88. Ashir A, Gray ML, Boutin RD, et al. Glycosaminoglycan in articular cartilage in vivo assessment with delayed Gd (DTPA) (2–1)-enhanced MRI. *Radiology.* 1997;205:551–558.
89. Maroudas A, Venn M. Chemical composition and swelling of normal and osteoarthritic femoral head cartilage. II, swelling. *Ann Rheum Dis.* 1977;36:399–406.
90. Bashir A, Gray ML, Hartke J, et al. Nondestructive imaging of human cartilage Glycosaminoglycan concentration by MRI. *Magn Reson Med.* 1999;41:857–865.
91. Tideruis CJ, Jessel R, Kim YJ, et al. Hip dGEMRIC in asymptomatic volunteers and patients with early osteoarthritis: The influence of timing after contrast injection. *Magn Reson Med.* 2007;57:803–805.
92. Boesen M, Jensen KE, Qvistgarrd E, et al. Delayed gadolinium enhanced MRI (dGEMRIC) of hip joint cartilage: Better cartilage delineation after intra-articular than intravenous gadolinium injection. *Acta Radiol.* 2006;4:391–396.
93. Gray AJ, Villar RN. The ligamentum tears of the hip: An Arthroscopic classification of its pathology. *Arthroscopy.* 1997;13:575–578.
94. Byrd JW, Jones KS. Traumatic rupture of the ligamentum tears as a source of hip pain. *Arthroscopy.* 2004;20:385–391.
95. Osinsi T, Malfair D, Steinbach L. Magnetic resonance arthrography. *Orthop Clin N Am.* 2006;37:299–319.
96. Keene GS, Villar RN. Arthroscopic anatomy of the hip: An in vivo study. *Arthroscopy.* 1994;10:392–399.
97. Gaunche CA, Sikka RS. Acetabular labral tears with underlying chondromalacia: A possible association with high level running. *Arthroscopy.* 2005;21:580–585.
98. Garbuz DS, Masri BA, Haddad F, et al. Clinical and radiographic assessment of the young adult with symptomatic hip dysplasia. *Clin Orthop.* 2004;418:18–22.
99. Hickman JM, Peters CL. Hip pain in the young adult: Diagnosis and treatment of disorders of the acetabular labrum and acetabular displasia. *Am J Orthop.* 2001;30:459–467.
100. Leunig M, Podeszwad D, Beck M, et al. Magnetic resonance arthrography of labral disorders in hips with dysplasia and impingement. *Clin Orthop.* 2004;418:74–80.
101. Watson RM, Roach NA, Dalinka MK. AVN and bone marrow edema syndrome. *Radiol Clin N Am.* 2004;42:207–219.
102. Hayes CW, Conway WF, Daniel WW. MRI of bone marrow edema pattern: Transient osteoporosis, transient bone marrow edema syndrome, or osteonecrosis. *Radiographics.* 1993;13:1001–1011.
103. Bloem JL. Transient osteoporosis of the hip: MR imaging. *Radiology.* 1988;167:753–755.
104. Wilson AJ, Murphy WA, Hardy DC, et al. Transient osteoporosis: Transient bone marrow edema? *Radiology.* 1988;167:757–760.
105. Schils J, Piraino D, Richmond BJ, et al. Transient osteoporosis of the hip: Clinical and imaging features. *Cleve Clin J Med.* 1992;59:483–488.
106. Balakrishman A, Schemitsch EH, Pearce D, et al. Distinguishing transient osteoporosis of the hip from AVN. *Can J Surg.* 2003;46:187–192.
107. Vande Berg BC, Malghem JJ, Lecouvet FE, et al. Idiopathic bone marrow edema lesions of the femoral head: Predictive value of MRI findings. *Radiology.* 1999;212:527–535.
108. Radke S, Rader C, Kenn W, et al. Transient marrow edema syndrome of the hip: Results after core decompression. *Arch Orthop Trauma Surg.* 2003;123:223–227.
109. Radke S, Kirschner S, Seipel V, et al. Treatment of transient bone marrow oedema of the hip-A comparative study. *Int Orthop.* 2003;27:149–152.
110. Lazarus ML, Rao VA. *Bone Marrow, Clinical MRI,* 3rd Ed. 108:3545–3575 Philadelphia, PA: W.B. Saunders, 2006.
111. Assouline-Dayan Y, Chang C, Greenspan A, et al. Pathogenesis and natural history of osteonecrosis. *Semin Arthritis Rheum.* 2002;32(2):94–124.
112. Robinson HJ, Hartleben PD, Lund G, et al. Evaluation of MRI in the diagnosis of osteoporosis of the femoral head: Accuracy compared with radiographs, core biopsy and intraosseous pressure measurements. *J Bone Joint Surg AM.* 1989;71:650–663.
113. Glimcher MJ, Kenzora JE. The biology of osteonecrosis of the human femoral head and its clinical implications. *Clin Orthop Relat Res.* 1977;138:284–308.
114. Glimcher MJ, Kenzora JE. The biology of osteonecrosis of the human femoral head and its clinical implications (II). *Clin Orthop Relat Res.* 1978;139:283–312.
115. Glimcher MJ, Kenzora JE. The biology of osteonecrosis of the human femoral head and its clinical implications (III). *Clin Orthop Relat Res.* 1979;140:273–312.
116. Jergensen HE, Lang P, Moseley M, et al. Histologic correlation in MRI of femoral head osteoneurosis. *Clin Orthop Rel Res.* 1990;253:150–163.
117. Beltran J, Herman LJ, Burk JM. Femoral head AVN: MRI with clinical pathologic and radionuclide correlation. *Radiology.* 1988;166:215–220.
118. Zurlo JV. The double-line sign. *Radiology.* 1999;212:541–542.
119. Ficat RP. Idiopathic bone necrosis of the femoral head. *J Bone Joint Surg.* 1985;67:3–9.
120. Steinberg ME, Hayken GD, Steinberg DR. A quantitative system for staging AVN. *J Bone Joint Surg BR.* 1995;77:34–41.
121. Mitchel DG, Rao VM, Dalinka MK, et al. Femoral head AVN: Correlation of MRI, radiographic staging, radionuclide imaging, and clinical findings. *Radiology.* 1987;162:709–715.
122. Khanna AJ, Yoon TR, Mont MA, et al. Femoral head osteonecrosis: Detection and grading by using a rapid MRI protocol. *Radiology.* 2000;217:288–292.
123. Cherian SF, Laorr A, Saleh KJ, et al. Quantifying the extent of femoral head involvement in osteonecrosis. *J Bone Joint Surg Am.* 2003;85:(2):309–315.
124. Shimizu K, Moriya H, Akita T, et al. Prediction of collapse with MRI of AVN of the femoral head. *J Bone Joint Surg Am.* 1994;76:215–223.
125. Bogost GA, Lizerbram EK, Crues JV. MRI in evaluation of suspected hip fracture: Frequency of unsuspected bone and soft-tissue injury. *Radiology.* 1997;197:263–267.
126. Lee JK, Yao L. Stress fractures: MRI. *Radiology.* 1988;169:217–220.
127. Deutsch AL, Mink JH, Wayman AD. Occult fractures of the proximal femur: MRI. *Radiology.* 1989;170:113–116.
128. Quinn SF, McCarthy JL. Prospective evaluation of patients with suspected hip fracture and indeterminant radiographs: Use of TI weighted images. *Skeletal Radiol.* 1998;27:199–204.
129. Kneeland JB. MRI of sports injuries of the hip. *Magn Reson Imaging Clin N Am.* 1999;7:105–115.
130. Pfirrmann CW, Chung CB, Theumann NH, et al. Greater Trochanter of the hip: Attachment of the abductor mechanism and a complex of three bursae-MRI and MR bursography in cadavers and MRI in asymptomatic volunteers. *Radiology.* 2001;221:469–477.
131. Robinson P, Barron D, Parsons W, et al. Adductor-related groin pain in athletes: Correlation of MRI with clinical findings. *Skeletal Radiol.* 2004;33:451–457.
132. Robinson P, White LM, Agur A, et al. Obturator externus bursa: Anatomic origin and MRI features of pathologic involvement. *Radiology.* 2003;228:230–234.
133. Vacarro JB, Sauser DD, Beals RK. Iliopsoas bursa imaging: Efficacy in depicting abnormal iliopsoas tendon motion in patients with internal snapping hip syndrome. *Radiology.* 1995;197:853–856.
134. Pelsser V, Cardinal É, Hobden R, et al. Extra-articular snapping hip: Sonographic findings. *Am J Roentgenol.* 2001;176:67–73.
135. Albers S, Spritzer C, Garrett W, et al. MR findings in athletes with pubalgia. *Skeletal Radiol.* 2001;30:270–277.
136. Taylor D, Meyers W, Moylan J, et al. Abdominal musculature abnormalities as a cause of groin pain in athletes: Inguinal hernias and pubalgia. *Am J Sports Med.* 1991;19:239–243.
137. Muckle DS. Associated factors in recurrent groin and hamstring injuries. *BR J Sports Med.* 1982;16:37–39.
138. Nelson EN, Kassarjian A, Palmer WE. MRI of sports-related groin pain. *Magn Reson Imaging Clin N Am.* 2005;13:727–742.
139. Orchard J, Read J, Verrall G, et al. Pathophysiology of chronic groin pain in the athlete. *Int J Sports Med.* 2000;1:1.
140. da Rocha RC, Chopard RP. Nutrition pathways to the symphysis pubis. *J Anat.* 2004;204(3):209–215.
141. Gibbon WW, Hession PR. Diseases of the pubis and pubic symphysis: MRI appearances. *AJR.* 1997;169:849–853.
142. Gray H, Pick P, Howden R. *Anatomy of the Human Body.* Philadelphia, PA: Lea & Febiger; 1985.
143. Fon LJ, Spence RA. Sportsman's hernia. *Br J Surg.* 2000;87:545–552.
144. Kemp S, Batt M. The sports hernia. *Br J Surg.* 2000;87:545–550.
145. Van de Berg J. Inguinal hernias: MRI and ultrasound. *Semin Ultrasound CT MR.* 2002;23(2):156–173.
146. Legeu MB, Rochet WL. Les cellulites perivesicales et pelviennes après certaines cystostomies du prostatectomies sus-pubiennes. *J Urol Med Chir.* 1923;15:1–11.
147. Williams P, Thomas D, Downes E. Osteitis pubis and instability of the pubic symphysis: When non-operative measures fail. *Am J Sports Med.* 2000;28:350–355.
148. Brennan D, O'Connell M, Ryan M, et al. Secondary cleft sign as a marker of injury in athletes with groin pain: MR image appearance and interpretation. *Radiology.* 2005;235:162–167.
149. Major N, Helms C. Pelvic stress injuries: The relationship between osteitis pubis (symphysis pubis stress injury) and sacroiliac abnormalities in athletes. *Skeletal Radiol.* 1997;26:711–717.
150. Paulis FD, Cacchio A, Michelini O, et al. Sports injuries in the pelvis and hip: Diagnostic imaging. *Eur J Radiol.* 1998;27:549–559.
151. Rupp TJ, Purcell C. Groin injury. Available at: http://www.emedicine.com/sports/topic/62htm. Accessed June 20, 2005.
152. Holmich P, Uhrskou P, Ulnits L, et al. Effectiveness of active physical training as treatment for long-standing adductor-related groin pain in athletes: Randomized trial. *Lancet.* 1999;353:439–443.
153. Anderson K, Strickland S, Warren R. Hip and groin injuries in athletes. *Am J Sports Med.* 2001;29:521–533.
154. Gilmore OJA. Gilmore's groin. *Sportsmed Soft Tissue Trauma.* 1992;3:12–14.
155. Malycha P, Lovell G. Inguinal surgery in athletes with chronic groin pain: Sportsman's hernia. *Aust N Z J Surg.* 1992;62:123–125.
156. Polglase AL, Frydman GM, Farmer KC. Inguinal surgery for debilitating chronic groin pain in athletes. *Med J Aust.* 1991;155:674–677.
157. Llauger J, Palmer J, Roson N, et al. Nonseptic arthritis: Imaging features with clinical and histo pathologic correlation. *Radiographics* 2000;20(Spec No):5263–5278.
158. Mengiardi B, Pfirrmann CW, Hodler J. Hip pain in adults: MRI appearance of common causes. *Eur Radiol.* 2007;17:1746–1746.

159. Byers PD, Cotton RE, Deacon OW, et al. The diagnosis and treatment of pigmented villonodular synovitis. *J Bone Joint Surg Br.* 1968;50:290–305.
160. Dorwart RH, Genant HK, Johnston WH, et al. Pigmented villonodular synovitis of synovial joints: Clinical, pathologic and radiologic features. *Am J Roentgenol.* 1984;143:877–885.
161. Kalil RK, Unni KK. Malignancy in pigmented villonodul synovitis. *Skeletal Radiol.* 1998;27(7):392–395.
162. Newman JS, Newberg AH. MRI of the painful hip in athletes. *Clin Sports Med.* 2006;25:613–633.
163. Cotton A, Flipo RM, Chastanet P, et al. Pigmented villonodular synovitis of the hip: Review of radiographic features in 58 patients. *Skeletal Radiol.* 1995;24(1):1–6.
164. Bancroft LW, Peterson JJ, Kransdorf MJ. MRI of tumors and tumor-like lesions of the hip. *Magn Reson Imaging Clin N Am.* 2005;13(4):757–774.
165. Maurice H, Crone M, Watt I. Synovial chondromatosis. *J Bone Joint Surg BR.* 1988;70(5):807–811.
166. Kim SH, Hong SJ, Park JS, et al. Idiopathic synovial osteochondromatosis of the hip: Radiographic and MR appearances in 15 patients. *Korean J Radiol.* 2002;3(4):254–259.
167. Kattapuram SV, Kushner DC, Phillips WC, et al. Osteoid osteoma: An unusual cause of articular pain. *Radiology.* 1983;147:383–387.
168. Hayes CW, Balkisoon AA. MRI of the musculoskeletal system: In the hip. *Clin Orthop Relat Res.* 1996;322:297–309.
169. Kransdorf MJ, Stull MA, Gilkey FW, et al. Oseoid osteoma. *Radiographics.* 1991;11:671–696.
170. Assoun J, Richardi G, Railhac J, et al. Osteoid osteoma: MRI vs CT. *Radiology.* 1994;191:217–223.
171. Lui PT, Chivers FS, Roberts CC, et al. Imaging of osteoid osteoma with dynamic gadolinium-enhanced MRI. *Radiology.* 2003;227:69–700.
172. Morel-Lavallee VAF. Decollements traumatiques de la peau et des couches sous-jacentes. *Arch Gen Med* 1863;1:20–38, 172–200, 300–332.
173. Letournel E, Judet R. *Fractures of the Acetabulum,* 2nd Ed. Berlin: Springer-Verlag; 1993.
174. Mellado JM, Bencardino JT. Morel-Lavallee Lesion: Review with emphasis on MRI. *Magn Reson Imaging Clin N Am.* 2005;13:775–782.
175. Collince C, Tornetta P III. Soft Tissue injuries associated with pelvic fractures. *Orthop Clin North Am.* 2004;35(4):451–456.
176. Hakdj, Olson SA, Matta JM. Diagnosis and management of closed internal degloving injuries associated with pelvic and acetabular fractures: The Morel-Lavallee lesion. *J Trauma* 1997;42:1046–1051.
177. Hudson DA, Knottenbelt JD, Krice JE. Closed degloving injuries: Results following conservative surgery. *Plast Reconstr Surg.* 1992;89(5):853–855.
178. Kittmeier SA, Wilson SC, Born CT, et al. Surgical management of soft tissue lesions associated with pelvic ring injury. *Clin Orthop Relat Res.* 1996;329:46–53.
179. Gregory P, Sanders R. The management of severe fractures of the lower extremities. *Clin Orthop Relat Res.* 1995;318:95–105.
180. Parra JA, Fernandez MA, Encinas B, et al. Morel-Lavallee effusions in the thigh. *Skeletal Radiol.* 1997;26(4):239–241.
181. Nakano M, Kondoh T, Igarashi J, et al. A case of chronic expanding hematoma in the tensor fascia lata. *Dermatol Online J.* 2001;7:6.

CHAPTER

3

Adam C. Zoga
George P. Hobbs

Imaging of the Pelvis

INTRODUCTION

Imaging studies dedicated to the pelvis are a mainstay of the hospital wards, primary care clinic, emergency medicine department, and sports medicine clinic in the 21st century. From the outset, it is extremely important that the referring clinician or subspecialist possess a basic understanding of differences between not only imaging modalities but also different protocols within a single modality that can drastically alter expected sensitivities and specificities when a study is requested. Most health care providers are comfortable with the idea that a magnetic resonance imaging (MRI) is likely to show soft tissue, visceral, and even osseous lesions that would be occult to even the highest-quality radiographic series. But equally important is the acceptance that an "MRI pelvis" will likely not approach the sensitivity for suspected pathologies that an appropriately ordered "MRI gyn pelvis" or "MRI pelvis, athletic pubalgia protocol" would. Further, some clinical indications warrant imaging techniques and protocols not available in all radiology practices, and the referrer must be knowledgeable enough in the science of imaging to recognize these instances, as radiology practices rarely direct patients to a competitor that might offer a more specialized imaging study. While imaging techniques dedicated to issues including gynecological pathologies in the visceral pelvis, spondyloarthropathies of the bony pelvis, or enteric disorders such as inflammatory bowel disease and appendicitis generally fall outside the scope of this chapter, both the clinician and the imager must acknowledge the numerous confounders for sports injury as a cause of pelvic, hip, and groin pain. In this chapter, we will detail available imaging modalities and protocols to be considered when dealing with the musculoskeletal pelvis, and hopefully provide a working guide for ordering the appropriate radiological examination. We will also review common, and occasionally uncommon, imaging patterns and pathologies associated with groin pain that might be encountered in the sports medicine, general surgery, or primary care clinic. Finally, as radiology is an ever-evolving field with regard to both techniques and observations, we will offer occasional insights and glimpses at where imaging may be headed in diagnosis and therapeutic guidance for some of these injuries over the next decade.

IMAGING MODALITY OPTIONS

When considering this question, the answer is likely to be different for clear mechanical hip pain than it would be for nebulous, activity-induced groin pain. Nonetheless, the clinical overlap between internal derangements of the hip and groin as well as the concomitance of hip and groin lesions generally make a radiographic series including a true anterior to posterior (AP) view of the pelvis a wise and economical first study. But many of the lesions and syndromes we will discuss in this chapter are entirely occult to plain radiographs. Diagnoses that can be suggested with a radiographic series of the pelvis include chronic osteitis pubis, subacute or chronic soft tissue hematomas, chronic stress fractures, and traumatic osseous avulsions. Confounding causes of groin pain visible on radiographs include sacroiliitis, lumbar spondyloarthropathy, some uterine fibroids and adnexal lesions, and femoroacetabular malalignments. For clinical athletic pubalgia, the pubic symphysis should be carefully scrutinized for eburnation (subchondral sclerosis), osteophyte formation, subchondral cysts (geodes), and erosions, any of which can be an indicator of chronic instability reflecting a tendinous lesion.[1] For unilateral groin pain and hip pain, the same lesions should be noted at the hip, as well as any asymmetry or variant femoroacetabular alignment.

Computerized tomography (CT or CAT scan) examinations have become so popular in clinical practice, that even a modest size emergency department will generate 25 to 50 CTs a night. It is probably safe to say, at this point, that the majority of patients seeking subspecialty sports medicine or general surgery consult for chronic pelvic or groin pain will have some sort of CT covering the pelvis in their medical record or radiology jacket (Fig. 3.1). CT protocols vary widely. In the emergency department, primary considerations typically center on emergent pathologies such as appendicitis, abscess, or urinary tract obstruction. Unfortunately, these types of CT studies generally offer little insight into musculoskeletal sources of pain. When reviewing a CT for a patient with chronic pelvic or groin pain, its inherent exquisite osseous detail should be utilized to evaluate articular surfaces at the hips, sacroiliac joints, and pubic symphysis for degenerative and posttraumatic lesions. But be wary, regardless of CT resolution and quality of two- and three-dimensional reformats, nondisplaced fractures are often occult to CT. If stress or insufficiency fracture is a primary differential consideration, then radiographs followed by MRI if necessary are a better imaging choice than CT. But even noncontrast CT is an excellent tool for evaluating the inguinal ring and canal, and infiltration of the fat surrounding enteric structures within the inguinal canal is a good indicator of strangulation. More often than not, however, the value of CT in the evaluation of

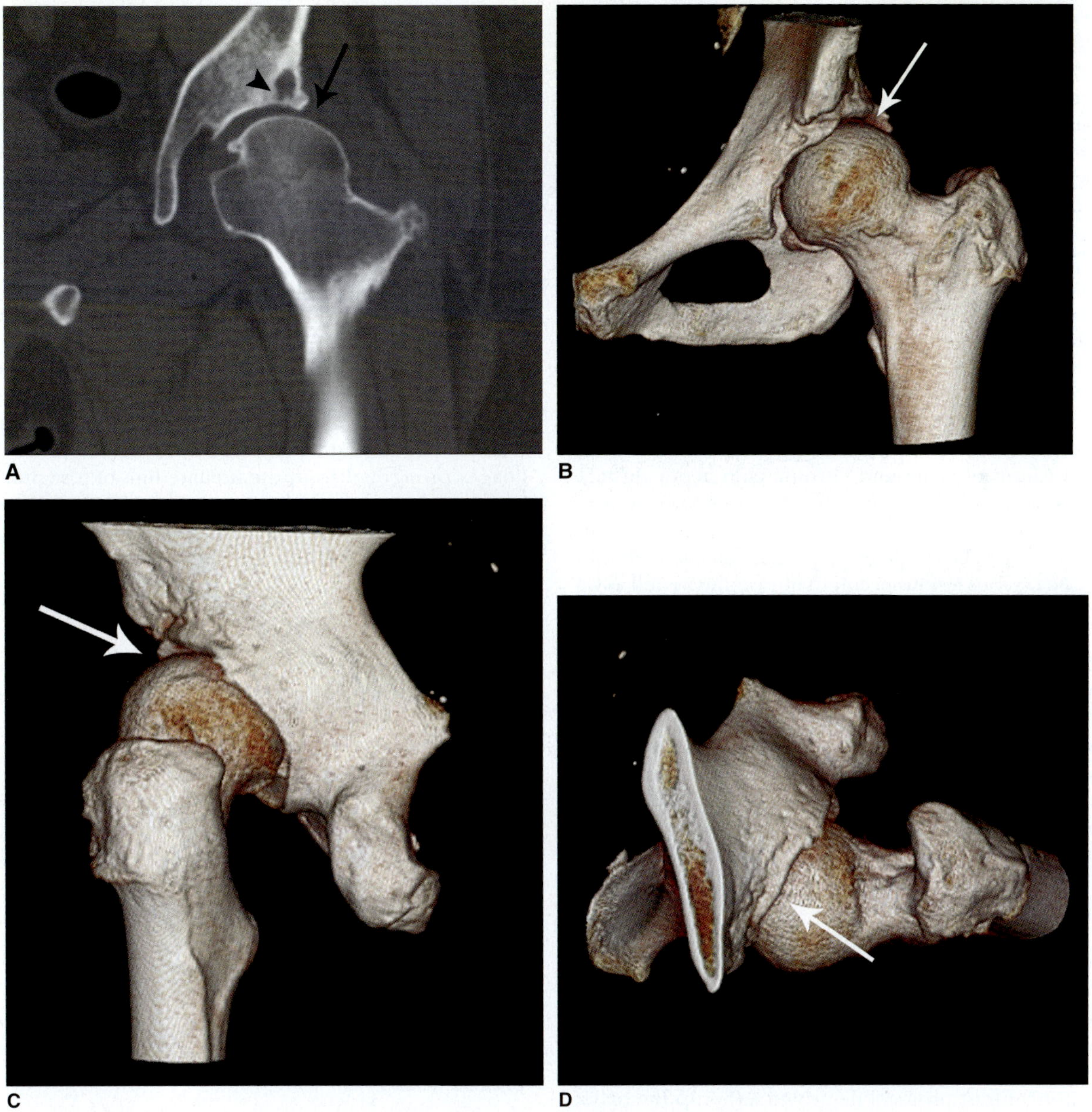

Figure 3.1. Ipsilateral hip pathology. Coronal CT image (**A**) and three-dimensional reformatted images of the left hip in the anterior (**B**), posterolateral (**C**), and superior (**D**) orientation demonstrate uncovering of the superior femoral head, typical for developmental acetabular dysplasia (*arrow*). Coronal CT image (**A**) demonstrates superior joint space loss with subchondral sclerosis and cystic change (*arrowhead*), consistent with osteoarthritis.

musculoskeletal pelvic pain is in the exclusion of confounding lesions, such as ureteral calculi, adnexal inflammatory processes, and enteric processes. In the outpatient clinic, CT is rarely the best choice as a first-line imaging examination if the problem is felt to be musculoskeletal.

Scintigraphy (bone scan, nuclear scan) was popular for a period as an indicator of osseous remodeling. Technetium injected intravenously will be avidly bound by osteoclastic and osteoblastic activity, making a bone scan sensitive for stress fracture, osteomyelitis, and osseous neoplasms. Unfortunately, too frequently a nuclear medicine bone scan is interpreted as "consistent with stress fracture, osteomyelitis, or neoplasm." While technetium bone scan remains the imaging study of choice in the assessment of osseous disease extent, as in metastases and hematogenous spread of multifocal osteomyelitis, its use in the evaluation of stress fracture, osteitis pubis, sacroiliitis, and other athletics-induced pelvic injuries has been replaced by MRI. Musculoskeletal ultrasound has become a niche in the imaging world over the past decade, and many myotendinous injuries typically assessed with MRI can be identified with equal sensitivity using ultrasound all the while taking the extremity or joint through a dynamic biomechanical axis. The term "pelvic ultrasound" inherently lends itself to a connotation of either transabdominal or transvaginal sonographic examination of gynecological structures. But a dedicated musculoskeletal ultrasound of pelvic tendinous and myotendinous structures can diagnose many nongynecologic causes of pelvis and groin pain related to muscles, tendons, bursae, and the inguinal rings.[2,3]

However, even among academic radiology departments, very few centers in North America offer dedicated musculoskeletal ultrasound clinic on a routine basis. These examinations are relatively labor intensive in terms of procedure time and direct patient interaction when compared with the outpatient MRI, and there is a worldwide paucity of ultrasound technologists trained in musculoskeletal applications. Another shortcoming of this modality is its limited assessment of osseous and articular structures. To date, the authors feel that ultrasound can be an extremely useful problem-solving tool in patients with myotendinous and teno-osseous pathologies about the pelvis, but it is most useful when performed in the hands of a skilled, subspecialized ultrasonographer, in conjunction with other imaging such as MRI for assessment of dynamic or biomechanical function or integrity of an injured structure, or for the purpose of image guidance during interventional procedures.

MRI has become the standard imaging modality for musculoskeletal causes of acute and chronic pain about the pelvis, when history and physical examination are nondiagnostic. MRI offers the unique combination of sensitivity for soft tissue injury that might not be visible by CT and the ability to identify nondisplaced osseous lesions occult to ultrasound as well as CT and plain radiography. In fact, in experienced hands, a noncontrast MRI examination frequently not only identifies the source of pain, but also the biomechanical cause for the lesion that has become the source of pain. MRI protocols are widely variable similar to CT, and the level of examination quality as well as interpretation can vary greatly similar to musculoskeletal ultrasound. For these reasons, the authors feel strongly that subspecialists referring patients for MRI should go beyond simply providing a prescription but get to know their potential MRI facilities and develop interpersonal relationships with interpreting radiologists whenever possible. An MRI examination of the pelvis ordered to evaluate uterine fibroids certainly warrants a vastly different protocol than an MRI of the pelvis ordered to evaluate potential causes of athletic pubalgia, yet they might have the same ordering or billing codes. Intravenous and intra-articular contrast can significantly add to the cost of an MRI, and is not always useful in establishing a diagnosis. For suspected musculoskeletal sources of pain, we support a noncontrast protocol dedicated either to the pelvic osseous and myotendinous structures remote from the pubic symphysis or to the pubic symphysis and its attachments while still imaging the entire pelvis. For if a finding on noncontrast MRI necessitates further evaluation, additional sequences can be acquired with or without contrast at the same visit or, if the study is acquired off hours without radiologist supervision, at a later date. The authors advocate that three short "survey" sequences covering the entire pelvis be acquired at the onset of each noncontrast pelvis MRI using the built in body coil as a receiver. A short tau inversion recovery (STIR) sequence in the coronal plane maximizes fat suppression and thus fluid sensitivity. It is a low resolution sequence and will not be adequate for delineation of small soft tissue lesions, but no fractures or destructive lesions will be missed and apophyses even as peripheral as the anterior superior iliac spine can be interrogated effectively. A nonfat suppressed T1-weighted spin echo (SE) is an important part of each of our MRI protocols, as it is specific for infiltrative bone marrow processes including metastases, myeloma, and infection that might otherwise be overlooked. And an axial T2-weighted fast spin echo (FSE) fat suppressed image is useful for assessing the symmetry of muscles, tendons, bursae, and osseous structures. After these three sequences, protocols vary based upon the clinical indication. If the suspicion is occult fracture, regardless of location, these three acquisitions should be diagnostic. For spondyloarthropathies, additional smaller field of view images in a coronal oblique plane angled with the sacrum allow for dedicated assessment of sacroiliac joint articular surfaces. In the setting of athletic pubalgia, we have developed a protocol designed to maximize specificity for teno-osseous injuries about the pubic symphysis, as well as sensitivity for the many potential confounding lesions remote from the symphysis that may contribute to pain. With an athletic pubalgia protocol, after the three survey sequences covering the entire pelvis, a surface receiver coil positioned on the lower abdomen ventral to the pubic symphysis is turned on and additional sequences are acquired with a smaller field of view ranging from 20 to 24cm (Table 3.1). Once this dedicated receiver coil is turned on, coronal oblique images prescribed from the arcuate line of a sagittal midline image or the anterior iliac crest off midline and centered at the pubic symphysis (Fig. 3.2) are obtained to open up the adductor tendon origins while showing the caudal rectus abdominis pubic attachment in plane.[1] Additionally, a true sagittal fat suppressed, fluid sensitive series centered at the symphysis delineated the rectus abdominis/adductor aponeurosis with its periosteal attachments on the anterior and anteroinferior aspect of the superior pubic ramus. The beauty of this athletic pubalgia MRI protocol is that it maximizes specificity for common musculoskeletal causes of groin pain as well as inguinal hernias, while offering enough imaging that many nonmusculoskeletal causes of pain will be at least noticed such that a more appropriate study can be undertaken. Ultimately, with MRI, the more information delivered to the imager the better and the best imagers tailor each examination to its specific differential considerations.

IMAGING FINDINGS IN COMMON CONDITIONS

FRACTURES

All clinicians treating musculoskeletal causes of pain about the pelvis must accept that some fractures involving the osseous pelvis or hips will be radiographically occult or not visible on conventional radiographs. To minimize this incidence, providing a clinical suspicion to the injury can frequently assist the imager in tailoring the radiographic examination with specific projections or views, such as the Judet view for acetabular fractures or the sacroiliac obliques for sacral ala fractures. Nonetheless, if a clinical suspicion for nondisplaced stress fracture of the pubic rami, insufficiency fracture of the sacrum, or subcapital fracture of the hip exists and radiographs are nondiagnostic or normal, then further imaging with a more tertiary modality is warranted. The authors feel that, in 2009, the indicated imaging for occult fracture about the pelvis is almost invariably MRI. A "fast" noncontrast MRI protocol including only three or four sequences can be acquired in less than 15min and should approach 100% sensitivity for fractures. At our institution, such a protocol is implemented with both emergency department patients and outpatients. A fracture will manifest on MRI as an intense focal high signal on fluid sensitive, fat suppressed sequences,

TABLE 3.1 MRI Protocol: Athletic Pubalgia

Primary Sequences	*Plane*	*Sequence*	*Coil*	*FOV*	*Slice*	*Matrix Nex*	*TR*	*TE*	*TI*	*Flip Angle*	*Band*	*ETL*	*Fat Supp?*	*Other*	*Est. Time (min)*
Localizer	3 plane	FSPGR	Body	36–48										Parameters set by system	2
1	Coronal	FSE-STIR	Body	24	4/1	256 × 1923	>2,000	20–40	150	—	16	8	—	Scan from pubic symphysis through ischial tuberosities	3–4
2	Coronal	T1 SE	Body	24	4/1	256 × 1922	400–800	Minimum	—	—	16	—	N	As above	3–4
3	Axial	T2 FSE	Body	20	4/1	256 × 1922	>2,000	50–60	—	—	16	8	Y	Scan from superior acetabulum through pubic symphysis	3–4
4	Sagittal	T2 FSE	Phase array surface	20–24	4/1	256 × 1922	>2,000	50–60	—	—	16	8	Y	Scan from right through left ischial tuberosities	3–4
5	Axial oblique	PD FSE	Phase array surface	20	4/1	256 × 2562	3,000	25	—	—	16	8	N	Prescribe plane to line paralleling anterior ilio-pubic cortex	3–4
6	Axial oblique	T2 FSE	Phase array surface	20	4/1	256 × 1922	>2,000	50–60	—	—	16	8	Y	As above	3–4

Special instruction: Empty bladder prior to imaging.

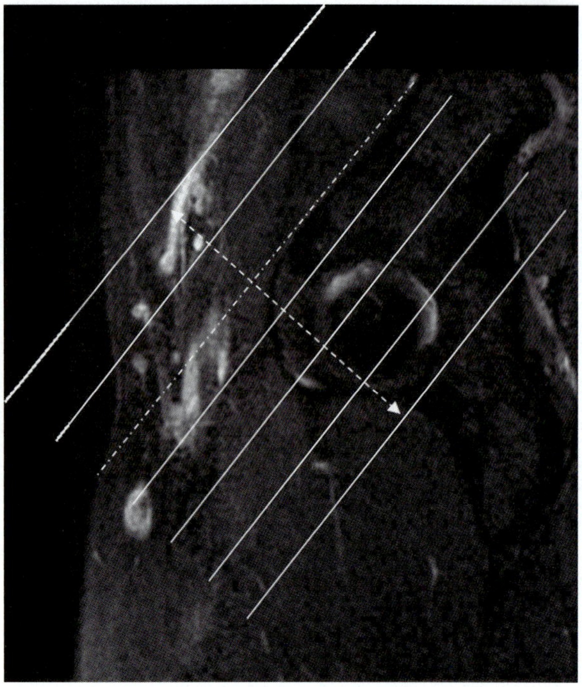

Figure 3.2. Axial oblique sequence acquisition. The axial oblique image is prescribed from a plane tangent to the arcuate line of the pelvis or the anterior iliac crest (*white lines*) as demonstrated on a sagittal image near the medial acetabulum.

whether STIR or T2 FSE. Frequently, an actual fracture line is seen on the nonfat suppressed T1-weighted sequence, but this finding is not a requirement to diagnose fracture (Fig. 3.3). Stress fractures occur in typical locations of biomechanical stress and generally show exuberant callus formation with periostitis and sclerosis at the fracture site reflecting repetitive injury.[4] Insufficiency fractures frequently occur in reproducible locations, including the sacral alae, the parasymphyseal pubic rami, the supra-acetabular regions, and the proximal femoral diaphyses. There is less periostitis and callus formation, but MRI findings are still highly sensitive and specific (Fig. 3.4). One caveat to confidently classify fractures by MRI is the accurate identification of pathologic fractures. Eroded, moth-eaten, and destroyed cortical margins in the setting of a primary osseous tumor are better demonstrated on plain radiography and on CT than they are on MRI. If there is any cause to suspect a fracture may be pathologic on MRI, then a full imaging workup is recommended, including radiographs, CT, or both for evaluation of lesion margins and matrix as well as a total body technetium bone scan to identify any additional osseous lesions. For isolated fractures, while scintigraphy is sensitive, its specificity does not approach that of MRI, and fractures, metastases, and osteomyelitis can have a similar appearance on bone scan. In the setting of trauma, if a patient is being imaged in the CT suite for intracranial, intrathoracic, or visceral injury, continuing the scan through the pelvis and then performing coronal, sagittal, and three-dimensional reformats from the helical acquisition can often provide useful additional information for osseous injury, including delineation of fracture extent and malalignment, even though nondisplaced fractures and osseous contusions may remain occult.

MYOTENDINOUS STRAINS

Muscle and tendon injuries about the pelvis, excluding osseous avulsions, are the domain of MRI and musculoskeletal ultrasound. As with fractures, noncontrast MRI protocols using a large field of view and fluid sensitive and fat suppressed sequences are generally adequate for injury identification and grading. Asymmetry is a useful tool in identifying focal soft tissue injuries among the numerous pelvic muscle groups. If the imager acquires three STIR or T2 FSE fat suppressed sequences in conventional coronal, sagittal, and axial planes centered at midline (the pubic symphysis is a good landmark), most myotendinous strains are easily and accurately identified. One of

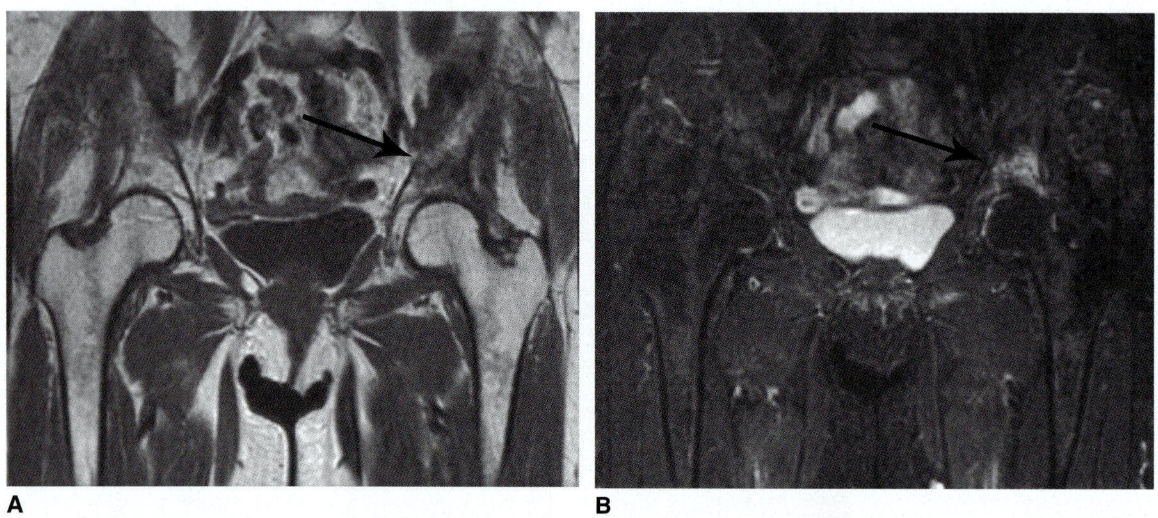

Figure 3.3. Acetabular stress fracture. Coronal T1-weighted (**A**) and STIR (**B**) images of the pelvis show linear signal abnormality in the left supra-acetabular region along the biomechanical weight-bearing axis (*arrows*) in a marathon runner, typical for a stress fracture.

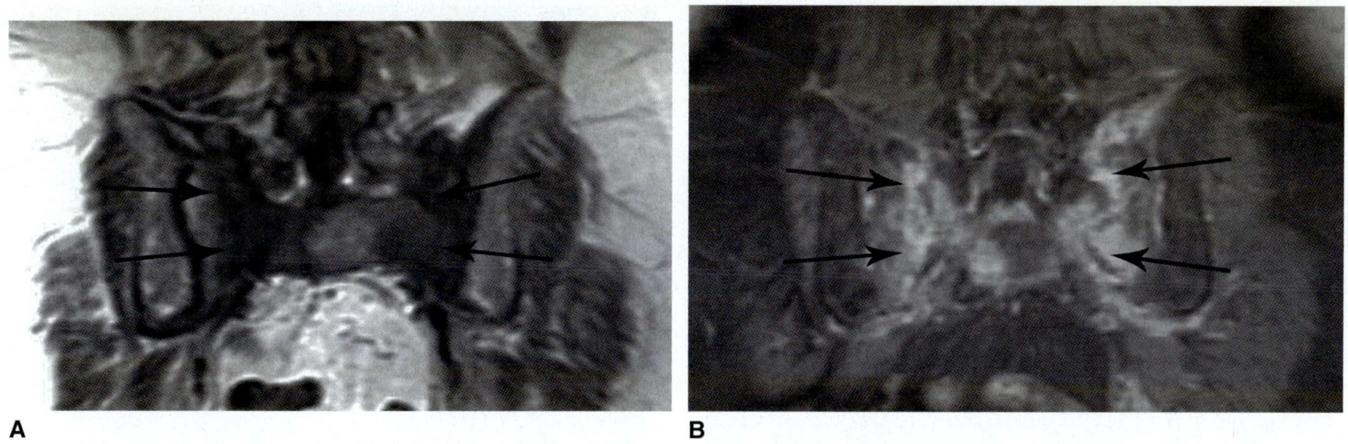

Figure 3.4. Sacral insufficiency fractures. Coronal T1-weighted (**A**) and STIR (**B**) images of the sacrum demonstrate linear signal abnormality with associated marrow edema within the bilateral sacral ala (*arrows*) in a middle aged female. This pattern on MRI is typical for sacral ala insufficiency fractures.

the planes is likely to image the muscular structure along with its contralateral counterpart in short axis, allowing for proper identification, sometimes with the help of an online or textbook atlas. Then, another plane is likely to delineate the lesion on long axis where it can be appropriately graded. The authors utilize a grading system based upon the configuration and extent of fluid signal replacing a muscle belly or about a myotendinous unit. With a grade I strain, fluid simply surrounds the muscle belly or myotendinous junction without replacing it, in a configuration resembling a "V." In a grade III strain or essentially a complete tear, the fluid signal replaces a portion of the muscle or tendon and the T2 hyperintense configuration resembles an inverted triangle. A grade II lesion is somewhere between the two, and my best interpretation of the morphology on MRI is a "V" with a meniscus filling its apex. This system works for most muscles throughout the body and can help predict recovery time and response to therapy.

In the pelvis, common myotendinous strains include the thigh adductors where the adductor longus is most frequently involved, the hip external rotators, the proximal hamstrings, the hip flexors, and the lower abdominal trunk flexors and rotators (Figs. 3.5–3.10). In some instances, the imager must be aware of common relationships between muscle injuries and specific activities (rectus femoris with kicking, sartorius with yoga, adductor longus with soccer, and pectineus with hockey), while in other situations, the imager must remember biomechanical axes that lead to a second antagonistic muscle group injury (rectus abdominis and thigh adductors).[5] Higher grade myotendinous injuries may lead to hematoma formation and consequential delayed healing (Fig. 3.11). Hematomas are

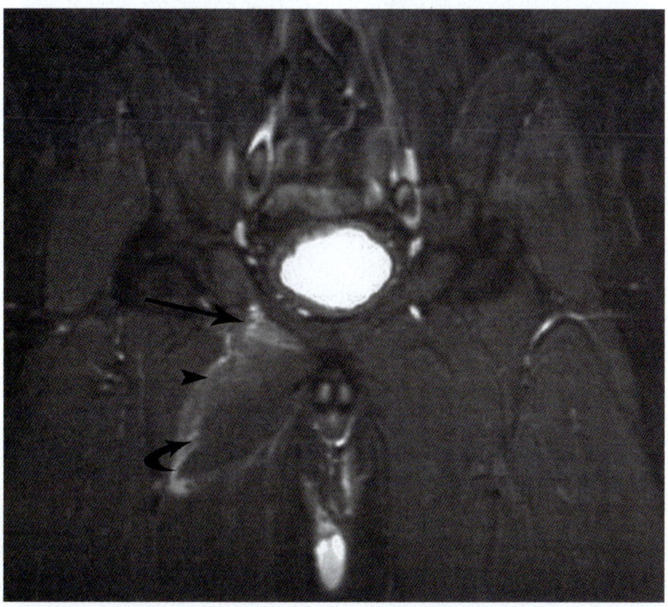

Figure 3.5. Coronal STIR image of the pelvis from a professional hockey player with pain on acceleration demonstrates intramuscular and perimuscular edema along the right external oblique (*arrow*), adductor magnus, adductor brevis (*arrowhead*), and pectineus (*curved arrow*) muscles, consistent with muscle strains throughout the adductor compartment.

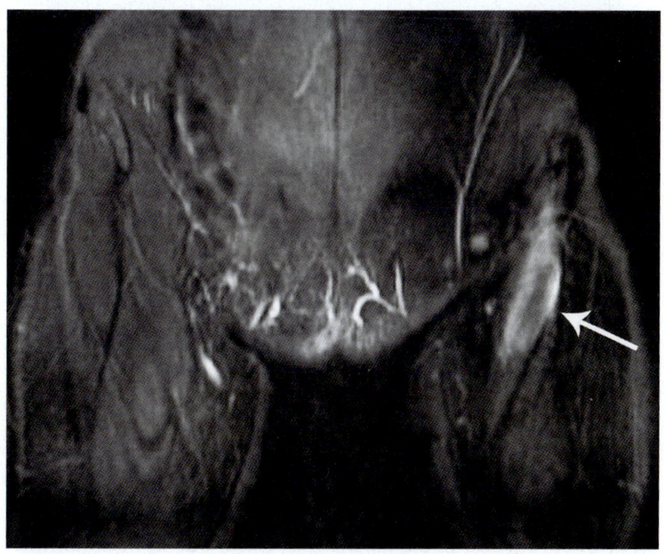

Figure 3.6. Left sartorius strain. Coronal STIR image of the pelvis in a yoga enthusiast with apprehension on hip flexion demonstrates intramuscular and perimuscular edema along the left sartorius (*arrow*).

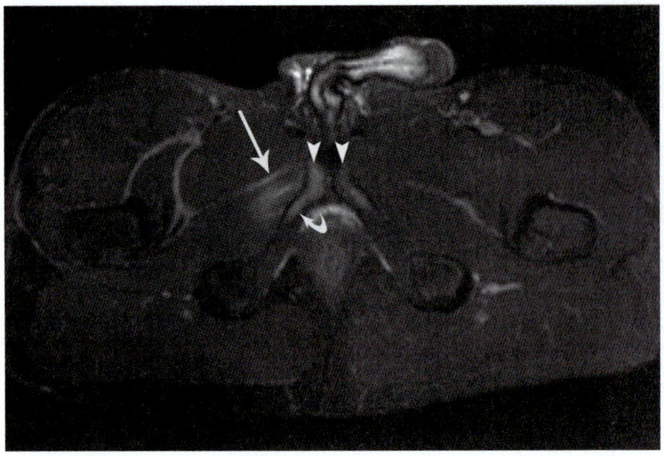

Figure 3.7. Axial T2-weighted fat suppressed image of the pelvis in a hockey professional forward with pain on hip external rotation and abduction demonstrates intramuscular and perimuscular edema isolated to the right obturator externus muscle (*arrow*), consistent with a muscle strain. Marrow edema within the pubic bodies (*arrowheads*) is indicative of osteitis pubis, and bony edema extending into the right inferior pubic ramus (*curved arrow*) indicates osseous stress response likely unrelated to the acute muscle injury.

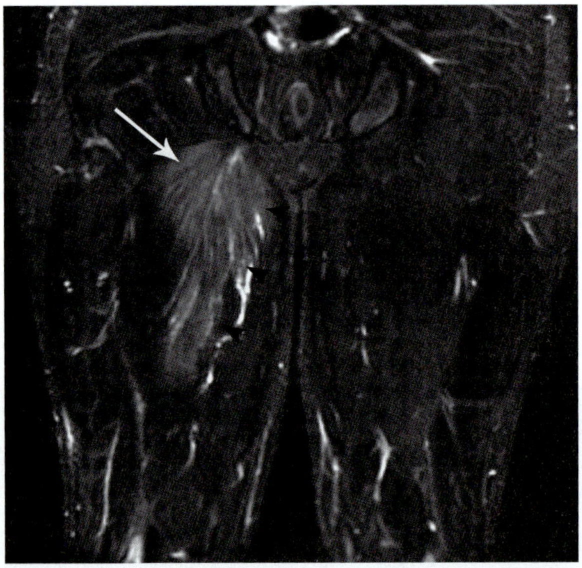

Figure 3.8. Adductor magnus and semimembranosus muscle strains. Coronal STIR image of the pelvis from a national football league (NFL) player with an acute injury demonstrates intramuscular edema within the adductor magnus (*white arrow*) and semimembranosus (*black arrowheads*).

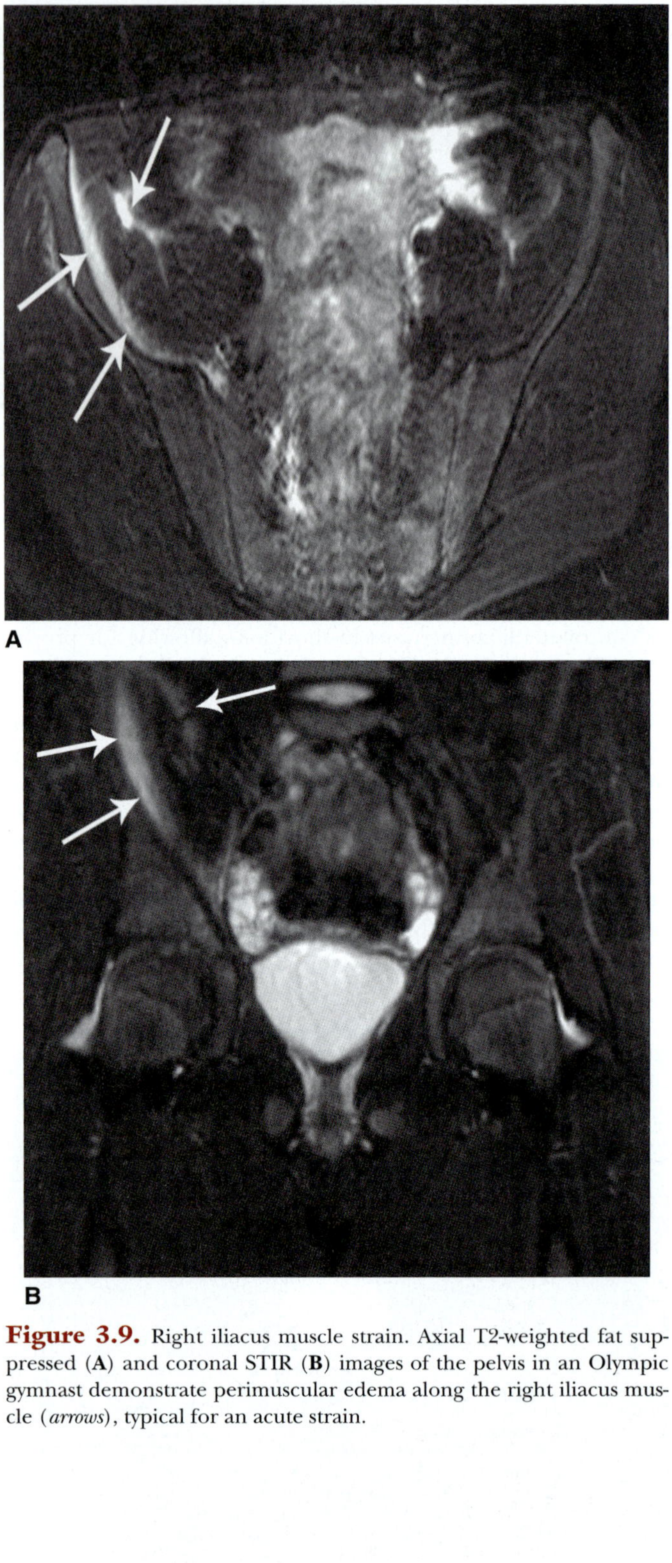

A

B

Figure 3.9. Right iliacus muscle strain. Axial T2-weighted fat suppressed (**A**) and coronal STIR (**B**) images of the pelvis in an Olympic gymnast demonstrate perimuscular edema along the right iliacus muscle (*arrows*), typical for an acute strain.

extremely variable and heterogeneous in signal on MRI, and the images can inaccurately call a hematoma any number of atraumatic lesions if not aware of the recent trauma. Further, an effort to further categorize a post-traumatic hematoma with intravenous contrast almost invariably leads to an incorrect diagnosis such as soft tissue sarcoma. For this reason, it is very important for the imager to recognize a myotendinous injury as a potential hematoma source, and it is equally as important for a referrer to alert the imager to recent trauma or a suspicion for strain.

Accurate identification of tendinous avulsions from bone has taken on increasing importance in recent years with technical

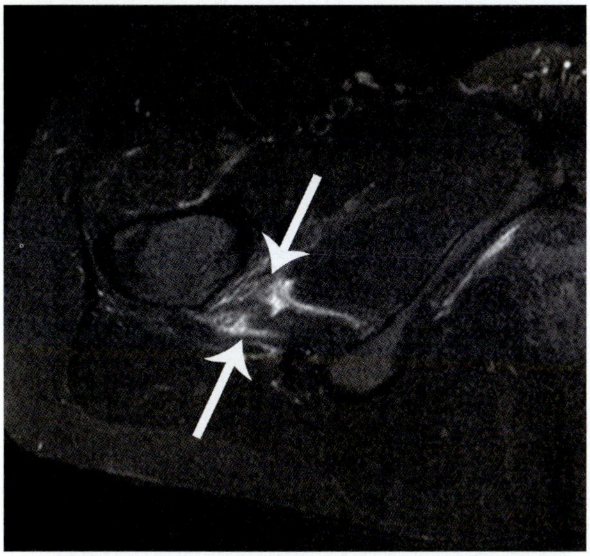

Figure 3.10. Quadratus femoris muscle strain. Axial T2-weighted fat suppressed image dedicated to the right thigh in a recreational soccer player shows perimuscular and intramuscular edema along the right quadratus femoris muscle.

advances in primary repair of such lesions, especially at the hamstring origins and the thigh adductor origins. While MRI is highly sensitive for such lesions, specificity can be lacking in some instances. If an MRI does not clarify whether or not the tendon is avulsed from its osseous origin, radiographs or CT may be helpful in searching for a displaced fragment of periosteum. But many lesions can be accurately classified by MRI on the basis of the integrity of the hypointense (black) bony cortex on nonfat suppressed T1-weighted images (Figs. 3.12 and 3.13).

APOPHYSITIS

In a young athlete, repetitive stress across immature ossification centers frequently leads to a set of painful musculoskeletal disorders that can be lumped together as apophysites. This diagnosis should be readily identified by MRI and is occasionally visible on a radiographic series. The key to diagnosis is an understanding of osseous maturity and biomechanical axes that may stress immature growth plates. While the appearance and maturation of growth centers in the bones of the elbow are well documented and memorized by most radiologists, pelvic ossification centers are more nebulous in textbooks and the imaging literature. Traumatized apophyses at the anterior superior iliac spine, anterior inferior iliac spine, ischial tuberosities, and pubic symphysis are frequent sources of pain in a young athlete.[6] Skeletally immature, kicking athletes are particularly prone to physeal injury at the site of the rectus femoris origin from the anterior inferior iliac spine ipsilateral to their dominant kicking leg. With osseous maturity occurring earlier in life, young female athletes are more likely to develop a similar condition at the anterior superior iliac spine related to either the Sartorius or the tensor fascia lata.

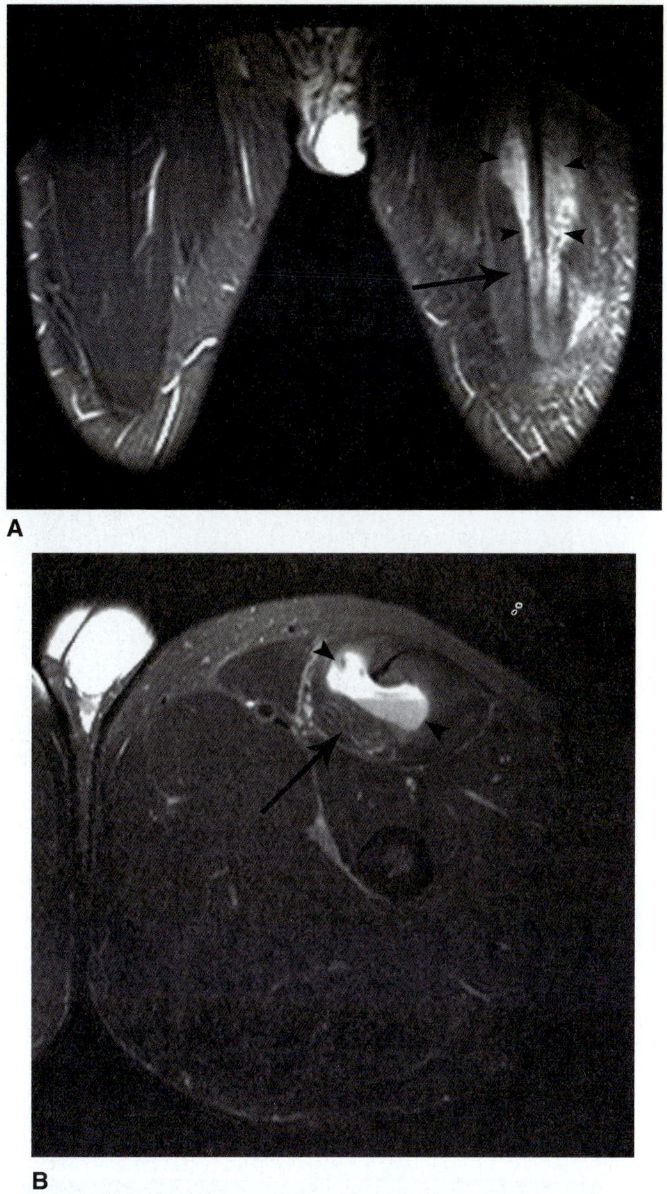

Figure 3.11. Left rectus femoris muscle strain with hematoma. Coronal STIR (**A**) and axial T2-weighted fat suppressed (**B**) images of the left thigh in a professional baseball player, 3 weeks after a thigh strain, show intramuscular edema within the left rectus femoris muscle (*arrows*) with an associated hematoma along the musculotendinous junction (*arrowheads*). Note the hematocrit level layering in this supine patient suggesting a subacute hematoma.

Regardless of location, hallmark MRI findings include subenthesial bone marrow edema and asymmetry of the physis itself in both morphology and signal (Fig. 3.14). Occasionally, in severe cases, soft tissue edema will extend into or about the involved tendon. With chronic proximal hamstring pain in a teen, the imager should always compare bone marrow signal in the ischial tuberosities, as an apophysitis can manifest simply as asymmetric bone marrow edema (Fig. 3.15). Tendon origin injuries in the vicinity of the pubic symphysis are common, so apophysitis type injuries certainly occur here related to the thigh adductors, but a thorough imaging description

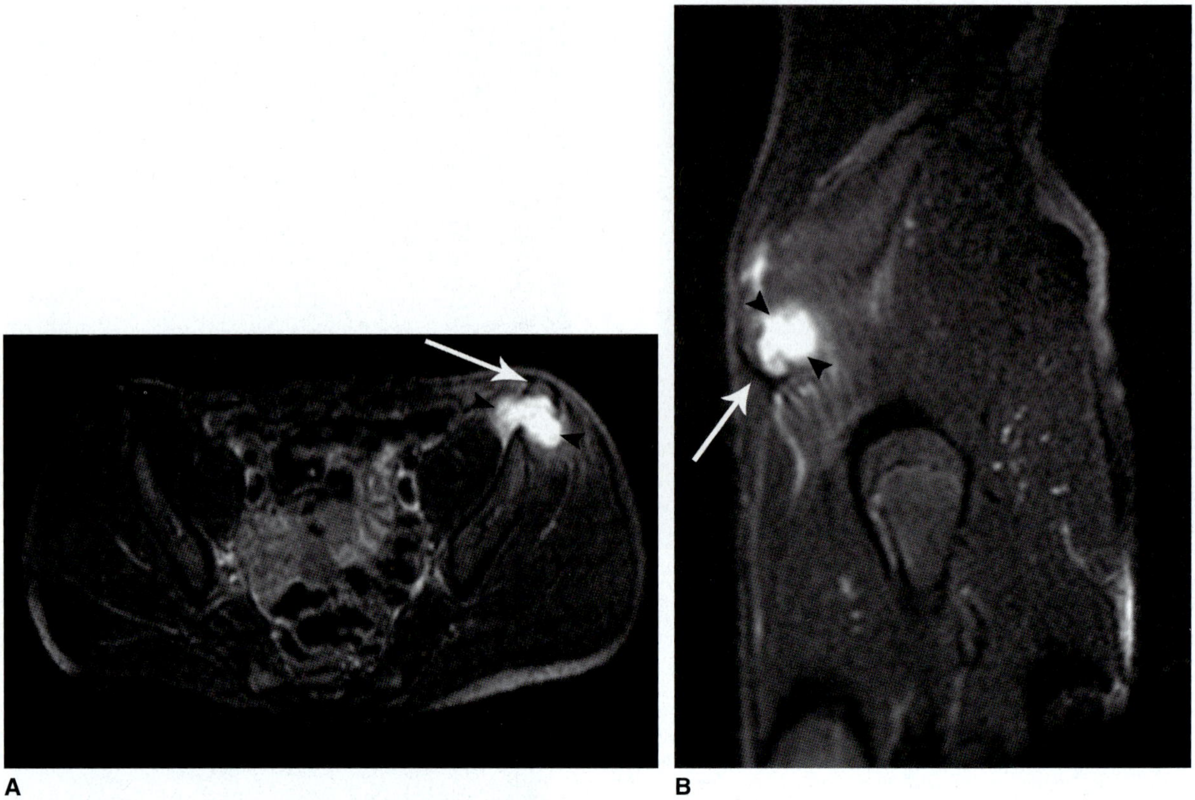

Figure 3.12. Anterior superior iliac spine avulsion. Axial (**A**) and sagittal (**B**) T2-weighted fat suppressed images of the pelvis in this skeletally mature recreational runner demonstrate a cortical avulsion at the left anterior superior iliac spine (*white arrow*) with an intervening hematoma (*black arrowheads*).

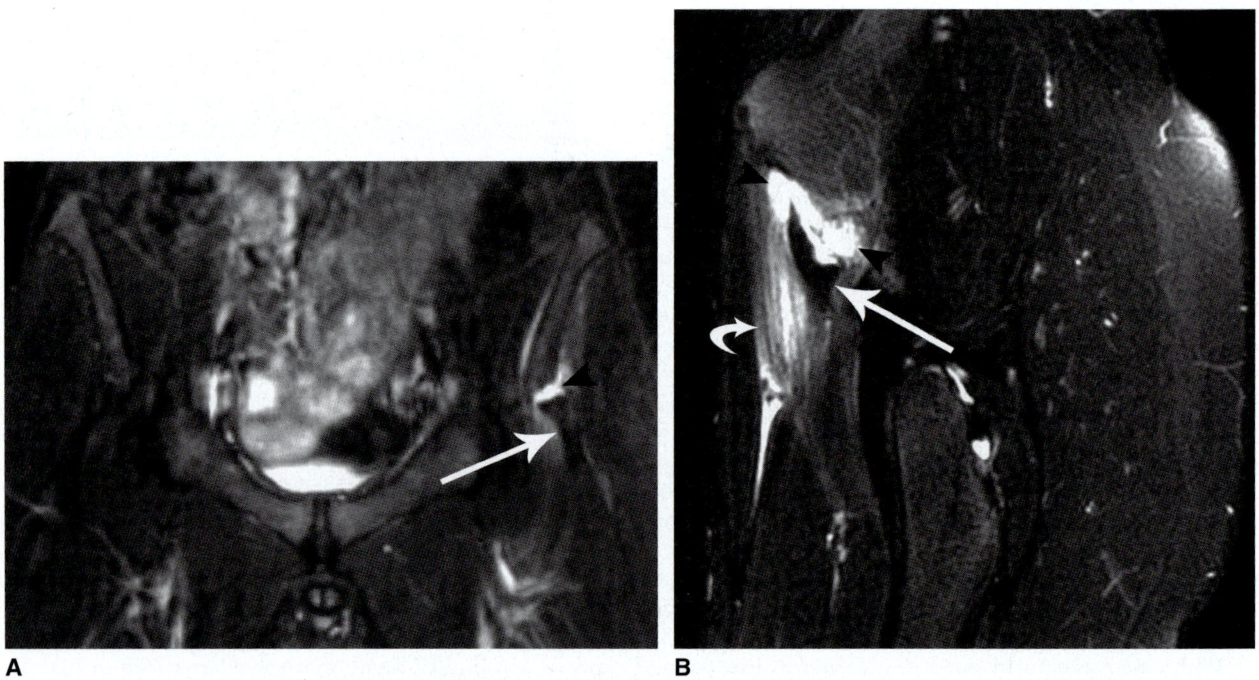

Figure 3.13. Anterior inferior iliac spine avulsion. Axial (**A**) and sagittal (**B**) T2-weighted images of the pelvis in a skeletally mature soccer player demonstrate cortical avulsion at the left anterior inferior iliac spine (*white arrow*) with an intervening hematoma (*black arrowheads*). The sagittal image (**B**) also demonstrates intramuscular edema within the left rectus femoris muscle (*curved arrow*).

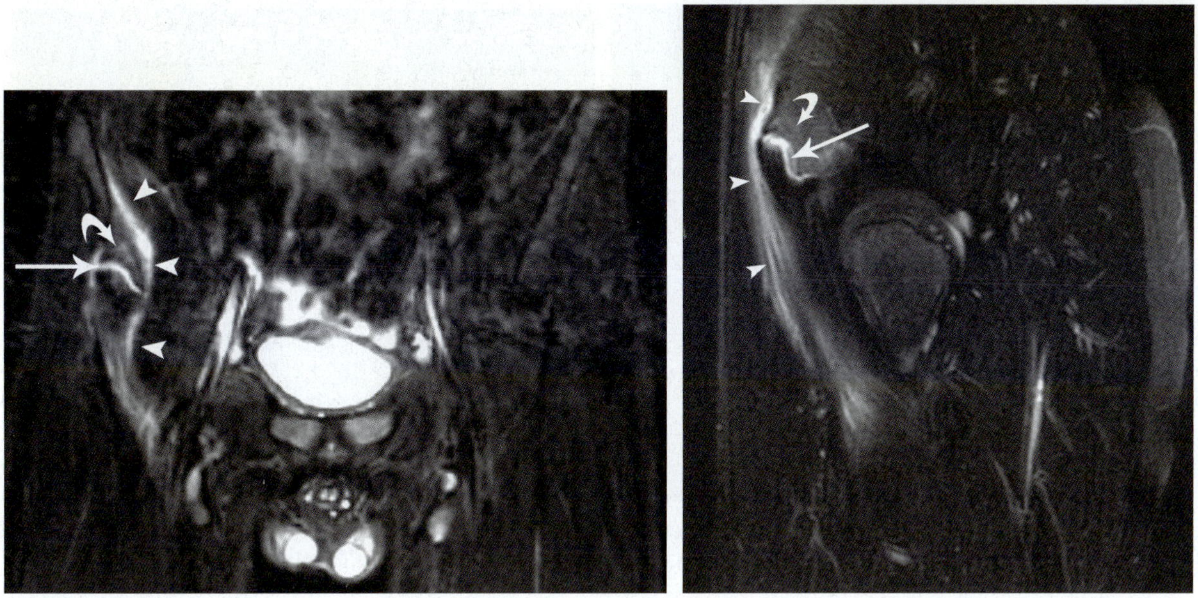

A B

Figure 3.14. Anterior inferior iliac spine apophysitis. Coronal STIR (**A**) and sagittal T2-weighted fat suppressed (**B**) images of the pelvis demonstrate edema within the physis of the right anterior inferior iliac spine (*straight arrow*) with associated subenthesial bone marrow edema (*curved arrow*) in a skeletally immature collegiate football kicker. Perimuscular and intramuscular edema are also noted along the adjacent right iliacus muscle (*arrowheads*).

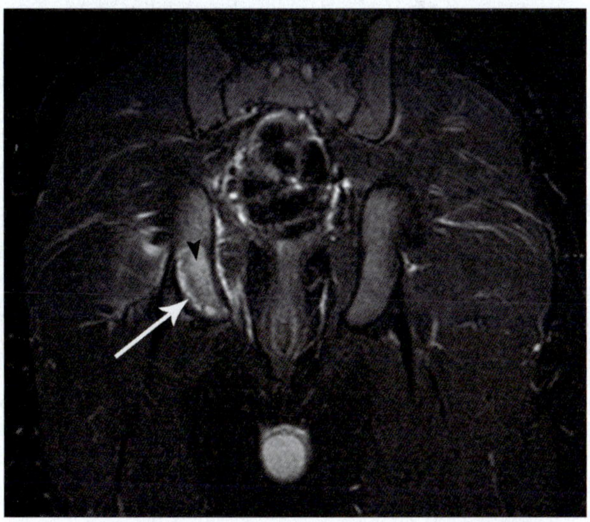

Figure 3.15. Ischial apophysitis. Coronal STIR image of the pelvis in a 15-year-old soccer player with loss of foot speed shows focal bone marrow edema within the right ischial physis (*arrow*) with subenthesial bone marrow edema (*arrowhead*).

does not currently exist. While MRI is certainly the standard for imaging apophyseal overuse injuries, an unexpected diagnosis can be made using radiographs or CT based upon ossification center asymmetry. And, while not generally the modality of choice, scintigraphic bone scans should offer excellent sensitivity for these injuries even if lacking the specificity of MRI.

ATHLETIC PUBALGIA SYNDROME

A number of the injuries already discussed might present clinically as athletic pubalgia. But several reproducible patterns of musculoskeletal injury about the pubic symphysis on MRI have been reported as highly associated with clinical athletic pubalgia or the diagnosis of "sports hernia."[7–12] If the goal is to find the lesion causing athletic pubalgia, then MRI is the imaging examination of choice and a noncontrast study utilizing a dedicated pubalgia protocol as discussed above is strongly encouraged. After image acquisition, review should follow a dogmatic algorithm with emphasis on grouping injuries into syndromes based upon MRI findings but directed toward appropriate treatment plans.[13–17] In this sense, review of athletic pubalgia MRI examinations is very similar to review of a study dedicated to the knee or the shoulder. First, the pubic symphysis articulation should be interrogated for osseous edema including its location in the bone and any asymmetry, as well as any degenerative arthopathic changes such as eburnation (subchondral sclerosis), subchondral cysts, and osseous erosion. Frequently, these osseous findings will lead to identification of the salient soft tissue lesions. At this point, any MRI secondary cleft should be noted, as its situs will serve as a strong indicator of the side of pain (Figs. 3.16 and 3.17).[18] Next, the imager should examine the morphology and signal of the caudal rectus abdominis attachments on the superior pubic rami. Then, adductor tendon origins should be reviewed, followed by a careful examination of inguinal canal anatomy with an emphasis on symmetry. Finally, care must be taken to assess more remote structures on the larger field of view sequences that might be a source of referred pain, including the sacroiliac joints, the hips, pelvic apophyses, and the visceral pelvis. Using this algorithm, the

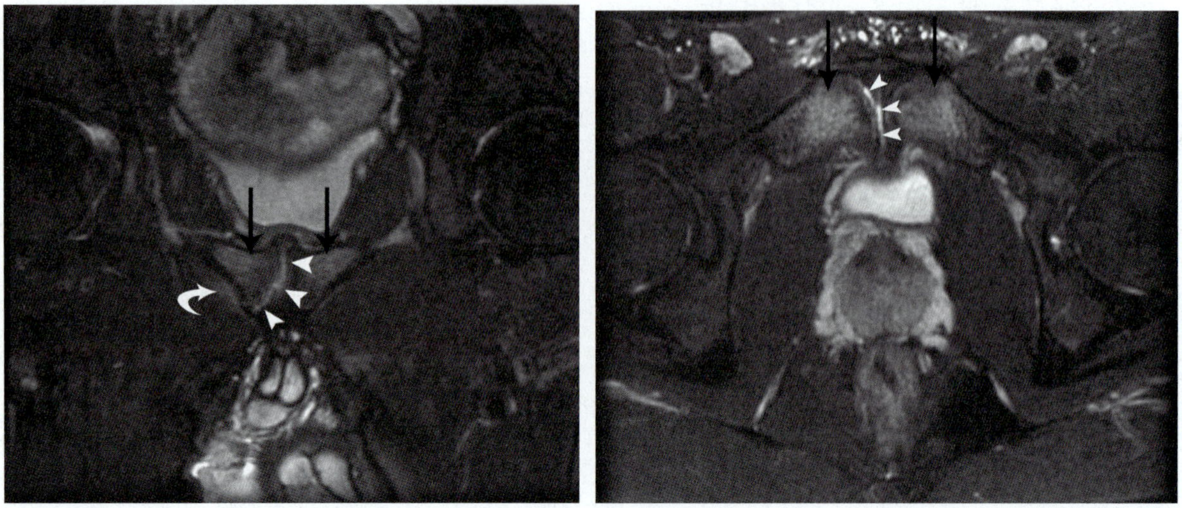

Figure 3.16. Unilateral secondary cleft sign. Coronal (**A**) and axial (**B**) T2-weighted fat suppressed images of the pelvis in a hockey player with unilateral groin pain demonstrate fluid intense signal (*arrowheads*) extending from the pubic symphysis along the anterior/inferior margin of the medial pubic body at the attachment of the rectus abdominis/adductor aponeurosis. Also present are osteitis pubis (*black arrows*) and a strain of the right obturator externus (*curved arrow*).

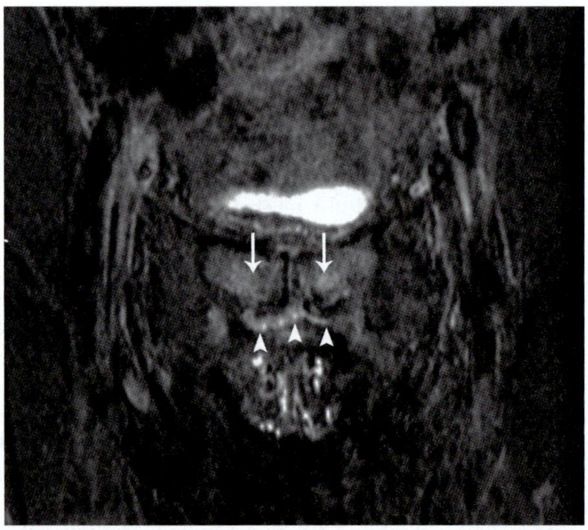

Figure 3.17. Bilateral secondary cleft sign. Coronal STIR image of the pelvis in a female professional distance runner demonstrates fluid intense signal (*arrowheads*) extending from the pubic symphysis along the anterior/inferior margin of the both pubic bodies at the attachment of the rectus abdominis/adductor aponeurosis. Also present is bilateral osteitis pubis (*arrows*).

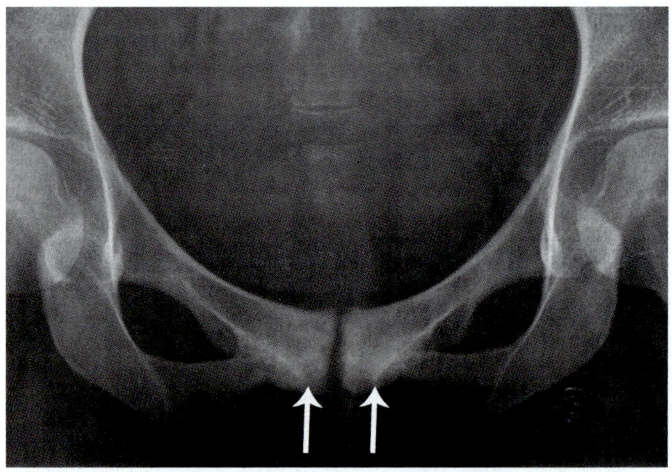

Figure 3.18. Radiographic appearance of osteitis pubis. Frontal image of the pelvis demonstrates sclerosis within the bilateral pubic bodies with subarticular irregularity about the pubic symphysis (*arrows*).

majority of patients with true athletic pubalgia will have one of the following MRI injury patterns:

Osteitis pubis: At MRI, osteitis pubis manifests as bone marrow edema resembling osteoarthritis of any other joint. Marrow edema is present on both sides of the symphysis in a subchondral location (Figs. 3.18 and 3.19), distinct from isolated subcortical marrow edema related to tendinous avulsive stress and to linear foci of marrow edema in fractures. While bone marrow edema must be present bilaterally on osteitis pubis, it is frequently asymmetric, with more extensive or intense edema on the side of dominant pain. Other findings seen with osteitis pubis in some cases include geode formation, eburbation, and resorption of subchondral bone (Fig. 3.20).[19–22] All of these suggest an element of chronicity and are likely to be bilateral. While isolated osteitis pubis at MRI has been reported, in the great majority of cases, a regional soft tissue lesion is identifiable, suggesting that osteitis pubis may be a secondary event analogous to osteoarthritis of the glenohumeral joint related to a long-standing labral tear and instability.[23,24]

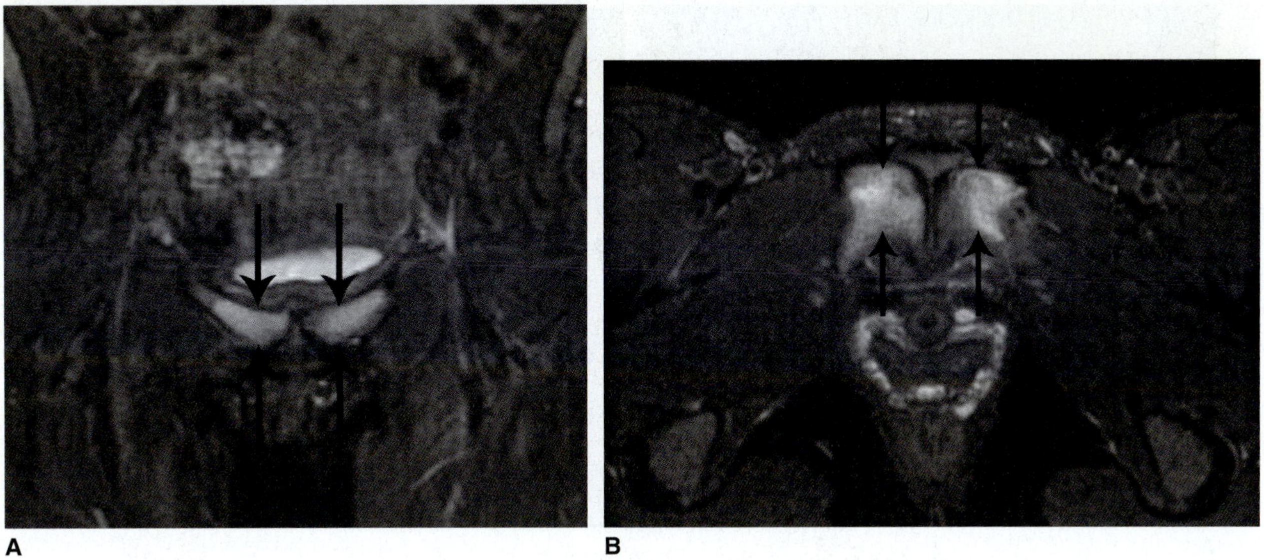

Figure 3.19. MRI appearance of acute osteitis pubis. Coronal (**A**) and axial (**B**) T2-weighted fat suppressed images dedicated to the pubic symphysis in a professional female sprinter demonstrate extensive marrow edema spanning the entire AP distance of both pubic bodies (*between arrows*).

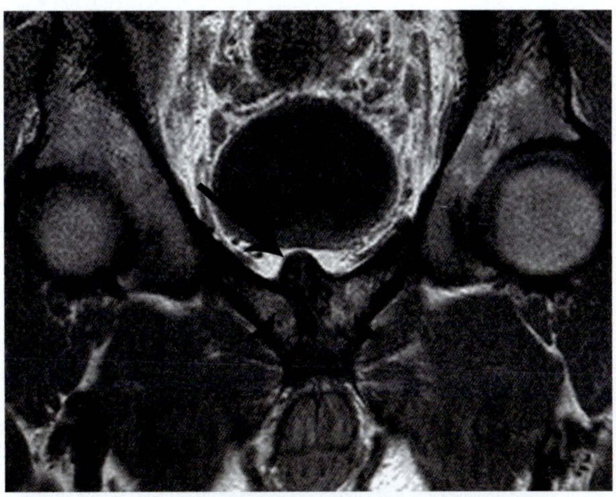

Figure 3.20. MRI appearance of chronic osteitis pubis. Coronal T1-weighted image of the pubic symphysis in a 23-year old male basketball player shows extensive subchondral sclerosis (eburnation), osteophytosis, and articular surface irregularity with mild marrow edema (*arrowheads*) within the pubic bodies.

Rectus abdominis strain: The caudal rectus abdominis muscle and tendon should be evaluated for abnormal T2 hyperintense signal, an indicator of acute injury, or either hypertrophic or atrophic morphology, suggesting a more chronic lesion. Thankfully, the contralateral rectus abdominis will be in view for direct comparison on all coronal and axial sections (Fig. 3.21). Specific attention must be directed to the elongated tenoperiosteal attachment of the caudal rectus abdominis tendon on the anteroinferior aspect of the superior pubic ramus, as a disruption here is frequently a pain stimulator and may also lead to instability at the pubic symphysis and secondary osteitis pubis. Distally, the lateral edge of the most caudal rectus abdominis helps to reinforce the posteromedial aspect of the superficial inguinal canal, so any deficiency here should be noted and reported. Frequently, distal rectus abdominis lesions confluently extend either into the ipsilateral adductor longus tendon origin or the contralateral rectus abdominis pubic attachment. Variations in injury include detachment without tear, myotendinous strain, and frank tear.[25]

Adductor tendon syndromes: Some lesions are isolated to the thigh adductor compartment, involving one or more tendons or muscles. Proximal adductor tendinopathies are analogous to these seen in the distal supraspinatus or Achilles at MRI, with tendon enlargement and abnormal signal as typical observations. More acute adductor injuries visible at MRI include proximal myotendinous strains, osseous avulsions at the tendon origins, and even calcific tendinosis (Fig. 3.22). All of these exhibit MRI findings similar to tendinous injuries elsewhere in the body. Numerous adductor variants have been described in the surgical literature and most can be seen at MRI.[26,27] One with a distinct pattern is "baseball pitcher–hockey goalie syndrome," often manifesting on MRI as isolated proximal adductor myotendinous edema and thickening or redundancy of the muscle sheath or epimysium at the same level (Fig. 3.23).[28–30] Occasionally, an adductor tendon is frankly torn and retracted near its origin without avulsing subjacent bone (Fig. 3.24). This lesion is highly associated with ipsilateral rectus abdominis injury. Less common thigh adductor syndromes visible at MRI include myotendinous hematomas and primary soft tissue neoplasms.

Rectus abdominis/adductor aponeurosis injury: As the most caudal rectus abdominis fibers blend with the adductor longus

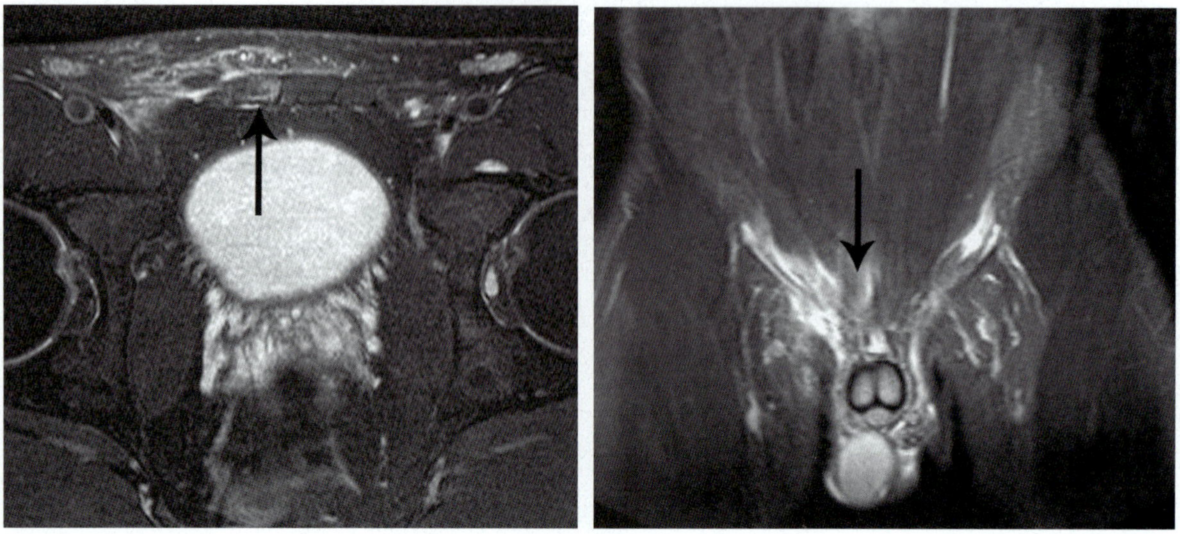

A B

Figure 3.21. Rectus abdominis strain. Axial T2-weighted fat suppressed (**A**) and coronal STIR (**B**) images of the pelvis in a major league baseball catcher demonstrate extensive intramuscular edema in the caudal right rectus abdominis to its attachment on the superior pubic ramus.

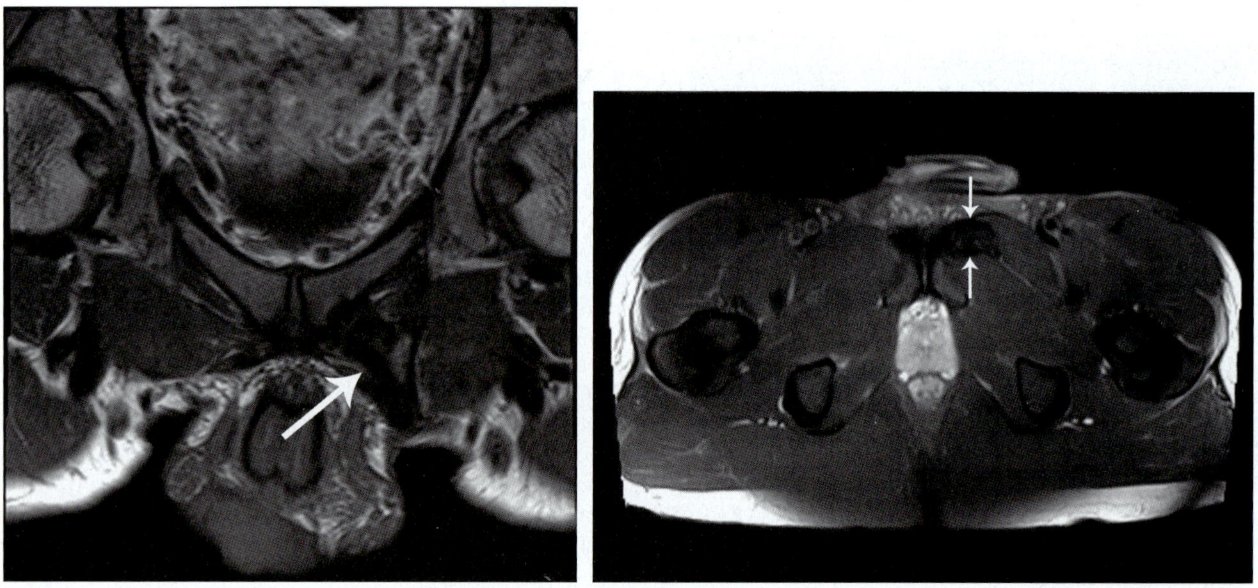

A B

Figure 3.22. Adductor calcific tendinopathy. Coronal (**A**) and axial (**B**) T1-weighted images of the pelvis in a recreational kickboxer demonstrate right adductor tendon enlargement with a heterogeneous intratendinous low signal consistent with calcium hydroxyapetite deposition (calcific tendinosis).

origin as well as the anterior and arcuate ligaments of the pubic symphysis, the symphyseal capsule and the pubic rami periosteum, injury often spans several of these structures. When describing these injuries at MRI review, it is impractical and seems shortsighted to simply log the injured structures as individual lesions. In an effort to provide a better image of the actual injury, some lesions are named more for their MRI appearance than for presentation or surgical findings. When a region of the distal rectus abdominis is detached from the pubic ramus confluently with partial or complete avulsion of the adductor longus origin, it can be described as an ipsilateral rectus abdominis/adductor detachment.[1] A frank tear involving both these

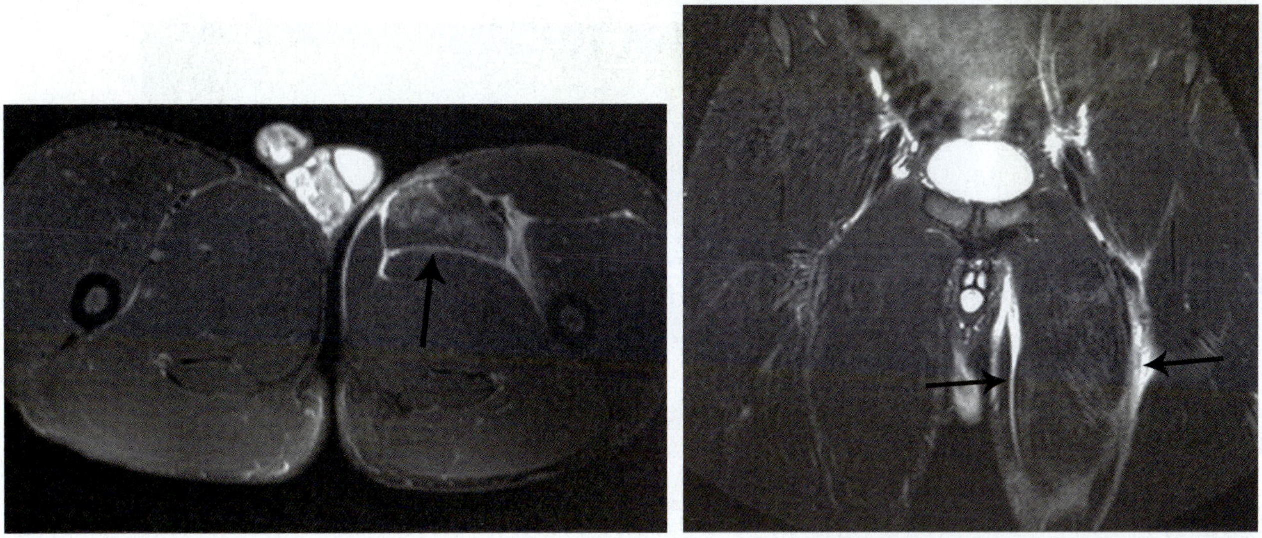

A B

Figure 3.23. Baseball pitcher–hockey goalie syndrome. Axial T2-weighted (**A**) and coronal STIR (**B**) images show edema and subtle bulging of the adductor longus due to herniation through a myofascial defect in a professional football tight end with a previous pelvic floor repair for a rectus abdominis tear.

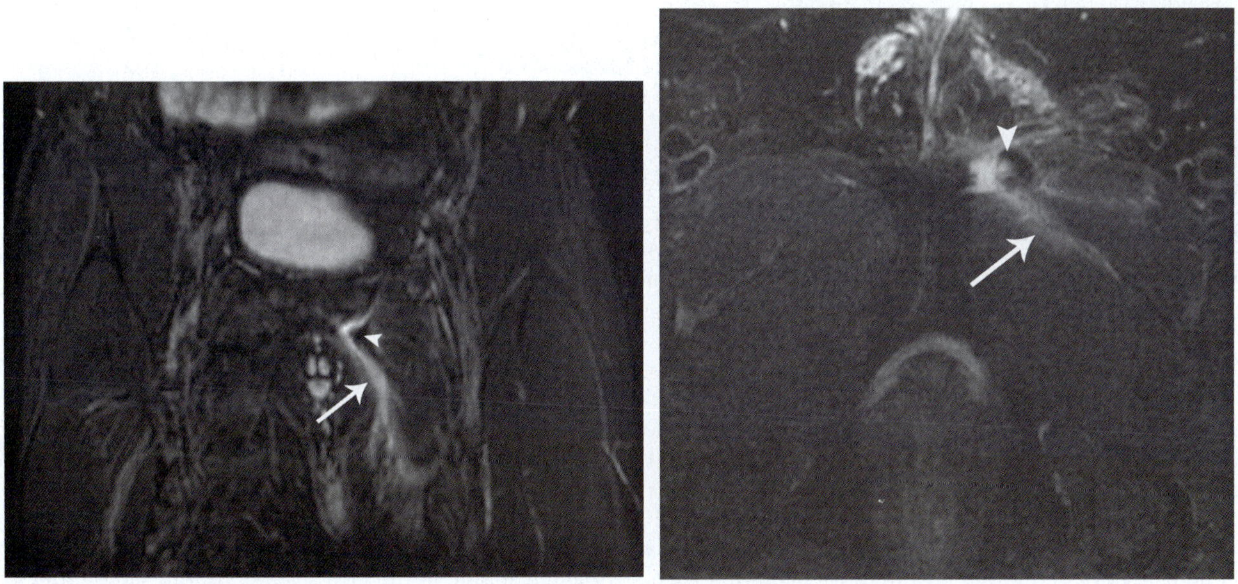

A B

Figure 3.24. Adductor tendon avulsion. Coronal STIR (**A**) and axial T2-weighted fat suppressed (**B**) images of the pelvis in a major league baseball pitcher show an osseous avulsion (*arrowhead*) of the adductor longus tendon from its origin at the left lateral pubic body with a more distal adductor muscle strain (*arrow*).

structures can be described in a similar fashion (Fig. 3.25). In fact, this pattern of rectus abdominis/adductor aponeurosis injury is likely to be the most frequent finding on pelvic MRI in the setting of athletic pubalgia. Further, this unilateral and confluent lesion involving the caudal rectus abdominis attachment and adductor tendon group origins at MRI is most likely to reflect the clinical diagnosis of a "sports hernia" or "sportsmans hernia."

Rectus abdominis/adductor aponeurotic plate disruption: In another common injury pattern in the setting of an athlete with groin pain, the caudal rectus abdominis detachment from its pubic attachment spans midline to involve both left and right, resembling a plate like delamination.[31] This pattern clearly reflects a bilateral lesion and can be called a rectus abdominis/ adductor aponeurotic plate disruption (Fig. 3.26). With these patterns, the presence and morphology of an MRI secondary

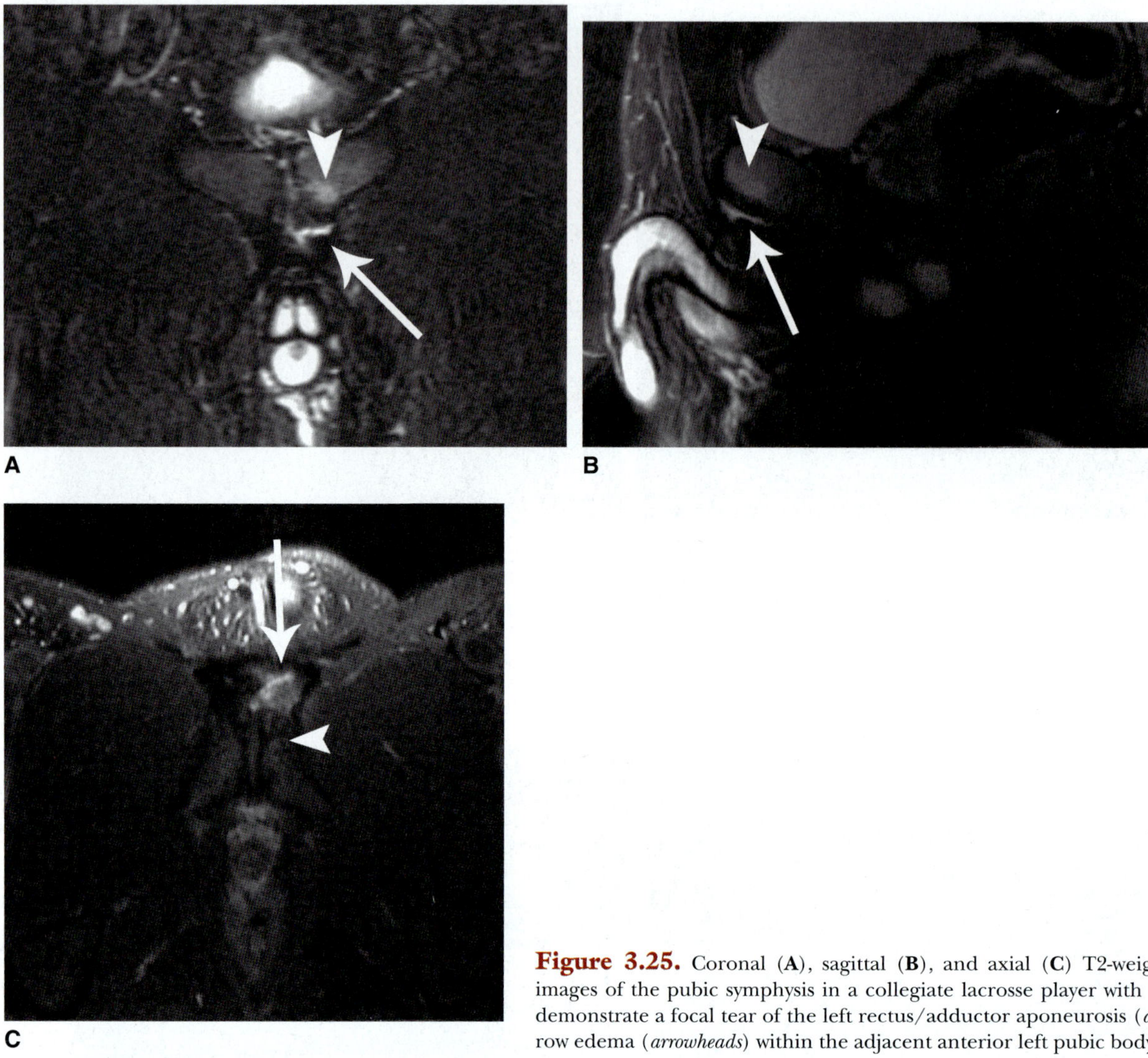

Figure 3.25. Coronal (**A**), sagittal (**B**), and axial (**C**) T2-weighted fat suppressed images of the pubic symphysis in a collegiate lacrosse player with left-sided groin pain demonstrate a focal tear of the left rectus/adductor aponeurosis (*arrow*) with mild marrow edema (*arrowheads*) within the adjacent anterior left pubic body.

cleft can be very helpful. A unilateral secondary cleft generally indicates an ipsilateral rectus abdominis/adductor detachment or tear, and a confluent, bilateral secondary cleft indicates a rectus abdominis/adductor aponeurotic plate disruption.[18,24,32] Osteitis pubis is commonly associated with each of these lesions and should be reported. Another MRI finding encountered frequently in the setting of a rectus abdominis/adductor aponeurosis lesion is atrophy of the rectus abdominis muscle, tendon, or both (Fig. 3.27). It is unclear whether this pattern of myotendinous atrophy reflects a chronic tendinous lesion at the pubic symphysis, a previous rectus abdominis muscle strain, or perhaps a post-traumatic denervation injury. But, at least in two of the series recording MRI findings in athletes with groin pain, the situs of rectus abdominis muscle atrophy tended to match that of ipsilateral groin pain.[7,33]

INGUINAL HERNIAS

Imaging inguinal and lower abdominal hernias with MRI as well as understanding the modalities limitations when it comes to hernias is quite simple. The inguinal canals will generally be presented in long axis on coronal oblique acquisitions prescribed from the arcuate line of the pelvis. The canals should be symmetric and no portion of the canal should contain enteric visceral structures. Further, there should be no focal, masslike fat, fluid, or fibrosis (Fig. 3.28). If an inguinal hernia is self-reducing, it is almost certain to reduce with the patient supine in the MRI scanner. In this setting, the dynamic nature of ultrasound with provocative maneuvers renders it the imaging modality of choice. But any sustained abdominal wall or inguinal hernia should be accurately identified by either CT or MRI, as fat is almost invariably involved and is readily visible with both modalities. Some innovative dynamic MRI techniques have been described utilizing ultrafast acquisitions during valsalva and with relaxation sequentially, but ultrasound is a less expensive and more practical modality. It should be acknowledged that several series have clearly concluded that true hernias are rare in the setting of clinical athletic pubalgia where MRI remains the preferred modality.[34–36]

CONFOUNDING PATHOLOGIES

A myriad of visceral, gastrointestinal, and gynecological diseases can manifest as musculoskeletal type pelvic, hip, and

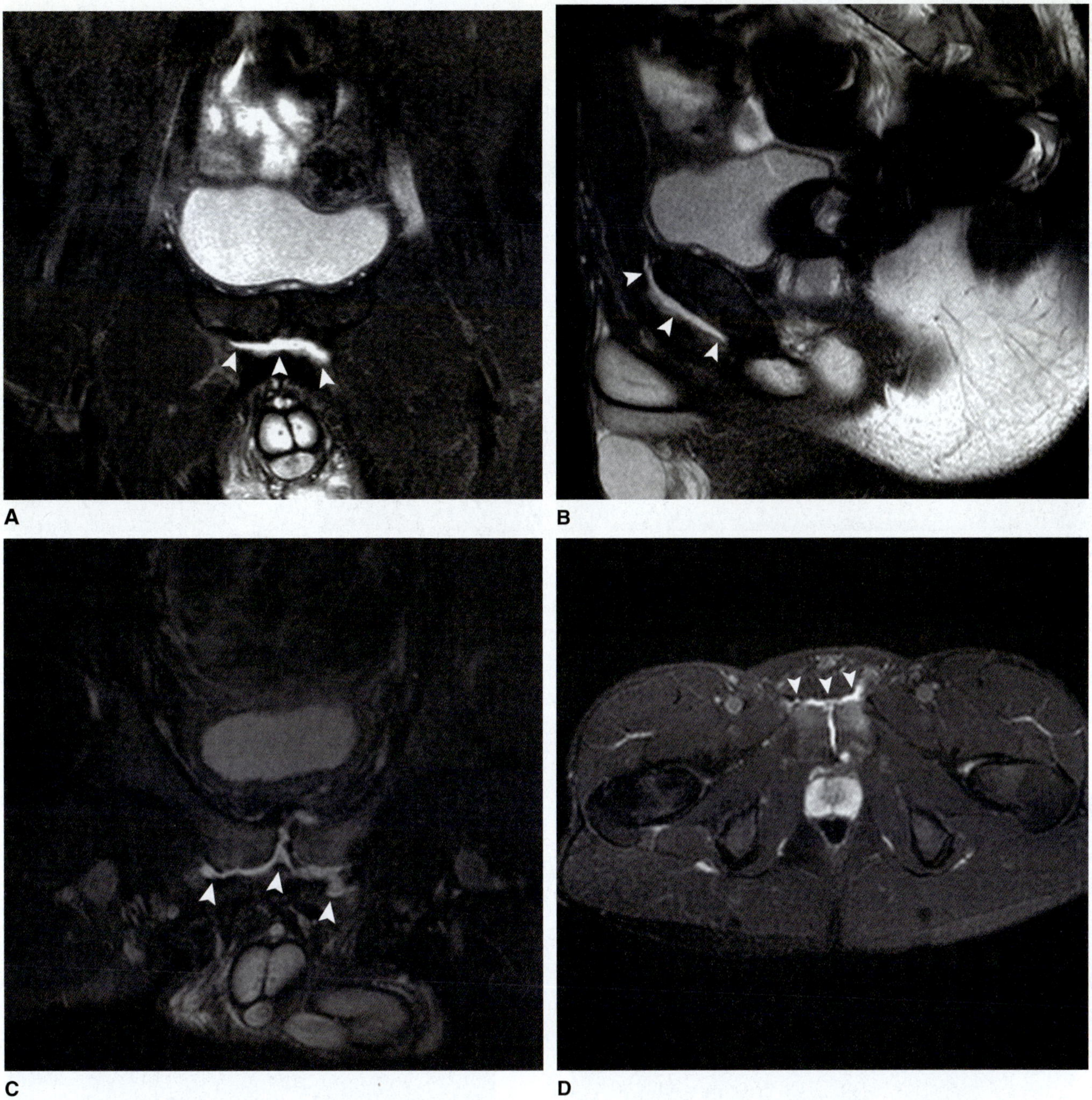

Figure 3.26. Rectus abdominis/adductor aponeurotic plate disruption. Coronal (**A**) and sagittal (**B**) T2-weighted fat suppressed images of the pelvis in a collegiate football player with groin pain upon activity resumption after 3 months of rest and coronal (**C**) and axial (**D**) T2-weighted fat suppressed images of the pelvis in an NFL punter with chronic groin pain both demonstrate detachment of the midline, left, and right aspects of the rectus abdominis/adductor aponeurosis (*arrowheads*) from its pubic attachment. This pattern often resembles a plate of soft tissue attachments lifting off the osseous structures at the anteroinferior pubic symphysis and has been termed a rectus abdominis/adductor aponeurotic plate disruption.

groin pain. This issue underlies the importance of prescribing and imaging technique with views dedicated to the structure most likely to be injured, as well as views covering other regional pelvic structures that may be a source of referred pain. Each imaging examination of the pelvis should provide at least a limited assessment of the sacroiliac joints, as arthropathies here may present with various patterns of referred pain. A unilateral sacroiliitis in a young patient is always concerning for a septic joint, as it is a favorite location for hematogenous spread of bacteremia. A bilateral sacroiliac process should raise

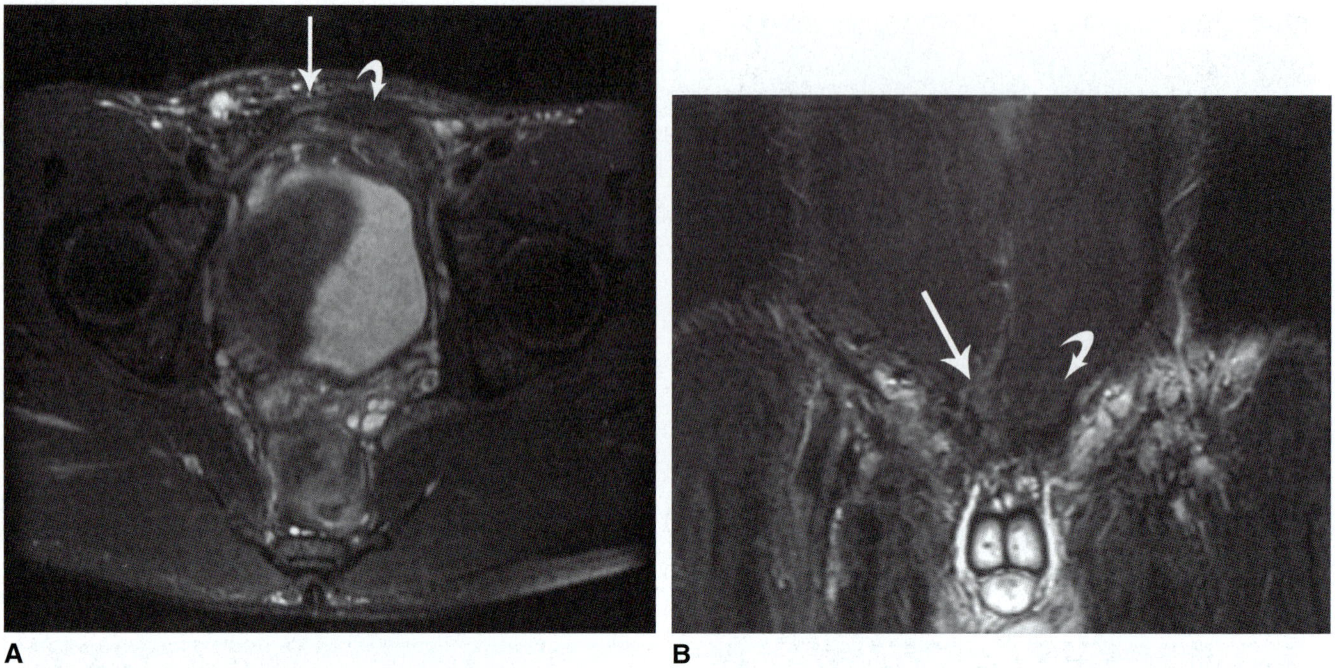

Figure 3.27. Right rectus abdominis muscle atrophy. Axial (**A**) and coronal (**B**) T2-weighted fat suppressed images of the pelvis demonstrate high signal and with decreased bulk of the caudal right rectus abdominis muscle and tendon (*straight arrow*) relative to a normal appearing left rectus abdominis (*curved arrow*).

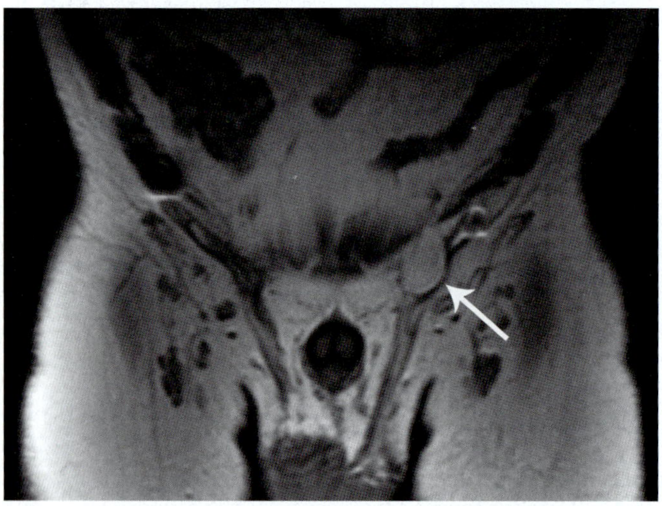

Figure 3.28. Inguinal hernia in a patient with left-sided groin pain. Coronal T1-weighted nonfat suppressed image of the pelvis demonstrates a fat-containing left inguinal hernia. Dedicated images of the pubic symphysis showed no tendinous or osseous injury.

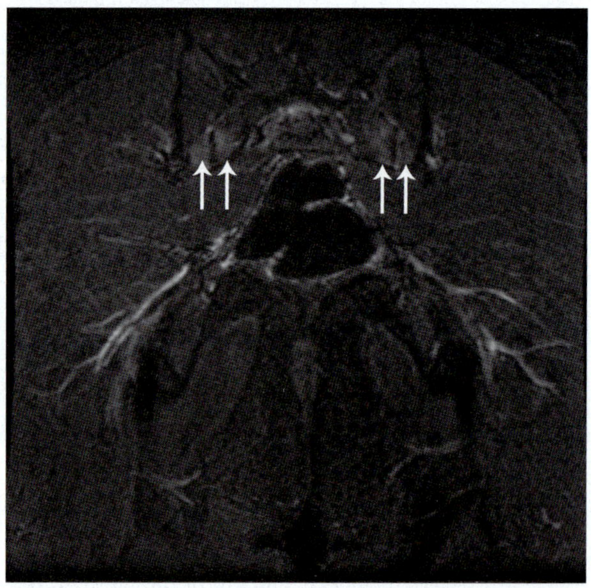

Figure 3.29. Bilateral sacroiliitis. Coronal STIR image of the sacrum in a 14-year-old male pentathlete demonstrates subchondral marrow edema (*arrows*) in a symmetric distribution along the caudal aspect of both sacroiliac joints. This patient was ultimately diagnosed with ankylosing spondylitis.

concern for early spondyloarthropathies including ankylosing spondylitis and juvenile rheumatoid arthritis, as well as systemic processes including inflammatory bowel disease (Fig. 3.29). The distal iliopsoas tendons should be followed carefully as asymmetric edema along the undersurface of the tendons may indicate iliopsoas bursitis, a common cause of groin/hip pain, especially with active flexion (Fig. 3.30). At the same time, the lower lumbar disc levels should at least be acknowledged on X-ray, CT, and MRI examinations for pelvic pain, and femoral-acetabular alignment should be checked for symmetry and any

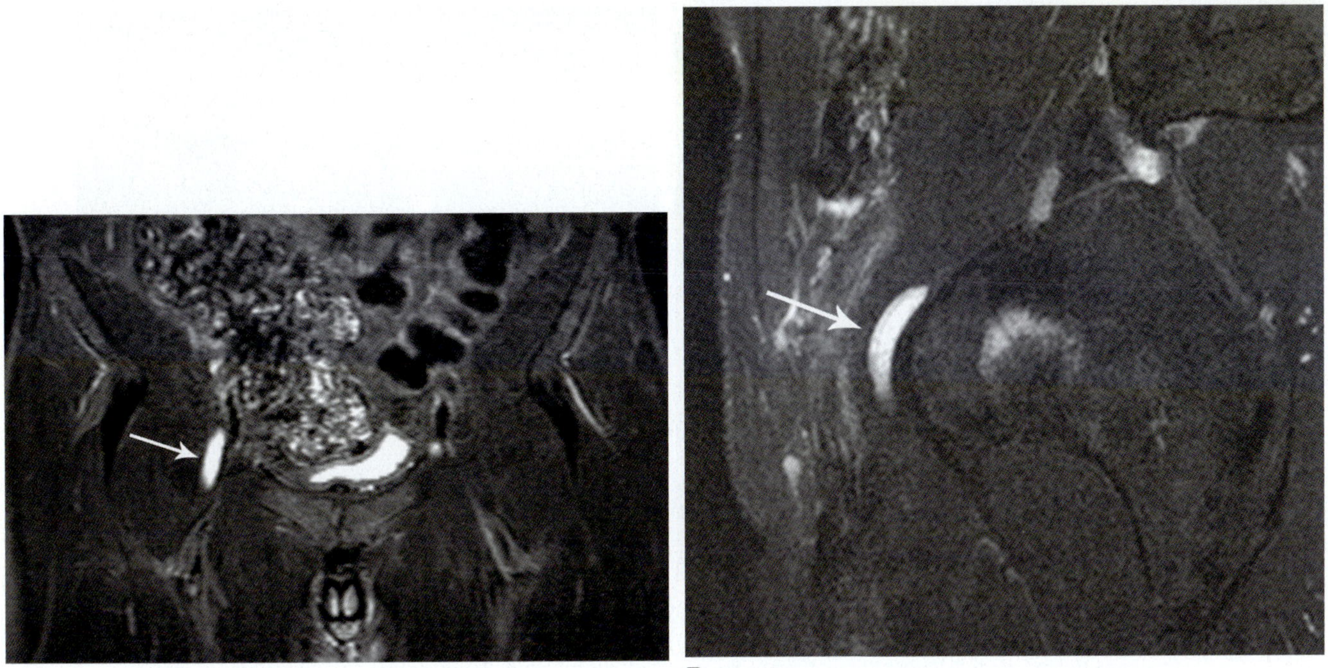

A B

Figure 3.30. Right iliopsoas bursitis. Coronal STIR (**A**) and sagittal T2-weighted fat suppressed (**B**) images of the pelvis in a national hockey league (NHL) goalie with pain upon hip flexion demonstrate linear fluid signal (*arrow*) along the undersurface of the right iliopsoas tendon, typical for iliopsoas bursitis.

of the patterns of impingement or dysplasia reviewed in the hip imaging chapter.

In young females, potential gynecologic sources of pain should be considered, even when musculoskeletal injury is suspected. Ovarian follicles tend to wax and wane in both size and symptomatology, so follow-up imaging at a different point in the menstrual cycle (6 weeks) is often a reasonable option when a symptomatic cyst is suspected. But other visceral sources of pain in females including adenomyosis, endometriosis, and uterine fibroids may be more occult to diagnosis and should always be remembered when reviewing imaging studies (Fig. 3.31). The syndrome of chronic groin or lower abdominal pain and suspected athletic pubalgia in a young nonathlete is always a worrisome scenario. In this setting, the imager should always remember to consider less common pathologies including nerve entrapment and soft tissue masses (Figs. 3.32 and 3.33).

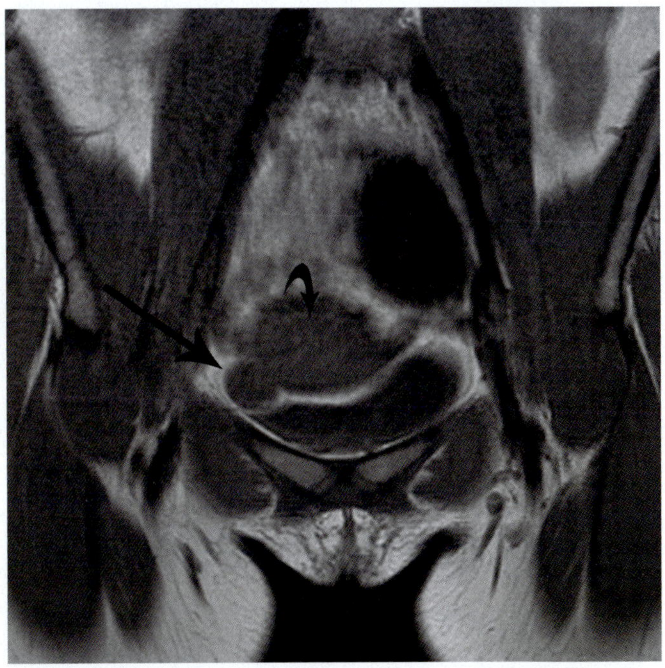

Figure 3.31. Uterine pathology. Coronal T1-weighted image of the pelvis in a 30-year-old recreational athlete with right-sided lower abdominal pain shows a rounded exophytic mass (*straight arrow*) extending from the right anterior aspect of the uterine fundus, typical for a subserosal fibroid (*curved arrow*). Her pubic symphysis structures were normal at MRI.

CONCLUSION

Imaging studies, and in particular MRI, clearly play an integral role in the assessment and treatment of pelvic and groin pain in a young patient and an athlete. While imaging interpretation is important, choosing the best imaging examination and imaging protocol may be even more important in this patient population. Noncontrast MRI examinations are generally the most useful modality in the setting of

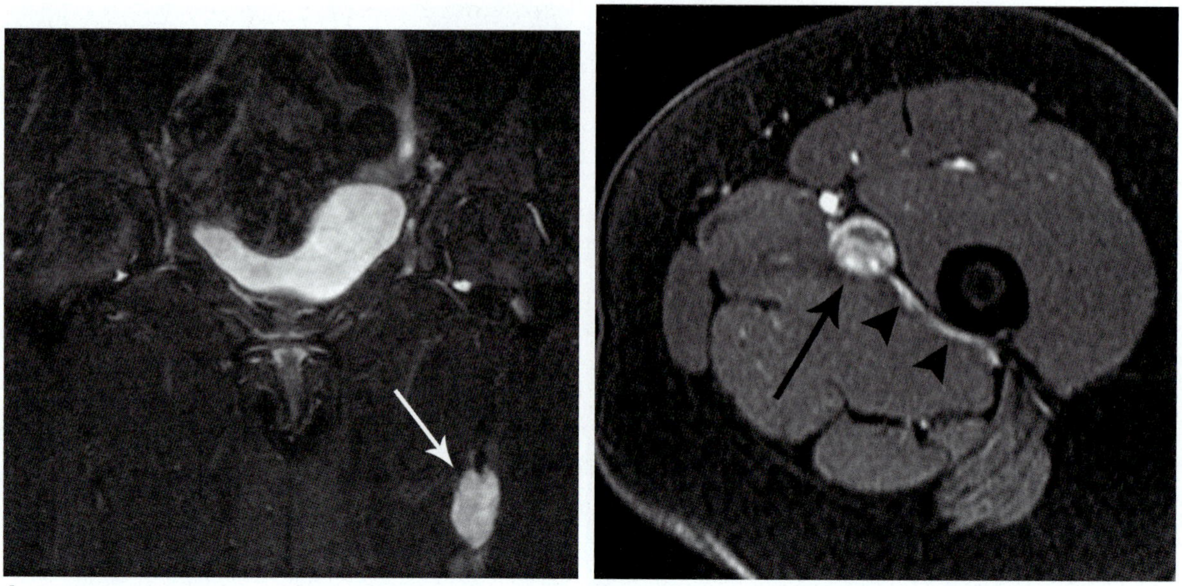

A B

Figure 3.32. Soft tissue masses. Coronal STIR (**A**) and axial postcontrast T1-weighted fat suppressed (**B**) images of the left thigh in a nonathletic 15-year-old female with groin pain demonstrate a circumscribed enhancing mass (*arrows*) within the left adductor compartment. Postcontrast axial image also demonstrates a prominent feeding artery (*arrowheads*). This mass had a histologic diagnosis of a synovial cell sarcoma in the thigh adductor compartment. While the initial study was performed using an athletic pubalgia protocol, the patient was called back to the imaging center for postcontrast sequences when the unexpected lesion was identified.

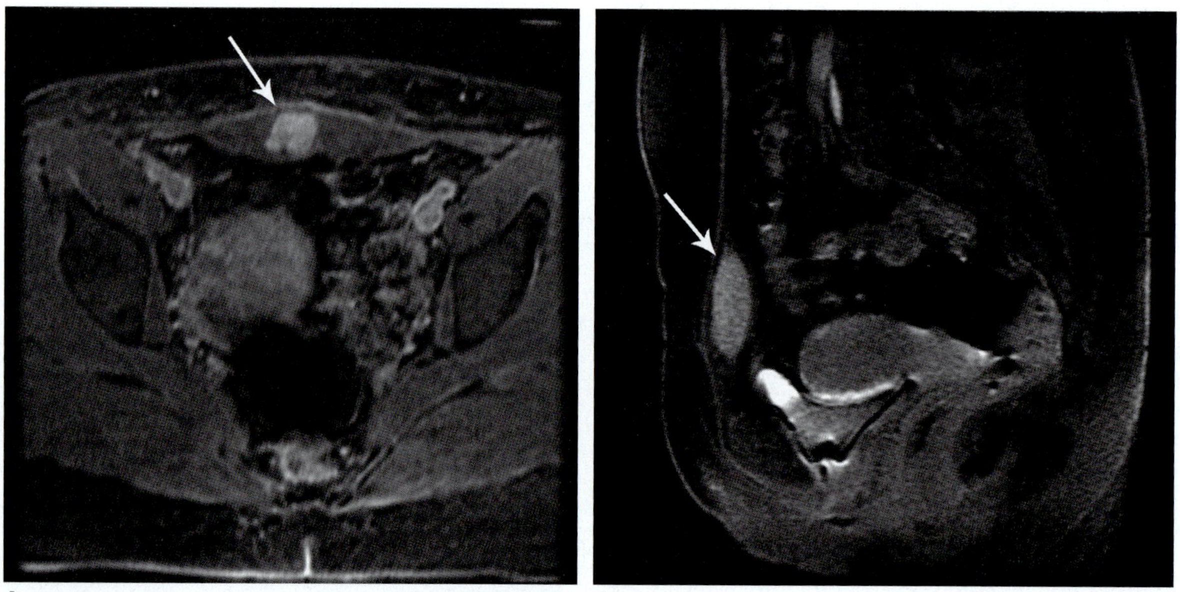

A B

Figure 3.33. Soft tissue masses. Axial (**A**) and sagittal (**B**) postcontrast T1-weighted images of the pelvis demonstrate a circumscribed, enhancing mass (*arrows*) within the right rectus abdominis muscle. This mass had a histologic diagnosis of a synovial cell sarcoma within the rectus abdominis at a site of previous caesarian section scar.

musculoskeletal injury, but CT and contrast-enhanced MRI are indicated for specific visceral indications and in the setting of infection and neoplasm. Reproducible patterns of MRI findings have been well described in the imaging and surgical literature and should be recognized. In a subset of patients, focused ultrasound examinations or CT may serve as appropriate first-line imaging tests. Communication between clinicians performing physical examination and clinicians performing imaging is vital in ultimately creating an effective treatment plan.

REFERENCES

1. Omar IM, Zoga AC, Kavanagh EC, et al. Athletic pubalgia and "sports hernia": Optimal MR imaging technique and findings. *Radiographics.* 2008;28(5):1415–1438.
2. Orchard JW, Read JW, Neophyton J, et al. Groin pain associated with ultrasound finding of inguinal canal posterior wall deficiency in Australian Rules footballers. *Br J Sports Med.* 1998;32:134–139.
3. Robinson P, Barron DA, Parsons W, et al. Adductor-related groin pain in athletes: Correlation of MR imaging with clinical findings. *Skeletal Radiol.* 2004;33:451–457.
4. LeBlanc KE, LeBlanc KA. Groin pain in athletes. *Hernia.* 2003;7:68–71.
5. Garrett WE Jr. Muscle strain injuries. *Am J Sports Med.* 1996;24(6 Suppl):S2–S8.
6. Peck DM. Apophyseal injuries in the young athlete. *Am Fam Physician.* 1995;51: 1891–1895,1897–1898.
7. Albers SL, Spritzer CE, Garrett WE Jr, et al. MR findings in athletes with pubalgia. *Skeletal Radiol.* 2001;30:270–277.
8. Caudill P, Nyland J, Smith C, et al. Sports hernias: A systematic literature review. *Br J Sports Med.* 2008;42:(12):954–964.
9. Taylor DC, Meyers WC, Moylan JA, et al Abdominal musculature abnormalities as a cause of groin pain in athletes: Inguinal hernias and pubalgia. *Am J Sports Med.* 1991;19:239–242.
10. Smodlaka VN. Groin pain in soccer players. *Physician Sportsmed.* 1980;8:57–61.
11. Hackney RG. The sports hernia: A cause of chronic groin pain. *Br J Sports Med.* 1993;27:58–62.
12. Kavanagh EC, Koulouris G, Ford S, et al. MR imaging of groin pain in the athlete. *Semin Musculoskelet Radiol.* 2006;10:197–207.
13. Meyers WC, McKechnie A, Philippon MJ, et al. Experience with "sports hernia" spanning two decades. *Ann Surg.* 2008;248(4):656–665.
14. Ziprin P, Prabhudesai SG, Abrahams S, et al. Transabdominal preperitoneal laparoscopic approach for the treatment of sportsman's hernia. *J Laparoendosc Adv Surg Tech A.* 2008;18(5):669–672.
15. Meyers WC, Foley DP, Garrett WE, et al. Management of severe lower abdominal or inguinal pain in high-performance athletes. PAIN (Performing Athletes with Abdominal or Inguinal Neuromuscular Pain Study Group). *Am J Sports Med.* 2000;28:2–8.
16. Malycha P, Lovell G. Inguinal surgery in athletes with chronic groin pain: The "sportsman's" hernia. *Aust NZ J Surg.* 1992;62:123–125.
17. Joesting DR. Diagnosis and treatment of sportsman's hernia. *Curr Sports Med Rep.* 2002;1:121–124.
18. Cunningham PM, Brennan D, O'Connell M, et al. Patterns of bone and soft-tissue injury at the symphysis pubis in soccer players: Observations at MRI. *Am J Roentgenol.* 2007;188:W291–296.
19. Vix VA, Ryu CY. The adult symphysis pubis: Normal and abnormal. *Am J Roentgenol Radium Ther Nucl Med.* 1971;112:517–525.
20. Gibbon WW, Hession PR. Diseases of the pubis and pubic symphysis: MR imaging appearances. *Am J Roentgenol.* 1997;169:849–853.
21. Verrall GM, Slavotinek JP, Fon GT. Incidence of pubic bone marrow oedema in Australian rules football players: Relation to groin pain. *Br J Sports Med.* 2001;35:28.
22. Kunduracioglu B, Yilmaz C, Yorubulut M, et al. Magnetic resonance findings of osteitis pubis. *J Magn Reson Imaging.* 2007;25(3):535–539.
23. Rodriguez C, Miguel A, Lima H, et al. Osteitis pubis syndrome in the professional soccer athlete: A case report. *J Athl Train.* 2001;36:437–440.
24. O'Connell MJ, Powell T, McCaffrey NM, et al. Symphyseal cleft injection in the diagnosis and treatment of osteitis pubis in athletes. *Am J Roentgenol.* 2002;179:955–959.
25. Moore KL, Dalley AF, Agur AMR. *Moore's Clinically Oriented Anatomy.* 5th Ed. Philadelphia, PA: Lippincott Williams & Wilkins; 2005.
26. Robinson P, Barron DA, Parsons W, et al. Adductor-related groin pain in athletes: Correlation of MR imaging with clinical findings. *Skeletal Radiol.* 2004;33:451–457.
27. Nicholas SJ, Tyler TF. Adductor muscle strains in sport. *Sports Med.* 2002;32:339–344.
28. Meyers WC, Lanfranco A, Castellanos A. Surgical management of chronic lower abdominal and groin pain in high-performance athletes. *Curr Sports Med Rep.* 2002;1:301–305.
29. Gokhale S. Three-dimensional sonography of muscle hernias. *J Ultrasound Med.* 2007;26:239–242.
30. Mellado JM, Perez del Palomar L. Muscle hernias of the lower leg: MRI findings. *Skeletal Radiol.* 1999;28:465–469.
31. Walheim G, Olerud S, Ribbe T. Mobility of the pubic symphysis: Measurements by an electromechanical method. *Acta Orthop Scand.* 1984;552:203–208.
32. Brennan D, O'Connell MJ, Ryan M, et al. Secondary cleft sign as a marker of injury in athletes with groin pain. MR image appearance and interpretation. *Radiology.* 2005;235: 162–167.
33. Zoga AC, Kavanagh EC, Omar IM, et al. Athletic pubalgia and the "sports hernia": MR imaging findings. *Radiology.* 2008;247(3):797–807.
34. Gullmo A. Herniography. The diagnosis of hernia in the groin and incompetence of the pouch of Douglas and pelvic floor. *Acta Radiol Suppl.* 1980;361:1–76.
35. Van den Berg JC, de Valois JC, Go PM, et al. Groin hernia: Can dynamic magnetic resonance imaging be of help? *Eur Radiol.* 1998;8:270–273.
36. Van den Berg JC, de Valois JC, Go PM, et al. Detection of groin hernia with physical examination, ultrasound, and MRI compared with laparoscopic findings. *Invest Radiol.* 1999;34:739–743.

CHAPTER

4

Benjamin G. Domb
Adam G. Brooks
Carlos A. Guanche

Physical Examination of the Hip

INTRODUCTION

As our understanding and treatment of hip pathology improves, a systematic, consistent, and reproducible means of clinically evaluating the hip is imperative. While a limp, groin pain, and limited internal rotation are often indicators of hip pathology,[1] the hip is overlooked as the original source of pain or pathology in 60% of primary hip disorders.[2] Hip pain can be ambiguous in its nature and origin, and pathologies of the hip and low back interact with one another and are easily confused. Hip problems can stem from disorders of the paravertebral muscles, which cause soft tissue instability and irregular tension on the hip.[3] Hip pain can also cause back pain by way of muscle contractures of the iliopsoas and the hamstrings or through secondary leg length discrepancy.[1] A systematic and reproducible physical examination of the hip is therefore a necessity for correct diagnosis as well as longitudinal follow-up.

The hip is a focal point of initiation for running and walking and can bear forces equal to over five times body weight during running or jumping.[4] Because the hip is almost universally subjected to high loads and extremes of motion during sport, hip pain is a common complaint in athletes. In one study, pathology of the hip accounted for 2.5% of adult athletic injuries and 5% to 9% of high school athletic injuries.[5] Hip pain is especially frequent in sports such as soccer, ballet, hockey, martial arts, rugby, and running.[5] A recent study of injuries in the National Basketball Association over 17 years found a total of 1,340 hip-related injuries causing 4,753 games missed.[6]

This chapter will focus on techniques to assess hip pathology in several dimensions: location (intra-articular vs. extra-articular), compartment (posterior, anterior, or lateral), and tissue (bony, ligamentous, or musculotendinous). The physical examination will also aid in differentiating between pain originating from the hip versus the back. This chapter comprises six sections. The first section will describe the patient history, and the subsequent five sections will correspond to the five positions in which the physical examination will be conducted: standing, sitting, supine, lateral, and prone.

PATIENT HISTORY

As with all clinical encounters, a detailed history is essential to the final diagnosis and should begin in a traditional manner with the patient's age, chief complaint, and the presence or absence of trauma.[7] Much detail about the hip pain should be elicited, including the location and severity of the pain, time of onset, specific quality, alleviating, aggravating, or associated factors, whether the pain is focal or diffuse. Additionally, similar pains, popping or locking symptoms, night pain, and any accompanying numbness or weakness are important to document. Back pain and hip pain will often coexist, so care should be taken to note the severity of one pain relative to the other. Radicular pain may exist with either hip or lumbar spine pathology and is unreliable as a differentiating factor. However, weakness, numbness, and paresthesias in the lower extremity are suggestive of neural compression, often occurring in the lumbar spine.

An inquiry should also be made into any treatment the patient has had and its effectiveness. This treatment may include pharmaceuticals such as nonsteroidal anti-inflammatory drugs (NSAIDs), physical therapy, or the use of assistive device.

To further aid in the diagnosis, the patient's activity level should be delineated. Specifically, the ability to complete activities of daily living, work responsibilities, and higher-impact activities should be documented. Participation in certain sports (running, soccer, ballet, hockey, golf, tennis, martial arts, and rugby) can be important since these sports are often associated with specific hip disorders.[8,9]

A thorough past medical and family history is critical. Past medical considerations should include hip disorders or dislocation during birth or infancy, past surgeries or major illnesses, and any history of trauma. Family history should include hip dislocations or any hip disorder, degenerative joint disease, rheumatologic disorders, and cancer. Also, the physician should be keenly aware of "red flags" such as fever, malaise, night sweats, weight loss, night pain, intravenous drug use, cancer history, or known immunocompromised state.[10] These "red flags" may indicate systemic problems, and further diagnostic tests may be necessary. Hip conditions can also be related to general medical conditions within the gastrointestinal, genitourinary, neurological, or vascular systems, making a complete, general physical examination an important component of the hip examination.

PHYSICAL EXAMINATION

Any orthopaedic physical examination should begin with an evaluation of the patient's general appearance, which may provide clues to the source of pain. The patient may then be brought to the standing position for the first portion of the exam.

STANDING

The standing examination consists of four parts: gait, alignment, Trendelenburg test, and the laxity test. Because the hip is essential to walk, hip pathologies will often visibly affect a patient's gait.[7] Six to eight full strides should be observed from both the frontal and sagittal planes, paying close attention to stride length, internal or external rotation of the foot, pelvic rotation, and the stance phase.[11] Any snapping or clicking should be noted since these noises may imply psoas contractures, iliotibial (IT) band tightness, or intra-articular pathology. The patient should be asked to rotate his or her hip to recreate the noise in order to differentiate between internal and external snapping.[8]

One of several types of abnormal gaits related to hip pain including antalgic gait, pelvic wink, Trendelenburg gait, excessive pelvic internal or external rotation, and true or false leg length discrepancies may be noted. An antalgic gait is one during which the patient limps to minimize the stance phase on the painful side thus limiting weight bearing. This gait pattern may indicate pain in the hip, pelvis, or lower back.[12,13] A pelvic wink is rotation in excess of 40° in the axial plane toward the affected hip when terminally extending the hip. This dysfunction can signify hip flexion contractures when lumbar lordosis or a forward-stooping posture is present or can indicate an internal hip pathology. Trendelenburg gait, or abductor lurch, is characterized by a lurching of the trunk toward the affected side during stance phase. The abductor muscles are responsible for stabilizing the pelvis during stance phase. If those muscles are compromised, the patient will compensate by lurching to the ipsilateral side to prevent the pelvis from sagging. In the case of intra-articular hip pathology, patients will frequently walk with a Trendelenburg gait in order to avoid increased joint reactive forces that occur with abductor contraction. Excessive internal or external rotation of the hip should be noted during the gait examination and will be discussed in the section "Sitting". Finally, a short leg limp during gait may imply either IT band pathology or true or false leg length discrepancy.

The alignment portion of the examination focuses on leg length discrepancy and spinal alignment. Several methods exist to assess possible true or false leg length discrepancy, which is especially important if a short leg limp is noted during the gait exam. First, examine the height of the shoulders relative to the ipsilateral iliac crest. Second, assess pelvic tilt, a condition that may indicate leg length discrepancy. Third, measure the distance from the anterior superior iliac spine (ASIS) to the ipsilateral medial malleolus. Differences in these measurements suggest a true leg length discrepancy in which the proportions of the bones are different on each side of the body.[14] If there is a short leg limp but no true leg length discrepancy is noted, conditions such as scoliosis, muscle spasms, or pelvic deformities may contribute.[8]

The assessment of spinal alignment involves inspection from two positions. First, the patient stands in front of the examiner and bends forward while the back is inspected for trunk rotation consistent with scoliosis, a contributing factor in functional leg length discrepancy. Second, the patient is viewed laterally for excessive lumbar lordosis or paravertebral muscle spasms. Hip flexor contractures can cause increased lumbar lordosis, and paravertebral muscle spasms can cause hip pain by placing abnormal tension on the hip.[3]

The next part of the standing examination is the Trendelenburg test (Fig. 4.1). A positive test consists of sagging of the pelvis greater than 2 cm while the patient lifts the contralateral leg off the floor. By lifting the right leg, one is testing the left abductor muscles and neural loop. A positive sign therefore suggests incompetence of abductor function. The maneuver should be performed first on the unaffected side to establish a comparative norm.

Finally, laxity can be assessed by checking for hyperextension of the knee and elbow, along with the thumb-to-wrist exam. The thumb-to-wrist exam involves an attempt to touch the anterior forearm with the thumb (Fig. 4.2). A positive thumb-to-wrist exam along with hyperextension of the knee and elbow beyond 5° is suggestive of generalized hyperlaxity of the ligaments.[9]

SITTING

The sitting examination consists of three parts: circulatory, neurological, and rotational. As with all aspects of the physical examination, bilateral evaluation in the seated position is essential. The circulatory examination requires checking the dorsalis pedis and posterior tibial pulses and inspecting the skin and lymphatics around the hip. This pulse is absent in 2% to 3% of normal, healthy young adults, so its absence alone would not be sufficient to conclude a vascular pathology.[15] Both sides should be compared for any scarring of the skin or lymphadenopathy.

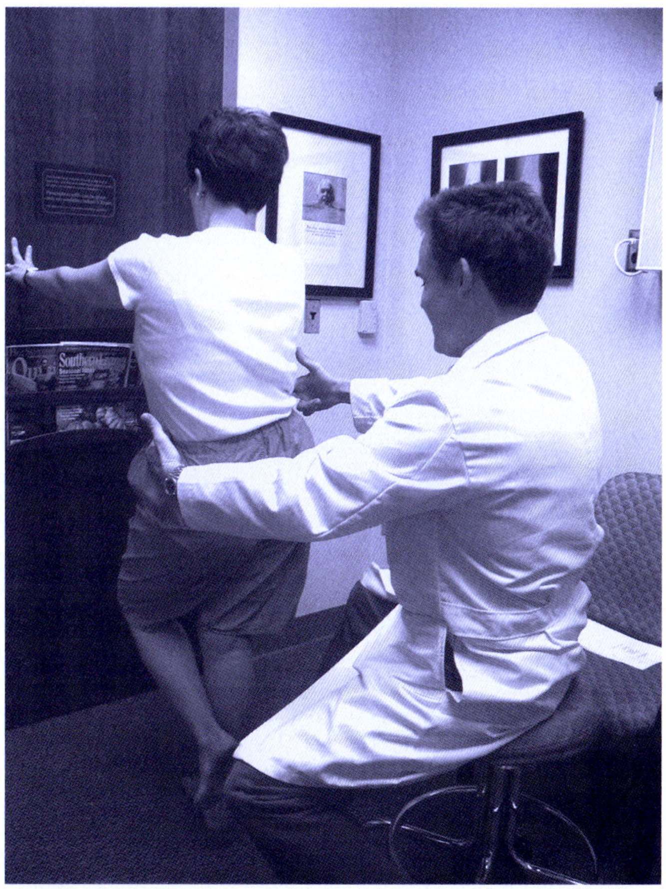

Figure 4.1. Trendelenburg sign is a test of the contralateral leg abductors. The patient lifts the leg and the pelvis is assessed for at least 2 cm of sag. (From Berry D, Steinman S. *Orthopaedic Surgery Essentials: Adult Reconstruction.* Philadelphia, PA: Lippincott Williams & Wilkins; 2007, with permission.)

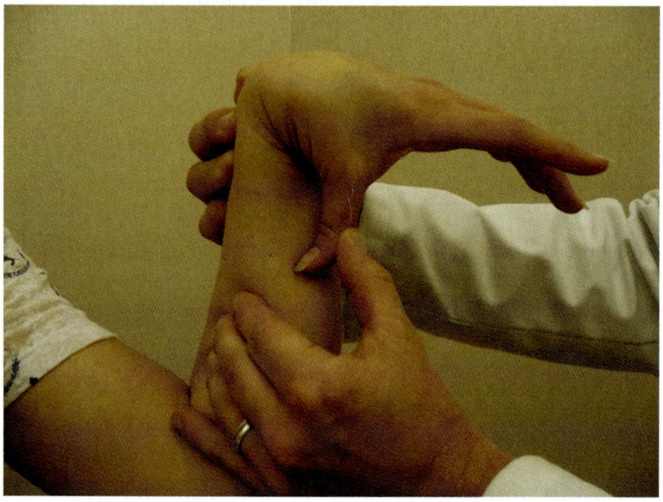

Figure 4.2. The thumb-to-wrist laxity test will determine if the patient has ligament hyperlaxity. A positive test occurs if the patient can touch the anterior forearm with the thumb.

The neurological examination will include motor and sensory components with a focus on the L2 through S1 spinal nerves. The motor component will test muscles innervated by the superior gluteal (L4–S1), obturator (L2–4), femoral (L2–4), and sciatic (L4–S3) nerves. To test the superior gluteal nerve (leg abductors), abduct both legs against force. For the obturator nerve (leg adductors), adduct against resistance. To test the femoral nerve (quadriceps femoris), extend the legs at the knee joint against resistance. Finally, to check the sciatic nerve (hamstrings and lower leg muscles), flex the legs at the knee joint and then dorsiflex, plantar flex, invert, and evert the foot, all against resistance.

Dermatomal sensation should be assessed bilaterally at the upper anterior thigh (L2), mid-anterior thigh (L3), knee (L4), middle three toes (L5), and lateral part of foot (S1) (Fig. 4.3). Special attention should be paid to the anterior thigh, a frequent site of neuralgia caused by compression of the lateral femoral cutaneous nerve as it passes through the pelvis over the psoas muscle and under the inguinal ligament.[16–19]

Deep tendon reflexes include the patellar and Achilles tendon reflexes. Patellar reflex is assessed by tapping the leg just below the patella at the patellar tendon with leg hanging freely. If the leg extends at the knee, the reflex is present. Ankle reflex, or Achilles reflex, is tested by holding the ankle in dorsiflexion and tapping the calcaneal tendon. If the foot plantar flexes, the reflex is present.

The last component of the neurological evaluation is the straight leg raise. The leg is passively raised with the knee held in extension. If the patient feels pain in the lower back or leg, lower the leg 10° and dorsiflex the foot to recreate the radicular pain (Fig. 4.4). A positive test within 0° to 30° indicates a compressed nerve root; a positive test within 30° to 60° suggests sacroiliac disease and greater than 60° suggests a lumbosacral disorder.[20,21] If the patient leans back at any point during this examination to avoid pain, the test is considered positive.

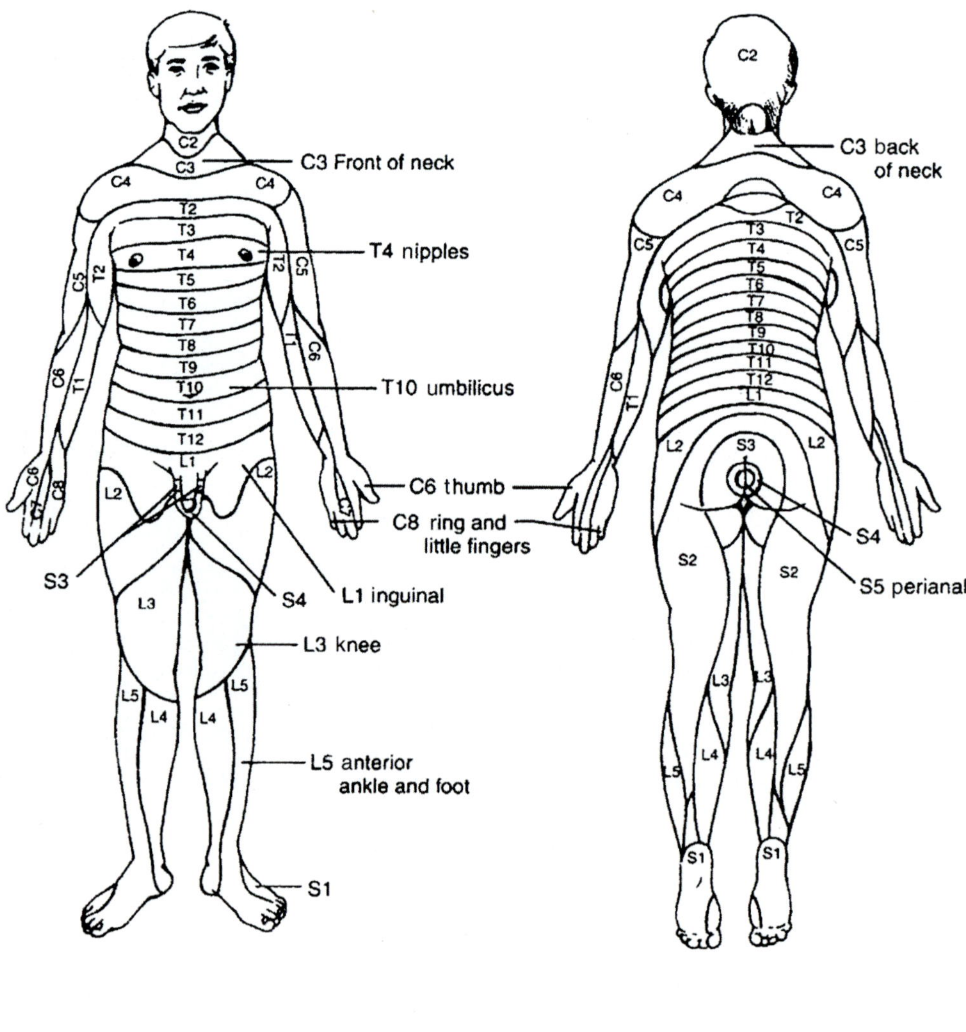

Figure 4.3. The dermatome map shows where to compare sensory function on both legs to assess neurological deficit to the corresponding spinal nerve. (From Berry D, Steinman S. *Orthopaedic Surgery Essentials: Adult Reconstruction.* Philadelphia, PA: Lippincott Williams & Wilkins; 2007, with permission.)

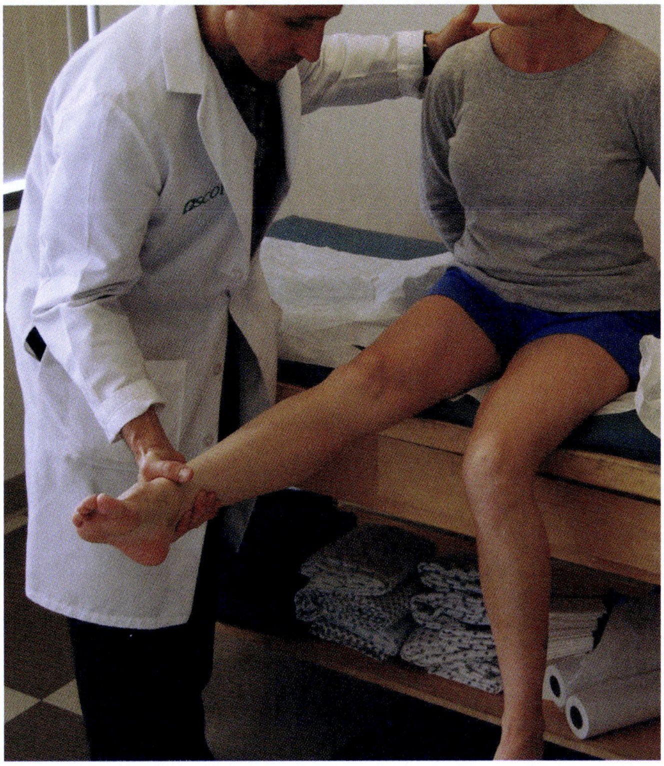

Figure 4.4. The straight leg raise test. Raise straight leg until pain is felt, then lower the leg 10° and dorsiflex to recreate the pain.

The final part of the seated examination involves evaluation of internal and external rotation of the hip. Rotation is best evaluated in the seated position because the hip is stabilized at a 90° angle, avoiding variability due to changes in flexion angle.[10] In addition, the seated position stabilizes the pelvis, which is difficult to accomplish in the supine position. The normal range for internal rotation of the hip is within 20° to 35°, and for external rotation is within 30° to 70°. Additionally, the terminally extended hip should internally rotate at least 10°. Loss of internal rotation is one of the initial signals for such problems as arthritis, effusion, and other internal derangements, as well as for slipped capital femoral epiphysis and muscular contractures.[22] Excessive internal rotation coupled with diminished external rotation suggests increased femoral anteversion.[14] Significant differences in rotational measurements from one side to another, whether or not in normal range, can indicate FAI or abnormal femoral or acetabular version.[1]

SUPINE

The supine examination includes the continued assessment of a range of motion, an abdominal exam, and a trauma assessment followed by provocative testing. To examine flexion, have the patient flex his or her knees and hips toward his or her chest and observe both sides at once. The limit of normal flexion is around 120°; significant loss of flexion can limit the patient's ability to perform activities of daily living.[7] When evaluating abduction and adduction range of motion, one should reference the position of the shaft of the femur to the midline of the pelvis. To test abduction, hold the ankle while supporting the leg and manually abduct the leg. Normal abduction is approximately 45°. Adductor contractures can cause a diminished abduction range of motion. Bringing the leg across the opposite leg tests adduction. Normal range is 20° to 30°, but may be diminished in the setting of abductor contracture.

Next in the supine examination is the assessment of the abdominal/ilioinguinal area, which begins with the palpation of several landmarks. Palpate the femoral pulse at the femoral triangle. Search for any fascial hernias or other masses in the abdominal region by having the patient contract the rectus abdominus and oblique muscles. Palpate any masses or hernias, if present. Palpate the adductor tubercle (Fig. 4.5) as the patient adducts the leg; reproduction of pain may indicate adductor tendonitis. Palpate the pubic symphysis (Fig. 4.5); if there is tenderness, one or more of several issues may be present including fracture, trauma, calcification, or osteitis pubis, and further investigation is required. Pelvic stability is assessed by pushing down on the bilateral iliac crests, looking for independent motion of the hemipelvises. Finally, attempt to elicit the Tinel sign at the femoral nerve by percussing the femoral nerve at the level of the ilioinguinal ligament. A positive Tinel sign occurs with tingling along the femoral nerve, possibly indicating a neurological pathology.

A generalized hip trauma examination includes log roll, heel strike, and the Stinchfield tests. All should cause marked pain in the presence of a hip fracture but may also be painful with intra-articular derangement. Rotating the leg internally and externally in the supine position performs the log roll. Striking the fist against the heel, creating an axial load on the hip, performs the heel strike. With the Stinchfield test, the patient must raise the fully extended leg against the pressure of the examiner's hand upon the thigh. Pressure is gradually increased as the leg is raised. The recreation of hip pain constitutes a positive test and suggests intra-articular or iliopsoas pathology.[14] In the setting of fracture, the patient will normally be unable to perform this test due to pain.

The supine examination concludes with provocative testing. The FADDIR test is performed by bringing the hip into maximal flexion, adduction, and internal rotation (Fig. 4.6). This test may be accentuated by adding an axial load with downward pressure over the knee. Pain in this position constitutes a positive FADDIR test, which may be the most sensitive indicator of FAI. The FADDIR test may also be conducted in the lateral position.

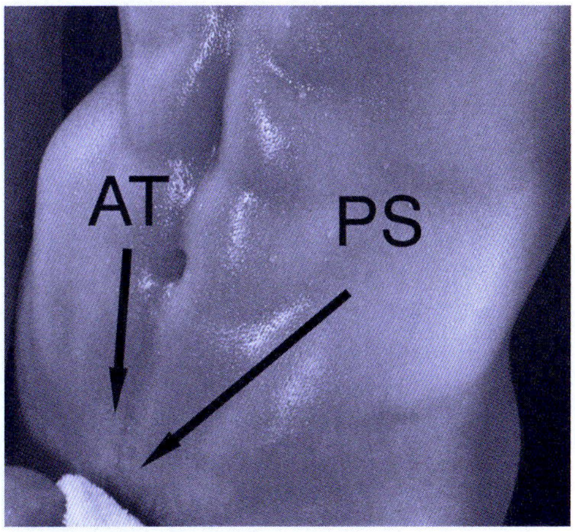

Figure 4.5. Palpation of the adductor tubercle (AT) or the pubic symphysis (PS) can help localize the source of pain. The pubic symphysis is directly in the midline, whereas the adductor tubercle is more lateral on either side of the symphysis.

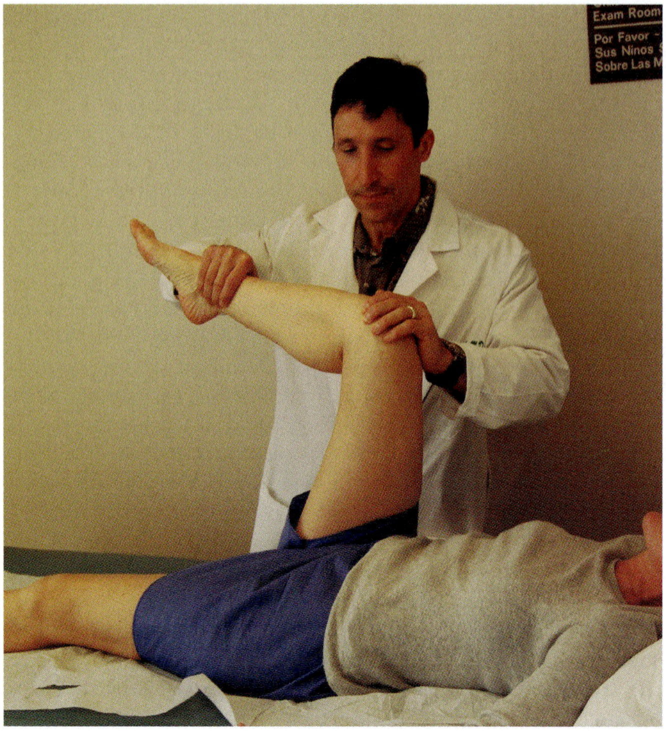

Figure 4.6. Supine FADDIR test. Bring the hip into maximal flexion, adduction, and internal rotation. This can be done in conjunction with an axial load applied at the knee.

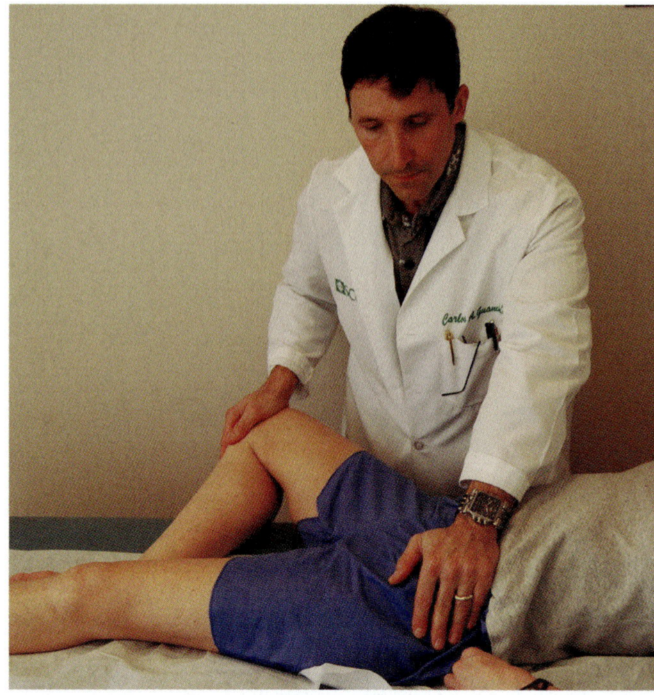

Figure 4.7. The Patrick/FABER test. Have the patient lie in a "figure four" position, with the affected extremity. Press on the affected knee to elicit pain in the sacroiliac region.

To perform the Patrick/FABER test, have the patient lie in a "figure four" position with the affected ankle lying on the thigh of the unaffected leg and then press on the affected knee to cause sacroiliac joint stress (Fig. 4.7). This stress may manifest itself in different types of pain, each delineating a different pathology. Groin pain implicates the iliopsoas as the origin of pain[14]; lateral hip pain suggests lateral FAI; and posterior pain may indicate sacroiliac joint pathology. To assess lateral FAI, move the leg through the full range of flexion and extension while abducted. Pain during this process signifies lateral rim impingement.

The Thomas test requires pulling the unaffected leg to the chest, flexed at the hip and knee, while lowering the affected leg to the table (Fig. 4.8). The Thomas test is positive if the patient cannot lower the affected thigh all the way to the table and may signify an iliopsoas contracture. A clicking sound during the Thomas test implies a labral tear.[10]

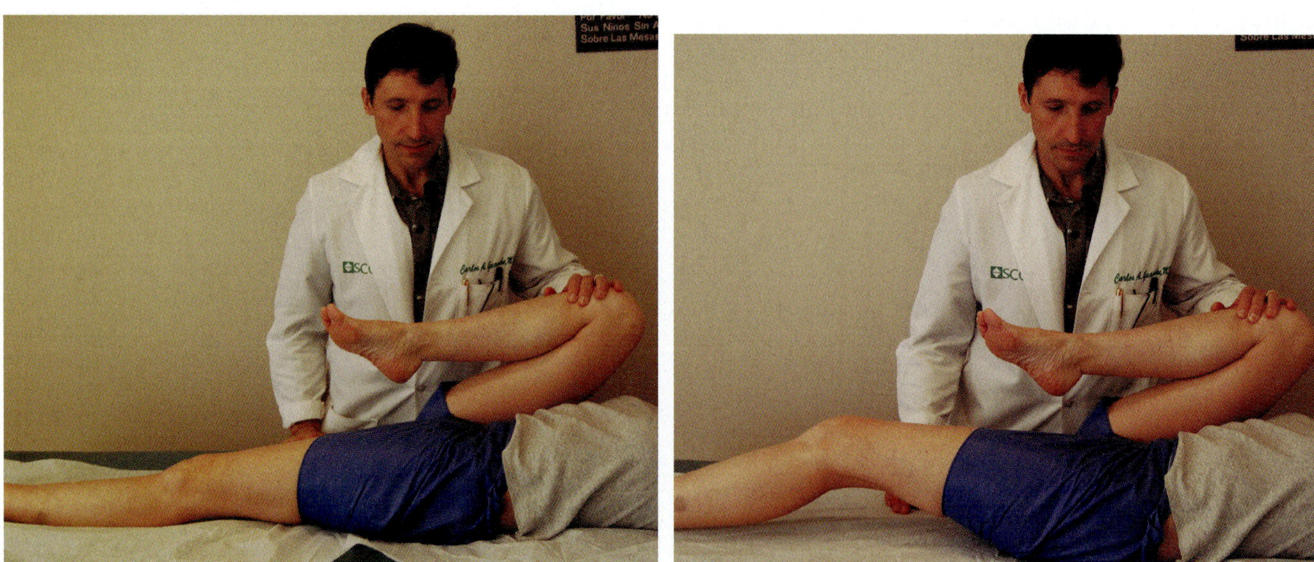

Figure 4.8. The Thomas test. The patient holds the unaffected leg flexed while attempting to lower the affected leg to the table. An inability to lower the affected leg constitutes a positive test, indicating iliopsoas contracture.

The McCarthy test is performed by rolling the hip through full flexion, extension, and internal/external rotation. The goal of this rotation is to emulate the patient's initial pain in order to localize it by finding sites of bony impingement.[23] A positive McCarthy test occurs with reproduction of the original pain and is most common in cases of an acetabular labrum tear.[23–26]

The final part of the supine exam is the Scour test, which can further delineate whether the hip pain is of an intra-articular or extra-articular nature. First, flex the hip and knee completely so that the knee is pointing to the shoulder. Next, rotate the hip around its arc of motion paying special attention to any bumps, catches, or irregularities during this motion (Fig. 4.9). The presence of any bumps or catches is a positive Scour test and suggests FAI.

LATERAL

The lateral examination takes place with the patient lying on his or her unaffected side. During the lateral examination, palpate several landmarks including the ischial tuberosity, the tensor fascia lata, the IT band, the sciatic nerve, the greater trochanteric bursa, the piriformis, the origin of the gluteus maximus along the ilium, sacrum, coccyx, and the sacroiliac joint (Fig. 4.10). Tenderness in any of these areas implies pathology and should be evaluated more closely. More specifically, tenderness at the ischial tuberosity is associated with biceps femoris contractures, avulsion fracture, or bursitis.[10] Tenderness at the sacroiliac joint would favor a diagnosis of sacroiliac inflammation, which may frequently mimic low back pathology. Pain in

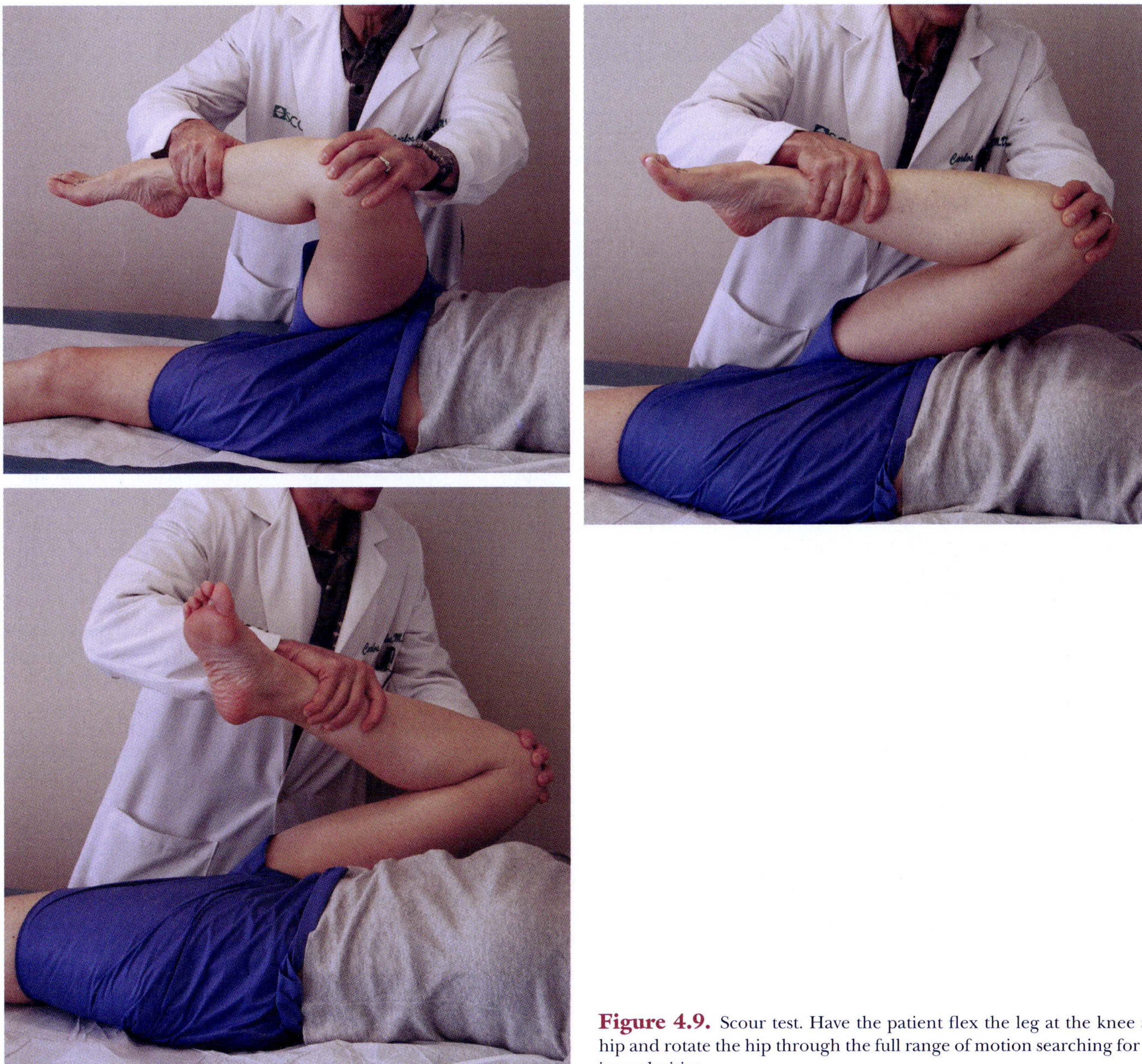

Figure 4.9. Scour test. Have the patient flex the leg at the knee and hip and rotate the hip through the full range of motion searching for any irregularities.

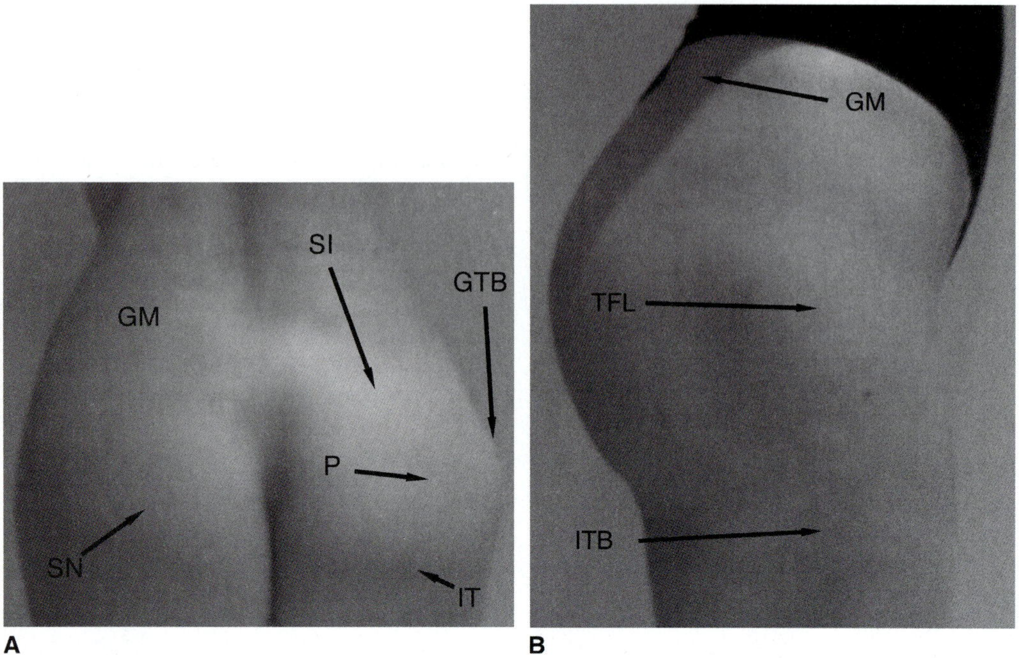

Figure 4.10. **A,B:** Palpation of several points during the lateral examination is important to localize pain origin. IT, ischial tuberosity; TFL, tensor fascia lata; ITB, iliotibial band; SN, sciatic nerve; GTB, greater trochanteric bursa, P, piriformis; GM, gluteus maximus origin; SI, sacroiliac joint.

the greater trochanteric bursa is associated with bursitis or IT band contractures.

The Ober test consists of three parts: extension, neutral, and flexion (Fig. 4.11). To perform the extension test abduct the affected leg and extend it at the hip while flexing the ipsilateral knee. When allowing the leg to fall, note if the leg adducts immediately or if a slight pause or any difficulty in adduction occurs. To perform the neutral test, abduct the leg while the knee is flexed but the hip is in the neutral position, and then allow the leg to fall into adduction. To perform the flexion test rotate the torso to lay both shoulders on the table while both legs are still in the lateral position. Abduct the unaffected leg with the knee fully extended and the hip flexed, and then allow the leg to fall into adduction. In all three tests, the examiner abducts the leg in the specific position and then releases the leg. If the leg maintains its abducted position longer than expected, the Ober test is positive. A positive extension Ober test indicates tensor fascia lata contracture, while a positive neutral test indicates gluteus medius contracture or tear. A positive flexion test indicates gluteus maximus contracture.

To perform the FADDIR test in the lateral position stand behind the patient and place a supporting hand under the patient's knee while using the other hand to palpate the hip (place the index finger on the anterior portion of the hip with the thumb pointing toward the posterior). Have the patient flex, adduct, and internally rotate the leg to elicit pain or discomfort (Fig. 4.12). If any pain or discomfort occurs, the test is thought to be positive.

The final part of the lateral examination is the abduction–extension–external rotation test (Fig. 4.13). With the knee fully extended, abduct the leg 30° with no rotation, and flex the hip 10°. Externally rotate the leg and place forward pressure on the greater trochanter while bringing the leg from 10° flexion to full extension. If pain occurs with the anterior pressure and abates in its absence, the test is positive. A positive abduction–extension–external rotation test may indicate anterior acetabular anteversion, iliofemoral ligament strain, or anterior instability of the hip. Patients who are positive for this test should also be assessed for generalized ligamentous laxity.

PRONE

The final component of the examination takes place in the prone position. Most of the tests and examinations in this position are performed as follow-up to earlier positive findings. Such examinations include palpation of the sacroiliac region, a modified Thomas test, and the Ely test. If indicated, knee and ankle examination may also be performed in this position. If previous examination has produced sacroiliac pain, palpate the three different areas in the sacroiliac region to specify which area is the origin of pain. These three areas are the suprasacroiliac region, the infrasacroiliac region (near the gluteus maximus), and the lower lumbar vertebral spinous processes (L4–L5).

The next part of the prone examination will help differentiate between iliopsoas and rectus femoris contractures. The modified Thomas test is used for the former while the Ely test is used to test the latter. To perform the modified Thomas test have the patient lie in the prone position and see if the pelvis rises off the examination table, indicative of an iliopsoas contracture. The Ely test is performed by flexing the leg at the knee until the lower leg is as close to the thigh as possible. If the pelvis and buttocks move upward in this position the test is positive, indicating rectus femoris contracture. Because the rectus femoris crosses both the hip and knee joints, the Ely test would only indicate contractures of that muscle as the bending of the knee stretches the rectus femoris across the knee.

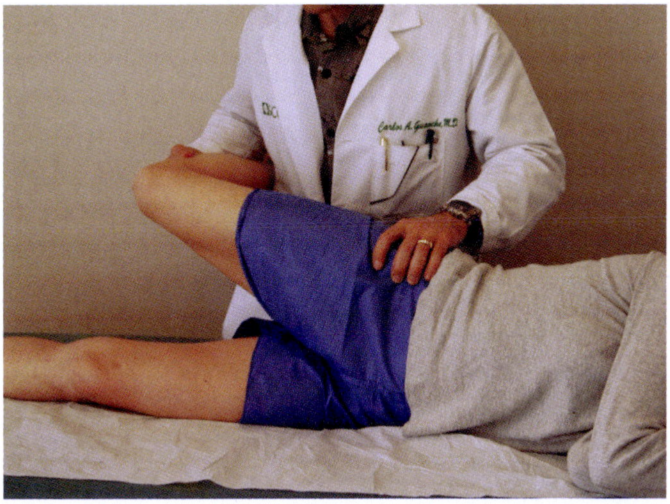

A

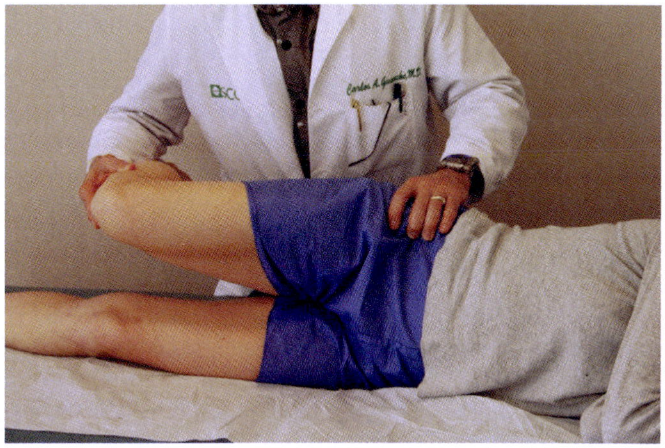

B

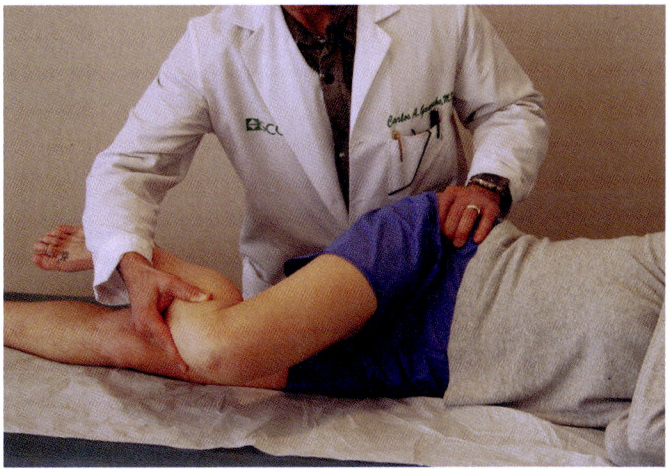

C

Figure 4.11. The Ober test is performed with the hip extended **(A)**, in a neutral position **(B)**, and flexed **(C)**. The knee is flexed in the extended and neutral test, but extended in the flexed test. Additionally, the patient's shoulders should be on the table during the flexed test.

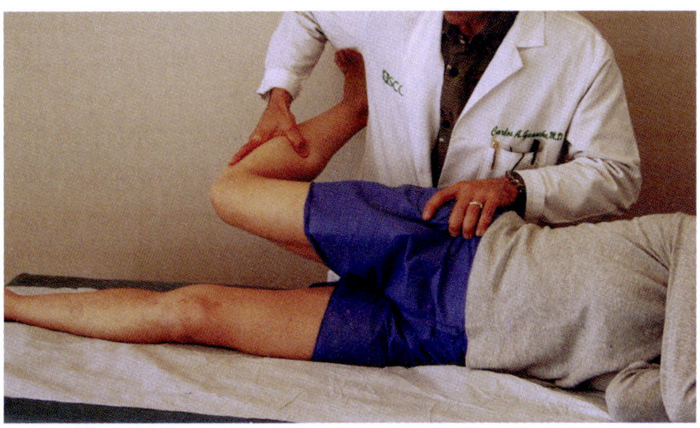

Figure 4.12. Lateral FADDIR test. Flex, adduct, and internally rotate the leg while placing one hand on the knee and the other hand on the hip to test for FAI.

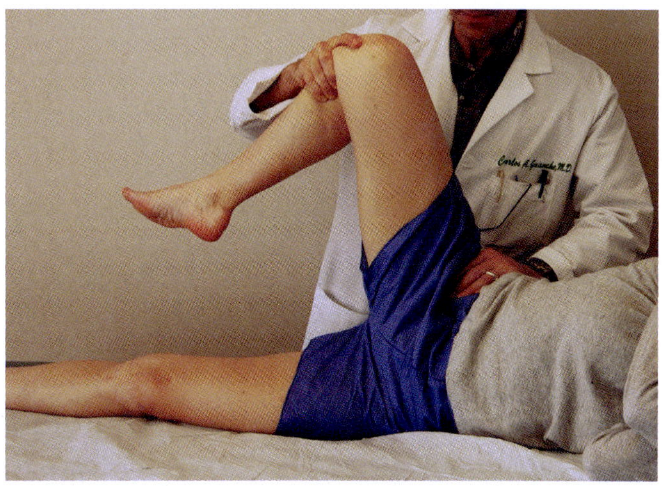

Figure 4.13. Abduction–extension–external rotation test. Extend the knee, abduct the leg 30°, and then externally rotate the leg while placing pressure on the greater trochanter and bringing the leg from 10° flexion to full extension.

CONCLUSION

The examination of the hip can be a confusing and challenging exercise. However, with a systematic approach, the myriad of possible diagnoses can be narrowed down. The conclusions reached through this examination should be used along with the patient's age, lifestyle, aspirations, and physical requirements in making treatment recommendations.

It is also important to keep an open mind regarding the coexistence of pathology that may be concurrent with hip-related pain. Avoiding "tunnel vision" is crucial and concomitant problems must be recognized and addressed along with any hip pathology. If the patient has both hip and back pathology and both are not addressed in the treatment plan, the outcome can be very poor.[1] Furthermore, superfluous radiographic investigation should be avoided. After a good history and physical examination, only 16% of hip complaints necessitate further radiographic study.[10]

As with any other physical examination, knowledge of the anatomy of the hip is crucial. The ultimate clarifying factor during the physical examination is a detailed understanding of the anatomy underlying every step. With this understanding, the examiner can unify all parts of the examination and arrive at a clear and correct diagnosis.

REFERENCES

1. Brown MD, Gomez-Martin O, Brookfield KF, et al. Differential diagnosis of hip disease versus spine disease. *Clin Orthop Relat Res.* 2004;419:280–284.
2. Byrd JWT. Hip arthroscopy. Presented at the 2005 Meeting of the Arthroscopic Association of North America. April 8–10, 2005.
3. Longjohn D, Dorr LD. Soft tissue balance of the hip. *J Arthroplasty.* 1998;13(1):97–100.
4. Boyd KT, Peirce NS, Batt ME. Common hip injuries in sports. *Sports Med.* 1997;24:273–288.
5. DeAngelis NA, Busconi BD. Assessment and differential diagnosis of the painful hip. *Clin Orthop Relat Res.* 2003;406:11–18.
6. Domb BG, Drakos M, Starkey C, et al. Injury and illness in the National Basketball Association: A 17-year overview. Submitted to *Am J Sports Med.*
7. Scopp JM, Moorman CT. The assessment of athletic hip injury. *Clin Sports Med.* 2001;20(4):647–659.
8. Braly BA, Beall DP, Martin HD. Clinical examination of the athletic hip. *Clin Sports Med.* 2006;25:199–210.
9. Martin HD. Clinical examination of the hip. *Oper Tech Orthop.* 2005;15:177–181.
10. Margo K, Drezner J, Motzkin D. Evaluation and management of hip pain: An algorithmic approach. *J Fam Pract.* 2003;52(8):607–617.
11. McCarthy J. *Early Hip Disorders: Advances in Detection and Minimally Invasive Treatment.* Boston, MA: Springer; 2003.
12. Magee DJ. Hip. In: Magee DJ, ed. *Orthopedic Physical Assessment.* 3rd Ed. Philadelphia, PA: W.B. Saunders; 1997, p. 460.
13. Hickman JM, Peters CL. Hip pain in the young adult: Diagnosis and treatment of disorders of the acetabular labrum and acetabular dysplasia. *Am J Orthop.* 2001;30:459–467.
14. Reider B, Martel JM. Pelvis, hip and thigh. In: Reider B, Martel JM, eds. *The Orthopedic Physical Examination.* Philadelphia, PA: W.B. Saunders; 1999, pp. 159–199.
15. Robertson GS, Ristic CD, Bullen BR. The incidence of congenitally absent foot pulses. *Ann R Coll Surg Engl.* 1990;72(2):99–100.
16. Hoppenfeld S, Hutton R. Physical examination of the hip and pelvis. In: Hoppenfeld S, Hutton R, eds. *Physical Examination of the Spine and Extremities.* Upper Saddle River, NJ: Prentice Hall; 1976, pp. 143–169.
17. Jakubowicz M. Topography of the femoral nerve in relation to components of the iliopsoas muscle in human fetuses. *Folia Morphol (Praha).* 1991;50(1–2):91–101.
18. Ritter JW. Femoral nerve "sheath" for inguinal paravaxcular lumbar plexus block is not found in human cadavers. *J Clin Anesth.* 1995;7(6):470–473.
19. Robinson DE, Ball KE, Webb PJ. Iliopsoas hematoma with femoral neuropathy presenting a diagnostic dilemma after spinal decompression [case reports]. *Spine.* 2001;26(6):E135–E138.
20. Evans RC. *Illustrated Essentials in Orthopedic Physical Assessment.* St Louis, MO: Mosby; 1994.
21. Hoppenfeld S. *Physical Examination of the Spine and Extremities.* San Mateo, CA: Appleton & Lange; 1976.
22. Troum OM, Crues JV. The young adult with hip pain: Diagnosis and medical treatment, circa 2004. *Clin Orthop Relat Res.* 2004;418:9–17.
23. McCarthy JC, Noble PC, Schuck M, et al. The role of labral lesions to development of early degenerative hip disease. *Clin Orthop Relat Res.* 2001;393:25–37.
24. Lage LA, Patel JV, Villar RN. The acetabular labral tear: An arthroscopic classification. *Arthroscopy.* 1996;12:269–272.
25. Farjo LA, Glick JM, Sampson TG. Hip arthroscopy for acetabular labral tears. *Arthroscopy.* 1999;15:132–137.
26. Fitzgerald RH Jr. Acetabular labrum tears: Diagnosis and treatment. *Clin Orthop Relat Res.* 1995;311:60–68.

CHAPTER

5

James Bond
Kevin S. Caperton
Andrew Ebert
Carlos A. Guanche

Arthroscopic Anatomy of the Hip

INTRODUCTION

Even though arthroscopy of the hip was introduced as early as 1931,[1] its clinical application has developed rather slowly.[2,3] Recent advancements in arthroscopic technique and equipment, however, have revolutionized the diagnosis and treatment of hip injuries. Currently, there is an unprecedented enthusiasm for hip arthroscopy. Clinical assessment of the hip is improving, and therefore arthroscopic indications are expanding. As hip arthroscopy becomes more common, it is vital that a precise knowledge of hip anatomy and common portal placement is coupled with proper patient selection, sound preoperative planning, and a consistent arthroscopic technique in order to maximize clinical outcomes.

INDICATIONS AND CONTRAINDICATIONS

The current indications for hip arthroscopy include loose body removal,[4–7] symptomatic acetabular labral tears,[8,16] chondral lesions,[17,18] iliopsoas bursitis,[2,19] osteochondritis dissecans,[20] ligamentum teres injuries,[21,22] internal and external snapping hip syndrome,[23–26] femoroacetabular impingement,[27,28] synovial abnormalities,[6,29–31] and infection.[32,33]

The clearest contraindication to hip arthroscopy is ankylosis of the hip joint.[34] Similarly, arthrofibrosis of the hip may preclude adequate positioning and distraction necessary for arthroscopic intervention. Open wounds and superficial infections around the hip also place the joint at unnecessary risk and should be avoided. A relative contraindication to hip arthroscopy is the patient with a stable osteonecrosis of the femoral head, as there have been reports of progression of the disease state following arthroscopy.[35,36]

SURGICAL TECHNIQUE: ARTHROSCOPIC SETUP

Although many studies have confirmed that hip arthroscopy can be effectively performed with the patient in the supine or the lateral decubitus position,[37–40] the discussion in this chapter will assume that the patient is in the supine position.

Both 30° and 70° video-articulated cameras are necessary for optimal visualization of the hip joint. We utilize the 70° arthroscope for our diagnostic exam. If any pathology is noted during the diagnostic exam, a different perspective from the 30° arthroscope usually increases the understanding of the pathology and commonly provides an easier working view for treatment of the pathology. Special 6-in., 16-gauge spinal needles are also very useful in hip arthroscopy. They aid in joint distraction via insufflation of the joint and also allow for the placement of a guide wire that can subsequently direct sharp obturators safely into the hip joint. Flexible probes, extra-long cannulas, shavers, burs, drills, and loose body retrievers have all increased the ability to arthroscopically treat a wide variety of hip pathology, and therefore should be utilized when indicated. Figure 5.1 shows all of the instruments we use for hip arthroscopy as they are laid out on the back table.

SURGICAL TECHNIQUE: PORTAL PLACEMENT

After the extremity is appropriately suspended in traction, the bony landmarks of the anterior and lateral hip are defined with a skin marker (Fig. 5.2). The principal landmarks include the greater trochanter, the anterior superior iliac spine (ASIS), and the pubic symphysis. The anterior, posterior, and superior aspects of the greater trochanter should be identified first and then a transverse line drawn from the superior aspect of the trochanter to the superior aspect of the pubic bone, which is represented in (Fig. 5.3) by the transverse dotted line. The ASIS is then identified and a sagittal line is drawn distally down the anterior thigh. In order to protect the medial neurovascular structures of the lower extremity, no portals should be placed medial to this sagittal line.

Three portals are routinely established in hip arthroscopy. These include the anterolateral (AL), the anterior (ANT), and the posterolateral (PL) portals. The anterolateral, portal is utilized as the introductory portal for virtually all routine hip arthroscopy and is positioned at the superior margin of the greater trochanter in line with its anterior border. This portal allows for a relatively straight line of entry into the central compartment of the hip joint as long as the hip is maintained in neutral rotation. Internal or external rotation of the hip can significantly alter the relationship between the greater trochanter and the femoral head and therefore should be avoided.[37,41]

The anterior portal has been described with slight variations by numerous authors.[37,39,41–43] Our anterior portal is typically 1 cm lateral and 1 cm distal from the intersection of the two lines previously described. The spinal needle is aimed approximately

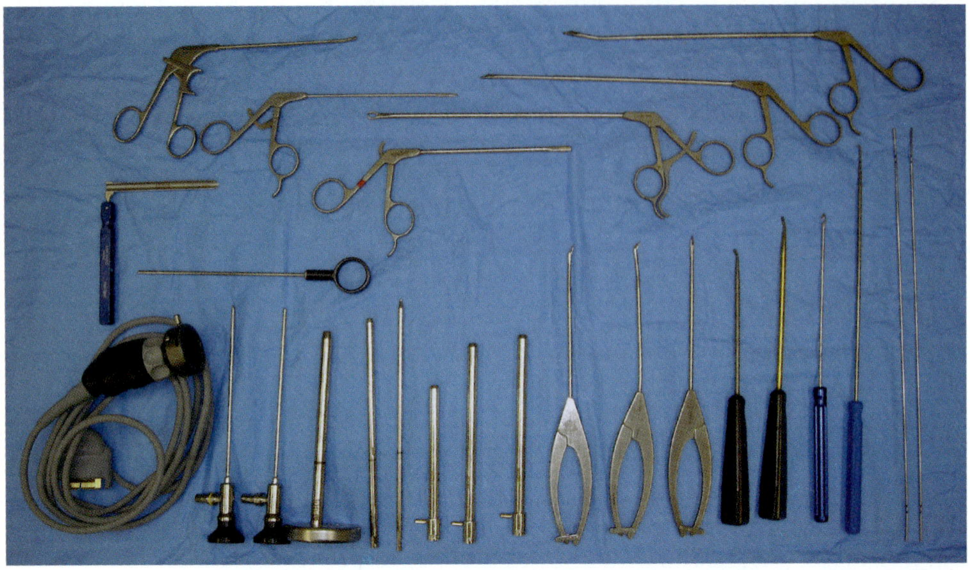

Figure 5.1. The basic back table setup with the instruments necessary for hip arthroscopy: A 30° and 70° arthroscope; two 6-in., 16-gauge spinal needles; two Nitinol guide wires; cannulated dilators and trochars for portal placement; 4.5, 5.0, and 5.5 mm cannulas; an extra-long probe, graspers, a loose body retriever; and routine suture passing and retrieving instruments.

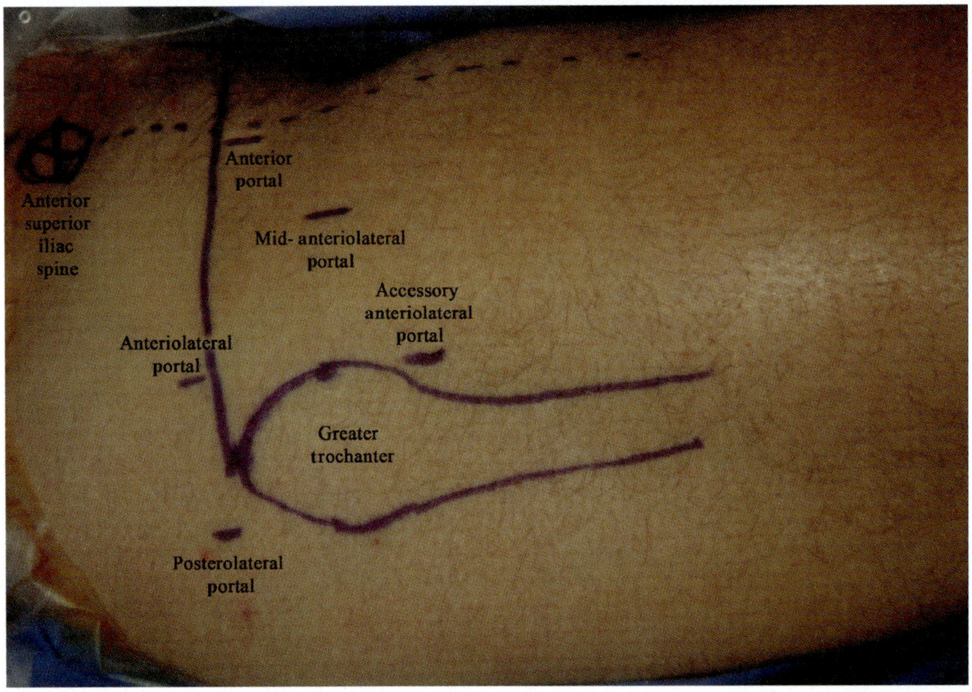

Figure 5.2. The common portals used for hip arthroscopy. The anterolateral portal is the most common introductory portal. This portal is positioned at the superior margin of the greater trochanter in line with its anterior border. The anterior portal is typically 1 cm lateral and 1 cm distal from the intersection of a sagittal line drawn down the middle of the anterior thigh and a transverse line drawn from the superior aspect of the greater trochanter to the superior aspect of the pubic bone. This portal is established under direct visualization from the anterolateral portal with the spinal needle aimed approximately 45° cephalad and 30° toward the midline from the skin entry site. The posterolateral portal is placed at the superior margin of the greater trochanter in line with its posterior border. Establishment of this portal is also facilitated by direct visualization. The midanterolateral portal is halfway between the anterior and anterolateral portals, about 2 cm distal to a line connecting the two portals. It is typically used in labral repairs, allowing for a better angle when placing anchors. The accessory anterolateral portal (AALP) is positioned approximately 3 to 5 cm distal to the anterolateral portal along the anterior border of the greater trochanter and allows for additional access to the peripheral compartment and debridement of the femoral neck.

45° cephalad and 30° toward the midline from the skin entry site,[37] but differing anatomic variations necessitate the aid of direct visualization from the arthroscope in the anterolateral portal when establishing the anterior portal. In particular, where excessive retroversion is encountered, the position of this portal may be more lateral and more distal. The nick and spread technique should also be utilized when creating this portal to protect the medial branch of the lateral femoral cutaneous nerve (LFCN).

The posterolateral portal is placed at the superior margin of the greater trochanter in line with its posterior border. Establishment of this portal is also facilitated by direct visualization, as this portal is approximately 3 cm from the sciatic nerve at the level of the

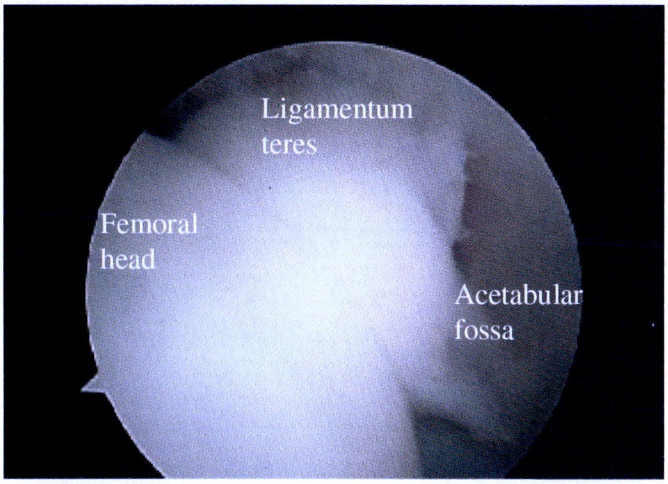

Figure 5.3. The medial wall of the acetabulum, the pulvinar, and the ligamentum teres of a left hip viewed from the anterolateral portal.

posterior hip capsule. It is important to avoid external rotation and excessive hip flexion during utilization of this portal as these positions can place the sciatic nerve at significant risk of injury.[42]

The accessory anterolateral portal (AALP) is positioned approximately 3 to 5 cm distal to the anterolateral portal along the anterior border of the greater trochanter. This portal is not utilized for the routine examination of the central compartment but does allow access to the peripheral compartment.

The midanterolateral portal (MAL) is halfway between the anterior and anterolateral portals, about 2 cm distal to a line connecting the two portals. It is typically used in labral repairs since it gives a better angle for anchor placement. In addition, it is also a good portal for debridement of the femoral neck. It can be used for both the resection as well as the visualization of the lesion while the anterolateral portal is used for the debridement.

Although these portals are planned for each arthroscopic procedure, it is important to note that because of the limited maneuverability within the hip joint, slight variations of these portals or even additional portals may be necessary to provide adequate exposure of the hip joint, reemphasizing the necessity of a precise knowledge of hip anatomy before performing an arthroscopic examination.

SURGICAL TECHNIQUE: DIAGNOSTIC ARTHROSCOPY

A SYSTEMATIC ARTHROSCOPIC EXAM OF THE HIP

We utilize a systematic arthroscopic examination of the central and peripheral compartments of the hip to increase the accuracy and reproducibility within each hip arthroscopy (Table 5.1). This standard approach ensures that all components of the hip are carefully inspected and allows for proper documentation that can be reviewed in the future. Additionally, a methodical technique allows us to compare arthroscopic findings with clinical presentations, further enhancing our diagnostic capabilities.

As previously mentioned, the anterolateral portal is always established as the introductory portal. Beginning with the 70° arthroscope our viewing progression is from the central to the anterior and then to the posterior aspects of the joint. With this progression, the structures visualized are the acetabular fossa, the posteromedial acetabular cartilage and labrum, the anterior triangle, the anterior labrum and paralabral sulcus, the posterolateral labrum, the posterior capsule, and the femoral head.

TABLE 5.1 Systematic Arthroscopic Examination of the Hip

Anterolateral portal
- Acetabular fossa
- Posteromedial acetabulum and labrum
- Anterior triangle
- Anterior labrum
- Posterolateral labrum
- Posterior capsule
- Femoral head

Anterior portal
- Ligamentum teres
- Posterior transverse ligament
- Anterior transverse ligament
- Superior acetabulum
- Lateral labrum
- Posterolateral capsule

Posterolateral portal
- Posterior gutter
- Weight-bearing acetabulum
- Anterolateral labrum
- Femoral head

Peripheral compartment
- Medial femoral neck
- Medial femoral head
- Anterior femoral head
- Lateral femoral head
- Lateral femoral neck
- Anterior femoral neck

After the arthroscope is introduced into the central compartment, the first landmark is easily attained by slowly withdrawing the arthroscope to gain perspective on the constituents of the medial wall of the acetabulum, which include the acetabular or cotyloid fossa, pulvinar, and ligamentum teres (Fig. 5.3). It is important to utilize this point for general orientation, but synovitis of the acetabular fossa and tears of the ligamentum teres are commonly seen from this perspective.[44]

The camera is then moved to visualize the posterior medial horn of the acetabular cartilage and labrum. With adequate distension, the posterior capsular reflection can also be observed in the background. The lens is then rotated superiorly and the camera is raised and retracted gently to visualize the anterior triangle, which is composed of the anterior capsule, anterior labrum, and femoral head (Fig. 5.4).

This structure is a very helpful landmark allowing for direct visualization of the spinal needle when establishing the anterior portal. Once the anterior portal is established, the camera is further retracted and the anterior labrum and paralabral sulcus are noted. Normally, the triangular anterior labrum blends with the acetabular cartilage inferiorly and paralabral sulcus superiorly. This is a common area to find labral tearing and degeneration.[9–16]

After further retraction of the arthroscope, the lens can be rotated inferiorly to view the lateral labrum and its attachment to the capsular sulcus. Pushing the camera inferiorly and rotating the lens superiorly helps visualize the posterior capsule

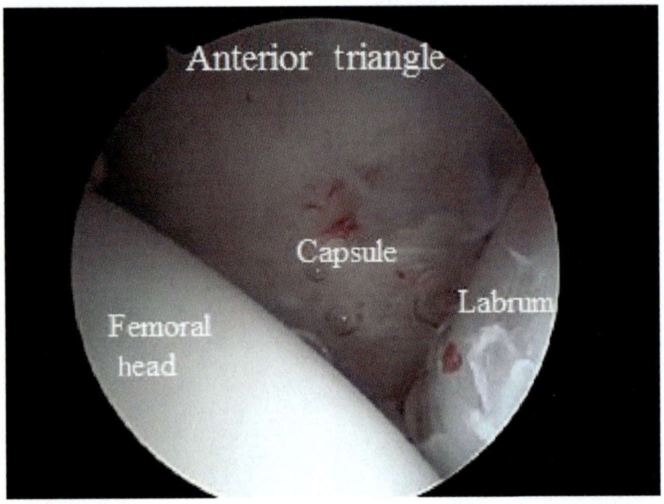

Figure 5.4. The anterior triangle of a left hip as seen from the anterolateral portal. The anterior triangle is composed of the anterior capsule, anterior labrum, and femoral head.

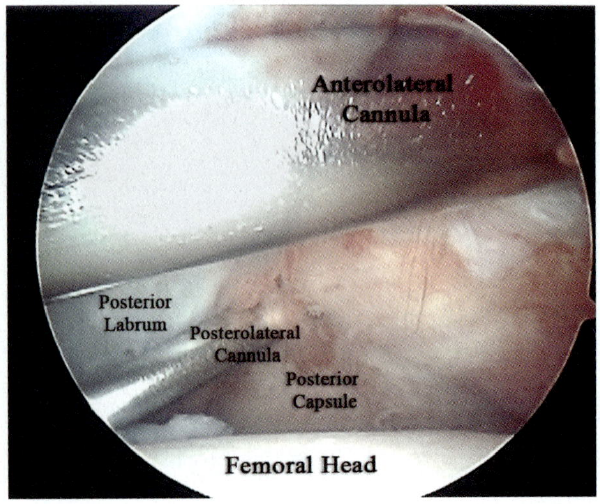

Figure 5.5. Establishment of the PL portal while viewing from the anterior portal of a left hip.

from its acetabular attachment to the concentric fibers of the zona orbicularis at the junction of the femoral head and neck. The last landmark through the anterolateral portal is obtained by pulling back the camera so that the cartilage of the femoral head can be examined from its inferior to superior margins. The leg is gently rotated internally and externally during this view to provide as much perspective as possible.

The 70° arthroscope is removed and placed over a guide wire into the joint from the previously established anterior portal. With the camera in the anterior portal, the joint is again inspected with an anteromedial-to-posterolateral viewing progression.

Similar to the anterolateral portal, the anterior examination begins in the medial fossa of the acetabulum. From this vantage point, the best view of the ligamentum teres can be obtained as it arises from the posteroinferior margin of the acetabulum and inserts onto the medial aspect of the femoral head.[2,37] Even subtle tears can be diagnosed with gentle rotation of the lower extremity. With adequate distraction, the camera can be gently maneuvered posteriorly into where the posterior aspect of the transverse ligament blends into the posteromedial labrum. This can be a place where articular loose bodies might reside.

Pulling the camera back and anterior to the ligamentum allows for a view of the next structure, which is the corresponding anterior aspect of the transverse ligament and its attachment to the anterior labrum. By rotating the lens laterally, the superior acetabular cartilage is seen. This inspection ends with the lateral labrum and point of entry for the anterolateral portal. This perspective provides an excellent viewpoint to aid in diagnosis, and debridement or repair of most labral tears.

The camera is then pushed past the anterolateral portal exposing the posterolateral capsule and allows for precise posterolateral portal placement under direct visualization (Fig. 5.5).

Once the placement of the posterolateral portal is satisfactory, the skin is incised and the arthroscope is placed over a guide wire into the posterolateral aspect of the joint. From this portal, the posterior capsule, the weight-bearing portion of the acetabulum, the AL labrum, and the femoral head can be visualized well.

From the medial notch, the arthroscope is slowly withdrawn and moved inferiorly over the posterior labrum into the inferior gutter, which runs from the capsular attachment on the posterior and medial acetabulum to the thickened cylindrical sleeve of the orbicular ligament that surrounds the femoral neck. The lens of the scope is then rotated cranially and advanced to see the weight-bearing dome of the acetabulum. This area is often where cartilage degeneration and cystic formation within the acetabulum is best appreciated. The camera is then translated superiorly to gain another vantage point of the AL labrum. Finally, by rotating the lens, the femoral head can be observed from the posterior aspect. The camera should slide tangentially along the cartilage surface in an effort to observe as much of the femoral head as possible.

After the appropriate treatment of any pathology diagnosed in the central compartment, the extremity is taken out of traction and the hip is positioned in approximately 45° of flexion. This relaxes the anterior capsule and ligaments and allows for an adequate inspection of the peripheral compartment. Similar to the method described by Dienst et al.,[45] a long spinal needle is directed from the anterolateral portal toward the medial physeal scar of the femoral head.

The visual flow once inside the peripheral compartment is from medial to lateral along the femoral head and then from lateral to medial along the femoral neck. There are six landmarks commonly inspected within the peripheral compartment, which include the medial femoral neck, the medial femoral head, the anterior femoral head, the lateral femoral head, the lateral femoral neck, and the anterior femoral neck.

Upon entering the peripheral compartment from the anterolateral portal, the initial view is typically of the medial neck. If the camera is oriented so that it is looking down upon the femoral neck, the first anatomic complex is a very consistent landmark, comprising the orbicular ligament, the medial synovial fold, and the femoral neck (Fig. 5.6).

Like the acetabular fossa and the ligamentum teres in the central compartment, the medial synovial fold and orbicular ligament serve as excellent orientation landmarks. This is very important, as correct orientation is the foundation of correct arthroscopic diagnosis and treatment.

From the medial neck, the camera is directed superiorly and slowly retracted as it is gently maneuvered under the orbicular

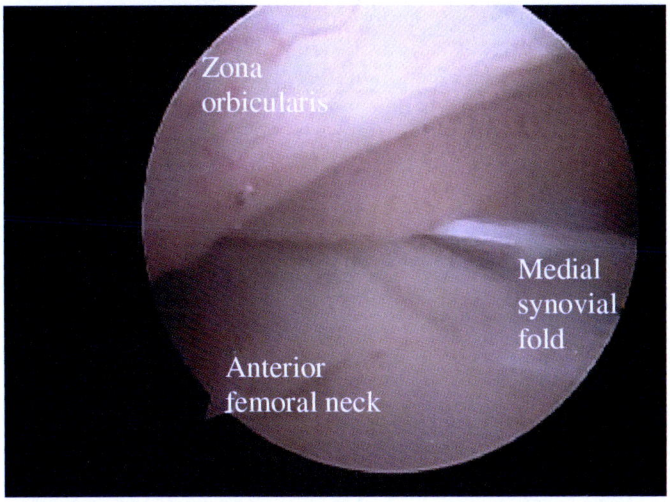

Figure 5.6. Anatomic landmark of the arthroscopic examination of the hip within the peripheral compartment of a left hip comprising the orbicular ligament, medial synovial fold, and femoral neck.

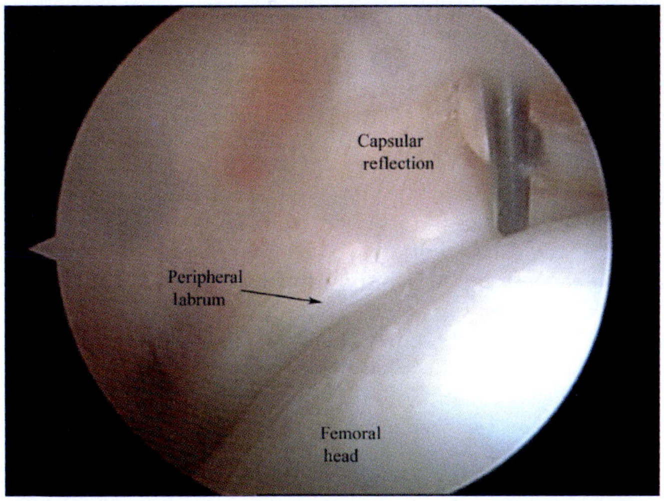

Figure 5.7. The lateral labrum and femoral head as viewed from the peripheral compartment of a left hip.

ligament, sliding into the medial gutter. It is not uncommon for loose bodies to hide in this area. After viewing the medial gutter, the scope can be rotated laterally, sliding along the entirety of the anterior femoroacetabular interface to visualize the anterior and lateral labrum and the femoral head.

The anterior capsule is usually too stiff to allow inspection past the lateral aspect of the labrum and femoral head. Therefore, the posterolateral aspect of the peripheral compartment is not a point on our routine examination. On rare occasions, however, the hip can be flexed and abducted to 45°, allowing the arthroscope to pass between the lateral synovial fold and the orbicular ligament into the posterolateral area. This area is small as the posterior joint capsule insertion is 2 to 3 cm proximal to that of the anterior capsule.[46] In our experience, this posterior area is easier to access after an adequate capsular release and femoral neck debridement.

From the lateral aspect of the femoral head, the camera is withdrawn distally to arrive at the lateral aspect of the femoral neck. From here, the fibers of the orbicular ligament can be seen from the peripheral compartment side and correspond nicely to the previous view from the central compartment (Fig. 5.7).

This is also the most common area for the cam lesion commonly seen with femoroacetabular impingement (Fig. 5.8).[27,47–50] With a view of the lateral femoral neck, the leg is flexed and internally rotated to document impingement of the femoral neck with the lateral acetabulum.

From the lateral neck the arthroscope is rotated medially to view the anterior neck. Unlike the medial and lateral synovial folds, the anterior synovial fold is tightly adherent to the anterior femoral neck and is rarely a distinct anatomic entity. The arthroscope is then pushed toward the medial neck where the orbicular ligament and medial synovial fold again come into view. This completes the round trip of the peripheral compartment and our systematic arthroscopic examination of the hip.

COMPLICATIONS

A meta-analysis of the literature detailing complications after 2,049 hip arthroscopies revealed a complication rate of

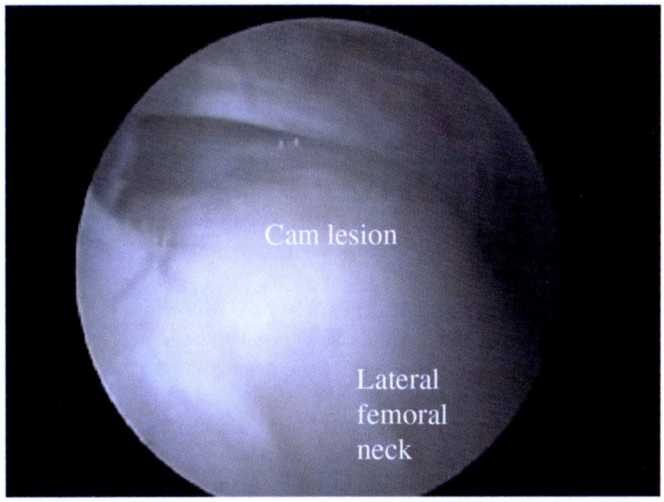

Figure 5.8. An example of a CAM lesion on the anterolateral aspect of the femoral neck.

2.2%.[51–56] Of these injuries, only 0.3% were permanent. Most of the injuries reported consisted of a transient neurapraxia that resolved within a few days. The pudendal nerve was the most common neurapraxia described, but transient neurapraxias of the femoral, sciatic, lateral femoral cutaneous, and peroneal nerves have all been reported. Eriksson et al.[51] also reported a case of pressure necrosis of the scrotum, and Rodeo et al.[55] described a case of pressure necrosis of the foot. In order to prevent these complications, meticulous attention must be paid to patient positioning and time of traction during each procedure. Traction should be intermittently released during prolonged procedures. It is important to note, however, that almost all of these reported injuries were prior to the adoption of the oversized, heavily padded perineal post that is currently available.[56]

Nerve injury can also occur secondary to direct laceration. Injury to the larger nerves surrounding the hip can be avoided by a precise knowledge of the anatomy and landmarks of the hip previously described.[56] The LFCN, however, is always at risk when establishing the anterior portal.[55] Therefore, a nick and spread technique should be utilized when creating this portal. Even with meticulous technique, however, reports of neurapraxia after forceful instrumentation and/or large, loose body removal have been reported.[56]

Although nerve injuries are the most commonly reported complication after hip arthroscopy, Byrd contends that the single most common complication is actually damage to the articular and labral surfaces, secondary to "scope trauma."[56] To avoid labral damage, it is important to re-enter the central compartment after initial insufflation of the joint. It is also important to note that from the anterolateral portal, instruments should always be angled so that they penetrate the capsule from underneath the labrum. The instruments can then be redirected superiorly to avoid scuffing of the femoral head. It is also possible for instruments to break secondary to vigorous levering against the sturdy envelope that surrounds the hip joint. Passing all arthroscopic instruments into the hip through sturdy metallic sheaths can help to minimize this complication.

Other rare but potential complications include heterotopic ossification (HO), avascular necrosis (AVN) of the femoral head, and fluid extravasation. HO is a relatively common complication of open hip and pelvis surgery. There is only one reported case, however, of HO along the anterior portal tract after hip arthroscopy.[48] The femoral head receives its blood supply from a tenuous vascular anastomosis.[47] Although there have been no reports of AVN as a direct consequence of hip arthroscopy, there are at least two reports of AVN progression following hip arthroscopy.[53,56] Whether this progression was secondary to the arthroscopic procedure or the natural history of the disease has not been determined. In light of these anecdotal reports, however, some contend that hip arthroscopy is contraindicated in patients with stable AVN.[2,53]

Fluid extravasation into the pelvis or abdominal regions is also an uncommon complication; but this can be potentially devastating. Bartlett reported a case of cardiac arrest resulting from the intra-abdominal extravasation of fluid during a loose body removal in a patient with an acetabular fracture. To reduce the risk of fluid extravasation, careful attention should be given to fluid management, especially when excessive surgery time is necessary and/or the hip joint and capsule are compromised.

Finally, although infection is a risk with any surgical procedure, the overall incidence of infection after hip arthroscopy is only 0.05%. In general, then, although surgeons should be keenly aware of the potential complications surrounding hip arthroscopy, they are relatively uncommon, especially if the early experiences with hip arthroscopy are extracted.

SUMMARY AND CONCLUSION

Currently, there is an unprecedented enthusiasm for hip arthroscopy, as this modality is transforming the management of hip injuries. Paramount to effective arthroscopy within any joint, however, is careful preoperative planning, precise portal placement, knowledge of the potential complications, and a methodical sequence of arthroscopic examination progressing from one part of the joint cavity to another systematically in each operative case.

Our systematic arthroscopic examination of the central and peripheral compartments ensures that all components of the hip are carefully inspected and increases the accuracy and reproducibility of diagnostic hip arthroscopy. This standard arthroscopic method also helps differentiate normal structures from their pathologic counterparts. Additionally, it allows us to correlate arthroscopic findings with clinical presentations, enhancing our diagnostic abilities and providing better clinical outcome studies. As new indications and techniques evolve within hip arthroscopy, this standardized approach to diagnostic hip arthroscopy provides a solid foundation.

REFERENCES

1. Burman M. Arthroscopy or the direct visualization of joints. *J Bone Joint Surg.* 1931;4:669–695.
2. Kelly BT, Riley JW III, Philippon MJ. Hip arthroscopy: Current indications, treatment options, and management issues. *Am J Sports Med.* 2003;31:1020–1037.
3. Byrd JWT. The role of hip arthroscopy in the athletic hip. *Clin Sports Med.* 2006;25:255–278.
4. Byrd JWT. Hip arthroscopy for post-traumatic loose fragments in the young active adult: Three case reports. *Clin Sport Med.* 1996;6:129–134.
5. Krebs VE. The role of hip arthroscopy in the treatment of synovial disorders and loose bodies. *Clin Orthop Relat Res.* 2003;406:48–59.
6. Okada Y, Awaya G, Ikeda T. Arthroscopic surgery for synovial chondromatosis of the hip. *J Bone Joint Surg.* 1989;71B:198–199.
7. Vakili F, Salvati EA, Warren RF. Entrapped foreign body within the acetabular cup in total hip replacement. *Clin Orthop Relat Res.* 1980;150:159–162.
8. Fitzgerald RH Jr. Acetabular labrum tears: Diagnosis and treatment. *Clin Orthop Relat Res.* 1995;311:60–68.
9. Mason JB. Acetabular labral tears in the athlete. *Clin Sports Med.* 2001;20:779–790.
10. Ueo T, Suzuki S, Iwasaki R, et al. Rupture of the labra acetabularis as a cause of hip pain detected arthroscopically, and partial limbectomy for successful pain relief. *Arthroscopy.* 1990;6(1):48–51.
11. Lage LA, Patel JV, Villar RN. The acetabular labral tear: An arthroscopic classification. *Arthroscopy.* 1996;12(3):269–272.
12. Philippon MJ. Debridement of acetabular labral tears with associated thermal capsulorrhaphy. *Oper Tech Sports Med.* 2002;10:215–218.
13. Dameron T. Bucket-handle tear of acetabular labrum accompanying posterior dislocation of the hip. *J Bone Joint Surg.* 1959;41A:131–134.
14. Santori N, Villar RN. Acetabular labral tears: Result of arthroscopic partial limbectomy. *Arthroscopy.* 2000;16(1):11–15.
15. Byrd JWT, Jones KS. Inverted acetabular labrum and secondary osteoarthritis: Radiographic diagnosis and arthroscopic treatment. *Arthroscopy.* 2000;16(4):417.
16. Ikeda T, Awaya G, Suzuki S. Torn acetabular labrum in young patients: Arthroscopic diagnosis and management. *J Bone Joint Surg.* 1988;70B:13–16.
17. Byrd JWT, Jones KS. Microfracture for grade IV chondral lesions of the hip. *Arthroscopy.* 2004;20(4):385–391.
18. Byrd JW. Lateral impact injury: A source of occult hip pathology. *Clin Sports Med.* 2001;20:801–815.
19. Philippon MJ. Arthroscopy of the hip: The management of the athlete. In: McGinty JB, ed. *Operative Arthroscopy.* 3rd Ed. Philadelphia, PA: Lippincott Williams & Wilkins; 2003, pp. 879–883.
20. Bowen JR, Kumar VP, Joyce JJ, et al. Osteochondritis dissecans following Perthes' disease: Arthroscopic-operative treatment. *Clin Orthop Relat Res.* 1986;209:49–56.
21. Gray AJ, Villar RN. The ligamentum teres of the hip: An arthroscopic classification of its pathology. *Arthroscopy.* 1997;13:575–578.
22. Rao J, Zhou YX, Villar RN. Injury to the ligamentum teres: Mechanism, findings, and results of treatment. *Clin Sports Med.* 2001;20:791–799.
23. Faraj AA, Moulton A, Sirivastava VM. Snapping iliotibial band: Report of ten cases and review of the literature. *Acta Orthop Belg.* 2001;67:19–23.
24. Jacobson T, Allen WC. Surgical correction of the snapping iliopsoas tendon. *Am J Sports Med.* 1990;18:470–474.
25. Dobbs MB, Gordon JE, Luhmann SJ. Surgical correction of the snapping iliopsoas tendon in adolescents. *J Bone Joint Surg.* 2002:84A:420–424.
26. Gruen GS, Scioscia TN, Lowenstein JE. The surgical treatment of internal snapping hip. *Am J Sports Med.* 2002;30:607–613.
27. Ganz R, Parvizi J, Beck M. Femoroacetabular impingement: A cause for osteoarthritis of the hip. *Clin Orthop.* 2003;417:112–120.
28. Guanche CA, Bare AA. Arthroscopic treatment of femoroacetabular impingement. *Arthroscopy.* 2006;22(1):95–106.
29. Janssens X, Van Meirhaeghe J, Verdonk R. Diagnostic arthroscopy of the hip joint in pigmented villonodular synovitis. *Arthroscopy.* 1987;3:283–287.
30. McCarthy JC, Bono JV, Wardell S. Is there a treatment for synovial chondromatosis of the hip joint? *Arthroscopy.* 1997;6(2):129–134.
31. Sim FH. Synovial proliferative disorders: Role of synovectomy. *Arthroscopy.* 1985;1(3):198–204.
32. Chung WK, Slater GL, Bates EH. Treatment of septic arthritis of the hip by arthroscopic lavage. *J Pediatr Orthop.* 1993;13:444–446.
33. Bould M, Edwards D, Villar RN. Arthroscopic diagnosis and treatment of septic arthritis of the hip joint. *Arthroscopy.* 1993;9(6):707–708.
34. Byrd JWT. Indications and contraindications. In: Byrd JWT, ed. *Operative Hip Arthroscopy.* 2nd Ed. New York: Springer; 2005, pp. 6–35.
35. Lavernia CJ, Sierra RJ, Grieco FR. Osteonecrosis of the femoral head. *J Am Acad Orthop Surg.* 1999;7:250–261.
36. Steinberg ME. Osteonecrosis of the hip: Summary and conclusions. *Semin Arthroplasty.* 1991;2:241–249.

37. Glick JM. Hip arthroscopy: The lateral approach. *Clin Sports Med.* 2001;20:733–747.
38. Glick JM. Hip arthroscopy using the lateral approach. *Instr Course Lect.* 1988;37:223–231.
39. Glick JM, Sampson TG, Gordon RB. Hip arthroscopy by the lateral approach. *Arthroscopy.* 1987;3:4–12.
40. Sweeney HJ. Arthroscopy of the hip: Anatomy and portals. *Clin Sports Med.* 2001;20:697–702.
41. Byrd JWT, Pappas, JN, Pedley MJ. Hip arthroscopy: An anatomic study of portal placement and relationship to the extraarticular structures. *Arthroscopy.* 1995;11(4):418–423.
42. Ide T, Akamatsu N, Nakajima I. Arthroscopic surgery of the hip joint. *Arthroscopy.* 1991;7(2):204–211.
43. Dorfmann H, Boyer T, Henry P, et al. A simple approach to hip arthroscopy. *Arthroscopy.* 1988;4(2):141–142.
44. Byrd JWT. Avoiding the labrum in hip arthroscopy. *Arthroscopy.* 2000;16(7):770–773.
45. Dienst M, Gödde S, Seil R, et al. Hip arthroscopy without traction: In vivo anatomy of the peripheral hip joint cavity. *Arthroscopy.* 2001;17(9):924–931.
46. Byrd JWT. Gross anatomy. In: Byrd JWT, ed. *Operative Hip Arthroscopy.* 2nd Ed. New York: Springer; 2005, pp. 69–83.
47. Lavigne M, Parvizi J, Beck M. Anterior femoroacetabular impingement. Part I: Technique of joint preserving surgery. *Clin Orthop Relat Res.* 2004;413:61–66.
48. Beck M, Leunig M, Parvizi J. Anterior femoroacetabular impingement. Part II: Midterm results of surgical treatment. *Clin Orthop Relat Res.* 2004;418:67–73.
49. Ito K, Minka M, Leunig M. Femoroacetabular impingement and the cam-effect. *J Bone Joint Surg Br.* 2001;83:171–176.
50. Murphy S, Tannast M, Kim YJ. Debridement of the adult hip for femoroacetabular impingement: Indications and preliminary clinical results. *Clin Orthop Relat Res.* 2004;429:178–181.
51. Eriksson E, Arvidsson I, Arvidsson H. Diagnostic and operative arthroscopy of the hip. *Orthopedics.* 1998;9:169–176.
52. Byrd JWT. Complications associated with hip arthroscopy. In: Byrd JWT, ed. *Operative Hip Arthroscopy.* 2nd Ed. New York: Springer; 2005, pp. 171–176.
53. Glick JM. Complications of hip arthroscopy by the lateral approach. In: Sherman OH, Minkoff J, eds. *Current Management of Complications in Orthopaedics. Arthroscopic Surgery.* Baltimore, MD: Williams & Wilkins; 1990, pp. 193–201.
54. Sampson TG. Complications of hip arthroscopy. *Clin Sports Med.* 2001;20:831–835.
55. Rodeo SA, Forster RA, Weiland AJ. Neurological complications due to arthroscopy. *J Bone Joint Surg.* 1993;75A:917–926.
56. Villar RN. *Hip Arthroscopy.* Oxford: Butterworth-Heinemann; 1992, pp. 1570–1575.

CHAPTER

6

Victor M. Ilizaliturri Jr.
Javier Camacho-Galindo

Position and Setup: The Lateral Approach

Arthroscopically, the hip joint can be divided into two separate compartments; the central compartment or iliofemoral joint and the peripheral compartment, which is the extra-articular but intracapsular portion of the hip joint.[1] Traction is necessary to provide access to the central compartment by separating the femoral head from the acetabulum. There are two different ways to position a patient for hip arthroscopy: supine and lateral. The first to be introduced was the supine position because it used existing operating room technology: fracture tables were utilized in hip arthroscopy as they were designed to provide traction for reduction of hip fractures.[2] The lateral position was introduced by Dr James Glick and Dr Thomas Sampson from San Francisco. They reported that it was especially useful in patients with morbid obesity.[3] This technique was adopted and further developed by Dr Joseph McCarthy in Boston.[4]

Parallel to the development of the lateral position for hip arthroscopy, Dr Thomas Byrd from Nashville became the champion of the supine position in hip arthroscopy and influenced many surgeons.[5] The supine position is the most commonly used position for hip arthroscopy in North America. It has the advantage of using standard fracture tables which are existing operating room equipment in almost every hospital. For the lateral position, special accessories for fracture tables or dedicated hip distractors are mandatory. Two of the most popular lateral hip distractors are the McCarthy hip distractor by Innomed (Savannah, GA) and the Smith & Nephew Lateral Hip Arthroscopy Distractor (Andover, MA).

The need for special traction equipment was a disadvantage of the lateral position, but the recent increase in the number of surgeons performing hip arthroscopy in addition to the fact that many procedures are being done in surgery centers may resume interest in the lateral position because dedicated distractors for the lateral position are economically more accessible than fracture tables and dedicated distractors for the supine position.

Most of the hip arthroscopy procedures in the 1990s were performed only at the central compartment.[4,6] Early in this decade, anatomy and access techniques to the peripheral compartment were popularized by Dr Michael Dienst in Germany[1] and the concept of femoroacetabular impingement[7] was introduced to the world of hip arthroscopy by Dr Thomas Sampson[8] which changed hip arthroscopy and introduced routine arthroscopy of the hip periphery. In both, the supine and the lateral approach, patient positioning should allow for a dynamic surgical procedure with steps with and without traction and some range of motion of the hip joint.[9,10]

ANESTHESIA

The procedure is performed with epidural anesthesia, which usually provides a good motor block and consequent muscle relaxation. Patients remain hospitalized for one day.

PATIENT POSITIONING

The patient is positioned lateral, resting on the nonoperative side on a fracture table with special accessories (Maquet, Rastatt, Germany). A horizontal perineal post of 10 cm in diameter is positioned horizontally on the operating table (Fig. 6.1). The perineal post is positioned laterally on the medial thigh and is elevated to provide a lateralization vector to the traction force (Fig. 6.2). The lateralization also distances the post from the pudendal nerve. The ipsolateral foot to the surgical side is fixed to the traction device of the fracture table. The nonoperative lower limb rests free on the table. When the lateral position for hip arthroscopy is utilized, the opposite limb is not fixed to a traction device because the body weight and the length of the nonoperative limb will stabilize and avoid pelvic tilt. In the case of the supine position, pelvic tilt is avoided by fixing the opposite foot to a traction device. Before traction is applied, the patients' genitalia should be inspected to verify that they are free of compression.

The hip is positioned in flexion of 20° to relax the anterior hip capsule. Flexion of more than 20° does not improve distraction of the hip joint and increases the possibility of injury to the sciatic nerve. Abduction is kept neutral to maximize separation of the iliofemoral joint. Neutral rotation is preferred while establishing arthroscopic portals to maximize the distance between the posterior edge of the greater trochanter and the sciatic nerve.[11]

The C-arm is positioned horizontally under the table to provide an anteroposterior view of the hip. A traction test is

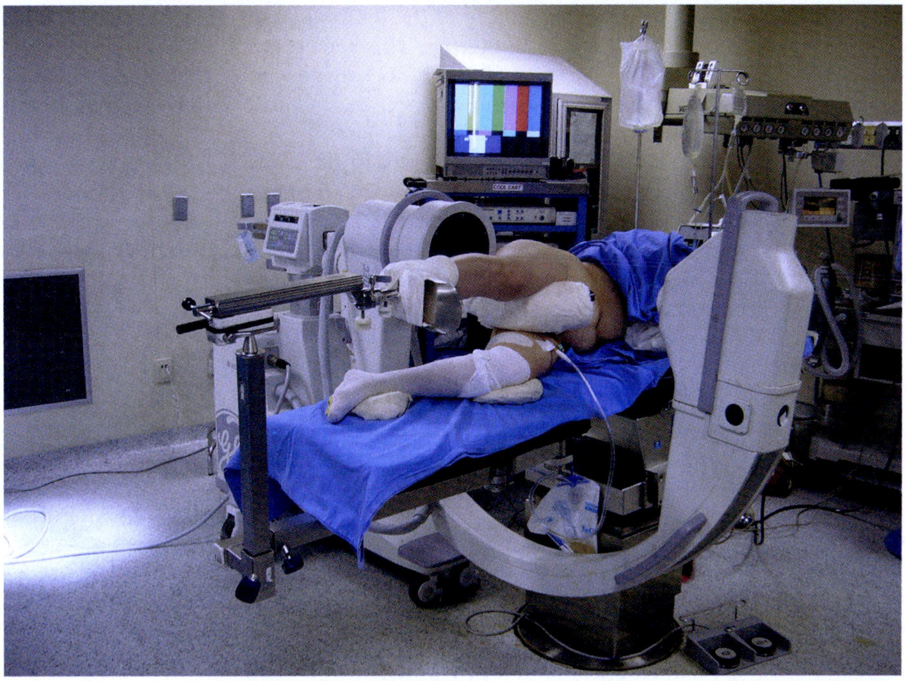

Figure 6.1. This photograph demonstrates a patient positioned for arthroscopy of the right hip in left lateral decubitus on a Maquet fracture table (Rastatt, Germany). Only the right foot is fixed to a traction device; pelvic tilt is avoided by the body weight and the opposite lower limb resting on the operating table. A horizontal perineal post is observed resting against the medial aspect of the right thigh. A C-arm is positioned horizontally under the operating table.

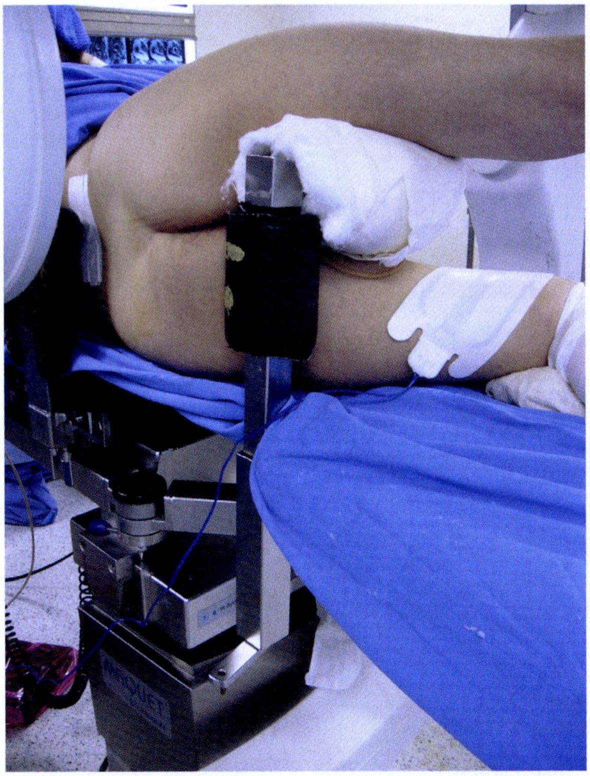

A

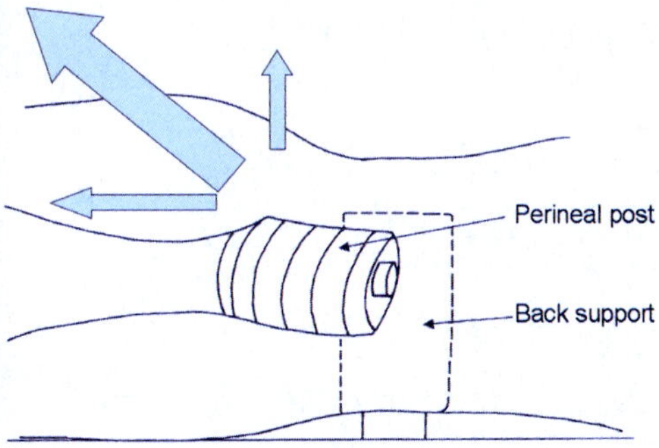

B

Figure 6.2. **A:** This photograph demonstrates a close-up of a patient positioned for arthroscopy of the right hip on left lateral decubitus. The perineal post has been "extra-padded" with cotton to increase the contact surface with the medial thigh and reduce the possibility of compression injury to the pudendal nerve. The perineal post has been elevated to rest against the medial thigh. The crank mechanism that elevates the post is at the bottom of the photograph. The posterior lumbosacral support prevents rollback on the perineal post especially when hip arthroscopy without traction is performed. **B:** Schematic representation of traction force. Note how the vector of traction is not straight distal but a combination of a distal and lateralizing force relative to the position of the hip. The traction vector roughly follows the direction of the femoral neck.

performed to confirm effective separation of the femoral head from the acetabulum at the image intensifier. This separation should be of at least 10 mm.[4] When separation does not occur, the foot fixation should be verified. In our experience, the most common reason for ineffective traction is loosening and migration of the foot in the traction device. The foot must be firmly fixed to the traction device and well padded to avoid compression injuries. There are different options available for foot fixation to the traction device. The "ski boot" design introduced by McCarthy provides a stable foot fixation and adequate padding. Most of the fracture tables provide boots with Velcro straps or belt-buckles. Velcro straps are usually better and more durable than belt-buckles. A low cost alternative is to use cotton wrapping on the foot for padding and firmly fix the foot to the traction device using ace bandages protected with surgical tape. If done adequately, this technique is effective and reproducible (Fig. 6.3). After a successful traction test is performed, the hip is flexed 35°, abducted and externally rotated to confirm mobility of the setup. This mobility will provide adequate access to the hip periphery (Fig. 6.4). The hip is brought back to neutral position and the surgical area prepared for surgery.

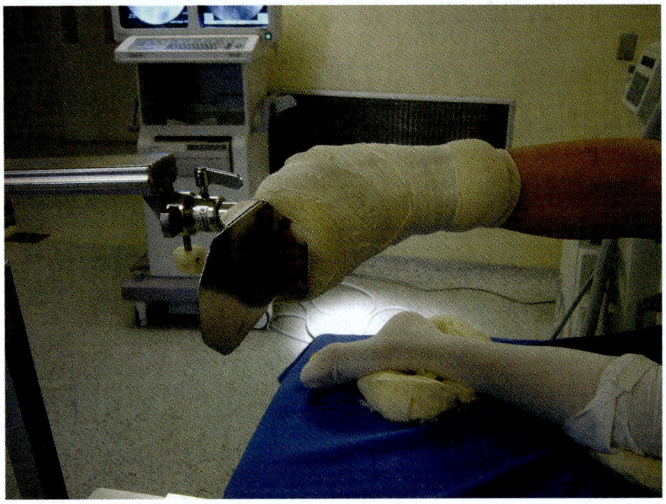

Figure 6.3. Cotton wrapping and Ace bandage-surgical tape fixation of the foot to the traction device.

When applying sterile drapes, we first start by covering both ends of the C-arm using sterile bags. Then waterproof adhesive sterile drapes are placed in a standard fashion. The surgeon should be careful not to cover portal sites with the drapes. The medial drape should be slightly medial to the anterior superior iliac spine. The posterior drape should be behind the posterior edge of the greater trochanter. The superior drape should be at the level of the anterior superior iliac spine and the distal drape should be 10 to 15 cm below the tip of the greater trochanter. After drapes are in position, a sterile gauze is placed over the area where the portals will be established and an adhesive transparent surgical drape is placed over the surgical area (including the gauze) (Fig. 6.5). This seal will prevent fluid from leaking under the drapes to the patient when the procedure starts.

After cables and tubes for arthroscopy are ready, traction is applied (traction starting time should be recorded to monitor its duration). With the traction established, the gauze is removed form the surgical area with the adhesive drape that covers it, landmarks are identified and marked on the skin with a skin marker (we prefer to mark the skin after traction is applied to avoid migration of the marks) (Fig. 6.6).

CHECKLIST FOR LATERAL PATIENT POSITIONING IN HIP ARTHROSCOPY

1. Horizontal perineal post with extra padding (10 cm diameter). The post is positioned against the medial thigh and elevated for lateralization and to protect the pudendal nerve.
2. Only the foot of the operative side is fixed to the traction device. Adequate padding and firm fixation are mandatory.

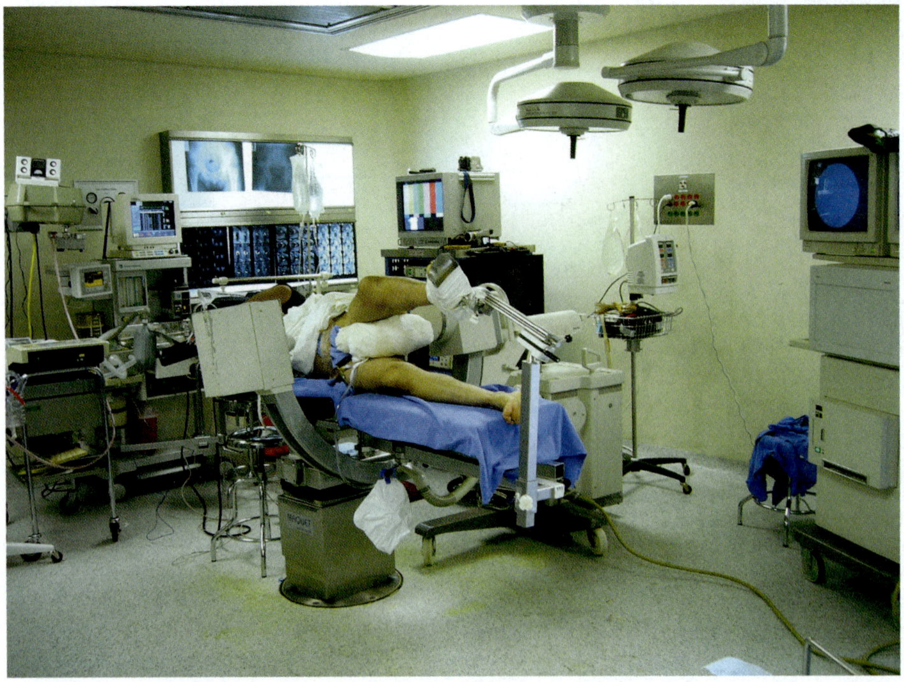

Figure 6.4. This photograph demonstrates a patient positioned for arthroscopy of the left hip in right lateral decubitus. The hip is flexed 35°, abducted, and externally rotated to relax the anterior hip capsule and provide access to the peripheral compartment. More abduction and external rotation will provide a lateral view of the hip at the image intensifier (a lateral view is needed when cam type femoroacetabular impingement is treated).

3. The hip must be in slight flexion (15° to 20°), neutral rotation, and 0° of abduction before traction.
4. The C-arm is positioned horizontally under the table. In obese patients, the C-arm may not be big enough to provide an AP view of the operative hip. If that is the case, it can be positioned over the patient with the arch inclined in the direction of the patient's head.

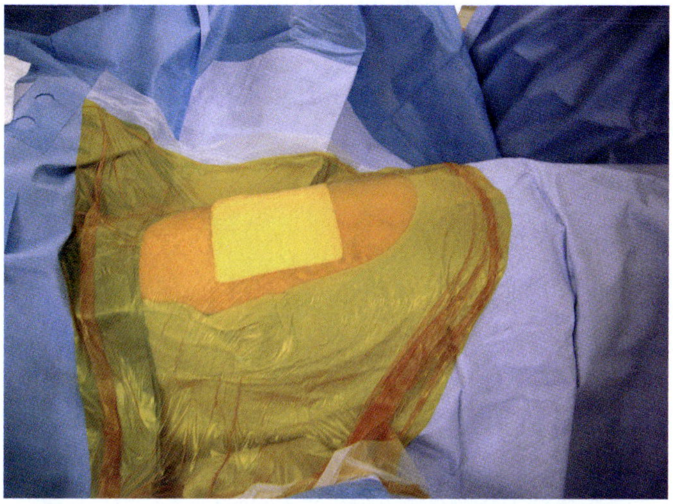

Figure 6.5. This photograph demonstrates a patient positioned for arthroscopy of the right hip in left lateral decubitus. The photograph was taken from the back side of the patient. Waterproof adhesive drapes are in position. The gauze is under the transparent adhesive surgical drape covering the portal sites.

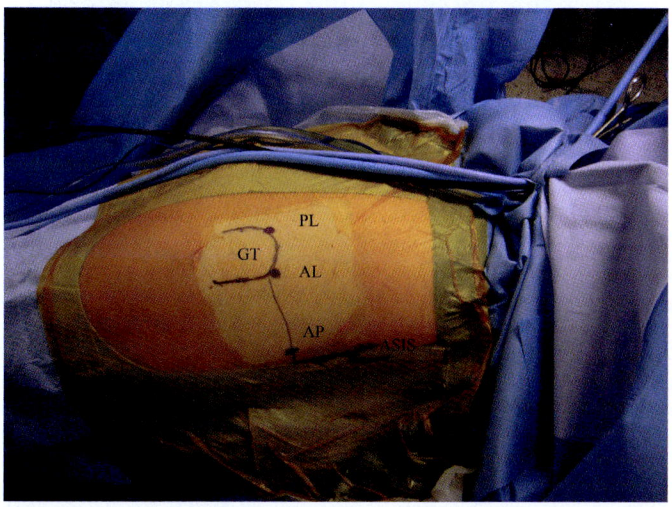

Figure 6.6. This photograph demonstrates a patient positioned for arthroscopy of the right hip in left lateral decubitus. The photograph was taken from the front side of the patient. The gauze was removed, leaving a window on the transparent adhesive surgical drape. The remaining surgical drape will create a waterproof seal to keep the patient dry during the operation. The greater trochanter (GT) and the anterior superior iliac spine (ASIS) have been marked on the skin. The anterolateral portal (AL) is at the anterior superior corner of the greater trochanter. The posterolateral portal (PL) is at the posterior superior corner of the greater trochanter. The anterior portal (AP) is 1 cm lateral to the crossing of a vertical line descending from the anterior superior iliac spine and a horizontal line directed anteriorly from the tip of the greater trochanter (we prefer to outline anatomical landmarks on the skin after traction has been applied to avoid migration of the skin marks).

5. A traction test is performed before preparing the surgical site. Separation of at least 10 mm between the acetabulum and femoral head should be achieved.
6. After the traction test, the hip is flexed to 35°, abducted, and externally rotated. A close-to-lateral view of the hip is confirmed at the image intensifier in this position.
7. The hip is brought to a neutral position.
8. The surgical area is prepared and draped for surgery.
9. After passage of cables and tubes for arthroscopy, traction is started.
10. Skin landmarks are identified and marked with the traction on.
11. The case is started.

ROOM SETUP AND EQUIPMENT

Arthroscopic access to the hip joint is not an outstanding technical achievement.[9] Safe and reproducible access depends on using an effective traction device properly, adequate fluoroscopic navigation, and specially designed hip arthroscopy instruments all combined with good surgical technique.

Because we position the patient lateral, in our setup, the surgeon stands in front of the patient to have better access to the anterior aspects of the hip (most of the pathology in the hip joint is anterior). The surgical assistant stands in front of the surgeon at the back side of the patient. This is a very convenient position for assisting during the operation. The arthroscopy tower is positioned at the back side of the patient, far to the side of the head, this allows the surgeon to have a direct and unobstructed view of the arthroscopy monitor and provides an adequate view to the assistant standing in front of the surgeon (Fig. 6.7). An arthroscopy suite with multiple monitors will provide an even better view to the assistant. The C-arm is under the operating table horizontally to provide an AP view of the hip throughout the case. If a lateral view is needed, it is achieved by moving the hip joint rather than the C-arm. The screens of the image intensifier are positioned at the back side of the patient, far to the side of the feet to provide a direct unobstructed view to the surgeon and an adequate view to the assistant standing in front of the surgeon. The scrub nurse is at the same side as the surgeon towards the feet of the patient. The anesthesiologist is at the usual position.

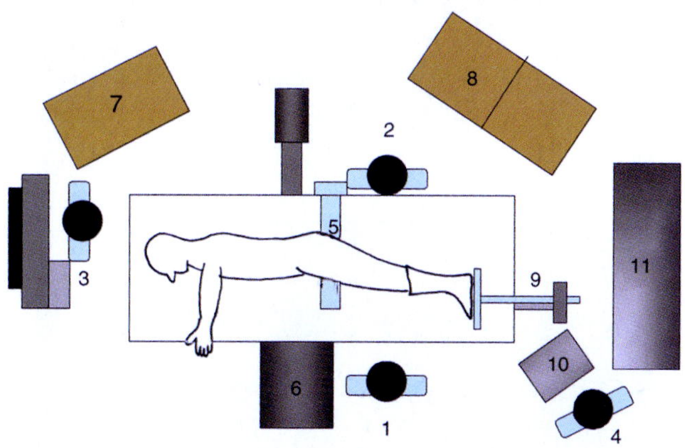

Figure 6.7. Schematic of the operating room setup. **1**: Surgeon, **2**: assistant, **3**: anesthesiologist, **4**: scrub nurse, **5**: perineal post, **6**: C-arm, **7**: arthroscopy tower, **8**: image intensifier monitors, **9**: traction device, **10**: Mayo stand, and **11**: back table.

We use a Maquet fracture table with special accessories for lateral traction (Rastatt, Germany), an image intensifier and an arthroscopy tower including the monitor, a digital camera, a high flow low pressure arthroscopy pump, saver and radiofrequency control console, and an image processing system.

We utilize the Hip Access System (Smith & Nephew, Andover, MA), which is a hip arthroscopy system based on a slotted cannula and designed to be used in combination with standard length 4.0 mm arthroscopes of 30° and 70°.

GENERAL TECHNIQUE

Three portals have been described to access the central compartment in hip arthroscopy: the anterolateral, posterolateral, and direct anterior.[12] The order in which these portals are established may vary between authors. The anterolateral portal, located at the anterior corner of the greater trochanter is always established first because it lies in the middle of the safety zone, which is limited posteriorly by the posterior edge of the greater trochanter. The sciatic nerve lies approximately 1.5 cm posterior to the femur.[12] The anterior limit is a vertical line descending from the anterior superior iliac spine, and the femoral neurovascular bundle lies medial to this line.[12]

With traction applied, the patient prepared, and landmarks marked on the skin, we start by introducing a 17-gauge spinal needle at the site of the anterolateral portal. The needle is navigated into the joint using fluoroscopy. Even though the anterolateral portal is at the center of the safe zone, it has the highest risk of iatrogenic injury to the intra-articular structures because it is done blindly without direct arthroscopic vision and guided only by fluoroscopy. Good separation of the femoral head and acetabulum is the first step to avoid iatrogenic injury. Separation depends on traction (Fig. 6.8). The spinal needle is introduced following the direction of the femoral neck as close as possible to the femoral head to avoid labrum penetration, with the tip of the needle in the opposite direction of the femoral head to contact the cartilage with the blunt side of the needle (Fig. 6.9). Access into the joint is confirmed by feeling the penetration of the hip capsule and not by "landing" the needle on the acetabulum to avoid injury to the acetabular cartilage. Once the capsule has been penetrated, the stylus can be removed from the needle and a nitinol (flexible metal) guide wire can be passed though the needle to "palpate" the acetabulum with its blunt tip and confirm intra-articular position of the needle. The guide wire is removed and 40 cc of saline is injected into the joint for distension. Distension increases separation of the acetabulum and the femoral head[11,13] (Fig. 6.10). Once the joint has been distended, a nitinol guide wire is reintroduced through the needle, the needle is removed, and a cannulated switching stick (Hip Access System; Smith & Nephew) is passed into the

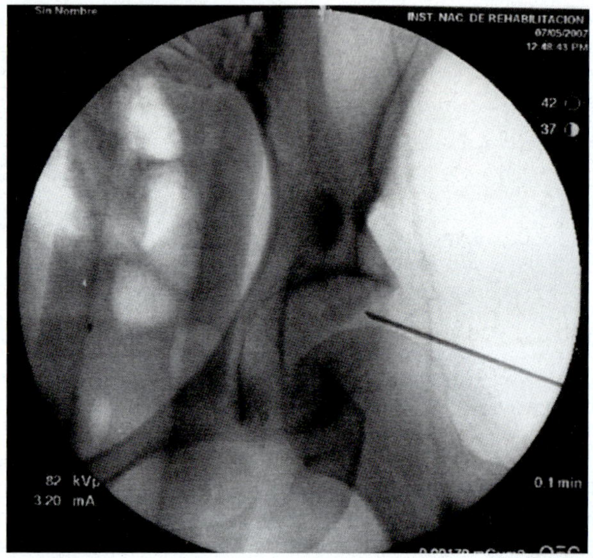

Figure 6.9. This image intensifier photograph demonstrates a spinal needle in position while the anterolateral portal is being established. Note how the needle is closer to the femoral head to avoid labral puncture. The tip of the needle is directed away from the head to avoid damaging the articular cartilage on the femoral head. The needle should not be "landed" on the acetabulum to confirm its intra-articular position. The needle should only be advanced to the point where perforation of the hip capsule is felt.

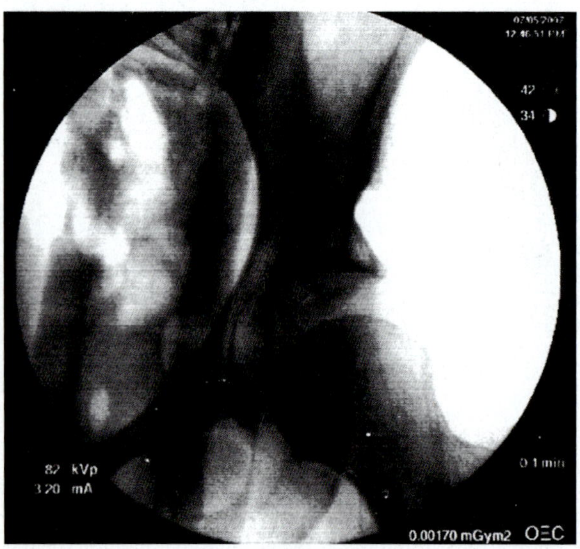

Figure 6.8. This image intensifier photograph demonstrates adequate separation of the acetabulum and femoral head when traction is applied.

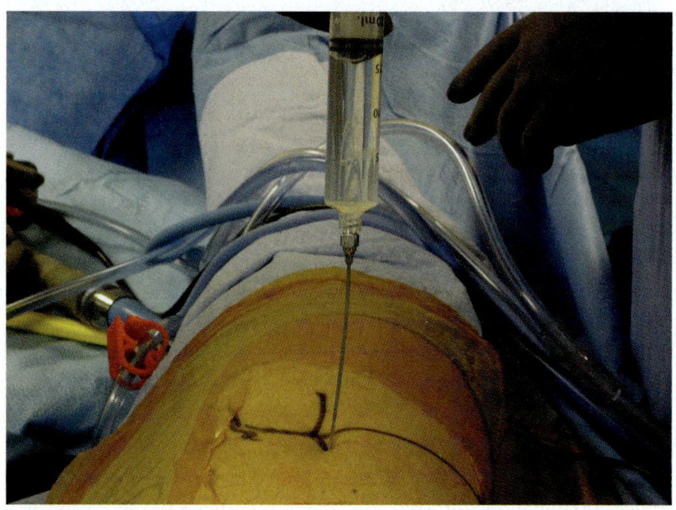

Figure 6.10. Anesthesiologist's view of a left hip. A spinal needle is in position at the anterolateral portal, saline is been injected to further distend the hip joint.

joint using the guide wire. The intra-articular placement of the switching stick can be confirmed using fluoroscopy and a standard rotatable double valve arthroscopy cannula for the 4.0 mm 30° arthroscope (Dyonics; Smith & Nephew) is passed over the switching stick. The latter is removed and a 4 mm 30° arthroscope (Dyonics; Smith & Nephew) is introduced.[14] One valve is used for inflow, which is set at 70 mm Hg and suction is placed at the second valve. The posterolateral portal is established next; it is located at the posterior corner of the greater trochanter. A 17-gauge spinal needle is introduced at the site of the posterolateral portal parallel to the direction of the arthroscope in the anterolateral portal (Fig. 6.11). The needle is visualized as it enters the joint through the lateral hip capsule between the free margin of the labrum and the femoral head. Fluoroscopy can also be used to assist in orienting the needle adequately for the establishment of this portal. The posterolateral portal is usually the second portal established when hip arthroscopy is done in the lateral decubitus. Supine position surgeons will usually establish the direct anterior portal second. With the needle in position, the stylus is removed, a nitinol guide wire introduced, and the needle is removed. The switching stick and a dilator (Hip Access System; Smith & Nephew) are assembled together and introduced into the joint using the guidewire; every step is done under direct arthroscopic vision to avoid damage to the articular cartilage or the labrum. A slotted cannula[15] (Hip Access System; Smith & Nephew) is slid around the dilator with its tip in close contact with the dilator to protect the labrum and articular cartilage when the slotted cannula enters the joint. With the slotted cannula in the joint, the switching stick-dilator assembly is removed and the slotted cannula is ready for instrument introduction (Fig. 6.12). The first instrument to be introduced is usually a hook probe. When the probe is in the joint, the slotted cannula is removed and the probe used "free-handed." When a different instrument is needed, the probe can be used as a guide to insert the slotted cannula and then removed. With the slotted cannula in position, the instrument or the portal can be exchanged.

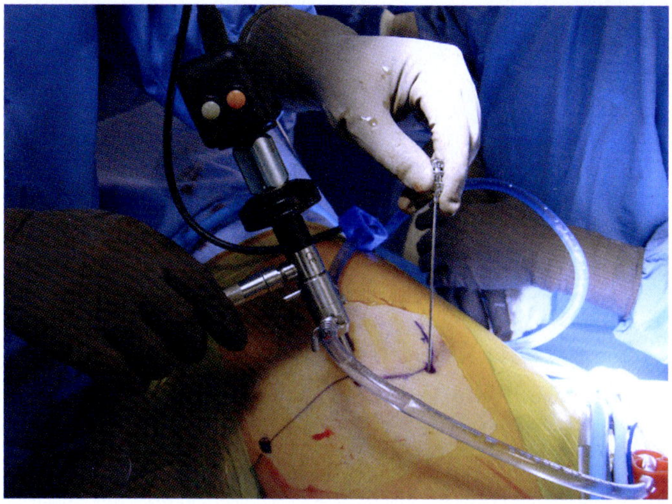

Figure 6.11. Anesthesiologist's view of a right hip. The arthroscope is at the anterolateral portal; a spinal needle is being introduced at the posterolateral portal under direct arthroscopic vision.

The direct anterior portal is located at the junction of a vertical line descending from the anterior superior iliac spine and a horizontal line from the tip of the greater trochanter. It is usually the third portal to be established when the lateral approach is used. The same technique described for the posterolateral portal is utilized to establish the direct anterior portal (Figs. 6.13 & 6.14). The anterolateral portal and the direct anterior portal are the most useful for arthroscopy of the central compartment.

When central compartment arthroscopy is concluded, instruments are taken out of the portals and traction is released, the hip is flexed 35°, abducted, and externally rotated. This position will relax the anterior hip capsule and facilitate access to the hip

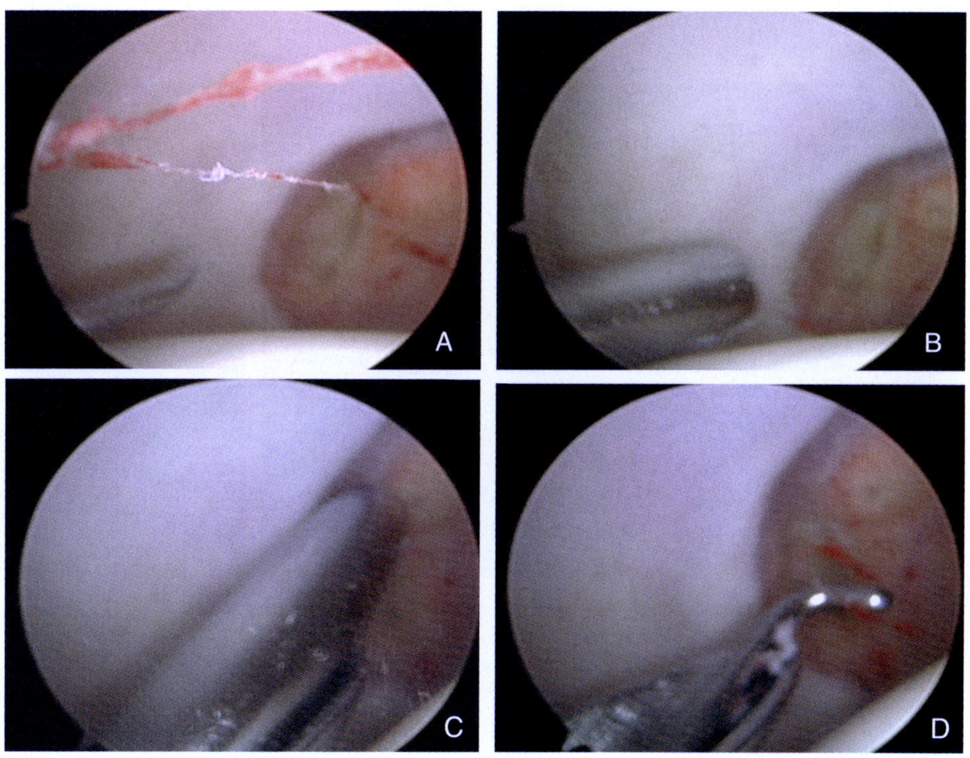

Figure 6.12. Arthroscopic series of photographs of the establishment of the posterolateral portal and introduction of a hook probe. The arthroscope is in the anterolateral portal. **A:** A spinal needle is in the posterolateral portal. The arthroscopic photograph demonstrates the needle in position between the femoral head and the labrum. **B:** A switching stick-dilator assembly has been introduced. **C:** A slotted cannula is in position around the dilator. **D:** A hook probe is introduced using the slotted cannula.

periphery. To access the hip periphery, the femoral neck is visualized at the image intensifier, and a spinal needle is introduced perpendicular to the direction of the femoral neck at the site of the anterolateral portal. The guide wire and cannulated instruments are utilized to establish the viewing portal and the arthroscope is introduced following the same technique as described before. Inferior accessory portals provide adequate access to the peripheral compartment (Figs. 6.15 & 6.16).

DISCUSSION

The lateral approach to hip arthroscopy is effective and reproducible. It depends on precise and adequate positioning of the patient. A checklist approach to follow every step for positioning a patient in the lateral decubitus for hip arthroscopy may be very helpful in achieving successful femoral head–acetabulum separation and access to the hip periphery.

After patient selection, patient positioning is the most important step in hip arthroscopy.

Because hip arthroscopy is a very sophisticated technical procedure, every element of operating room infrastructure and hip arthroscopy instruments should be always available.

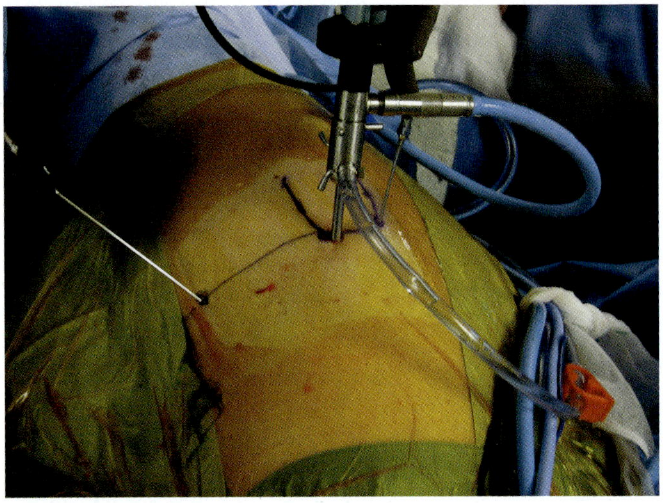

Figure 6.13. Anesthesiologist's view of a right hip. The arthroscope is at the anterolateral portal, a spinal needle is in position at the posterolateral portal. A second spinal needle is being introduced at the anterior portal triangulated toward the tip of the arthroscope at the tip.

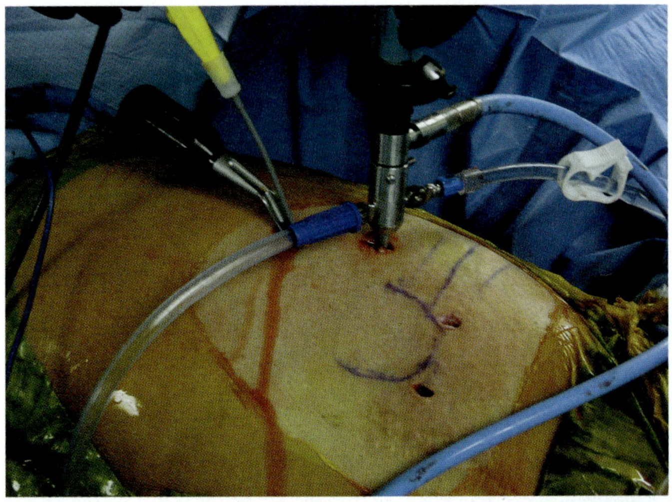

Figure 6.15. Posterior view of instruments being introduced into accessory portals to access the peripheral compartment. The arthroscope is at the anterior superior accessory portal. A slotted cannula and a radiofrequency device are at the anterior distal accessory portal. The anterolateral and posterolateral portals are seen at the superior and posterior corner of the outlined greater trochanter respectively (the position of the accessory portals may be adjusted depending of each case. They are usually located distal to the central compartment portals and between the anterior femur and a vertical line descending from the anterior superior iliac spine). The hip is flexed 35°, externally rotated, and abducted as shown in Figure 6.4.

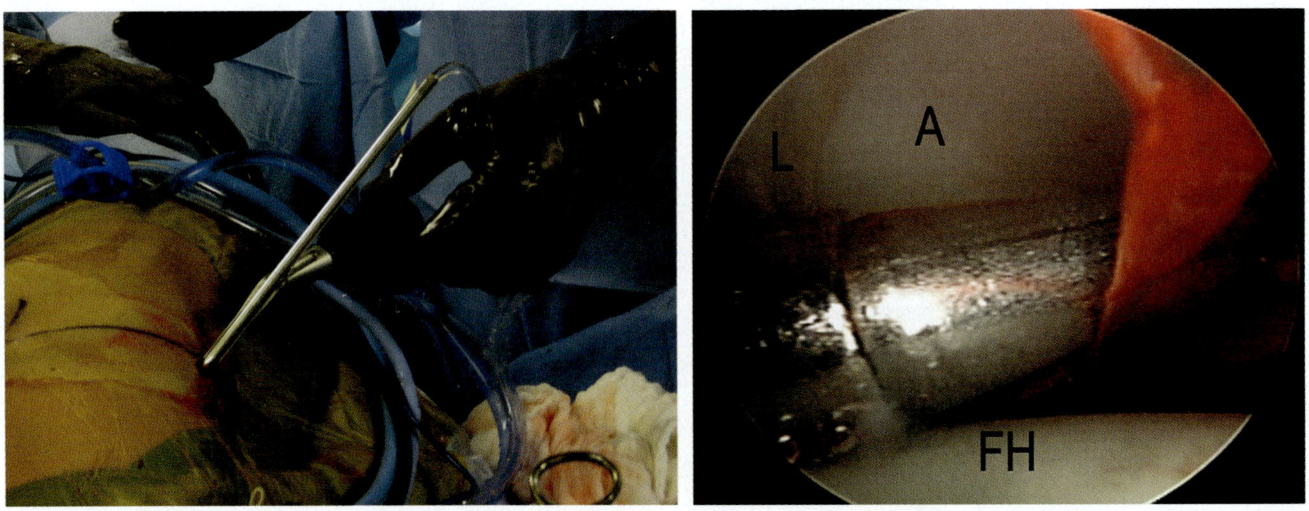

Figure 6.14. To the left: Anesthesiologist's view of a right hip. A dilator-switching stick assembly is in the direct anterior portal, a slotted cannula is being introduced around the dilator. To the right the dilator-switching stick assembly is visualized inside the joint through the anterior hip capsule betw een the anterior labrum (L) and the femoral head (FH), the acetabulum (A) is at the top of the photograph. The arthroscopic view is from the anterolateral portal.

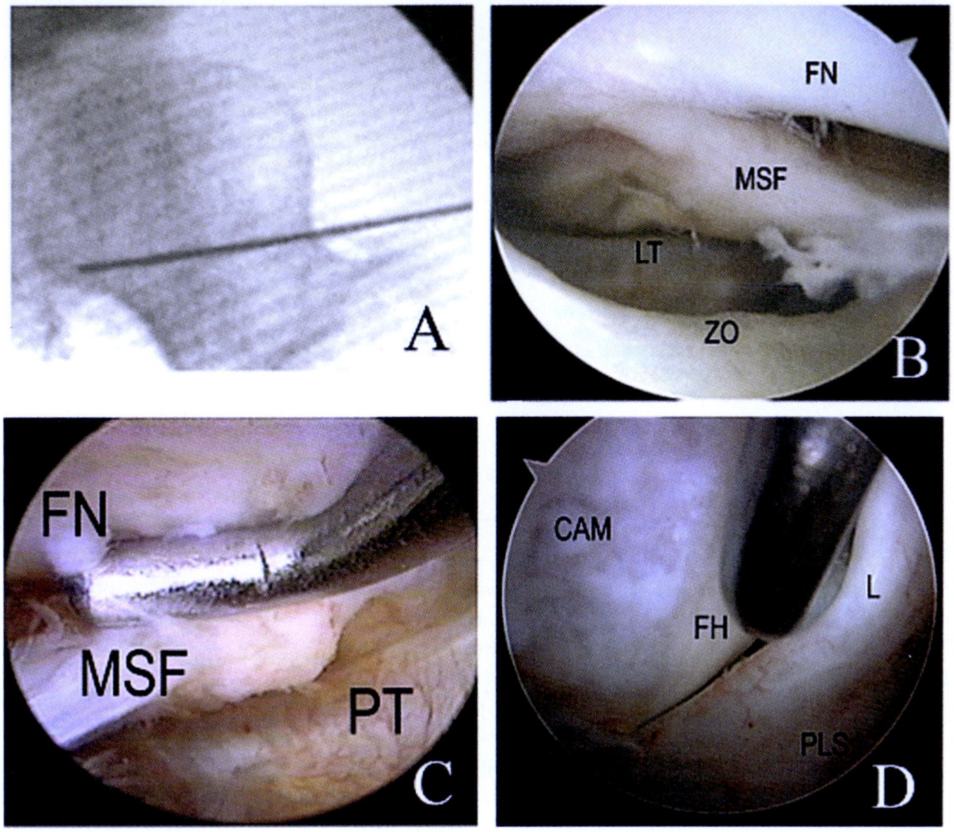

Figure 6.16. A series of photographs on access to the hip periphery is presented. **A:** Fluoroscopy photograph demonstrating introduction of the spinal needle into the hip periphery. Note the perpendicular direction of the needle relative to the femoral neck. **B**: Arthroscopic photograph of a left hip. A panoramic view of the anterior inferior peripheral compartment is presented. The femoral neck (FN) is at the top of the photograph. The medial synovial fold (MSF) is under the femoral neck. The zona orbicularis (ZO) is at the bottom of the photograph. The ligamentum transversum (LT) is at the center of the photograph. **C:** Arthroscopic photograph of a right hip. The femoral neck (FN) is at the top. The probe is on the medial synovial fold (MSF). Fibers of the psoas tendon (PT) can be seen through the anterior hip capsule. **D**: A right hip with a cam type femoroacetabular impingement (CAM). The probe is between the anterior labrum (L) and the femoral head (FH). The perilabral sulcus is at the bottom of the photograph.

REFERENCES

1. Dienst M, Godde S, Seil R, et al. Hip arthroscopy without traction in vivo anatomy of the peripheral joint cavity. *Arthroscopy.* 2001;17:924–931.
2. Eriksson E, Arvidsson L, Arvidsson H. Diagnostic and operative hip arthroscopy of the hip. *Orthopedics.* 1986;9:169–176.
3. Glick JM, Sampson TG, Gordon RB, et al. Hip arthroscopy by the lateral approach 1987;3:4–12.
4. McCarthy JC, Day B, Busconi B. Hip arthroscopy: Applications and technique. *J Am Acad Orthop Surg.* 1995;3:115–122.
5. Byrd JWT. Hip arthroscopy utilizing the supine position. *Arthroscopy.* 1994;10:275–280.
6. Clarke MT, Arora A, Villar RN. Hip arthroscopy: complications in 1054 cases. *Clin Orthop Relat Res.* 2003;406:84–88.
7. Beck M, Leunig M, Parvizi J, et al. Anterior femoroacetabular impingement: part II. Midterm results of surgical treatment. *Clin Orthop.* 2004;418:67–73.
8. Sampson TG. Arthroscopic treatment of femoroacetabular impingement. *Tech Orthop.* 2005;20:56–62.
9. Byrd JWT. The supine approach. In: Byrd JWT, ed. *Operative Hip Arthroscopy*, 2nd Ed. New York: Springer-Verlag New York; 2004, pp. 145–169.
10. Ilizaliturri VM Jr, Mangino G, Valero FS, et al. Hip arthroscopy of the central and peripheral compartment by the lateral approach. *Tech Orthop.* 2005;20:32–36.
11. Dienst M, Seil R, Godde S, et al. Effects of traction, distension and joint position on distraction of the hip joint: an experimental study in cadavers. *Arthroscopy.* 2002;18:865–871.
12. Byrd JWT, Pappas JN, Pedley MJ. Hip arthroscopy: an anatomic study of portal placement and relationship to the extraarticular structures. *Arthroscopy.* 1995;11:418–423.
13. Byrd JWT. Avoiding the labrum in hip arthroscopy. *Arthroscopy.* 2000;16:770–773.
14. Ilizaliturri VM Jr, Mangino G, Valero FS, et al. Special instruments and technique for hip arthroscopy. *Tech Orthop.* 2005;20:9–16.
15. Ilizaliturri VM Jr, Acosta-Rodriguez E, Camacho-Galindo J. A minimalist approach to hip arthroscopy: the slotted cannula. *Arthroscopy.* 2007;23:560.

CHAPTER

7

J. W. Thomas Byrd

Position and Setup: Supine

INTRODUCTION

Arthroscopy of the hip can be effectively performed with the patient in either the supine or lateral position. The choice is largely dictated by the surgeon's personal preference. The merits of the supine position are outlined as follows: Positioning of the patient is simple and can be accomplished in just a few minutes. The procedure can be performed on virtually any standard fracture table with an orientation to the joint that is familiar to orthopaedic surgeons accustomed to managing hip fractures. With this position, the layout of the operating room is user-friendly for the surgeon, assistants, and operating room staff. There is reliable access for all standard portal placements and it easily accommodates repositioning for arthroscopy of the peripheral compartment as well as iliopsoas bursoscopy to access the iliopsoas tendon. A final important advantage of the supine position regards intra-abdominal fluid extravasation. This is a potentially serious complication of hip arthroscopy and has been reported only in the lateral position.[1,2] With the patient on his or her side, the abdominal and pelvic cavities lie in a dependent position, creating a reservoir into which gravity flow will allow the fluid to collect.

The hip joint has both an intra-articular and a peripheral compartment. Most hip pathology is found within the intra-articular region; therefore, distraction is necessary to achieve arthroscopic access. Performing hip arthroscopy without traction has not been popular because it does not allow access to the intra-articular region. However, it is now recognized that this method can be a useful adjunct to the traction technique.[3,4] Hip flexion relaxes the capsule and allows access to the peripheral compartment, which is intracapsular, but extra-articular. Numerous lesions, such as synovial disease and free-floating loose bodies, are encountered in this area that may be overlooked with traction alone. Femoral sided impingement lesions (cam impingement) are best addressed from the peripheral compartment. Hip flexion also allows generous access to the capsule for plication or thermal modulation.

DICTUMS ON HIP ARTHROSCOPY

Regardless of the position or technique that is chosen for performing this procedure, there are several dictums that should be thoroughly understood. First, a successful outcome is most clearly dependent on proper patient selection. A technically well-executed procedure will fail when performed for the wrong reason. This may include failure of the procedure to meet the patient's expectations. Second, the patient must be properly positioned in order for the case to go well. Poor positioning will assure a difficult procedure. Third, simply gaining access to the hip joint is not an outstanding technical accomplishment. The paramount issue is accessing the joint in as atraumatic a fashion as possible. Due to its constrained architecture and dense soft tissue envelope, the potential for inadvertent iatrogenic scope trauma is significant and, perhaps to some extent, unavoidable. Thus, every reasonable step should be taken to keep this concern to a minimum. Perform the procedure as carefully as possible and be certain that it is being performed for the right reason.

OPERATING ROOM SETUP

ANESTHESIA

The procedure is performed on an outpatient basis under general anesthesia. Epidural is an appropriate alternative, but requires an adequate motor block to ensure muscle relaxation.

PATIENT POSITIONING

A fracture table can be used, or a versatile distractor has been developed that can be adapted to a standard operating room (OR) table. The patient is positioned supine. An oversized (12 cm outer diameter) formed urethane perineal post is used. This is positioned laterally against the medial thigh of the operative leg (Fig. 7.1). Lateralizing the perineal post adds a slight transverse component to the direction of the traction vector (Fig. 7.2). It also distances the post from the area of the pudendal nerve, lessening the risk of compression neurapraxia.

The operative hip is positioned in extension and approximately 25° of abduction. Slight flexion might relax the capsule and facilitate distraction, but excessive flexion should be avoided because it exerts tension on the sciatic nerve and may increase the risk of traction neurapraxia. Neutral rotation of the extremity during portal placement is important for proper orientation, but freedom of rotation of the foot plate during the procedure facilitates visualization of the femoral head.

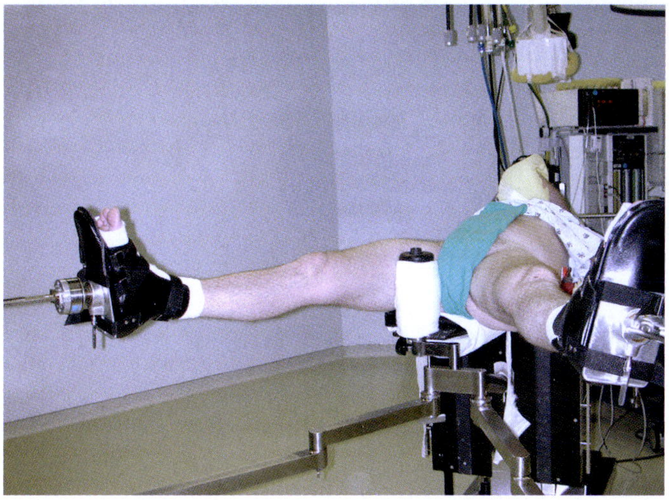

Figure 7.1. The patient is positioned on the fracture table so that the perineal post is placed as far laterally as possible toward the operative hip resting against the medial thigh. (Reprinted from Byrd JWT, MD, with permission.)

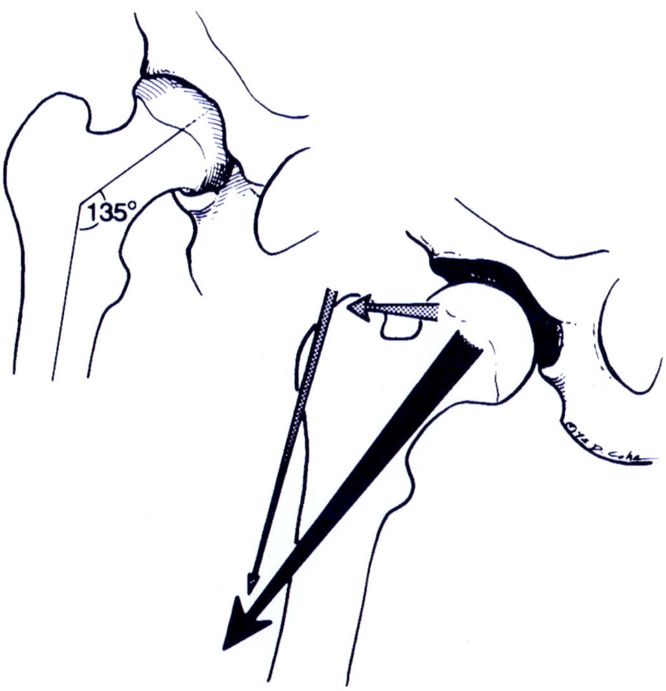

Figure 7.2. The optimal vector for distraction is oblique relative to the axis of the body and more closely coincides with the axis of the femoral neck than the femoral shaft. This oblique vector is partially created by abduction of the hip and partially accentuated by a small transverse component to the vector. (Reprinted from Byrd JWT, MD, with permission.)

The contralateral extremity is abducted as necessary to accommodate positioning of the image intensifier between the legs. Prior to distracting the operative hip, slight traction is applied to the nonoperative leg. This stabilizes the torso on the table and keeps the pelvis from shifting during distraction of the operative hip.

Traction is then applied to the operative extremity, and distraction of the joint is confirmed by fluoroscopic examination. Usually, about 50 pounds of traction force is adequate. Sometimes more force is necessary for an especially tight hip, but should be undertaken with caution.

If adequate distraction is not readily achieved, allowing a few minutes for the capsule to accommodate the tensile forces often results in relaxation of the capsule and adequate distraction without excessive force. Also, a vacuum phenomenon will be apparent fluoroscopically. This is created by the negative intracapsular pressure caused by distraction. This seal will be released when the joint is distended with fluid at the time of surgery and may further facilitate distraction. However, the effect is variable and should not be depended on to overcome inadequate traction.[5]

Once the ability to distract the hip joint has been confirmed, the traction is released. The hip is then prepped and draped, and traction is reapplied when ready to begin arthroscopy. The surgeon, assistant, and scrub nurse are positioned on the operative side of the patient. The monitor and arthroscopy cart with an attached sterile Mayo stand containing the video-articulated arthroscopes and power shaver are positioned on the contralateral side (Fig. 7.3).

EQUIPMENT

Most standard fracture tables can accommodate the few specific needs of hip arthroscopy. A tensiometer is a helpful tool that can be incorporated into the foot plate. This is especially useful for monitoring the intraoperative ability to maintain adequate distraction. A large-sized perineal post with generous padding distributes the pressure on the perineum more safely and facilitates lateralization of the operative hip.

An image intensifier is used for all cases. This is important for assuring precise portal placement. Simply accessing the joint is often not difficult. More important are care and precision in portal placement to minimize the risk of iatrogenic damage.

Both the 30° and 70° video-articulated arthroscopes are routinely used to optimize visualization. Interchanging the two scopes allows excellent visualization despite the limited maneuverability caused by the bony architecture of the joint and its dense soft tissue envelope. The 30° scope provides the best view of the central portion of the acetabulum and femoral head and the superior portion of the acetabular fossa, while the 70° scope is best for visualizing the outer edges of the joint, the acetabular labrum, the capsule, and the inferior portion of the fossa.

A fluid pump provides significant advantages in the hip. A high flow system can provide optimal flow without having to use excessive pressure. This is important for visualization and safety. Adequate flow is essential for good visualization in order to perform the procedure effectively and in an expedient manner. Flow cannot be as precisely modulated with a gravity system, creating difficulties both with visualization and extravasation. However, the surgeon must always be cognizant that the pump is functioning properly.

Extra-length cannulas are specifically designed to accommodate the dense soft tissue envelope that surrounds the hip (Fig. 7.4). The extra length has been accomplished by shortening the accompanying bridge which allows these cannulas to be used with a standard arthroscope. Special cannulated obturators also allow passage of the cannula/obturator assembly over a nitanol guide wire prepositioned in the joint through

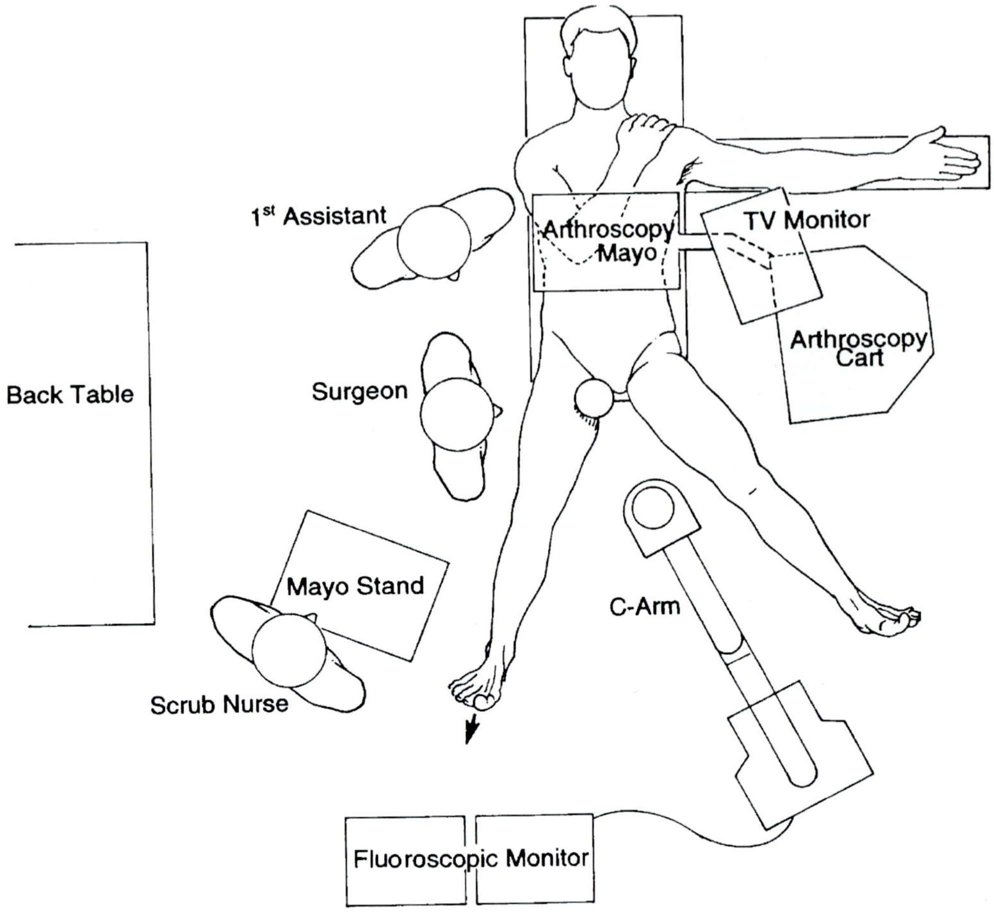

Figure 7.3. Schematic of the operating room layout showing the position of the surgeon, assistant, scrub nurse, arthroscopy cart, monitor, and Mayo, scrub nurse's Mayo, C-arm, and back table. (Reprinted from Byrd JWT, MD, with permission.)

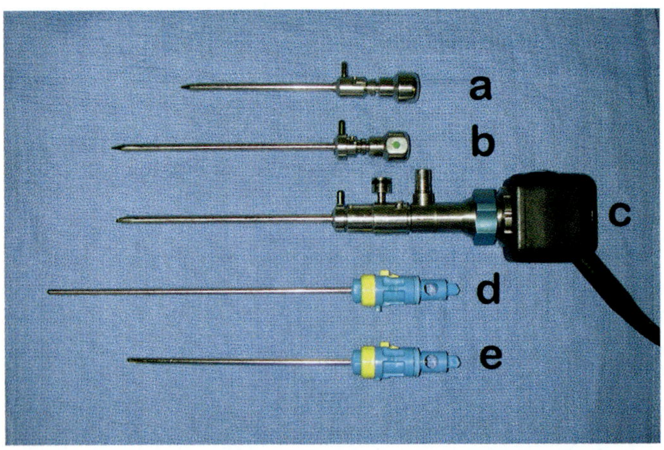

Figure 7.4. A standard arthroscopic cannula (*a*) is compared to the extra-length cannula (*b*). A modified bridge (*c*) has been shortened to accommodate the extra-length cannula with a standard length arthroscope. Extra-length blades (*d*) are also available compared to the standard length blades (*e*). (Reprinted from Byrd JWT, MD, with permission.)

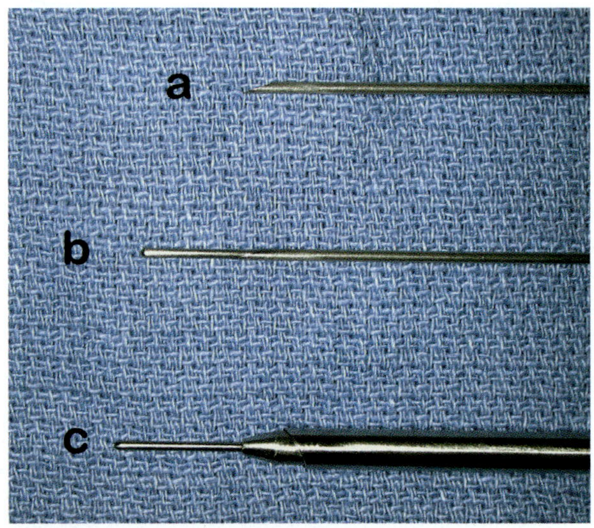

Figure 7.5. The cannulated obturator system allows for greater ease in reliably establishing the portals once proper positioning has been achieved with the spinal needle. The 6-in. 17-gauge spinal needle (***a* and *b***) accommodates the passage of a Nitanol wire (***b* and *c***). Specially treated, the wire is resistant to kinking. The cannulated obturator allows for passage of the obturator/cannula assembly over the guide wire (*c*). (Reprinted from Byrd JWT, MD, with permission.)

6-in. 17 gauge spinal needles (Fig. 7.5). The scrub nurse's Mayo stand contains the instruments routinely needed for each case (Fig. 7.6). The 5 mm cannula is used for initial introduction of the arthroscope while the inflow is attached. The diameter allows adequate flow for the fluid management system attached through the bridge. Once all three portals have been established, the inflow can be switched to one of the other cannulas and the 5 mm cannula is replaced with a 4.5 mm cannula. The use of three 4.5 mm cannulas allows complete interchangeability of the arthroscope, instruments, and inflow. The 5.5 mm cannula is available for larger shaver blades.

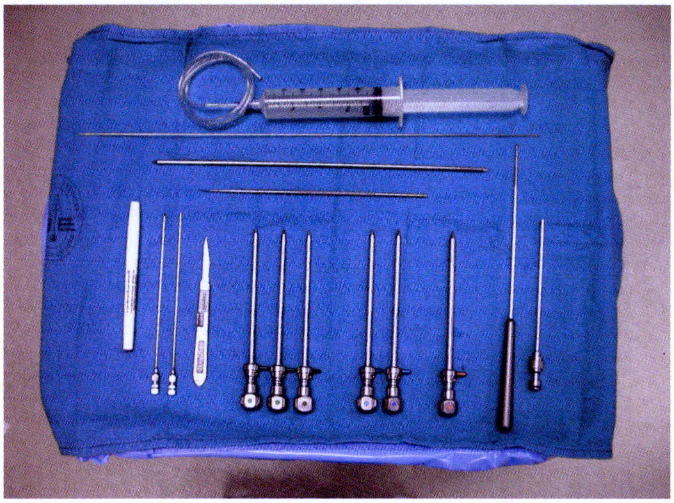

Figure 7.6. The scrub nurse's Mayo stand contains basic instruments necessary for initiating the arthroscopic procedure including: a marking pen; no. 11 blade scalpel; 6-in. 17-gauge spinal needles; 60 mL syringe of saline with extension tubing; a Nitanol guide wire; three 4.5, two 5.0, and one 5.5 mm cannulas with cannulated and solid obturators; a switching stick; a separate inflow adapter; and a modified probe. (Reprinted from Byrd JWT, MD, with permission.)

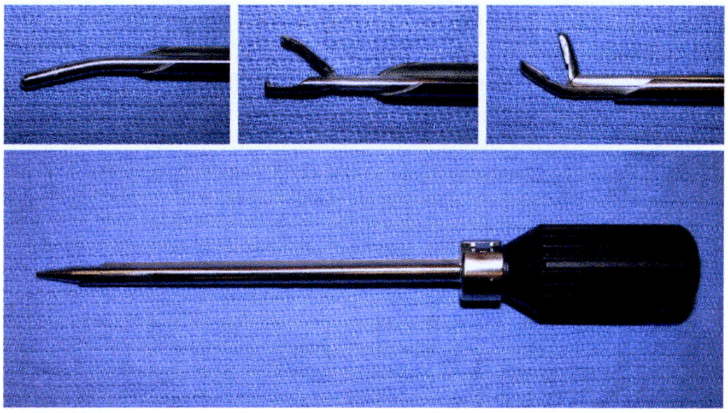

Figure 7.7. A slotted cannula with its accompanying cannulated obturator accommodates the passage of curved shaver blades and larger hand instruments into the joint. (Reprinted from Byrd JWT, MD, with permission.)

Extra-length blades are available. Curved designs are especially helpful for maneuvering within the spherical geometry of the joint. These can be passed through specially designed slotted cannulas (Fig. 7.7), which accommodate the curved shaver blades as well as other hand instruments. Specially designed hand instruments must be not only longer, but also of sturdy construction to minimize the risk of instrument breakage.

Thermal devices demonstrate specific advantages in the hip. The small diameter allows access to recesses within the joint that are difficult to access with mechanical blades. Also, because of the limits on maneuverability, it can be difficult for the shaver to excise damaged articular cartilage or labrum and create a stable edge. Thermal devices are often much more effective at creating a smooth transition zone, preserving more healthy tissue.

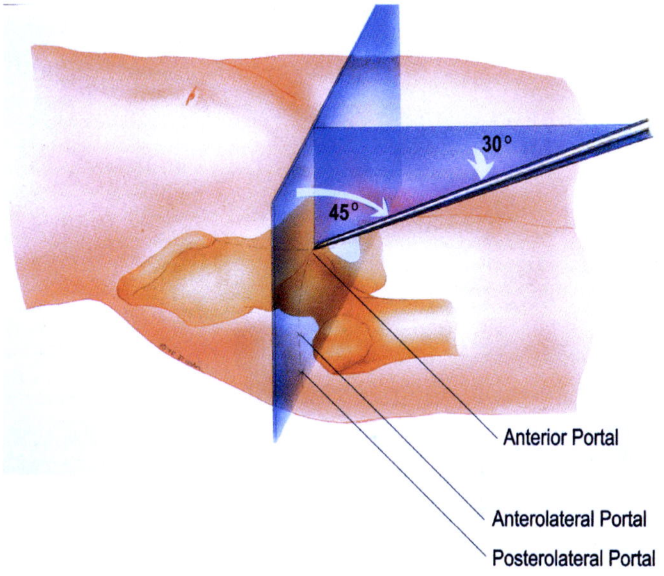

Figure 7.8. The site of the anterior portal coincides with the intersection of a sagittal line drawn distally from the anterior superior iliac spine and a transverse line across the superior margin of the greater trochanter. The direction of this portal courses approximately 45° cephalad and 30° toward the midline. The anterolateral and posterolateral portals are positioned directly over the superior aspect of the trochanter at its anterior and posterior borders. (Reprinted from Byrd JWT, MD, with permission.)

GENERAL TECHNIQUE

The technique described here has proved to be effective and reproducible.[6,7]

Portals

Three standard portals are utilized for arthroscopy of the intra-articular compartment: anterior, anterolateral, and posterolateral (Figs. 7.8 & 7.9).[8,9] The site of the anterior portal coincides with the intersection of a sagittal line drawn distally from the anterior superior iliac spine and a transverse line across the superior margin of the greater trochanter. The direction of this portal courses approximately 45° cephalad and 30° toward the midline. The anterolateral and posterolateral portals are positioned directly over the superior aspect of the trochanter at its anterior and posterior borders.

Anterior Portal

The pathway of the anterior portal penetrates the muscle belly of the sartorius and the rectus femoris before entering the anterior capsule (Fig. 7.10). At the portal level, the lateral femoral cutaneous nerve is usually divided into three or more branches. Consequently, the portal usually passes within several millimeters of one of these branches. Because of the multiple branches, the nerve is not easily avoided by altering the portal position. Rather, it is protected by utilizing a meticulous technique in portal placement. Specifically, the nerve is most vulnerable to a deeply placed skin incision which lacerates one of the branches. Therefore, the initial stab wound should be made carefully through the skin only. Passing from the skin to the capsule, the anterior portal runs almost tangential to the axis of the femoral nerve and lies only slightly closer to it at the level of the capsule, with an average minimum distance of 3.2 cm. The relationship of the ascending branch of the lateral circumflex femoral artery is variable but averages 3.6 cm inferior to the anterior portal.

Anterolateral Portal

The anterolateral portal penetrates the gluteus medius prior to entering the lateral aspect of the capsule at its anterior margin (Fig. 7.11). The superior gluteal nerve lies an average of 4.4 cm superior to the portal.

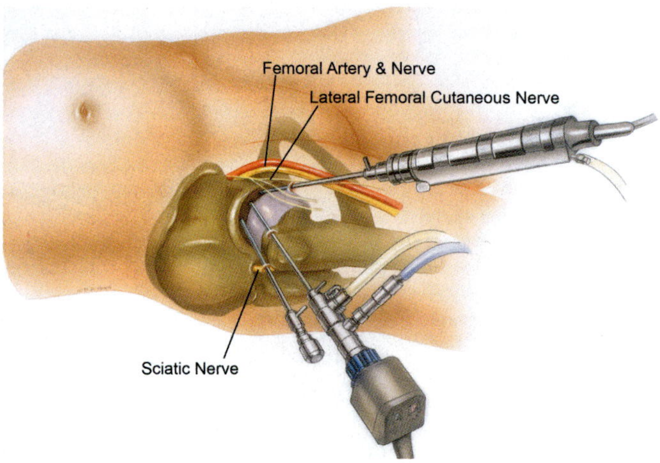

Figure 7.9. The relationship of the major neurovascular structures to the three standard portals is demonstrated. The femoral artery and nerve lie well medial to the anterior portal. The sciatic nerve lies posterior to the posterolateral portal. Small branches of the lateral femoral cutaneous nerve lie close to the anterior portal. Injury to these is avoided by utilizing proper technique in portal placement. The anterolateral portal is established first, since it lies most centrally in the safe zone for arthroscopy. (Reprinted from Byrd JWT, MD, with permission.)

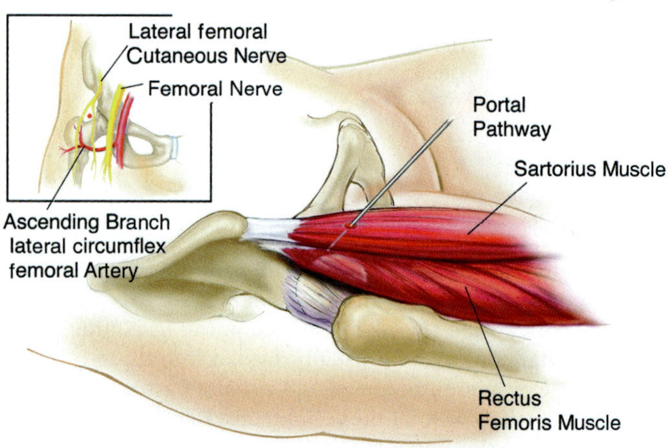

Figure 7.10. Anterior portal pathway/relationship to lateral femoral cutaneous nerve, femoral nerve, and lateral circumflex femoral artery. (Courtesy of Smith & Nephew Endoscopy, Andover, MA.)

Posterolateral Portal

The posterolateral portal penetrates both the gluteus medius and gluteus minimus prior to entering the lateral capsule at its posterior margin (Fig. 7.12). Its course is superior and anterior to the piriformis tendon. The portal lies closest to the sciatic nerve at the level of the capsule with the distance averaging 2.9 cm. An average distance of 4.4 cm separates the portal from the superior gluteal nerve.

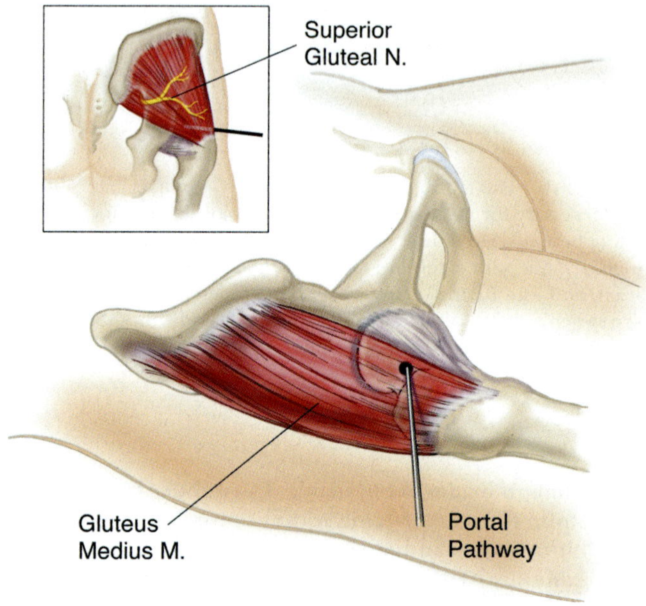

Figure 7.11. Anterolateral portal pathway/relationship to superior gluteal nerve. (Courtesy of Smith & Nephew Endoscopy, Andover, MA.)

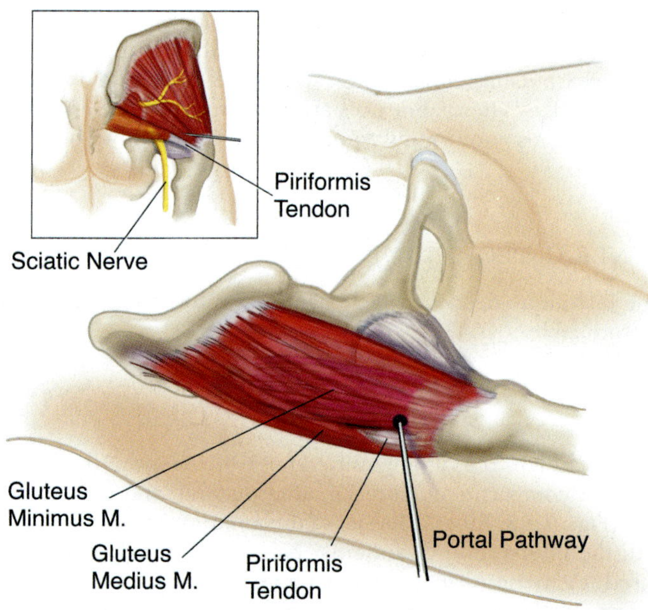

Figure 7.12. Posterolateral portal pathway/relationship to the sciatic nerve and superior gluteal nerve. (Courtesy of Smith & Nephew Endoscopy, Andover, MA.)

Portal Placement

The anterolateral portal lies most centrally in the "safe zone" for arthroscopy and thus the portal is placed first.[8,9] Subsequent portal placements are assisted by direct arthroscopic visualization. This initial portal is placed by fluoroscopic inspection in the AP plane. However, orientation in the lateral plane is equally important. With the leg in neutral rotation, femoral anteversion places the center of the joint just anterior to the center of the greater trochanter. Thus, the entry site for the anterolateral portal at the anterior margin of the greater trochanter corresponds with the entry of the joint just anterior to its midportion. This correct entry site of the joint is achieved by keeping the instrumentation parallel to the floor during portal placement (Fig. 7.13).

When distracting the hip, a vacuum phenomenon will usually be present (Fig. 7.14A). Prepositioning for the anterolateral portal is performed with a 6-in. 17 gauge spinal needle under fluoroscopic control. Careful positioning of this needle is essential because, with the cannulated arthroscopy system, the cannula/obturator assembly will enter exactly where the needle has been placed. Release of the vacuum seal, by insertion of the needle, creates an air arthrogram affect, which may assist in silhouetting the outline of the lateral labrum (Fig. 7.14B).[10] The tactile feel is important, because greater resistance is felt if the labrum is inadvertently penetrated, more so than when just penetrating the capsule. Once the needle has been placed, the joint is then distended with approximately 40 mL of fluid and the intracapsular position is confirmed by the backflow of the fluid. Distension of the joint enhances distraction (Fig. 7.14C). If it is felt that the needle may have pierced the labrum, once the joint has been distended, it is a simple process to back the needle out and re-enter the capsule below the level of the labrum.

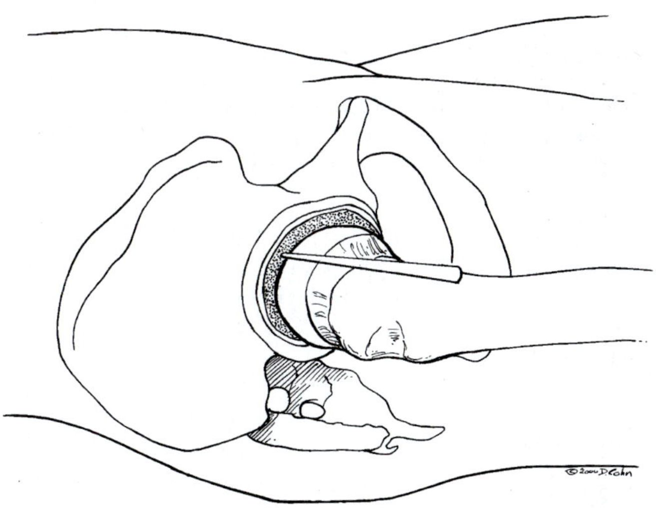

Figure 7.13. With the patient supine, the hip is in neutral rotation with the kneecap pointing toward the ceiling. A needle placed at the anterior margin of the greater trochanter (anterolateral position) is maintained in the coronal plane by keeping it parallel to the floor as it enters the joint. Due to femoral neck anteversion, the entry site will be just anterior to the joint's center. If the entry site is too anterior, it becomes crowded with the anterior portal. If it is too posterior, it becomes difficult to properly visualize the entry site for the anterior portal. (Reprinted from Byrd JWT, MD, with permission.)

A stab wound is made through the skin at the needle. The guide wire is placed through the needle and the needle is removed. The cannulated obturator with the 5 mm arthroscopy cannula is passed over the wire into the joint (Fig. 7.14D).

While establishing the portal, the cannula/obturator assembly should pass close to the superior tip of the greater trochanter and then directly above the convex surface of the femoral head. It is important to keep the assembly off the femoral head to avoid inadvertent articular surface scuffing.

Sometimes, blood will be present within the joint due to the traction force necessary to distract the surfaces. This is difficult to clear until a separate egress has been established. However, venting the fluid with the spinal needle from anterior will clear the field of view.

Once the arthroscope has been introduced, the anterior portal is placed next. Positioning is now facilitated by visualization from the arthroscope as well as fluoroscopy. The 70° scope works best for directly viewing where the instrumentation penetrates the capsule. Prepositioning is again performed with the 17 gauge spinal needle, entering the joint directly underneath the free edge of the anterior labrum. As the cannula/obturator assembly is introduced, it is lifted up to stay off the articular surface of the femoral head while passing underneath the acetabular labrum.

If proper attention is given to the topographical anatomy in positioning the anterior portal, the femoral nerve lies well medial to the approach.[8,9] However, the lateral femoral cutaneous nerve lies quite close to this portal. It is best avoided by utilizing proper technique in portal placement. The nerve is most vulnerable to laceration by a skin incision placed too deeply.

Lastly, the posterolateral portal is introduced. The fluoroscopic guidelines are similar to the anterolateral portal. Rotating the lens of the arthroscope posteriorly brings the entry site underneath the posterior labrum into view. Placement under arthroscopic control ensures that the instrumentation does not stray posteriorly, potentially placing the sciatic nerve at risk. The hip remains in neutral rotation during placement of the posterolateral portal. External rotation of the hip would move the greater trochanter more posteriorly and, since this is the main topographical landmark, the sciatic nerve might be more at risk for injury (Fig. 7.15).

Portal Placement for Peripheral Joint[3,4,7]

After completing arthroscopy of the interior of the hip, the instruments can be removed and traction released for access to the peripheral compartment. The hip is flexed approximately 45°, which relaxes the anterior capsule (Fig. 7.16). From the anterolateral entry site, the spinal needle penetrates the capsule on the anterior neck of the femur under fluoroscopic control (Fig. 7.17A & B). Using the guide wire, the cannula/obturator assembly is then placed (Fig. 7.17C). The 5 mm cannula is preferable with the inflow attached to the scope.

For instrumentation, an ancillary portal is placed 5 cm distal to the anterolateral portal. Once again prepositioning is performed with the 17 gauge spinal needle, directly observing through the arthroscope where the needle enters the peripheral compartment (Fig. 7.17D). Many loose bodies reside in this area and can be retrieved. Recontouring of the femoral head

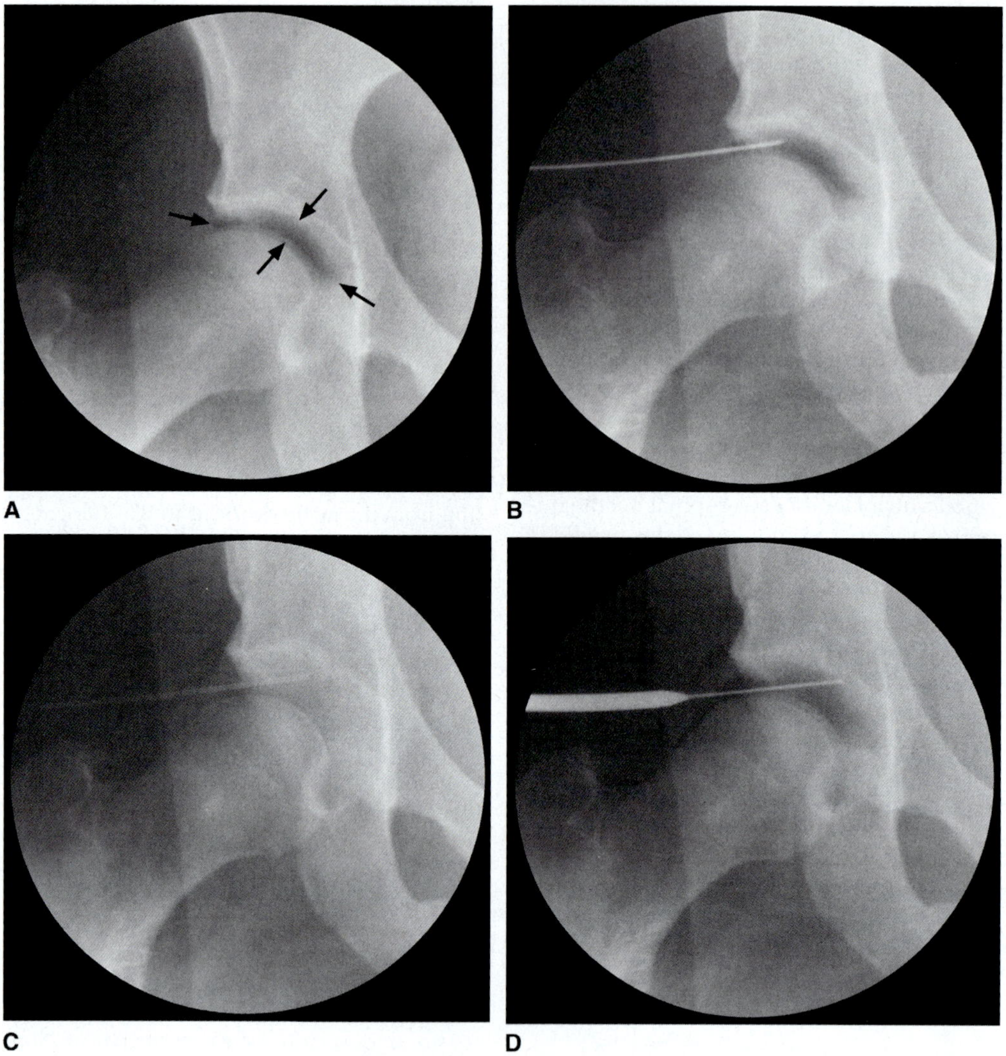

Figure 7.14. AP fluoroscopic view of a right hip. **A:** A vacuum effect is apparent due to the negative intracapsular pressure created by distraction of the joint (*arrows*). **B:** A spinal needle is used in prepositioning of the anterolateral portal. Venting the joint with the needle releases the vacuum effect creating an air arthrogram that silhouettes the free margin of the lateral labrum (*arrow*). **C:** Distension of the joint with the fluid further facilitates distraction. **D:** The cannula/obturator assembly is passed over the Nitanol wire that had been placed through the spinal needle. (Reprinted from Byrd JWT, MD, with permission.)

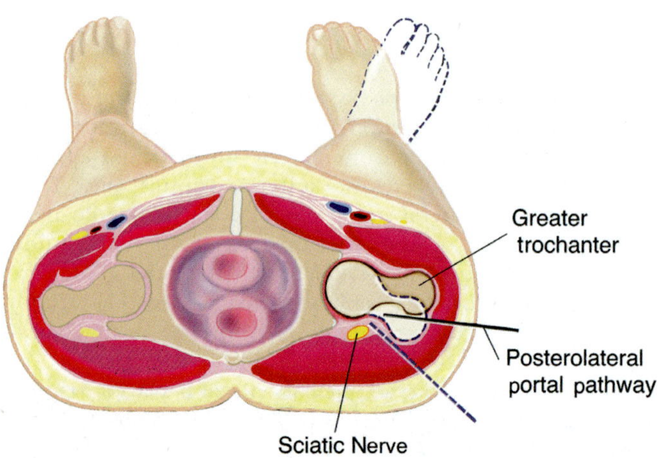

Figure 7.15. Neutral rotation of the operative hip is essential for protection of the sciatic nerve during placement of the posterolateral portal. (Courtesy of Smith & Nephew Endoscopy, Andover, MA.)

associated with cam impingement is best addressed from the peripheral compartment. This also provides superior access to the synovial lining and capsule, which is important for performing a thorough synovectomy and also aids when performing a thermal capsulorrhaphy.

Diagnostic Arthroscopy

When preparing for hip arthroscopy, the surgeon formulates a tentative treatment plan based on the preliminary diagnosis. However, the definitive treatment strategy will be dictated by the findings observed at arthroscopy. With the current limitations of investigative techniques, the arthroscopic findings may differ significantly from those implied by the preoperative studies. Thus, a systematic and thorough initial inspection of the joint is imperative. Once all aspects of the intra-articular pathology have been identified, the surgeon can then embark on intervention with appropriate time management to address all aspects

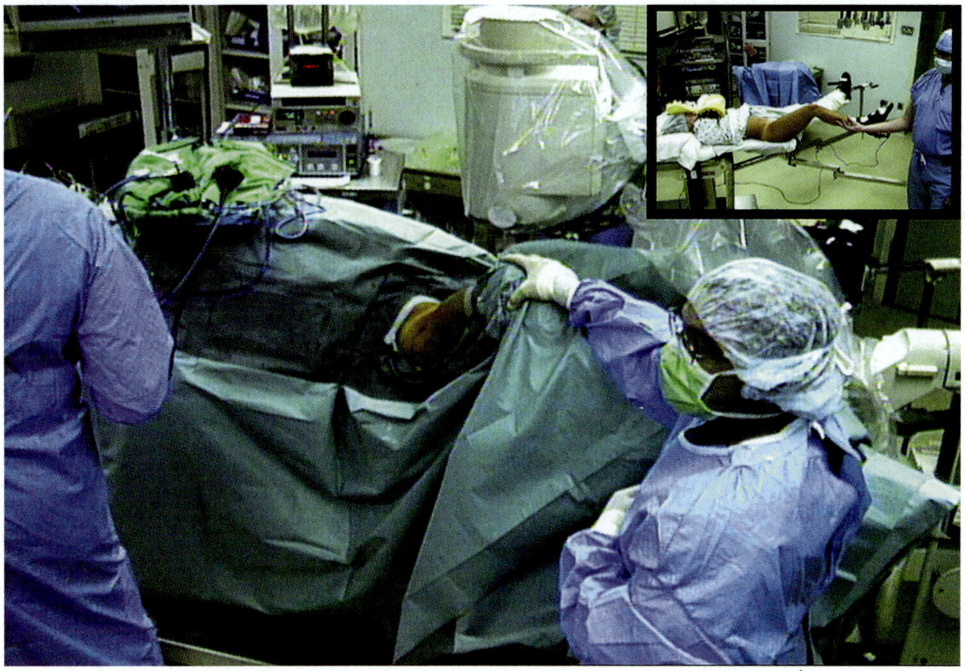

Figure 7.16. The operative area remains covered in sterile drapes while the traction released and the hip flexed 45°. Inset top right corner: Illustrates position of the hip without the overlying drape. (Reprinted from Byrd JWT, MD, with permission.)

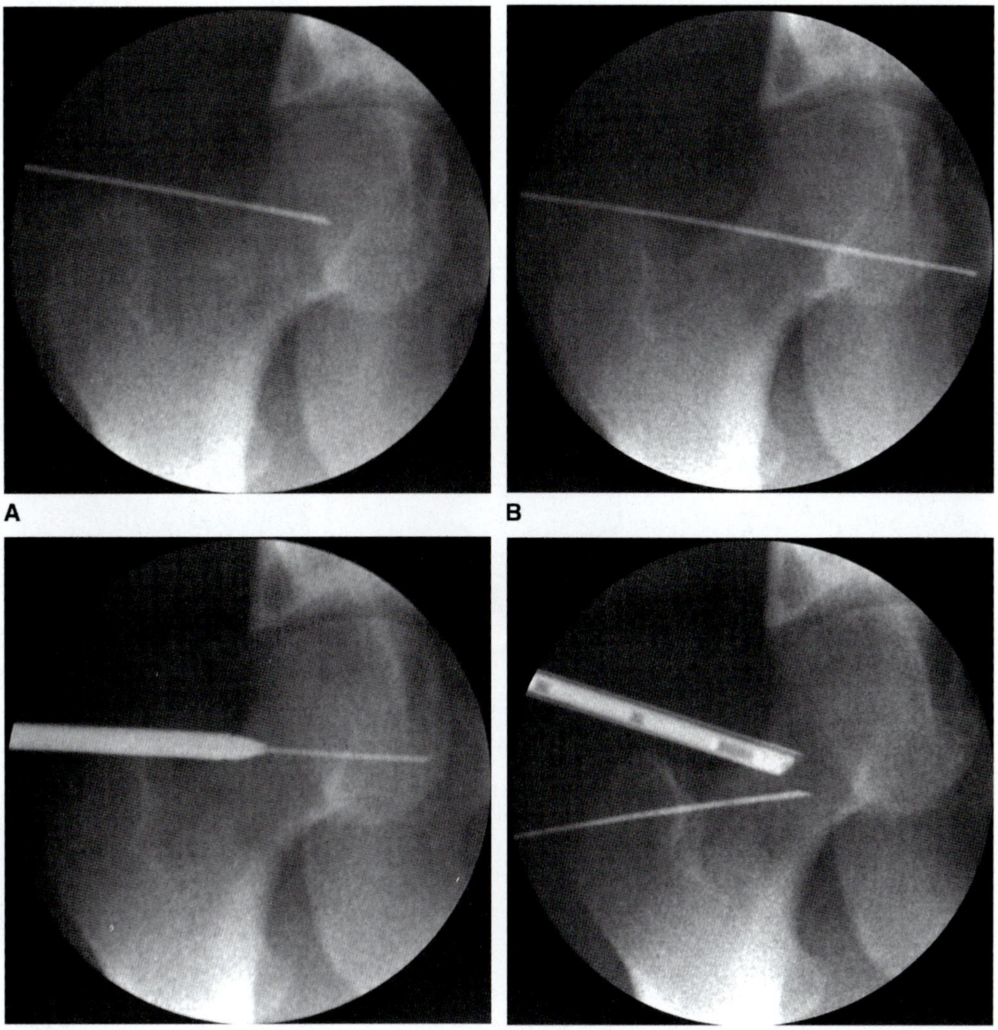

A B C D

Figure 7.17. AP fluoroscopic view of the flexed hip. **A:** From the anterolateral entry site, the 17-gauge spinal needle has been repositioned on the anterior neck of the femur. The spinal needle can be felt perforating the capsule before contacting the bone. **B:** The guide wire is placed through the spinal needle. It should pass freely to the medial capsule as illustrated. **C:** The cannula obturator assembly is placed over the guide wire. **D:** The position of the 30° arthroscope is shown while a spinal needle is placed for an ancillary portal. (Reprinted from Byrd JWT, MD, with permission.)

within the joint. The surgeon should avoid spending considerable time on one obvious aspect of the pathology to only then realize that there is other coexistent damage that needs to be addressed as well.

Using the three-portal technique (anterior, anterolateral, and posterolateral), inspection begins from the anterolateral portal (Fig. 7.9). This is the first portal established since it lies most centrally in the safe zone for arthroscopy. Inspection begins with the 70° scope as this provides the best view of the outer margins of the joint and is used for allowing direct arthroscopic visualization of where the other two portals are placed. The anterolateral portal provides the best view of the anterior portion of the joint (Fig. 7.18)

Next, the arthroscope is placed in the anterior portal. Viewing laterally, the relationship of the lateral two portals underneath the lateral labrum is seen (Fig. 7.19). The surgeon should be especially cognizant to critique the entry site of the anterolateral portal, since this is the portal that is placed only

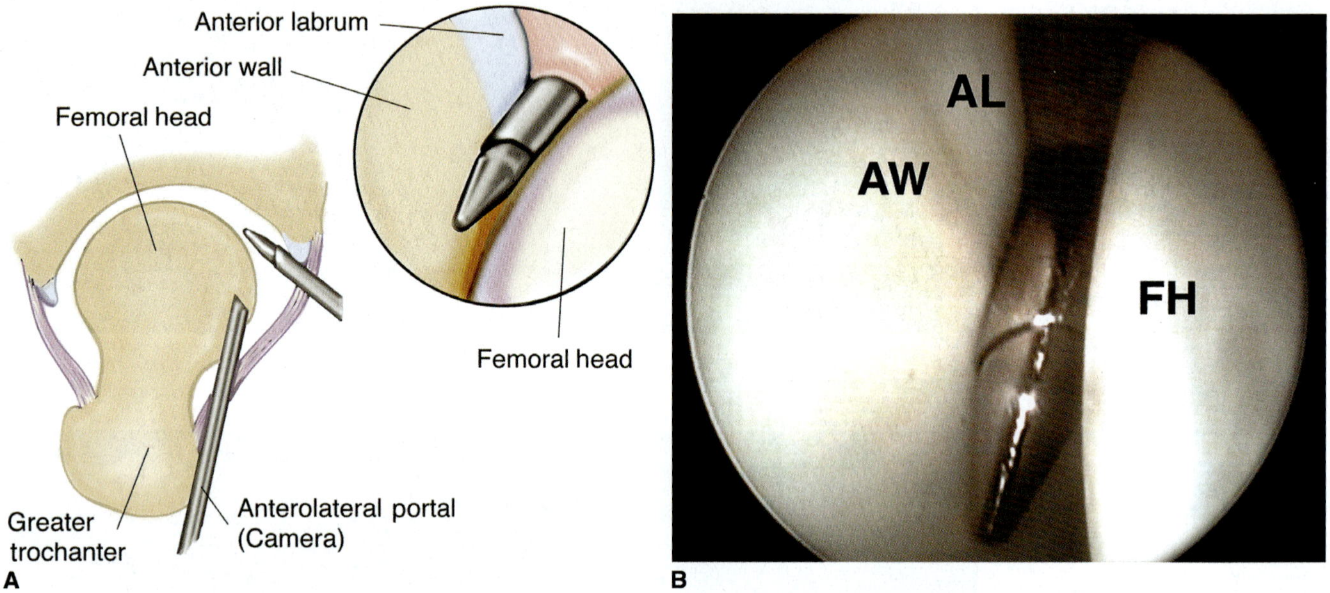

Figure 7.18. **A:** Arthroscopic view of the right hip from the anterolateral portal. (Courtesy of Smith & Nephew Endoscopy, Andover, MA.) **B:** Demonstrated are the anterior acetabular wall (AW) and the anterior labrum (AL). The anterior cannula is seen entering underneath the labrum and the femoral head (FH) is on the right. (Reprinted from Byrd JWT, MD, with permission.)

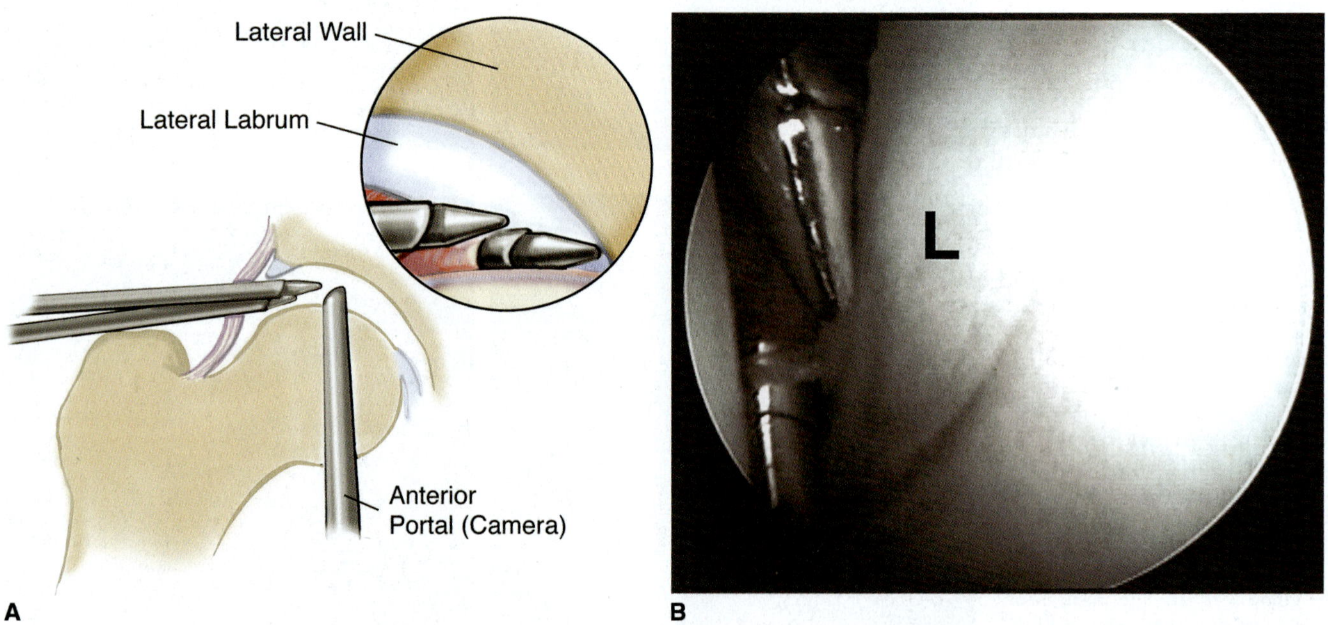

Figure 7.19. **A:** Arthroscopic view from the anterior portal. (Courtesy of Smith & Nephew Endoscopy, Andover, MA.) **B:** Demonstrated are the lateral aspect of the labrum (L) and its relationship to the lateral two portals. (Reprinted from Byrd JWT, MD, with permission.)

under fluoroscopic guidance without benefit of arthroscopic visualization of where the portal enters the joint. Viewing medially from the anterior portal, the surgeon can see the most inferior limit of the anterior labrum (Fig. 7.20).

The arthroscope is then placed in the posterolateral portal which provides the best view of the posterior regions of the joint, especially the posterior labrum (Fig. 7.21). The posterior labrum is the portion that is least often damaged and has the most consistent morphological appearance. Thus, viewing this area is often used as a reference in assessing variations of the anterior or lateral labrum and the accompanying pathology.

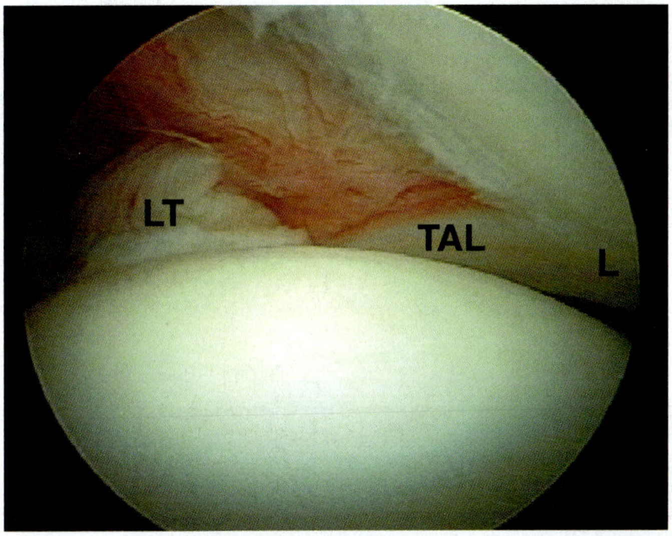

Figure 7.20. Viewing inferomedially from the anterior portal demonstrates where the inferior aspect of the anterior labrum (L) becomes contiguous with the transverse acetabular ligament (TAL) below the ligamentum teres (LT). (Reprinted from Byrd JWT, MD, with permission.)

Each of the three portals provides a different perspective on the acetabular fossa (Fig. 7.22). The 70° scope provides a direct view of the ligamentum teres which resides in the inferior portion of the fossa. The transverse acetabular ligament can also be partially viewed coursing underneath the ligamentum teres. After completing the inspection with the 70° scope, the 30° scope is then used, reversing the sequence of steps between the three portals. The 30° scope provides a better view of the central portion of the femoral head and acetabulum and the superior portion of the acetabular fossa.

Once the traction has been released and the hip flexed, the arthroscope is repositioned from the anterolateral portal on the anterior neck of the femur, providing an excellent perspective of the peripheral compartment (Figs. 7.23 & 7.24). This brings into view the structures that cannot be seen from inside the joint and also provides a different peripheral perspective on some of the intra-articular structures. The medial synovial fold is consistently visualized adjacent to the anteromedial neck of the femur.

Normal Variants

The lateral and the anterior portions of the labrum are the most variable. Sometimes this portion of the labrum is thin, poorly developed, and hypoplastic and, at other times, may appear enlarged. In the presence of acetabular dysplasia, the lateral labrum is especially hypertrophic having more of a stabilizing and weight-bearing role substituting for the absent lateral portion of the bony acetabulum. A labral cleft is sometimes present (Fig. 7.25).[11] This is a normal finding and should not be misinterpreted as a traumatic detachment. The distinguishing features are absence of damaged appearing tissue and absence

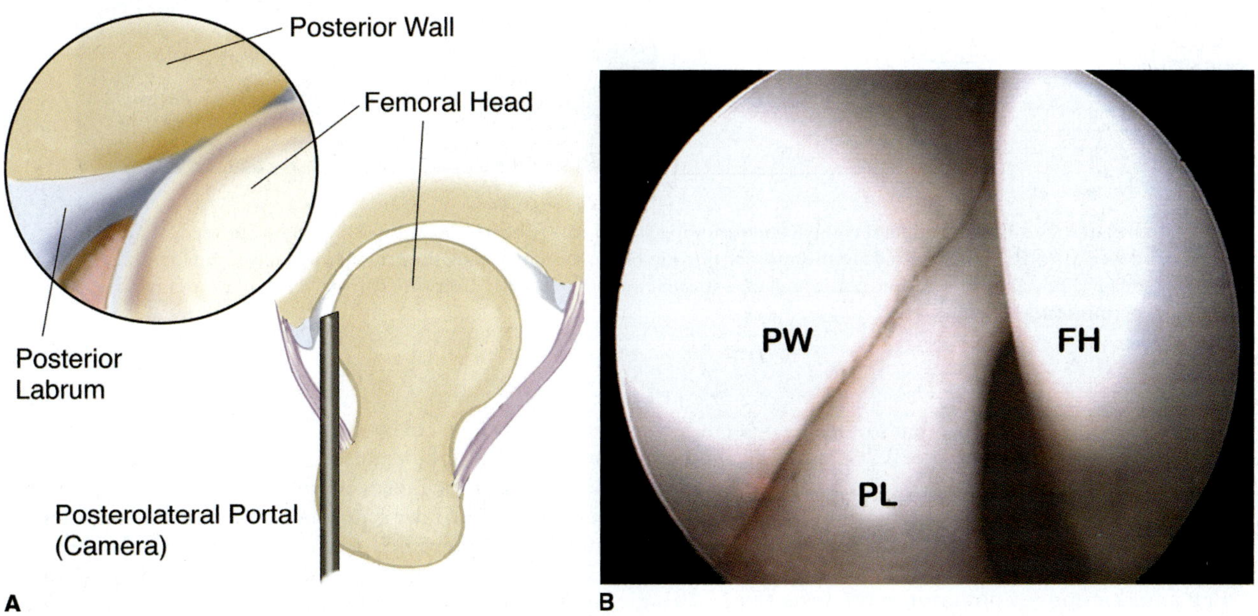

Figure 7.21. **A:** Arthroscopic view from the posterolateral portal. (Courtesy of Smith & Nephew Endoscopy, Andover, MA.) **B:** Demonstrated are the posterior acetabular wall (PW), posterior labrum (PL), and the femoral head (FH). (Reprinted from Byrd JWT. Hip arthroscopy—The supine position. In: McGinty JB, Caspari RB, Jackson RW, *et al.*, eds. *Operative Arthroscopy*. New York: Raven Press; 1996, pp. 1091–1099, with permission.)

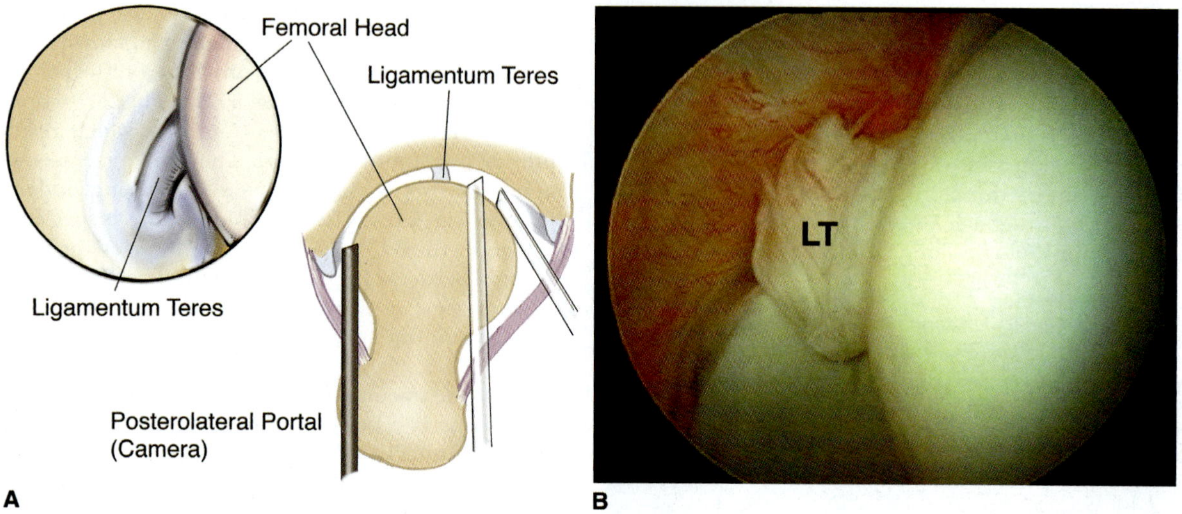

Figure 7.22. **A:** The acetabular fossa can be inspected from all three portals. (Courtesy of Smith & Nephew Endoscopy, Andover, MA.) **B:** The ligamentum teres (LT), with its accompanying vessels, has a serpentine course from its acetabular to its femoral attachment. (Reprinted from Byrd JWT, MD, with permission.)

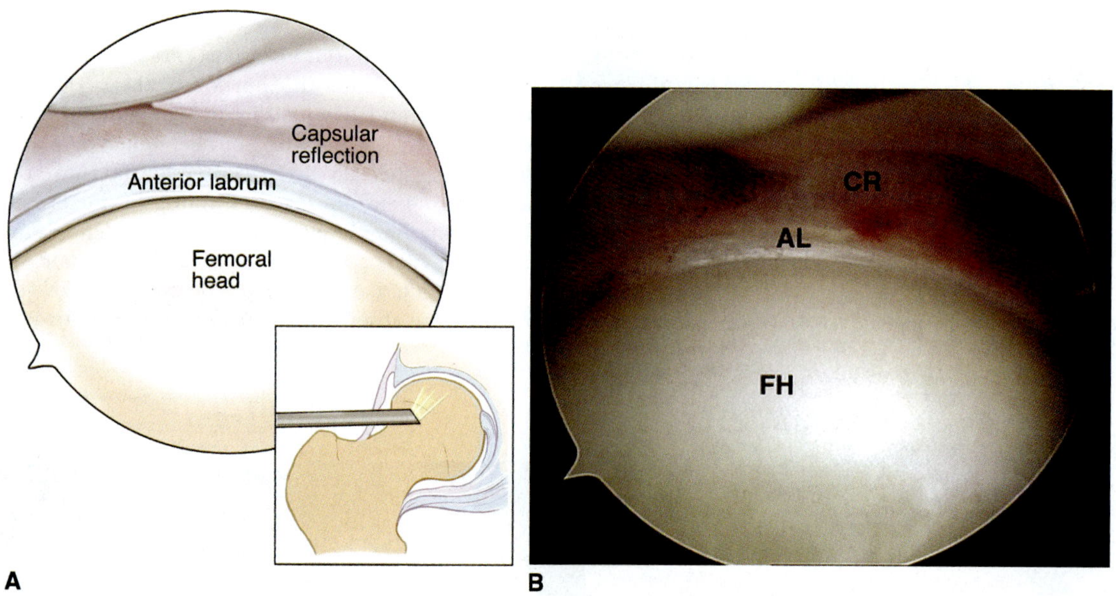

Figure 7.23. **A:** Peripheral compartment viewing superiorly. (Courtesy of Smith & Nephew Endoscopy, Andover, MA.) **B:** Demonstrated are the anterior portion of the joint including the articular surface of the femoral head (FH), anterior labrum (AL), and the capsular reflection (CR). (Reprinted from Byrd JWT, MD, with permission.)

of any attempted healing response that would be expected in the presence of a trauma.

Remnants of the triradiate cartilage may be evident in adulthood as a physeal scar, void of overlying articular cartilage, extending in a linear fashion along the medial aspect of the acetabulum anterior and/or posterior to the fossa (Fig. 7.26). This should not be misinterpreted as an old fracture line.

A commonly encountered observation in adults is a stellate articular lesion immediately above the acetabular fossa referred to as the stellate crease (Fig. 7.27).[12] When seen, it is unlikely to be of clinical significance as a contributing cause of pain and is of uncertain long-term prognostic significance regarding susceptibility to a future degenerative disease. Occasionally, this must be distinguished from traumatic articular lesions which can occur in this same area, especially from a lateral blow to the hip impacting the femoral head against the superomedial acetabulum.

Another variation that has not been previously described involves the supra-acetabular fossa and keyhole complex. A bony

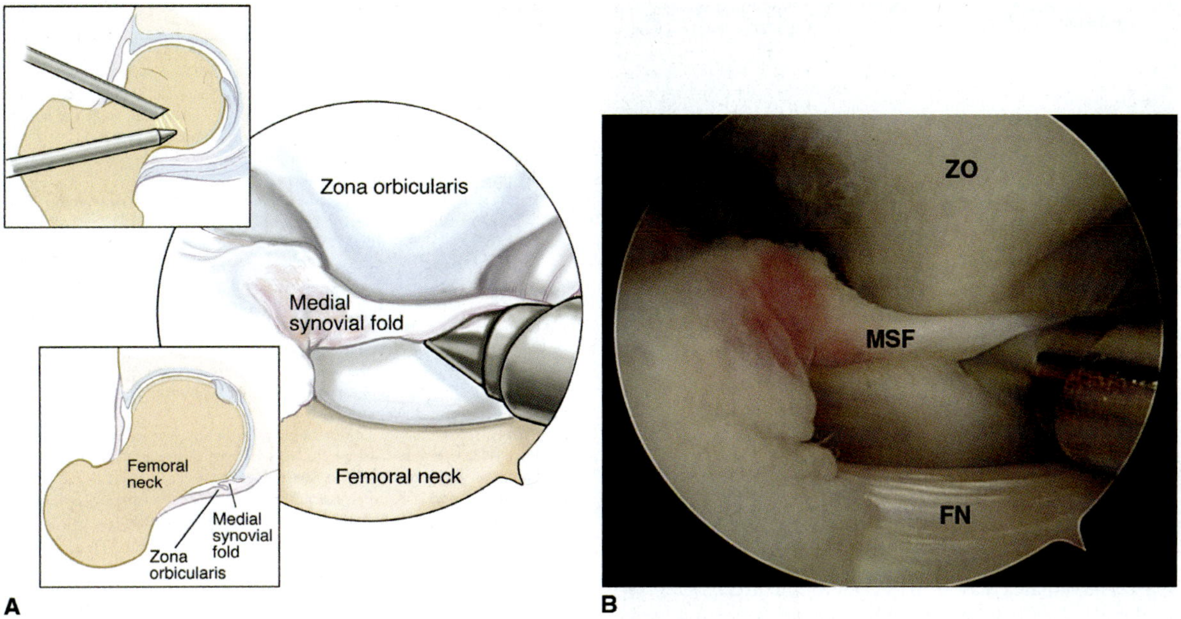

Figure 7.24. **A:** Peripheral compartment viewing medially. (Courtesy of Smith & Nephew Endoscopy, Andover, MA.) **B:** Demonstrated are the femoral neck (FN), medial synovial fold (MSF), and the zona orbicularis (ZO). (Reprinted from Byrd JWT, MD, with permission.)

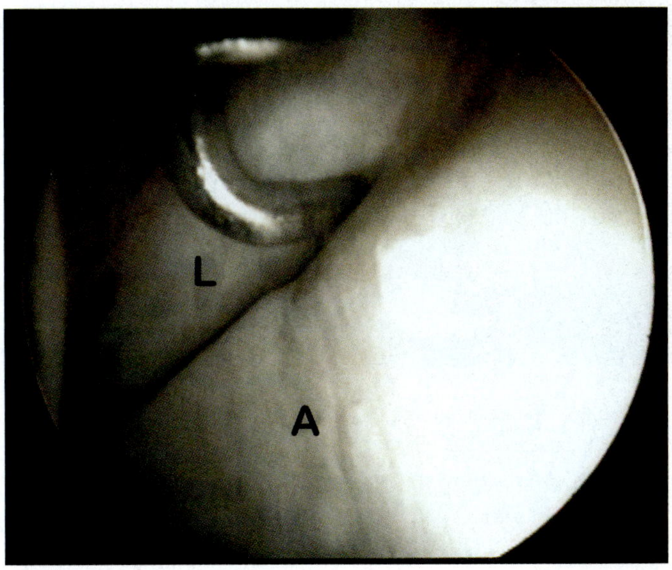

Figure 7.25. The cleft identified by the probe sometimes separates the margin of the acetabular articular surface from the labrum (L). This is a normal variant without evidence of trauma or attempted healing response. (Reprinted from Byrd JWT, MD, with permission.)

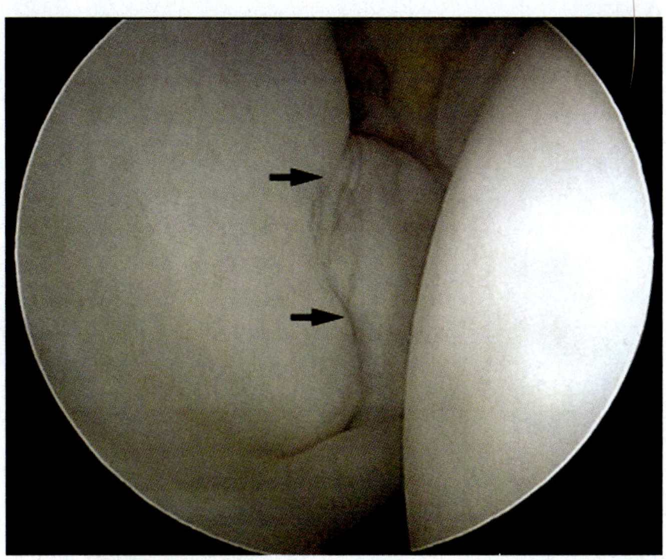

Figure 7.26. The physeal scar (*arrows*) is an area devoid of articular surface that may extend posteriorly from the acetabular fossa (as shown here), or anteriorly demarcating the area of the old triradiate physis. (Reprinted from Byrd JWT, MD, with permission.)

recess may be present and supramedial acetabular surface. This is usually evident on plain films, and on MRI will appear as a fluid-filled defect (Fig. 7.28A & B). This supra-acetabular fossa is filled with amorphous fibrous tissue and may display fibrous bands extending down to the formal acetabular fossa (Fig. 7.28C). This configuration demonstrates a "keyhole" shape when viewing through the arthroscope. Debridement of the fibrotic bands may be necessary to fully visualize the underlying acetabular architecture. Presently, it is unclear whether this contributes to the symptoms in some patients or is strictly an incidental finding.

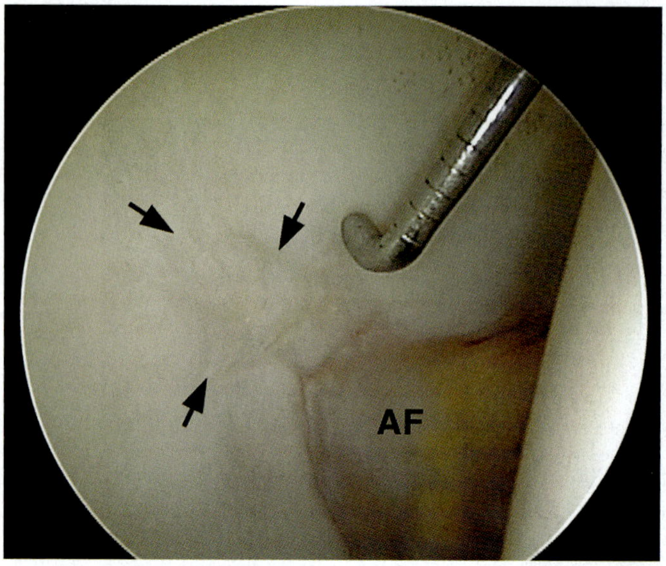

Figure 7.27. The stellate crease is frequently found directly superior to the acetabular fossa (AF) characterized by a stellate pattern of chondromalacia (*arrows*). This appears to be a normally occurring process, even in young adults, without clear prognostic significance. (Reprinted from Byrd JWT, MD, with permission.)

REFERENCES

1. Sampson TG. Complications of hip arthroscopy. *Clin Sports Med.* 2001;20(4):831–836.
2. Bartlett CS, DiFelice GS, Buly RL, et al. Cardiac arrest as a result of intraabdominal extravasation of fluid during arthroscopic removal of a loose body from the hip joint of a patient with an acetabular fracture. *J Orthop Trauma.* 1998;12(4):294–299.
3. Dienst M, Godde S, Seil R, et al. Hip arthroscopy without traction: In vivo anatomy of the peripheral hip joint cavity. *Arthroscopy.* 2001;17(9):924–931.
4. Dienst M. Hip arthroscopy without traction. In: Byrd JWT, ed. *Operative Hip Arthroscopy.* 2nd Ed. New York: Springer-Verlag; 2005, pp. 170–188.
5. Byrd JWT, Chern KY. Traction vs distension for distraction of the hip joint during arthroscopy. *Arthroscopy.* 1997;13(3):346–349.
6. Byrd JWT. The supine approach. In: Byrd JWT, ed. *Operative Hip Arthroscopy.* 2nd Ed. New York: Springer-Verlag; 2005, pp. 145–169.
7. Byrd JWT. Hip arthroscopy. *J Am Acad Orthp Surg.* 2005;14:433–444.
8. Byrd JWT, Pappas JN, Pedley MJ. Hip arthroscopy: An anatomic study of portal placement and relationship to the extra-articular structures. *Arthroscopy.* 1995;11(4):418–423.
9. Byrd JWT. Portal anatomy. In: Byrd JWT, ed. *Operative Hip Arthroscopy.* 2nd Ed. New York: Springer-Verlag; 2005, pp. 110–116.
10. Byrd JWT. Avoiding the labrum in hip arthroscopy. *Arthroscopy.* 2000;16(7):770–773.
11. Byrd JWT. Labral lesions, an elusive source of hip pain: Case reports and review of the literature. *Arthroscopy.* 1996;12(5):603–612.
12. Villar R, Santori N. Arthroscopic anatomy of the hip. In: Byrd JWT, ed. *Operative Hip Arthroscopy.* 2nd Ed. New York: Springer-Verlag; 2005, pp. 117–128.

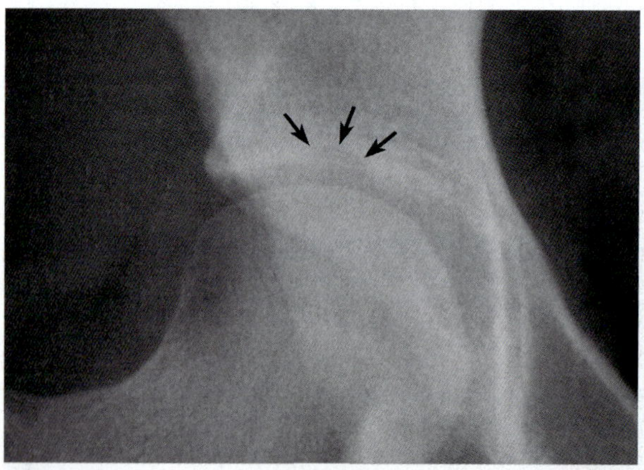

A

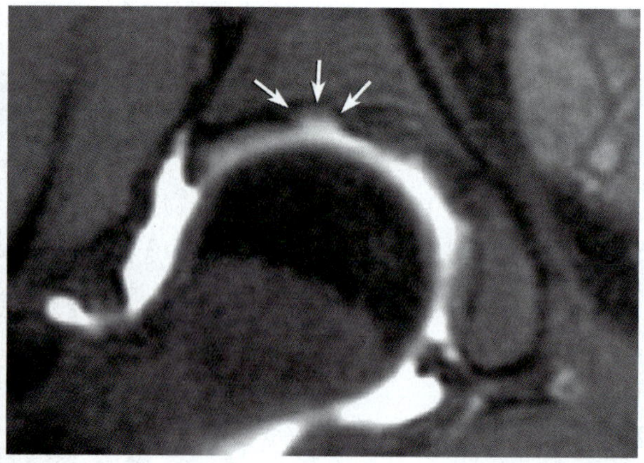

B

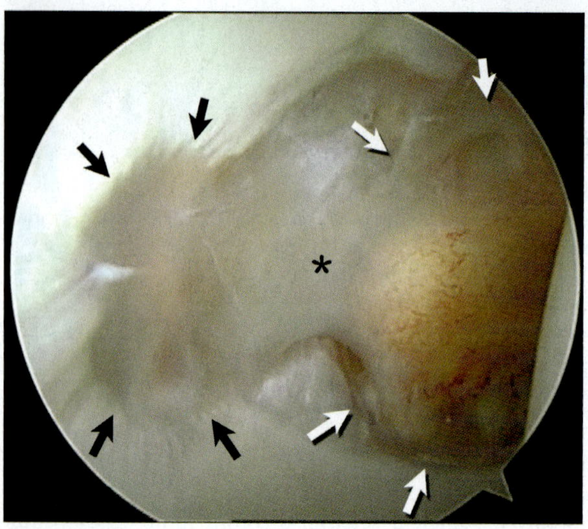

C

Figure 7.28. The supraacetabular fossa is a morphological variant. **A:** AP radiograph of a right hip illustrates the typical appearance (*arrow*). **B:** A coronal T1-weighted MRI image with gadolinium arthrography illustrates the typical defect (*arrows*) filled with contrast. **C:** An arthroscopic view illustrates the supraacetabular fossa (*black arrows*) with fibrotic bands (*) extending down into the acetabular fossa proper (*white arrows*). The configuration gives the appearance of a "keyhole." (Reprinted from Byrd JWT, MD, with permission.)

CHAPTER

8

Michael W. Geary
Carlos A. Guanche

Treatment of Labral Pathology

Our understanding of hip labral pathology as an etiology of hip pain is evolving. The various treatment interventions available are also in flux. This chapter will review the current knowledge of the anatomy and pathophysiology of the hip labrum and its impact on hip mechanics. A synopsis of current diagnostic and treatment algorithms will also be presented.

BASIC SCIENCE

The hip labrum is a fibrocartilaginous structure that surrounds the rim of the acetabulum in a nearly circumferential manner. It is contiguous with the transverse acetabular ligament across the acetabular notch. The vascularity and histology of the hip labrum has been well described in the literature.[1–3] The labrum is widest in the anterior half and thickest in the superior half and merges with the articular hyaline cartilage of the acetabulum through a transition zone of 1 to 2 mm.[2] The labrum is attached to the edge of the bony acetabulum via a thin tongue of bone that extends into the tissue via a zone of calcified cartilage and adheres directly to the outer surface of this bony extension without a zone of calcified cartilage. A group of three or four vessels are located in the substance of the labrum on the capsular side of this bony extension from the acetabulum. The labrum is separated from the hip capsule by a narrow synovial-lined recess.

In general, the vascular supply of the adult hip labrum is poor and regional differences in vascularity do exist. Kelly et al. used cadaveric injection studies to define the vascularity of the labrum and demonstrated that the capsular portion of the labrum is significantly more vascular than the articular side.[1] Furthermore, the capsular portion that is adjacent to the bony acetabulum has the highest mean vascularity (Fig. 8.1). Immunohistochemistry has also been used to describe the vascularity of the labrum.[3] These studies have shown that the blood supply is derived from the adjacent hip capsule and only the peripheral one third of the labrum has a vascular supply. Extrapolating from our understanding of the healing capacity of the meniscus and the results of these two studies, repair strategies should be considered in tears involving only the peripheral labrum.

The labrum functions to enhance the stability of the hip by maintaining the negative intra-articular pressure within the joint.[4] The structure also enhances joint stability and congruity.[5] Through a poroelastic finite element model it was delineated that the labrum functions to provide structural resistance to the lateral motion of the femoral head within the acetabulum. Furthermore, it has been demonstrated that it also functions to decrease contact pressures within the hip and decrease cartilage surface consolidation, probably as a result of its effect on maintaining the articular fluid in contact with the weight bearing cartilage through its joint sealing effect.[6,7]

ETIOLOGY OF LABRAL TEARING

There are several theories on the mechanism of pathologic labral tearing, reflecting the fact that the etiology is likely multifactorial in nature. Byrd[8] proposed general mechanisms where tearing of the hip labrum might occur. In the setting of a normal labrum, supraphysiologic loads would be required to produce a labral tear. Conversely, in the setting of an abnormal labrum, tearing could occur at physiologic loads.

More specifically, injury to the hip labrum could occur with a traction injury whereby failure would occur with excessive and repetitive external rotation of the hip on the anterior labrum. One obvious mechanism is posterior instability associated with significant trauma that could produce a labral lesion as a result of subluxation or dislocation of the femoral head. Atraumatic instability has also been attributed to a deficient labrum associated with the redundant capsular/ligament tissue.[9] This deficient complex can create an abnormal load distribution due to a transiently incongruent joint from subtle subluxation. Sports that require repeated hip rotation (football, golf, gymnastics, soccer, ballet, and baseball) are susceptible to overuse injuries to the labrum and capsuloligamentous complex.[9,10] Tears of the labrum or iliofemoral ligament can result in insufficiency of the buffer mechanism and increased tension on the joint capsule that can be further exacerbated by slight superior and lateral inclination of the acetabulum.[9] In addition, cadaveric analysis of hip stability following capsular venting and a 15 mm labral tear has shown that positions of hip extension, when combined with abduction or external rotation forces, result in large strains in the anterior labrum at the acetabulum–labrum interface.[11] A breach of the integrity of labral function was shown to permit increased displacement of the femur relative to the acetabulum during extreme ranges of motion.

Finally, compressive lesions to the anterior labrum could occur with excessive and repetitive flexion and/or internal rotation of the hip. This process could be accelerated in the

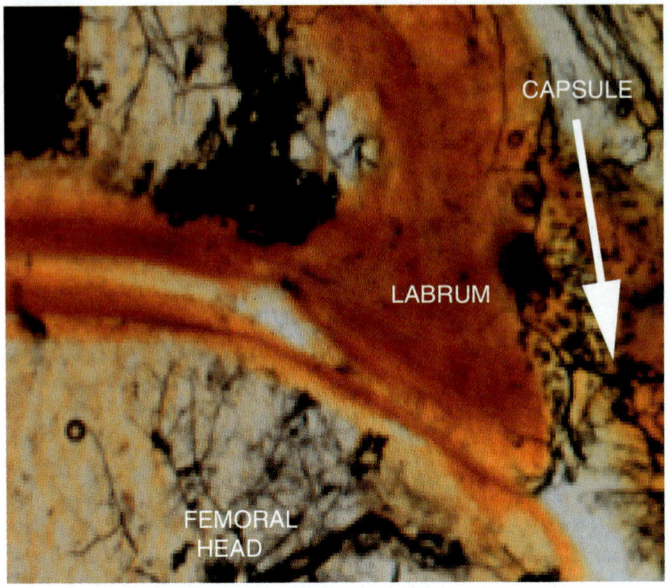

Figure 8.1. Vascularity of the hip labrum. Cross-sectional image of hip labrum prepared with Spalteholtz technique depicting the vascularity adjacent to the capsulolabral junction with a relative paucity of vascularity at the articular cartilage–labral junction. (Courtesy of Bryan Kelly, MD.)

setting of femoroacetabular impingement, where there exists an anatomic predisposition to trauma to the anterior labrum with flexion and internal rotation of the hip.

Regardless of the mechanism, the majority of labral tears encountered at the time of arthroscopy occur in the anterior quadrant. In a series by Fitzgerald,[12] 45 of 49 labral injuries were documented in the anterior marginal attachment of the acetabulum. These findings are supported by another study that reported that 96% of labral tears encountered in a series of 436 consecutive hip arthroscopies occurred in the anterior quadrant.[13]

EPIDEMIOLOGY

The exact prevalence of acetabular labral tears in the general population is not known. One study, however, has investigated the incidence of these injuries in athletes presenting with groin pain. A clinical assessment, in addition to magnetic resonance arthrography (MRA), on 18 patients, in an age range from 17 to 48, presenting to a sports clinic with complaints of groin pain revealed that in 4 out of the 18 athletes (22%) a labral tear was documented on MRA.[14]

DIAGNOSIS OF LABRAL TEARS OF THE HIP

The clinical presentation of patients with a tear of the labrum is variable and as a result, the diagnosis is often missed initially. Burnett et al.[15] reported on a series of 66 patients in whom the diagnosis of a labral tear had been made by arthroscopy. In this series, the mean time from onset of symptoms to diagnosis was 21 months. An average of 3.3 health care providers had seen each patient prior to being diagnosed with a labral tear. Groin pain was the most common complaint (92%), with the onset of symptoms most often insidious. The most common exam finding was a positive "impingement sign," which occurred in 95% of patients in this series. This sign consists of groin pain with flexion and internal rotation of the symptomatic hip. Therefore, in young active patients presenting with complaints of groin pain, with or without a history of trauma, the diagnosis of a labral tear of the hip should be suspected and investigated further.

Multiple studies have demonstrated the superior accuracy of MRA over standard magnetic resonance imaging (MRI) in diagnosing labral tears.[16,17] Intra-articular gadolinium has been shown to improve the sensitivity of diagnosing labral pathology from 25% to 92% using a small field of view.[17] Therefore, when clinical suspicion of a hip labral tear exists, MRA using a small field of view is the study of choice.

An intra-articular lidocaine injection is useful in situations where the diagnosis of labral pathology is equivocal or if a tear has been diagnosed by MRA, but it is uncertain whether symptoms are related to this finding. Similar to its use in diagnosing external impingement of the shoulder, if patients experience relief from their symptoms following the injection, the diagnosis of pain secondary to hip intra-articular pathology is more certain.

Finally, the most sensitive test for the documentation of labral pathology is arthroscopy of the hip. With symptoms and exam findings consistent with labral pathology, and where MRA fails to show a tear, it is not unreasonable to consider performing an arthroscopy for diagnostic and therapeutic reasons after a period of conservative management has failed. Surgical intervention, however, should not be entertained until all other forms of treatment including activity modification, physical therapy, and nonsteroidal anti-inflammatory medications have failed.

TREATMENT: NONOPERATIVE

CLASSIFICATION OF LABRAL TEARS

Lage et al.[18] have described an arthroscopic classification of labral tears. Four groups were described: radial flap, radial fibrillated, longitudinal peripheral, and mobile tears. Radial flaps were the most common, followed by radial fibrillated, longitudinal peripheral, and mobile tears. They also classified degenerative tears based on the location and the extent of the tear. Stage I degenerative tears are localized to one segment of an anatomic region, anterior or posterior. Stage II tears involve an entire anatomic region, and stage III tears are diffuse and involve more than one region. The extent of tearing correlated with the degree of degenerative changes including erosive changes.[19] The articular lesions are most often located adjacent to the labral tear, often at the labrochondral junction.[20]

Another classification is based on histologic analysis of cadaveric specimens.[2] Type 1 tears are detached from the labrum with displacement from the fibrocartilaginous labrum–cartilage junction. Type 2 tears involve one or more cleavage planes of variable depth within the substance of the labrum. Increased microvessel formation has been documented within both types of tear patterns. Based on these investigations, it was concluded that tears of the acetabular labrum are acquired conditions that are highly prevalent in aging adult hips and are likely to occur early in the arthritic process. This explains the fact that many of the tears that are diagnosed have no obvious traumatic etiology and may be attritional in nature.

Labral tears secondary to trauma are generally isolated to one quadrant depending on the direction of trauma and these may be amenable to an arthroscopic repair.[20] Recurrent torsional maneuvers subject the anterior portion of the articular–labral junction to recurrent microtrauma and tears as a result of capsular elongation, particularly at the level of the iliofemoral ligament.[21] Pivoting or twisting sports appear to predispose to these injuries.

Once the diagnosis of a labral tear has been made, a discussion is held with the patient regarding treatment options. Conservative treatment options include avoiding activities that cause symptoms and a supervised therapy program that emphasizes hip range of motion and core strengthening. While it is unlikely that the tear will heal over time, it is possible that symptoms may stabilize to the point that the patient no longer experiences problems. If conservative management is elected, the patient should understand the need to avoid activities that produce symptoms and the possibility that the tear may progress and potentially predispose to arthritic changes in the affected hip. To our knowledge, there are no published series detailing the results of physical therapy for the treatment of symptomatic hip labral tears.

TREATMENT: OPERATIVE

The decision to proceed with operative intervention should be heavily weighted on refractory, mechanical symptoms. The majority of labral tears are treated with debridement; however, some tears are amenable to arthroscopic repair. As discussed above and documented by Petersen, the blood supply to the labrum enters from the adjacent joint capsule.[3] Vascularity was detected in the peripheral one third of the labrum while the inner two-thirds of the labrum are avascular. Thus, peripheral tears have healing potential and repairs should be considered if this is observed at the time of surgery. However, McCarthy et al.[20] reported 436 consecutive hip arthroscopies including 261 labral tears, all of the tears were located at the relatively avascular articular junction.

TECHNIQUE FOR ARTHROSCOPIC LABRAL DEBRIDEMENT

The procedure can be performed in either the supine or lateral position, and it simply depends on the level of comfort that the physician has with the particular setup. The procedure should employ both a 30° and 70° arthroscope for a thorough assessment of the labrum as well as the associated pathology. Modified arthroscopic flexible instruments, extended shavers, and hip-specific instrumentation should be available to improve access to all areas of the hip joint.

A diagnostic arthroscopic examination of the central compartment can be done systematically not only to evaluate the labrum from anterior to posterior but also to locate possible cartilage lesions on both the acetabular and femoral side. In addition, the integrity of the ligamentum teres should be assessed. This area can be a source of pain as a result of impingement of the soft tissues between the femoral head and acetabulum. Any loose bodies should be noted and their source identified. Finally, an assessment should be made of any obvious capsular redundancy or laxity.

Many patients will have a significant synovitis associated with the labral tearing and an effort should be made to resect some of the inflamed tissue not only for visualization of the joint but also to decrease the associated pain. This should be undertaken with a radiofrequency (RF) probe to decrease the potential for bleeding and subsequent compromise of the surgical field.

The goal of the surgical procedure should be to preserve as much native tissue as is technically feasible while resecting the degenerative or damaged material. This is important to maintain the labrum's role as a secondary joint stabilizer and minimize the potential for arthrosis. Fraying from labral tears should be debrided with the use of either motorized shavers or RF probes. Placing absorbable suture through the defect and tying the suture through the capsule can stabilize the intrasubstance labral tears. It is important to delineate the areas of abnormal tissue that are identified both on radiographs (in the form of perilabral calcifications) and on MRI/A (abnormal signal intensity) to thoroughly address the labral pathology.

Adjacent cartilage damage should be searched for and thoroughly addressed. Superficial lesions can be gently debrided with mechanical shavers and perhaps stabilized with the use of RF probes. Grade IV Outerbridge lesions should be managed with a thorough debridement down to a bleeding bed and preparation with microfracture awls (Fig. 8.2).

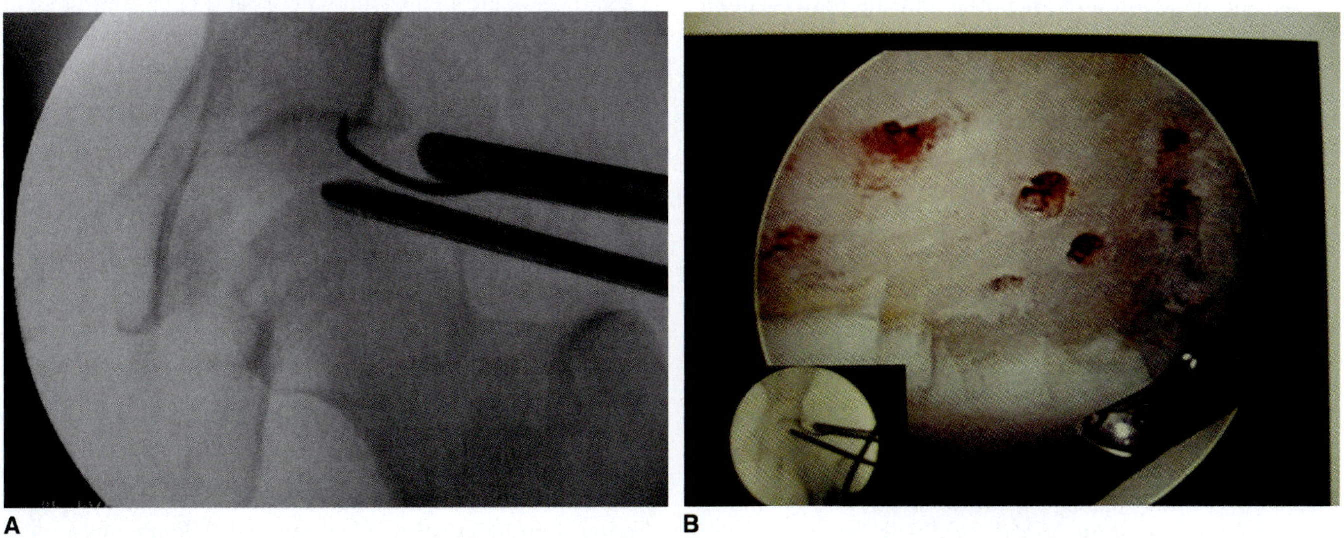

A B

Figure 8.2. Chondroplasty of articular cartilage lesions. **A:** Chondroplasty awl used in the preparation of significant chondral injuries of the acetabular and femoral cartilage. **B:** Final area of preparation.

REHABILITATION FOLLOWING DEBRIDEMENT

Formal therapy for range of motion and strengthening of the operative hip is begun 7 to 10 days following surgery. Weight bearing following an isolated arthroscopic labral debridement should be unrestricted with the use of crutches limited to the early postoperative period only (3 to 5 days). The standard protocol includes a gradual progression from increasing the range of motion to unrestricted strengthening. Aggressive hip flexor strengthening should be limited until full range of motion is obtained and hip mechanics are relatively normal. In cases where abnormal mechanics substitute the psoas and/or hip flexors abnormally, a significant tendonitis can develop which is difficult to eradicate. Explosive and rotational activities should also be limited for at least 6 weeks. The return to unrestricted activity is predicated on a full, painless range of motion and normal strength of the pelvic, abdominal, and lower extremity musculature.

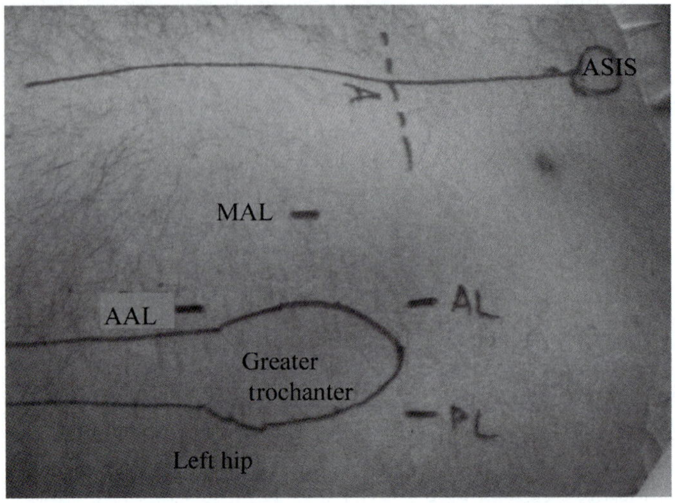

Figure 8.3. The standard arthroscopic portals employed for labral repairs. Accessory midanterolateral portal is useful as a result of its appropriate angle of approach to the acetabular bone. ASIS, anterior superior iliac spine; A, anterior portal; AL, anterolateral portal; PL, posterolateral portal; AAL, accessory anterolateral portal.

TECHNIQUE FOR ARTHROSCOPIC LABRAL REPAIR

The decision to perform a labral repair is still a process in its infancy. The current indications are tears that are symptomatic and have either obvious vascularity within their substance or they are repairable to the acetabular bony wall (or the adjacent capsule). In general, a tear less than 1 cm in length does not require repair since there is minimal associated instability and mechanical symptomatology. In addition, the decision to perform a repair should be predicated on having the appropriate instrumentation as well as adequate technical ability in the performance of the procedure.

Arthroscopic labral repairs can technically be performed with good short-term outcomes.[22,23] The long-term studies that are available are only with open techniques, but these also support labral repairs.[24] The arthroscopic techniques include the use of routine anterior and anterolateral portals as well as an accessory mid-anterior portal that is halfway between the two portals and about 2 cm distal (Fig. 8.3).[8] The routine use of several accessory portals is supported by the fact that the anterior anatomy allows for safe portal establishment anywhere between the standard anterior portal and the posterolateral portal.

As with the debridements described above, the surgical procedure includes a diagnostic arthroscopy with treatment of any associated pathology. In addition, most labral tears that are repaired will also require at least a partial debridement of the avascular and often degenerative tissue. Following completion of the debridement, preparation is made for the repair. Similar to the concept of arthroscopic labral repair in the shoulder, the use of suture anchors has been shown to be effective for fixation in those cases where a bony detachment has occurred. In situations where the tear is in the labrocapsular junction, the repair can be performed with the use of suture material that is placed around the labrum and repaired to the adjacent capsular tissue.[25]

Where the labral tear involves a detachment from the acetabulum, either as a result of trauma or attritional tearing as described in the Seldes classification, a suture anchor is required for stabilization of the tear.[2] The position of the anchor is critical in reestablishing the normal anatomy of the labrum. It should be placed on the acetabular rim, in order to achieve an appropriate angle of approach, while not penetrating into the articular cartilage. Avoiding chondral injury, both in the head (upon delivery of the anchor) and with respect to acetabular penetration, is important as it can become a factor in joint degeneration. Both endoscopic and fluoroscopic visualizations are essential. (Fig. 8.4) Options for repair include traditional suture anchors that include knot tying or, more recently, the use of knotless anchors (PushLock; Arthrex, Inc.; Naples, FL) that allow for relatively easier technical maneuvers within the tight confines of the hip joint (Fig. 8.5).

Once the anchor is placed, a suture-passing device should be employed for penetration of the labrum. A variety of devices exist for this purpose with some employing shuttle devices and some simply penetrating through the tissue (Fig. 8.6). Most of the instruments have been adapted from those employed in shoulder arthroscopy (Fig. 8.7).

In cases where an intrasubstance split is to be addressed, the cleavage plane in the labrum should be fully defined and debrided of nonviable tissue.[26] A suture shuttle device can be used to deliver a looped monofilament suture between the junction of the articular cartilage and the fibrocartilage labrum. A suture penetrator is then employed through the capsule to grasp the loop of the monofilament. The looped suture is then used to shuttle a monofilament suture around the labral tearing and through the capsule. The suture is then tied in an extra-articular position with the use of tactile feel and an automatic suture cutter (Fig. 8.8).

REHABILITATION FOLLOWING LABRAL REPAIR

Formal therapy for range of motion and strengthening of the operative hip is begun 7 to 10 days following the surgery. Early range of motion is initiated to limit the scarring in the joint associated with the surgical trauma. Weight bearing following an isolated arthroscopic labral debridement should be restricted to toe-touch with the use of crutches for the first 4 weeks. The most important principle is to limit the rotational

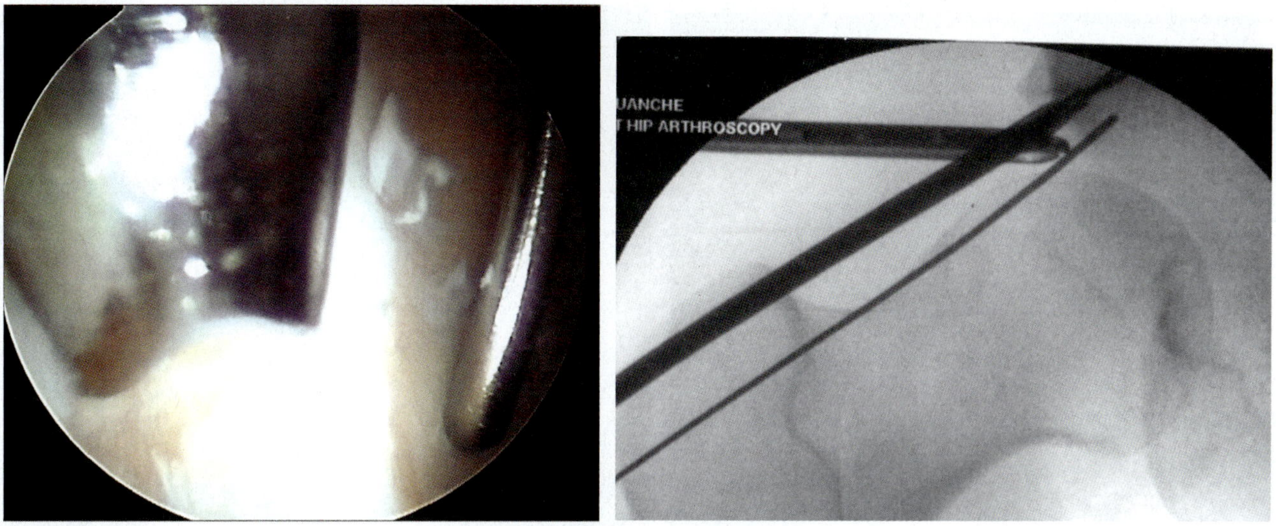

A B

Figure 8.4. Arthroscopic and endoscopic visualization of suture anchor insertion. **A:** An endoscopic view of suture anchor cannula prior to anchor delivery. **B:** Fluoroscopic image of cannula with its projected course away from the articular margin of the joint.

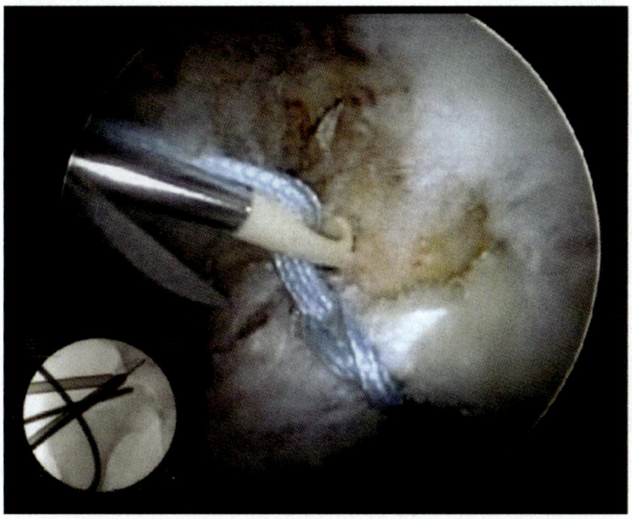

Figure 8.5. Insertion of knotless anchor in the superior acetabulum. (Push lock anchor: Arthrex, Inc; Naples, FL.)

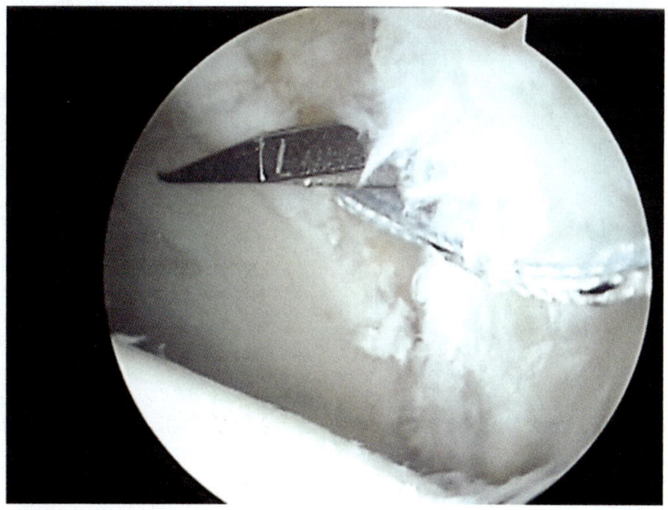

Figure 8.6. Suture penetrator in place within the substance of a labrum that is detached from the acetabular bony wall.

stresses that the repaired labrum experiences in the first few weeks. The ranges that put the repair at risk include flexion past 90°, abduction past 25°, and internal/external rotation limited to 25°.[27] Limitations are placed on flexion past 90° for 10 days while abduction and adduction are limited to 25° for 4 weeks. Beginning at 4 weeks, a gradual progression from increasing the range of motion to unrestricted strengthening is begun. The use of stationary bicycling is encouraged and instituted in the first 10 days. Aggressive hip flexor strengthening should be limited until full range of motion is obtained and hip mechanics are relatively normal. In cases where abnormal mechanics substitute the psoas and/or hip flexors abnormally, a significant tendonitis can develop which is difficult to eradicate. Explosive and rotational activities should also be limited for at least 12 weeks. The return to unrestricted activity is predicated on a full, painless range of motion and normal strength of the pelvic, abdominal, and lower extremity musculature. This typically occurs at approximately 4 to 6 months postoperatively.

RESULTS

There are numerous studies detailing the use of arthroscopy in treating lesions of the hip labrum. However, collective interpretation is confounded by the nonuniform use of outcome measures and a lack of validated outcomes for nonarthritic hip pain. Further complicating the matter is the fact that many published

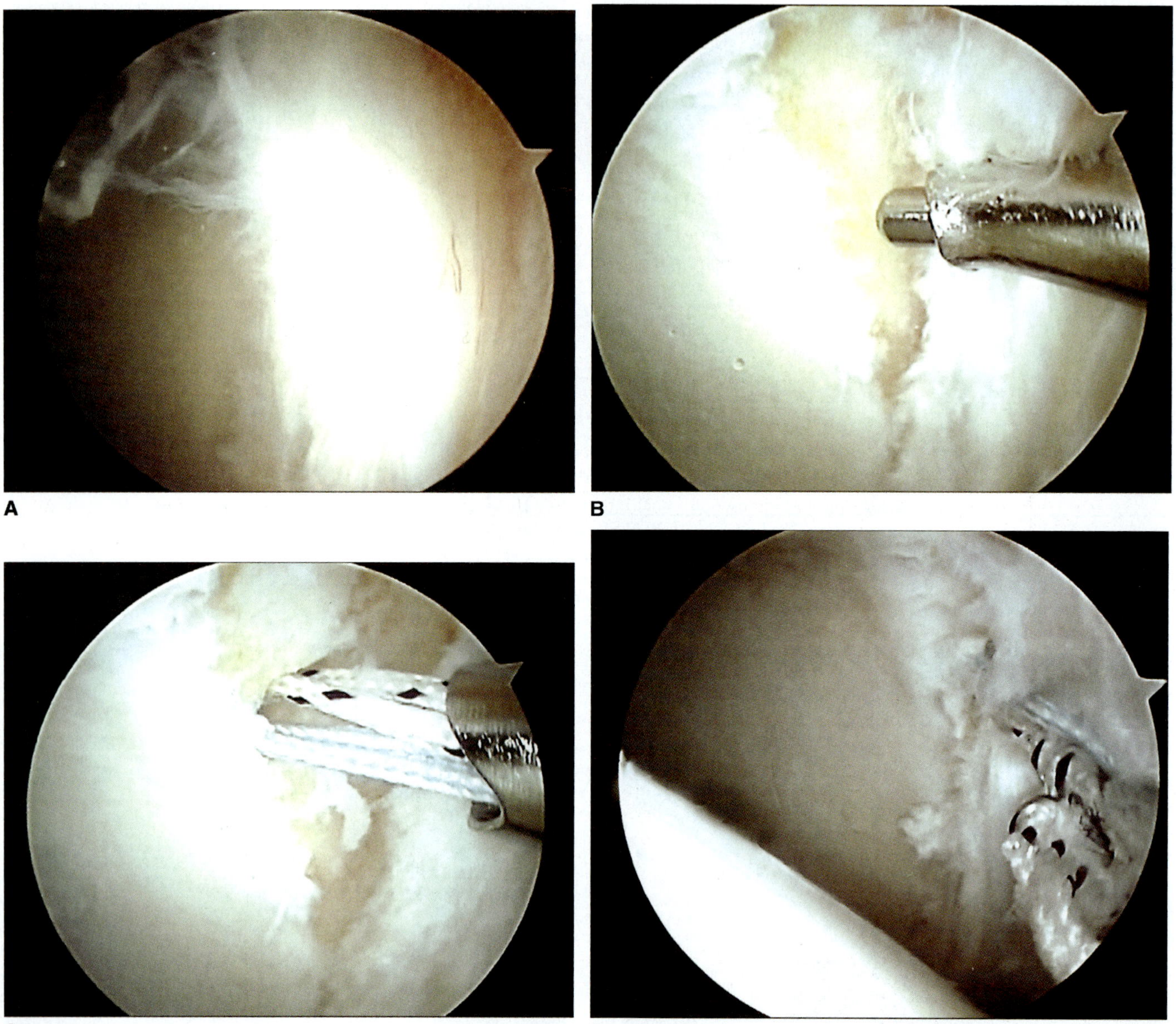

A B C D

Figure 8.7. Labral repair using a suture anchor with penetrator devices. **A:** Labral tear in a left hip, viewed from the anterolateral portal. **B:** Prepared bony bed. **C:** Anchor in place. **D:** Final repair.

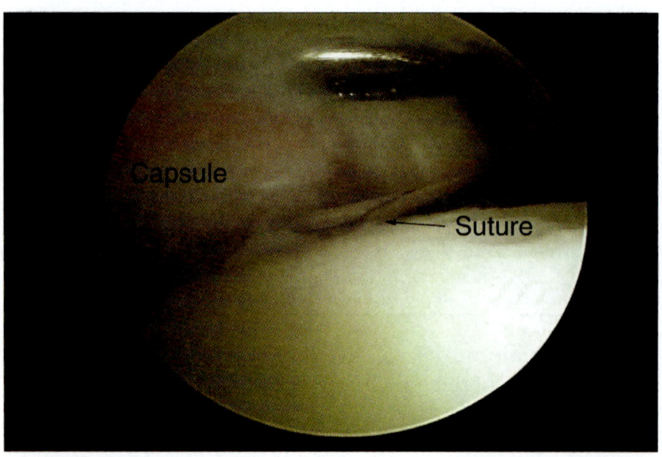

Figure 8.8. Repair of labrum with extracapsular suture positioning.

series contain heterogeneous study populations where subjects have associated hip pathology, such as arthritis, dysplasia, and femoroacetabular impingement, in addition to labral tearing.

Robertson et al.[28] recently reviewed the body of literature on this subject. Multiple databases were utilized to identify articles on the use of arthroscopy in the treatment of hip labral tears published between 1980 and 2005. Initially, 26 articles were identified. After review, it was found that only five focused on arthroscopic treatment of hip labral tears and provided sufficient outcome data with at least 2-year follow-up.[24,29,30–32] In analyzing these studies collectively, they concluded that patients with a symptomatic labral tear that failed conservative management were not claiming worker's compensation, did not have severe arthritis or acetabular dysplasia, and could expect the following results after undergoing arthroscopic labral debridement: A patient satisfaction rate of 67% at 3.5-year follow-up,

TABLE 8.1 Summary of Studies on the Results of Arthroscopic Debridement and Repair of Tears of the Hip Labrum

Study	*Labral treatment*	*Number of patients*	*Mean follow-up*	*Results*
Byrd and Jones[29]	D	35	2 year	Significant improvement in Harris Hip Score (HHS); Best in labral tears or loose bodies
Farjo et al.[24]	D	28	13–100 month	71% good/excellent without arthritis; 21% good/excellent with DJD
O'Leary et al.[30]	D	86	30 month	91% improvement with labral tears; 40% with osteonecrosis; 44% with DJD
Potter et al.[31]	D	40	13–55 month	70% overall patient satisfaction
Santorini and Vellar[3]	D	76	24–61 month	67% overall satisfaction; mean MHHS 89.8
Hines et al.[22]	R	52	9 month	85% good/excellent results
Ross et al.[23]	R	19	6 month	Significant improvement in MHHS, SF-36, nonarthritic hip, and VAS; 67% satisfied

D, debridement; R, repair.

good results by modified Harris Hip (MHH) Score in satisfied patients, and complete resolution of mechanical symptoms in 50% of the patients (Table 8.1).

To date, there are no published series on the long-term outcome of arthroscopic repair of hip labral tears. Indications for what lesions constitute a "repairable lesion" are currently evolving. Recently, outcome results on a series of 52 patients who underwent arthroscopic hip labral repair with a mean follow-up of 9 months were presented by Hines et al.[22] Patients experienced a significant improvement in all outcome measures at the time of follow-up. Outcome measures included the Hip Outcome Score, the Nonarthritic Hip (NAH) Score, and the MHH (Table 8.1).

Another study encompassing 19 patients has recently been published. Interestingly, the mechanism of injury was traumatic in seven patients (33%) and twisting in three patients (14%), with the remaining 52% reporting an insidious onset, lending credence to the concept of repetitive traction injury leading to tears.[33] At a minimum follow-up of 6 months, 12 of the 18 patients (67%) reported that they were satisfied with their procedure. Significant improvements were documented in MHH score, SF-36, VAS, and NAH score (Table 8.1).

FUTURE DIRECTIONS

In summary, the mechanical effects of the labrum appear to substantiate the need to preserve as much tissue as possible. The effects of a decrease in synovial fluid within the weight-bearing dome of the acetabulum, as a result of labral resection, are probably detrimental on a long-term basis. Therefore, treatment of patients having mechanical symptoms with underlying labral pathology needs to be undertaken in a conservative fashion to alleviate symptoms and also to prevent (or delay) the development of degenerative changes.

There are key questions that remain to be answered in the use of hip arthroscopy to treat lesions of the hip labrum. The first would be to determine the long-term results of arthroscopic debridement of tears of the hip labrum. Furthermore, how do these results compare to the natural history of tears of the hip labrum. Second, and in conjunction with the first question, how do short- and long-term results of arthroscopic repair of the torn hip labrum compare to those of arthroscopic debridement.

The available literature supports the concept that the labrum is important for both the stability of the joint as well as the cartilage protection.[34] The long-term effects of repair or excision clearly need to be further delineated before definitive management can be discerned. Intuitively, the preservation of as much relatively normal labral tissue with any surgical procedure is critical to the long-term preservation of the native hip joint.

REFERENCES

1. Kelly BT, Shapiro GS, Digiovanni CW, et al. Vascularity of the hip labrum: A cadaveric investigation. *Arthroscopy*. 2005;21(1):3–11.
2. Seldes RM, Tan V, Hunt J, et al. Anatomy, histologic features, and vascularity of the adult acetabular labrum. *Clin Orthop*. 2001;382:232–240.
3. Petersen W, Petersen F, Tillmann B. Structure and vascularization of the acetabular labrum with regard to the pathogenesis and healing of labral lesions. *Arch Orthop Trauma Surg*. 2003;123:283–288.
4. Takechi H, Nagashima H, Ito S. Intra-articular pressure of the hip joint outside and inside the limbus. *J Jpn Ortho Assoc*. 1982;56:529–536.
5. Ferguson SJ, Bryant JT, Ganz R, et al. The influence of the acetabular labrum on hip joint cartilage consolidation: A poroelastic finite element model. *J Biomech*. 2000;33:953–960.
6. Ferguson SJ, Bryant JT, Ganz R, et al. An in vitro investigation of the acetabular labral seal in hip joint mechanics. *J Biomech*. 2003;36:171–178.
7. Ferguson SJ, Bryant JT, Ganz R, et al. The acetabular labrum seal: A poroelastic finite element model. *Clin Biomech*. 2000;15:463–468.
8. Byrd JW. Arthroscopic acetabular labral repair: Indications, technique & early results. Presented at *2006 AANA Specialty Day Meeting*. Chicago, IL, March 25, 2006.
9. Philippon MJ. The role of arthroscopic thermal capsulorrhaphy in the hip. *Clin Sports Med*. 2001;20:817–829.
10. Bombelli R, ed. *Structure and Function in Normal and Abnormal Hips*. 3rd Ed. New York, NY: Springer-Verlag New York; 1993.
11. Crawford MJ, Dy CJ, Alexander JW, et al. The biomechanics of the hip labrum and the stability of the hip. *J Orthop Res*. 2007;465:16–22.
12. Fitzgerald RH. Acetabular labrum tears. Diagnosis and treatment. *Clin Orthop*. 1995;311:60–68.

13. McCarthy JC, Noble PC, Schuck MR, et al. The watershed labral lesion: Its relationship to early arthritis of the hip. *J Arthroplasty.* 2001;16(8 suppl 1):81–87.
14. Narvani AA, Tsiridis E, Kendall S, et al. A preliminary report on prevalence of acetabular labrum tears in sports patients with groin pain. *Knee Surg Sports Traumatol Arthrosc.* 2003;11:403–408.
15. Burnett RS, Della Rocca GJ, Prather H, et al. Clinical Presentation of patients with tears of the acetabular labrum. *J Bone Joint Surg Am.* 2007;88A:1448–1457.
16. Palmer WE. MR arthrography of the hip. *Semin Musculoskelet Radiol.* 1998;2:349–362.
17. Toomayan FA, Holman WR, Major NM, et al. Sensitivity of MR arthrography in the evaluation of acetabular labral tears. *Am J Roentgenol.* 2006;186(2):449–453.
18. Lage LA, Patel JV, Villar RN. The acetabular labral tear: An arthroscopic classification. *Arthroscopy.* 1996;12:269–272.
19. Neumann G, Mendicuti AD, Zou KH, et al. Prevalence of labral tears and cartilage loss in patients with mechanical symptoms of the hip: Evaluation using MR arthrography. *Osteoarth Cart.* 2007;15:909–917.
20. McCarthy J, Noble P, Aluisio FV, et al. Anatomy, pathologic features, and treatment of acetabular labral tears. *Clin Orthop Rel Res.* 2003;406:38–47.
21. Philippon MJ. Debridement of acetabular labral tears associated with thermal capsulorrhaphy. *Oper Tech Sports Med.* 2002;10:215–218.
22. Hines SL, Philippon MJ, Kuppersmith D, et al. Early results of labral repair. Presented at *2007 Annual AANA Meeting.* April 27, 2007, San Francisco, CA.
23. Ross AE, Javernick M, Freedman B, et al. Arthroscopic hip labral repair. *Arthroscopy.* 2006;22:e30.
24. Farjo LA, Glick JM, Sampson TG. Hip arthroscopy for acetabular labral tears. *Arthroscopy.* 1999;15:132–137.
25. Murphy KP, Ross AE, Javernick A, et al. Repair of the adult acetabular labrum. *Arthroscopy.* 2006;22:e3.
26. Kelly BT, Weiland DE, Schenker ML, et al. Current concepts: Arthroscopic labral repair in the hip: Surgical technique and review of the literature. *Arthroscopy.* 2005;21:1496–1504.
27. Ikeda T, Awaya G, Suzuki S, et al. Torn acetabular labrum in young patients: Arthroscopic diagnosis and management. *J Bone Joint Surg.* 1988;70(B):13–16.
28. Robertson WJ, Kadrmas WR, Kelly BT. Arthroscopic management of labral tears in the hip. A systematic review. *Clin Orthop.* 2006;455:88–92.
29. Byrd JW, Jones KS. Prospective analysis of hip arthroscopy with 2-year follow-up. *Arthroscopy.* 2000;16:578–587.
30. O'Leary JA, Bernard K, Vail TP. The relationship between diagnosis and outcome in arthroscopy of the hip. *Arthroscopy.* 2001;17:181–188.
31. Potter BK, Freedman BA, Andersen RC, et al. Correlation of short form-36 and disability status with outcomes of arthroscopic labral debridement. *Am J Sports Med.* 2005;33:864–870.
32. Santorini N, Villar RN. Acetabular labral tears: Result of arthroscopic partial limbectomy. *Arthroscopy.* 2000;16:11–15.
33. Crawford MJ, Dy CJ, Alexander JW. The biomechanics of the hip labrum and the stability of the hip. *Clin Orthop Rel Res.* 2007;465:16–22.
34. Espinosa N, Rothenfluh DA, Beck M, et al. Treatment of femoro-acetabular impingement: Preliminary results of labral refixation. *J Bone Joint Surg.* 2006;88A:925–935.

CHAPTER

9

Jason Kurian
Carlos A. Guanche

Hip Instability

Unlike the shoulder, which relies primarily on static and dynamic soft tissue restraints for its stability, the hip depends primarily on its osseous anatomy. The hip's unique soft tissue envelope also plays a role in its stability, particularly when there is any significant deviation from the normal.[1] When considering a patient with hip pain that is believed to be at least in some way the result of hip instability, both osseous and soft tissue anatomy must be considered. Acute events as well as chronic/congenital abnormalities must be entertained when developing a differential diagnosis.

The origin of hip instability can be either traumatic or atraumatic. Traumatic dislocation is typically accompanied by a history of an acute event. The spectrum of symptoms can range from frank dislocation to subtle subluxation, with or without concomitant injury. Atraumatic hip instability can result from repetitive rotational movements such as those required in golf or gymnastics. The hypothesized mechanism for this type of instability is a subclinical capsular laxity accompanied by mild hip dysplasia that may progress over time.[2] Generalized laxity and connective tissue disorders such as Marfan and Ehlers–Danlos syndromes are also causes of atraumatic instability.

Treatment of hip instability is largely based on the underlying cause. Diagnosing the etiology of the problem begins with a proper history and physical examination followed by plain radiographs. Specialized radiographs may be indicated as well as further imaging. Depending on the diagnosis, treatment may consist of conservative care involving temporary immobilization, activity modification, physical therapy, and eventual return to activity. In refractory cases, surgical capsular repair or labral/capsular treatment may be necessary. In the presence of severe dysplasia or with the progression to arthritis, periacetabular osteotomy or total joint arthroplasty may be considered. Traumatic dislocations may also require concomitant fragment excision/fixation.

ANATOMY

Although hip anatomy has been discussed previously, some important points need to be further delineated. Once fused, the acetabular surface is oriented approximately 45° caudally and 15° to 20° anteriorly. Significant alterations in acetabular version or inclination as well as its orientation relative to the femoral head/neck can affect the joint capsules and ligaments. In addition, the suction effect that relies on joint congruency for its function may be compromised.[1] These factors may become etiologic in the development of hip instability and need to be considered in the treatment algorithm.

While relying largely upon its bony anatomy, hip stability is complimented by the acetabular labrum and capsuloligamentous complex. In the neutral anatomic position, the anterior part of the femoral head is not engaged in the acetabulum. The acetabular labrum compensates for this by covering this portion of the femoral head. The labrum is attached to the transverse acetabular ligament anteriorly and at the base of the fovea posteriorly and proceeds to run around the circumference of the acetabular rim.[1] The labrum deepens the "socket" and aids in maintaining the suction effect that provides additional hip stability.[3] Absence of the labrum can lead to a loss of this suction effect as well as an increased cartilage surface consolidation and increased contact pressures of the femoral head on the acetabulum.[4–6] Proprioceptors and nociceptors have been identified within the labrum, which may explain the decreased proprioception and increased pain in the athlete with a torn labrum.[7] Much like the meniscus in the knee, the labrum is largely avascular except for the most peripheral portion near the capsule, diminishing its ability to heal.[8]

The labrum is not, however, a stand-alone structure. It functions in conjunction with the capsuloligamentous complex. The fibrous hip capsule and its ligaments are like a thick sleeve. Anteriorly, this complex primarily consists of the iliofemoral ligament, or the ligament of Bigelow.[1] The ligament of Bigelow, 12 to 14 mm thick and shaped like an inverted Y, provides resistance to the hip extension beyond neutral and resists external rotation.[1] The pubofemoral ligament, which arises from the pubic portion of the acetabular rim and passes below the neck of the femur to blend with the most inferior fibers of the iliofemoral ligament, reinforces the inferior and anterior capsule, resisting extension and abduction.[1] A third structure, the ischiofemoral ligament, reinforces the posterior surface of the capsule and has a spiraling pattern.[1] Finally, the zona orbicularis is a deep layer of fibers within the capsule that forms a circular pattern around the femoral neck, constricting the capsule and helping to maintain the femoral head within the acetabulum.[1]

The position of maximum hip joint stability is in full extension because it is in this position that the twisted orientation of the capsular ligaments causes a screw home effect.[1] However, the articular surfaces of the hip joint are not in optimal contact in this position (the "close packed" position). Optimal contact occurs in the loose packed position of flexion and lateral rotation as the ligaments uncoil.[1] The greatest risk of traumatic dislocation, then, is when the joint is in neither the close packed nor the maximally congruent position. This occurs in the flexed and adducted position.[1]

The ligamentum teres and psoas tendon are two extra-articular structures about the hip, which deserve additional discussion.[1] The ligamentum has no real stabilizing effect on the hip joint while the psoas protects the anterior intermediate capsule that is devoid of ligamentous protection.[1]

CLINICAL EVALUATION

Due to the nature of the hip anatomy previously described, it is easy to see why the evaluation of a patient with hip instability can be a diagnostic dilemma. Hip instability can manifest as overtly as frank traumatic dislocation or can be as obscure as occult groin pain or clicking. Hip pain, clicking, or "giving way" in the young adult patient may arise from any number of anatomic structures. The picture can be further complicated by referred pain from the lumbosacral region as well as the genitourinary tract and abdominal wall.[9] Age also plays a significant role in determining a differential diagnosis for hip pain.[10] In children, hip dislocation, bony avulsions, apophyseal injuries, fractures, SCFE, Perthes, DDH, and toxic and septic arthritis are all potential causes.[10,11] In the adult, the spectrum of potential injuries is equally wide.[9,10]

The history should include a qualitative assessment of the main complaint to determine if it is primarily a pain, a clicking, a catching or an instability. A golfer may describe weakness in the involved leg while swinging for power such as while using his driver. Pain may also occur after long periods of sitting, when getting out of a car, or rising from a chair. Timing of the onset of the complaint is also essential. Precipitating factors as well as potential referred or systemic causes must be assessed.[11]

Although the physical examination of the hip has been described previously, specific examination maneuvers should be considered in cases of possible instability. Antalgic gait patterns where there is shortening of the stance phase and step length on the affected side can result from instability. A Trendelenburg gait may indicate an attempt to bring the center of gravity over the affected side to decrease the moment arm across that hip joint.[12] The patient with atraumatic instability may be able to demonstrate subluxation or dislocation of the involved hip, although this is rare.

Traumatic hip instability can manifest with pain on prone extension/external rotation of the involved hip. A positive axial distraction test can be confirmed with a positive vacuum sign on dynamic fluoroscopy (Fig. 9.1).[1] Apprehension may also be elicited with the patient in the lateral decubitus position while suspending the affected leg in slight abduction.

Imaging should always begin with plain radiographs. The standard views are an AP pelvis as well as an AP and lateral of the affected hip.[13] Apart from being able to detect the common radiographic features of trauma, plain radiographs can also help detect femoroacetabular impingement by suggesting a deformed femoral neck or an overriding anterior acetabular rim.

Several radiographic indices have been described to differentiate normal from abnormal osseous anatomy based on the AP pelvis radiograph. The Tonnis angle is used to assess lateral subluxation of the femoral head and subsequent increased forces across the weight bearing acetabulum (Fig. 9.2). Three lines are used to define this angle. Line 1 is a horizontal line connecting the inferior aspects of the ischial tuberosities. The second line is a line parallel to line 1, drawn from the center of the femoral head to be assessed. Line 3 extends from a line drawn through the medial and lateral points of the sourcil (or roof) of the affected acetabulum. The angle this line creates as it intersects line 2 is the Tonnis angle. A measurement of less than 10° is considered normal.[14]

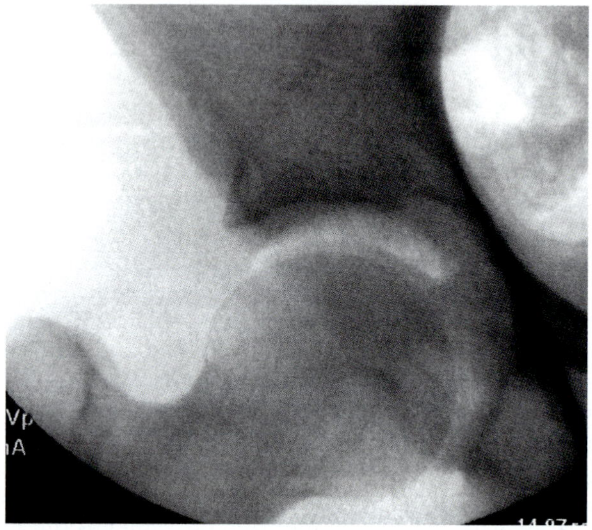

Figure 9.1. Suction seal effect of the joint: Intraoperative image of 16-year-old patient with repetitive use instability due to high-level gymnastics participation. Minor axial traction (20 lb) causes significant distraction and subluxation of the joint. (Adapted from Bellabarba C, Sheinkop M, Kuo K. Idiopathic hip instability. *Clin Orthop.* 1998;355:261–271.)

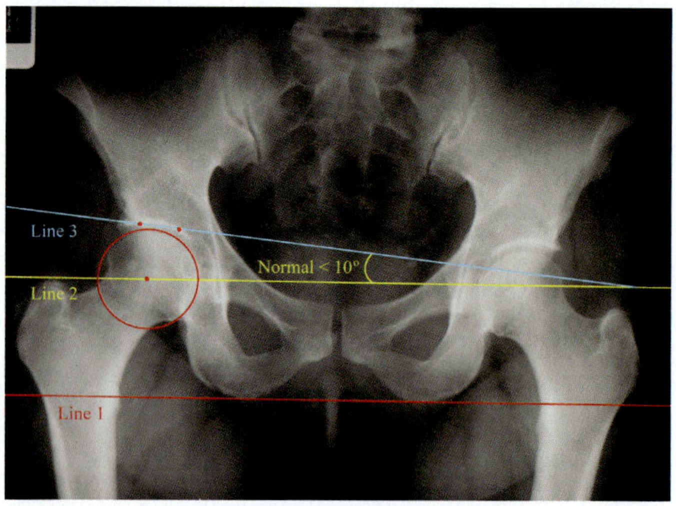

Figure 9.2. An AP radiograph showing the technique of measuring the Tonnis Angle (normal <10°). In this case, the red line (line 1), connecting the two ischial tuberosities, is the reference line upon which all other lines are based. The yellow line, line 2, is a line drawn parallel to line 1 through the center of the femoral head. The angle that is formed between line 2 and a line 3 connecting two points demarcating the "sourcil" or weight-bearing surface of the acetabulum is the Tonnis angle. (Adapted from Delaney S, Dussault RG, Kaplan PA, et al. Radiographic measurements of dysplastic adult hips. *Skeletal Radiol.* 1997;26:75–81.)

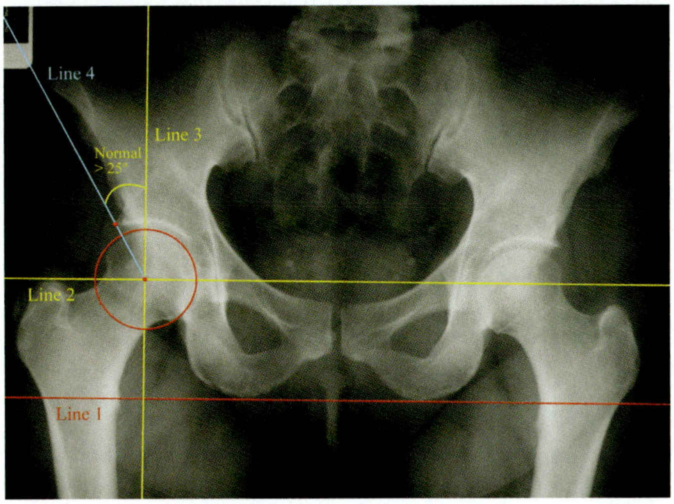

Figure 9.3. An AP radiograph showing the measurement technique for the center-edge angle of Wiberg. The red line represents the initial reference line through the tuberosities that provides the parallel line for line 2 through the femoral head. Line 3 is a line directly perpendicular to line 2 and the angle between this line and line 4 (a line from the center of the femoral head to the lateral edge of the acetabulum). This angle should be greater than 25°, with 20° to 25° being considered borderline. (Adapted from Delaney S, Dussault RG, Kaplan PA, et al. Radiographic measurements of dysplastic adult hips. *Skeletal Radiol.* 1997;26:75–81.)

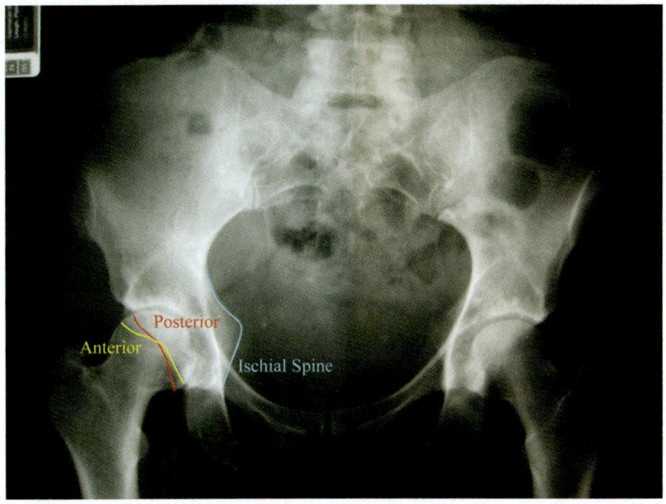

Figure 9.4. An AP radiograph demonstrating the crossover sign indicating acetabular retroversion. Note the red line (representing the anterior wall of the acetabulum) crosses the yellow line (representing the posterior wall of the acetabulum). Also of note is the visualization of the ischial tuberosity (blue line), which is normally superimposed by the acetabulum but easily visible in the retroverted acetabulum. (Adapted from Delaney S, Dussault RG, Kaplan PA, et al. Radiographic measurements of dysplastic adult hips. *Skeletal Radiol.* 1997;26:75–81.)

The center edge angle of Wiberg assesses the acetabular inclination. This angle requires four lines (Fig. 9.3). The first line is a line crossing the inferior aspects of the ischial tuberosities. A second line is drawn parallel to the first and begins at the center of the femoral head to be assessed. The third line is perpendicular to the second, beginning at the center of the femoral head. Finally, a fourth line is drawn, beginning at the center of the femoral head, through the lateral edge of the acetabulum. This angle should measure at least 20° to 25° to be considered normal.[15,16] One can estimate the acetabular version using the AP pelvis by looking for a "crossover sign" (Fig. 9.4). The two lines involved estimate the posterior and anterior rims of the acetabulum. The posterior rim is traced from the ischial tuberosity superolaterally to the roof of the acetabulum. The anterior rim is traced from the teardrop in a superior and lateral direction along the rim to the roof. If these lines cross, it is estimated that the acetabulum is retroverted[14,15,17]; if not, it is assumed that the acetabular version is within the normal 10° to 15° of the anterior version.

When evaluating a patient with potential residual dysplasia, the faux profile view is often used to evaluate the anterior and lateral coverage of the femoral head by the acetabulum. While plain radiographs are sufficient for diagnosis in a number of cases, there are pathologic entities that require further investigation. Among the choices for more advanced imaging are bone scan, ultrasound, computed tomography (CT), including CT arthrography and 3D reconstructions, magnetic resonance imaging (MRI), and MRI arthrography.[9,13,18]

Imaging of bony lesions about the hip is best accomplished using CT as it provides the greatest spatial resolution of bony structures. Cases of questionable hip dysplasia should employ CT in preoperative planning. The use of intra-articular contrast in CT arthrography can increase the contrast between the cartilage and the labral tissue.[9,13,19]

MRI has become the most reliable means of diagnosing unresolved hip pathology outside of direct visualization and is often useful in cases of instability. MRI has been shown to effectively demonstrate inflammatory arthropathies and joint effusions[13,20] but has been less accurate in assessing articular cartilage lesions.[21–24] Contrast MRI studies in patients with a torn labrum or torn iliofemoral ligament can result in a larger volume of intra-articular contrast and, thus, indirectly confirm the diagnosis of instability (Fig. 9.5).[1]

ATRAUMATIC INSTABILITY

As is the case in the shoulder, where numerous types of instability have been described, the separation between traumatic and atraumatic instability in the hip is often difficult. For the

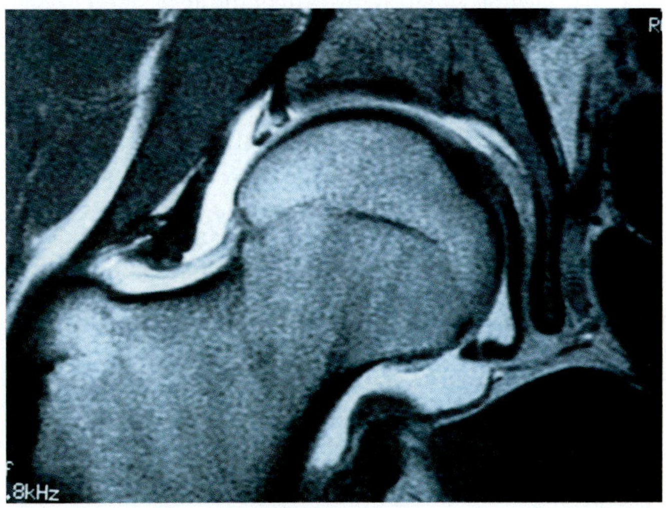

Figure 9.5. MRI image of patient with hip instability secondary to excessive capsular volume. Image is a T2 coronal image. Also note the large labral tear that is evident in this image.

purpose of this chapter, we will consider only those instability syndromes that are the direct result of a distinct, traumatic event that caused a discrete subluxation or frank dislocation as truly traumatic instability. All other congenital dysplasias and connective tissue disorders as well as repetitive use injuries and idiopathic syndromes will be considered atraumatic.

Congenital connective tissue disorders can predispose a patient to atraumatic hip instability. There have been very few reports in the literature of habitual hip dislocation which have not been accompanied by Ehlers–Danlos syndrome, arthrochalasis multiplex congenita, Marfan syndrome, Down syndrome, or congenital or acquired hip dysplasia.[1] As opposed to the frank episodes of subluxation or dislocation that may be seen in atraumatic shoulder instability, idiopathic hip instability often presents with a much more subtle pattern.

In a review of five cases of presumed coxa saltans, or snapping hip syndrome, Bellabarba et al.[2] described a syndrome of "idiopathic hip instability." In this series of five patients, all patients presented with a long history of snapping in the groin, gait disturbances and pain in the provocative position of hip flexion, adduction, and internal rotation that had escaped diagnosis. It seemed as if the patients should fit into one of the previously described categories of snapping hip: internal, external, and intra-articular.[25–39] These patients, by contrast, had physical examinations consistent with generalized ligamentous laxity and AP pelvis radiographs suggestive of mild dysplasia, as evidenced by a slightly lower center edge angle.[2] They complained of symptoms of popping and snapping when rising from a chair or in other instances when the hip was subjected to flexion adduction and internal rotation. Symptoms were alleviated by extension abduction and external rotation. Both the exacerbating and the alleviating maneuvers were analogous to the Barlow and Ortolani signs used in infants while diagnosing developmental hip dysplasia, suggesting a posterior direction to the instability. Furthermore, when the unanesthetized, nonsedated patient had the affected hip subjected to gentle manual traction without counter traction, 4 to 10 mm of inferior subluxation was seen. The force used to "subluxate" the hip in this instance was much less than the 400 N of axial force described by Arvidsson as necessary to create the radiographic vacuum sign that suggests subluxation.[40] All of the above evidence led the authors to postulate that subclinical hip dysplasia, combined with capsuloligamentous laxity, caused a break in the suction mechanism of the hip during gait, causing a popping sensation.[2] Presuming that the instability was largely posteriorly directed and the preoperative arthrography showed posterior capsular redundancy, one patient of the five underwent open posterior capsular plication. The posterior capsule was advanced proximally with suture anchors and the inferior capsule was imbricated superiorly. This tightening of the posterior capsule seemed to prevent the posterior subluxation until the patient fell and had a recurrence of symptoms after an interval of symptom free activity.[2]

Atraumatic instability has also been attributed to a deficient labrum associated with redundant capsular/ligament tissue.[1] This deficient complex can create an abnormal load distribution due to a transiently incongruent joint from a subtle subluxation. The previously mentioned screw home mechanism caused by the dynamic nature of the hip capsule and its associated ligaments may help explain why pelvic rotation and external rotation of the hip commonly elicit the symptoms of hip instability. Professional and high level athletes who participate in sports that require repeated hip rotation (football, golf, gymnastics, soccer, ballet, and baseball) are susceptible to overuse injuries to the labrum and capsuloligamentous complex.[1,41] Tears of the labrum or iliofemoral ligament can result in insufficiency of the buffer mechanism and increased tension on the joint capsule that can be further exacerbated by slight superior and lateral inclination of the acetabulum.[1] In addition, cadaveric analysis of hip stability following capsular venting and a 15 mm labral tear has shown that positions of hip extension, when combined with abduction or external rotation forces, result in large strains in the anterior labrum at the acetabulum–labrum interface.[42] In addition, a breach of the integrity of labral function was shown to permit increased displacement of the femur relative to the acetabulum during extreme ranges of motion.

Philippon, in 2001, described labral degeneration combined with subtle rotational hip instability secondary to redundant capsular tissue as a common injury pattern seen in elite athletes in his practice. Ten patients were treated with arthroscopic labral debridement and thermal capsulorrhaphy. Postoperatively, the patients were allowed to bear weight as tolerated and had rotation and extension precautions for 18 days. All patients had improvement in their Harris hip scores as compared to their preoperative state, with 83% of them having significant improvement in their symptoms at 12 to 24 months follow-up.[1] In contrast, Villar reported only 67.5% success in 58 cases at a mean of 3.5-year follow-up with labral debridement and without capsular treatment.[42] Alternatively, plication can also be performed by passing nonabsorbable, braided suture through the capsule, thus imbricating the capsular tissue (Fig. 9.6).[8]

Although the preliminary results of thermal capsulorrhaphy in the hip have been promising, more long-term follow-up is needed as is suggested by the shoulder literature. Basic science experiments involving thermal capsulorrhaphy were initially promising. These studies showed that the thermal energy delivered to tissue via laser or radiofrequency resulted in shrinkage of the tissue by disrupting the intramolecular cross-links in the collagen triple helix.[43,44] The amount of tissue shrinkage is directly related to the temperature applied, and the optimal temperature appears to be between 65 °C and 75 °C.[45–48] Thermal treatment causes immediate collagen and cell damage, resulting in decreased mechanical stiffness that lasts at least 2 weeks. After this, the tissue undergoes active repair and by 12 weeks, it has similar mechanical properties and cellular components to the native capsule.[49,50] Several studies in the shoulder have shown good results when anterior instability is treated by thermal capsulorrhaphy combined with anterior labral repair.[51–55] These studies are hard to interpret, however, as they combine two procedures.

Miniaci and McBirnie used only thermal capsulorrhaphy in the treatment of multidirectional instability and had 47% recurrent instability.[56] In addition to recurrent instability, complications such as capsule destruction, nerve injuries, and cartilage damage that can lead to massive chondrolysis and premature osteoarthritis can occur.[56–60] Heat capsulorrhaphy in the hip, therefore, should be used with caution at this time.

While subtle hip dysplasia combined with capsular laxity and labral pathology can lead to symptomatic hip instability amenable to arthroscopic treatment, care must be taken to recognize more significant hip dysplasias. Overtly dysplastic hips typically share common abnormalities that occur to a

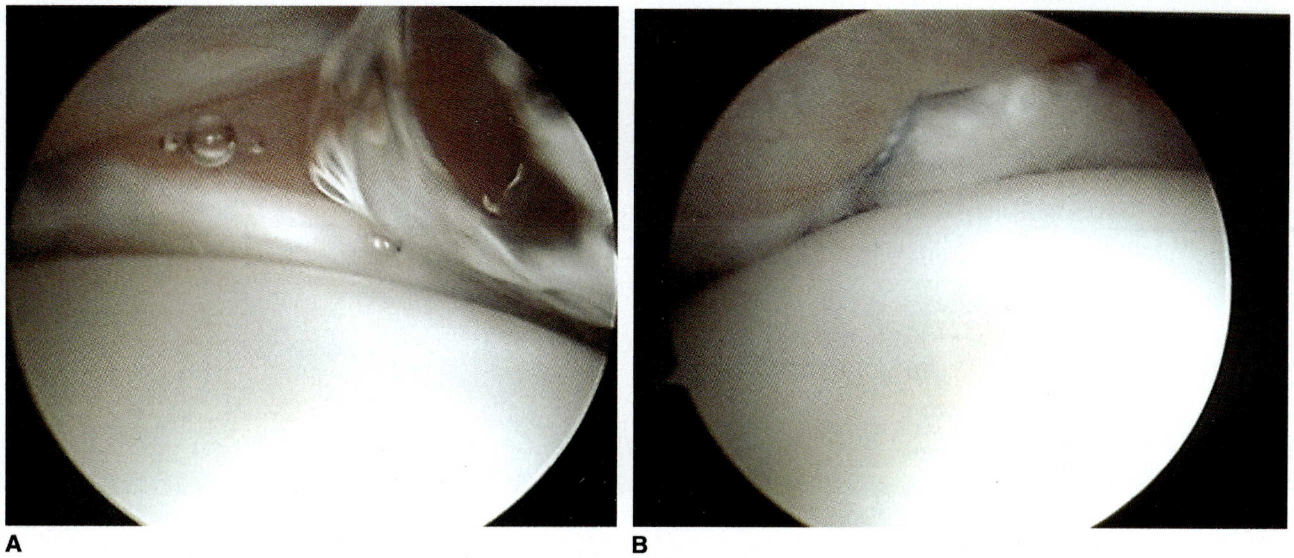

Figure 9.6. Capsular redundancy in a 16-year-old gymnast with no major macrotraumatic event. **A:** Arthroscopic view of right hip viewed from the anterolateral portal while in the peripheral compartment. The perilabral sulcus is seen to be large. The labrum is relatively normal. **B:** View following capsulorrhaphy using suture anchors. Note the obliteration of the perilabral sulcus, with the suture in place immediately proximal to the acetabular rim.

greater or lesser extent depending on the severity.[61] The true acetabulum is usually shallow, lateralized, and anteverted and deficient anteriorly and superiorly. There may be underdevelopment of the entire pelvis. On the femoral side, the femoral head is usually small and the neck is usually excessively anteverted and short with an increased neck-shaft angle. The greater trochanter may be displaced posteriorly and the femoral canal may be narrow.[62] The presence of significant hip dysplasia in the adult can be ascertained using primarily plain radiography. AP pelvis and false profile lateral plain films of the affected hip allow for the measurement of the anterior center-edge angle of Lequesne and de Seze,[63] the lateral center-edge angle of Wiberg,[64] the horizontal position of the hip joint center,[65] acetabular roof obliquity,[64,65] and the integrity of Shenton line.

A patient who presents with radiographic evidence of dysplasia but little or no symptomatology should be treated nonsurgically with strengthening and proprioceptive training of the hip and trunk musculature.[62] Nonsteroidal anti-inflammatories can be used and combined with cessation of high impact activities. The patient should be educated about the potential natural history of increasing instability and the potential development of degenerative arthritis. To this end, a re-examination and repeat radiographs should be documented at 1 to 2 year intervals.[62] Surgical intervention should be reserved for those patients that fail conservative management and have persistent symptoms. Arthroscopic treatment for mildly dysplastic hips has been discussed in detail and is not indicated in the patient with significant dysplasia. In addition, significant labral hypertrophy occurs in these patients. The role of this excess labral tissue has not been completely elucidated, but it may be significant in its effect on joint stability. Aggressive resection of this tissue can accelerate degenerative changes and possibly lead to early joint degeneration. Pelvic and femoral osteotomies, arthrodesis, resection arthroplasty, and replacement arthroplasties have all been described as potential treatment options.[62] Each patient needs to be evaluated individually and the treatment tailored to his or her specific pathology. Regardless of the method of treatment, the goals remain the same with pain relief being the first goal. Osteotomies that may be expected to slow the progression of degenerative changes by better distributing the weight bearing forces across the hip joint have been described. These procedures may also provide better preservation of bone stock for potential subsequent arthroplasty.[62]

Since the majority of pathology in hip dysplasia is acetabular in origin, the role of femoral osteotomies as a stand-alone procedure is minimal. Pelvic osteotomies can be segregated into two basic groups. The reconstructive osteotomies are indicated for patients in whom articular congruity is achievable and are intended to restore more normal hip anatomy and biomechanics with the goal of improving symptoms and preventing degenerative changes.[62] Patients for whom a pelvic osteotomy may be indicated include young patients with symptomatic dysplasia without excessive proximal migration of the center of rotation, reasonably well maintained range of motion, and no more than mild degenerative changes as classified by Tonnis.[61,62]

A commonly performed procedure is the Bernese periacetabular osteotomy. The procedure is indicated in patients with symptoms of hip mechanical overload, impingement, or instability resulting from insufficient acetabular coverage.[67] The advantages of the Bernese osteotomy include only one incision, the vascularity of the acetabulum remains intact via the inferior gluteal artery and the abductor mechanism is not violated.[68] The series of straight, reproducible, extra-articular cuts preserve the integrity of the posterior column while allowing for large corrections in lateral and anterior rotation as well as medialization.[68] The preservation of the posterior column allows for minimal internal fixation and early weight bearing without

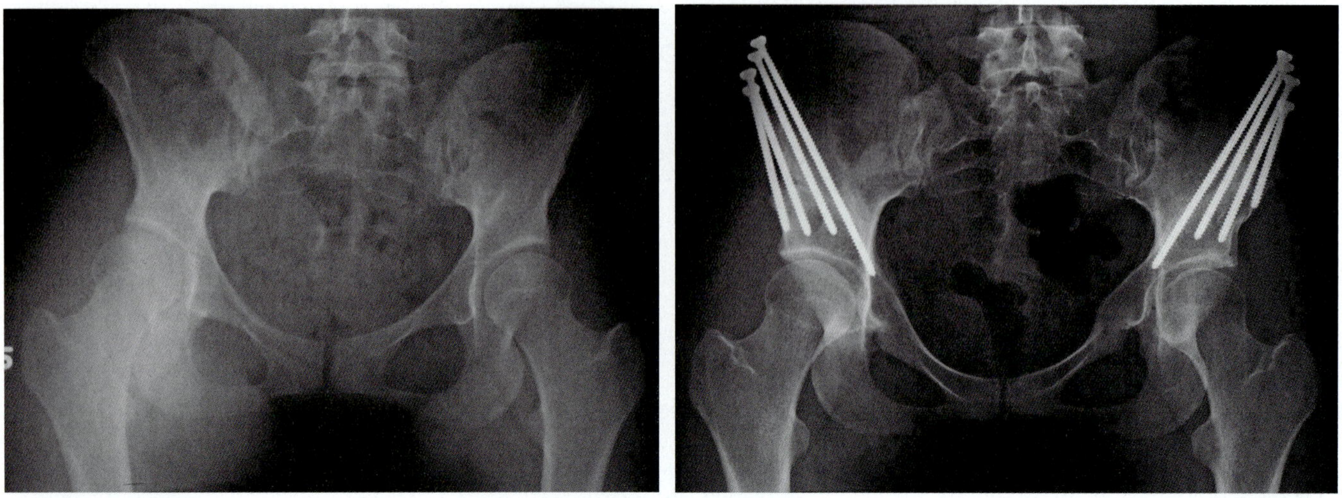

A B

Figure 9.7. Periacetabular osteotomy. **A:** 19-year-old female with history of hip pain and increasing disability. **B:** Postoperative radiograph following periacetabular osteotomy. (Adapted from Tonnis D, Legal H, Graf R, eds. *Congenital Dysplasia and Dislocation of the Hip in Children and Adults.* Berlin, Germany: Springer–Verlag; 1987.

external immobilization, and since the shape of the pelvis is unchanged, normal vaginal childbirth is possible postoperatively (Fig. 9.7).[69]

Siebenrock[70] updated the preliminary results initially reported by Ganz[67] to include an average follow-up of 11.3 years. Excellent correction was maintained and the hip joint was preserved in 82% of patients, while 73% of patients reported good to excellent results. In the 58 patients with preserved hip joints, flexion and internal rotation were decreased while the remaining patients underwent either total hip arthroplasty (THA) (12) or hip fusion (1).[70] Similar results have been obtained by several other authors.[68,69,71,72] Trousdale reported on 42 patients with a mean follow-up of four years, 15 of which had preoperative grade 1 Tonnis changes, 18 had grade 2, and 9 had grade 3. Results were good or excellent in 32 of 33 in those with preoperative Tonnis grade 1 or 2 changes; however, in those with grade 3 changes, eight of the nine underwent subsequent THA.[71] Another study reported on 21 procedures with an average of 3.2 years follow-up. Hip scores improved significantly as did the acetabular index and the anterior and lateral center-edge angles. At follow-up, 16 hips had similar degenerative changes while three had improved and two were worse. One of the two which fared worse required total hip replacement.[72]

Due to the complex nature of the operation, complications have been reported which include nerve injury (particularly to the lateral femoral cutaneous and peroneal branch of the sciatic nerve), inadvertent intra-articular extension of the osteotomy, and heterotopic ossification.[73–77] In addition, excessive anteriorization of the acetabulum can lead to femoroacetabular impingement that may require further treatment.[75]

Other reconstructive osteotomies have been described, including the Salter innominate. Wong-Chung et al.[78] reported favorable results with this procedure in children, but less promising results in adolescents and adults. A number of double and triple osteotomies have also been described in the literature but have largely been replaced by the Bernese.[79–84] Spherical osteotomies have shown the ability to provide good lateral coverage but are technically difficult and have limited ability to medialize the hip joint or provide anterior coverage.[84,85] Salvage osteotomies, such as the Chiari and Shelf osteotomies, are indicated in severely dysplastic hips with issues beyond the scope of this chapter.[62]

Femoral osteotomies are indicated in the rare incidence when the femur is the primary location of deformity or when pelvic osteotomy does not provide adequate coverage.[62] Combined femoral and acetabular osteotomies have been reported in up to 27% of cases.[66–72] Coxa valga is the most common indication for isolated femoral osteotomy in patients with hip dysplasia and mild acetabular deformity. A varus-producing femoral osteotomy can increase the joint congruency in these patients.[62]

A thorough discussion of arthroplasty options for patients with hip instability secondary to dysplasia is beyond the scope of this chapter. However, some knowledge of the subject is essential for educating patients regarding the natural history of instability due to dysplasia. Patients with residual dysplasia and instability may develop degenerative changes,[62] and when they do, early and mid-term results for THA have been promising.[86] THA in this population, however, is significantly more complex than the typical THA. When possible, reconstructing the socket near its anatomic location is ideal, but occasionally, medialization and elevation of the acetabulum and lateral bone grafting are needed to obtain adequate bony coverage. Noncemented acetabular components have shown better results than cemented components. On the femoral side, the location of the acetabular reconstruction and leg length play important roles in determining the type of femoral reconstruction. Femoral shortening via metaphyseal resection followed by greater trochanteric osteotomy and advancement is occasionally required due to leg length and sciatic nerve issues. In the femur, cemented and noncemented techniques have shown similar results.[62]

TRAUMATIC INSTABILITY

As discussed earlier, the spectrum of hip instability ranges from subtle changes such as snapping and pain to acute subluxations and frank traumatic dislocations. The most common mechanism for hip dislocation is a dashboard motor vehicle injury with a posteriorly directed force against a flexed knee

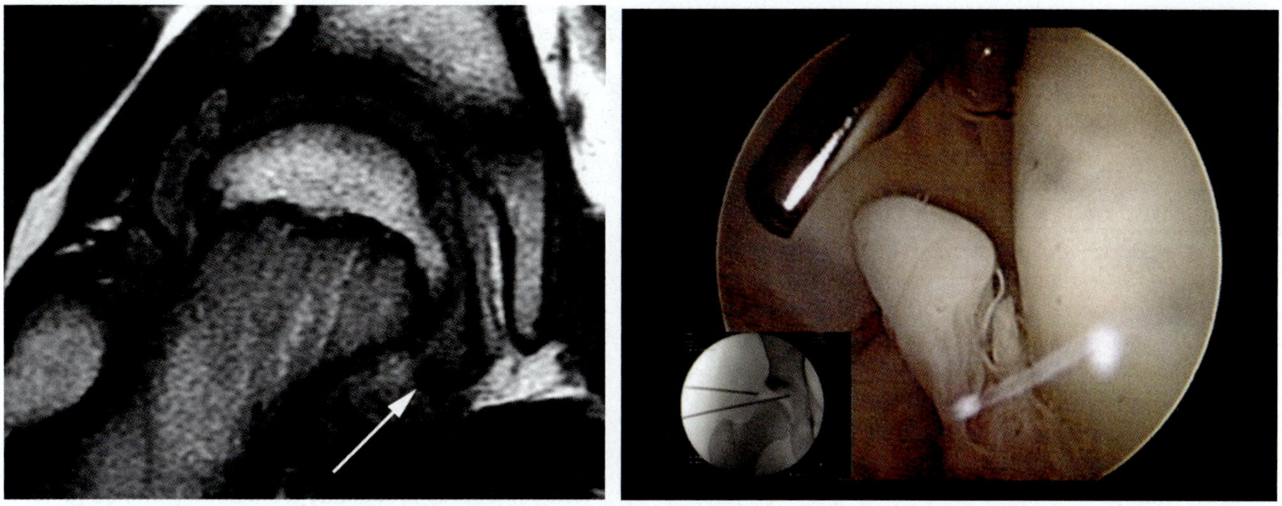

Figure 9.8. Tear of the ligamentum teres following hip instability. **A:** T2-weighted coronal image. The tear is seen at the inferior margin of the acetabulum (*arrow*). **B:** Arthroscopic view of ligamentum tear.

and hip. During athletics, dislocations may occur via a forward fall onto a flexed knee with the hip flexed or a blow from behind while down on all four limbs (Fig. 9.8).[87] Sports such as American football, skiing, jogging, gymnastics, basketball, biking, and soccer have all had reports of traumatic dislocations (Fig. 9.9).[87–90] Excessive capsular laxity has been associated with these types of dislocations.[28,38,91–96] Irrespective of the degree of initial trauma, if normal capsular healing fails to occur, persistent laxity may occur and predispose the patient to instability (Fig. 9.10). Two cases of posterior dislocation following minor trauma while playing soccer have been reported. The patients developed recurrent posterior dislocation with trivial incidents secondary to large posterior capsular redundancy.[97] Similarly, recurrent anterior dislocations have occurred as a result of excessive anterior capsular redundancy.[98] These patients have been treated nonoperatively with brief immobilization, physical therapy, and activity modification. Open capsular shift/repair has been particularly successful in preventing further dislocation.[99] Arthroscopic treatment of this type of capsular laxity using either thermal capsulorrhaphy or capsular plication combined with labral debridement has been discussed earlier in this chapter, and at least in the short term, it has provided promising results while potentially avoiding the complications of heterotopic ossification and osteonecrosis of the femoral head which may be encountered with open procedures.[1]

Hip arthroscopy has been shown to be an important part of the armamentarium in the effort to at least delay the onset of post-traumatic degenerative joint disease (DJD) following traumatic dislocation.[100–102] Residual intra-articular bony or osteochondral fragments may be responsible for the development of DJD in complex dislocations.[98,103–106] The incidence of osteoarthritis secondary to traumatic hip dislocation has been

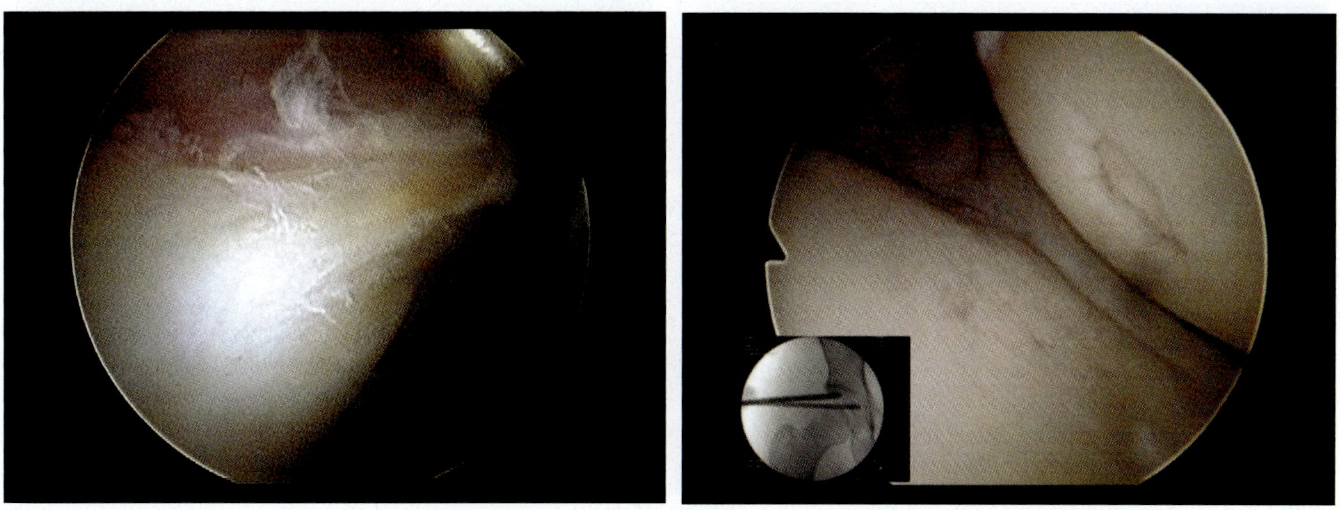

Figure 9.9. Labral tear following dislocation of the hip in a 19-year-old college basketball player. **A:** The view is of the right hip, from the anterolateral portal. Note the significant synovial reaction around the labral tearing. **B:** Focal femoral head defect in the same patient.

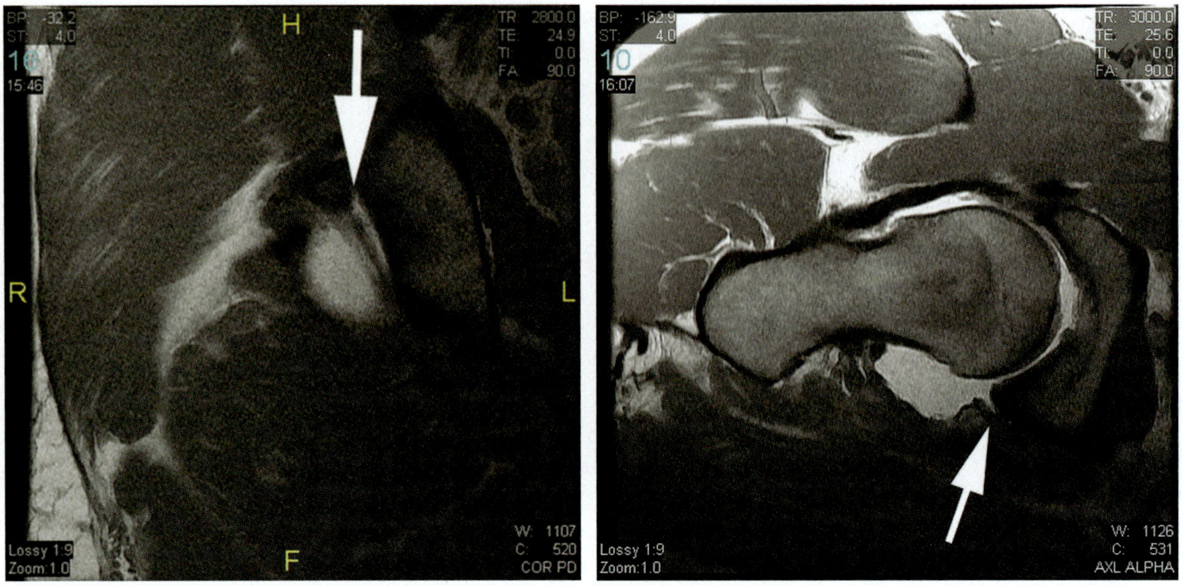

A B

Figure 9.10. MRI following hip dislocation with no bony involvement. **A:** Torn posterior capsule. Image is a T1 weighted, coronal image through the posterior aspect of the joint. The tear is seen longitudinally at the margin of the posterior labrum (*arrow*). To the right of the arrow is the posterior acetabular wall. **B:** T1-weighted axial image depicting a posterior capsulolabral avulsion (*arrow*).

reported between 24% and 57%, depending on the severity of the trauma.[107–111] Simple dislocations, or those without radiographic evidence of fracture, have been shown to have the lowest incidence of subsequent DJD. However, the incidence of post-traumatic DJD in these injuries is still 24%.[111]

Nonconcentric reduction after a traumatic dislocation is considered an absolute indication for operative intervention. The presence of loose bodies, however, has been considered a relative indication, particularly if the reduction is concentric and the loose bodies are located below the fovea.[112–114] An in vivo rabbit model has shown that free cartilaginous loose particles inside the joint increase chondrolytic enzyme activity and induce secondary arthrosis.[114] In the 1990s, hip arthroscopy was begun to be used to remove loose bodies seen on plain radiography or CT, largely due to the concern that these fragments could eventually lead to post-traumatic arthritis.[98,103–106] While performing these arthroscopies, previously unrecognized cartilaginous loose bodies were frequently found.[101] Since 24% of "simple" dislocations have been shown to develop subsequent DJD, the literature would support that these loose bodies that had been previously undetected could actually contribute significantly to the development of post-traumatic DJD and they should be addressed prophylactically with arthroscopic removal (Fig. 9.11).[101,111]

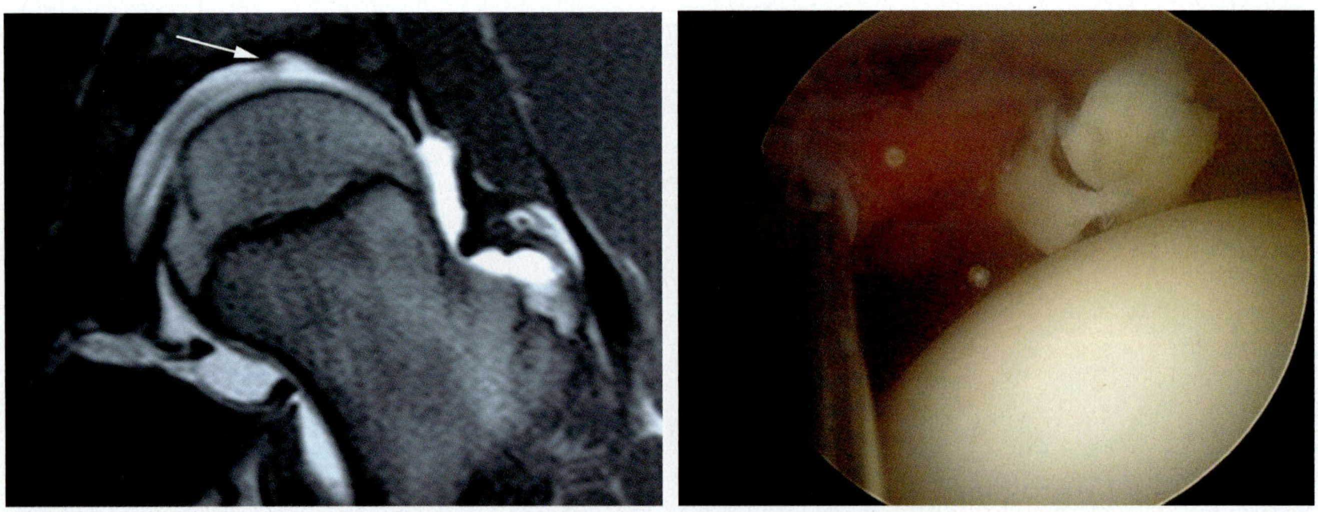

A B

Figure 9.11. Loose cartilaginous bodies in a hip following dislocation. **A:** MRI scan of loose bodies following a hip dislocation in a collegiate basketball player. Image is T1-weighted coronal image. Loose body is cartilaginous and not appreciated on plain film (*arrow*). **B:** Arthroscopic image of loose body.

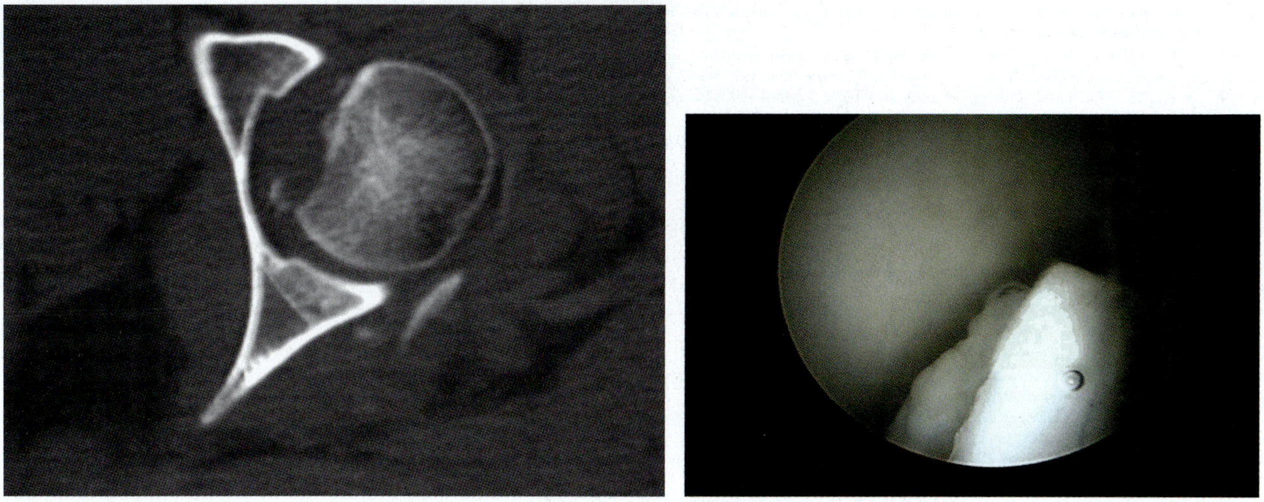

Figure 9.12. Loose bodies in the hip with nonconcentric reduction. **A:** CT scan through the center of the femoral head depicting multiple loose bodies within the joint. **B:** Intraoperative image of loose osteocartilaginous fragment that was removed.

Mullis and Dahners[102] reported on a series of 36 patients treated with hip arthroscopy following dislocation. Excluding the procedures in which a repeat arthroscopy was performed for retained loose bodies, the average time for arthroscopy was 15 days. Out of 36 (69%) patients, 26 had radiographic evidence of loose bodies (nonconcentric reduction and/or radiographically visible loose bodies). In nine patients, there was a concentric reduction without radiographic evidence of loose bodies. Intraoperatively, 33 of 36 (92%) patients were found to have loose bodies. Seven of the nine (78%) patients with no preoperative radiographic evidence of loose bodies had loose bodies found after arthroscopy (Fig. 9.12).

Yamamoto et al.[101] documented a 15-year experience with hip arthroscopy after traumatic dislocation. Ten joints in nine patients were treated 1 to 7 days post dislocation. Seven hips were classified as Thompson–Epstein (TE) I injuries, two type II, one type IV, and one central fracture dislocation. All dislocations had arthroscopic lavage and debridement. One TE I fracture underwent arthroscopic osteosynthesis of the femoral head fracture and one TE II had extraction of the fragment. The other TE II injury, two of the TE I injuries, as well as the TE IV injury had subsequent ORIF of the fragment. After arthroscopy, seven of ten (70%) joints revealed loose osteochondral fragments that were not recognized preoperatively with radiographs or CT scan. At a minimum of 5 years follow-up, eight of ten joints were asymptomatic. One joint (Pipken type 3 femoral head fracture) went on to develop femoral head avascular necrosis (AVN) that was not symptomatic. The one TE IV injury developed hip joint DJD at 1 year. These results prompted the authors to recommend arthroscopic debridement for all TE type I and type II dislocations but not types III and IV.

There has been some concern regarding the timing of arthroscopy after traumatic dislocation in terms of the risk of AVN,[114] prompting those concerned to recommend a 6 week waiting period postdislocation before performing arthroscopy. However, the two previously discussed arthroscopic surgeries were performed in the first 7 days by Yamamota and in the first 2 weeks by Dahners.[101,102] The complications observed in the Dahners study were three repeat procedures for retained loose bodies and some fluid extravasation into the gluteal compartment which resolved without incident.[101] Yamamoto et al.[101] had one case of AVN which developed in a patient with a Pipken type 3 injury.

CONCLUSION

The spectrum of hip instability is wide and includes symptomatology that ranges from one that is similar to a simple snapping hip to a complete dislocation that results in persistent repeated dislocations. A thorough history and physical examination combined with the appropriate imaging studies are essential in determining where on this spectrum the patient's complaints fit.

The treatment of these disorders also covers a wide range. Conservative care that includes temporary immobilization followed by activity modification, physical therapy, and the eventual return to activity can be effective for those with mild capsular or musculotendinous injuries. More significant instability that includes labral injury, capsular laxity, and possibly mild acetabular dysplasia can be treated effectively with open capsular plication, or more recently, arthroscopic capsular plication, thermal capsulorrhaphy, and labral debridement (or repair). Hip dysplasia that involves bony abnormalities that cannot be addressed by arthroscopic or open capsular means can be treated using periacetabular osteotomy while dysplasia that involves significant DJD is better treated with THA. Finally, traumatic dislocations with retained loose bodies and/or femoral head fractures can be treated with open or arthroscopic loose body removal as well as arthroscopic or open femoral head/acetabular fixation.

REFERENCES

1. Philippon MJ. The role of arthroscopic thermal capsulorrhaphy in the hip. *Clin Sports Med.* 2001;20:817–829.
2. Bellabarba C, Sheinkop M, Kuo K. Idiopathic hip instability. *Clin Orthop.* 1998;355:261–271.
3. Takechi H, Nagashima H, Ito S. Intra-articular pressure of the hip joint outside and inside the limbus. *J Jpn Orthop Assoc.* 1982;56:529–536.
4. Ferguson SJ, Bryant JT, Ganz R, et al. An in vitro investigation of the acetabular labral seal in hip joint mechanics. *J Biomech.* 2003;36:171–178.

5. Ferguson SJ, Bryant JT, Ganz R, et al. The acetabular labrum seal: A pro-elastic finite element model. *Clin Biomech.* 2000;15:463–468.
6. Ferguson SJ, Bryant JT, Ganz R, et al. The influence of the acetabular labrum on hip joint cartilage consolidation: A pro-elastic finite element model. *J Biomech.* 2000;33:953–960.
7. Kim YT, Azuma H. The nerve endings of the acetabular labrum. *Clin Orthop.* 1995;320:176–181.
8. Kelly BT, Wiliams RJ, Philippon MJ. Hip arthroscopy: Current indications, treatment options, and management issues. *Am J Sports Med.* 2003;316:1020–1037.
9. Kallas KM, Guanche CA. Physical examination and imaging of hip injuries. *Oper Tech Sports Med.* 2002;10:176–183.
10. Scopp JM, Moorman CT III. The assessment of athletic hip injury. *Clin Sports Med.* 2001;20:647–659.
11. Paletta GA Jr, Andrish JT. Injuries about the hip and pelvis in the young athlete. *Clin Sports Med.* 1995;14:591–628.
12. Hoppenfeld S. Physical examination of the hip and pelvis. In: Hoppenfeld S, ed. *Physical Exam of the Spine and Extremities.* Norwalk: Appleton and Lange; 1976, p. 143.
13. Erb RE. Current concepts in imaging the adult hip. *Clin Sports Med.* 2001;20:661–696.
14. Tonnis D, Heinecke A. Acetabular and femoral anteversion: Relationship with osteoarthritis of the hip. *J Bone Joint Surg Am.* 1999;81(12):1747–1770.
15. Delaunay S, Dussault RG, Kaplan PA, et al. Radiographic measurements of dysplastic adult hips. *Skeletal Radiol.* 1997;26(2):75–81.
16. Wenger DR, Bomar JD. Human hip dysplasia: Evolution of current treatment concepts. *J Orthop Sci.* 2003;8(2):264–271.
17. Reynolds D, Lucas J, Klaue K. Retroversion of the acetabulum: A cause of hip pain. *J Bone Joint Surg Br.* 1999;81(2):281–288.
18. DePaulis F, Cacchio A, Michelini O, et al. Sports injuries in the pelvis and hip: Diagnostic imaging. *Eur J Radiol.* 1998;27(suppl):S49–S59.
19. Kneeland JB. MR imaging of sports injuries of the hip. *Magn Reson Imaging Clin N Am.* 1999;7:105–115.
20. Beltran J, Caudill JL, Herman LA, et al. Rheumatoid arthritis: MR imaging manifestations. *Radiology.* 1987;165:153–157.
21. Edwards DJ, Lomas D, Villar RN. Diagnosis of the painful hip by magnetic resonance imaging and arthroscopy. *J Bone Joint Surg.* 1995;77B:374–376.
22. Hodler J, Trudell D, Pathria MN, et al. Width of the articular cartilage of the hip: Quantification by using fat suppression spin echo MRI in cadavers. *Am J Roentgenol.* 1992;192:351–355.
23. Potter HG, Montgomery KD, Heise CW, et al. MRI of acetabular fractures: Value in detecting femoral head injury, intraarticular fragments, and sciatic nerve injury. *Am J Roentgenol.* 1994;163:881–886.
24. Czerny C, Kramer J, Neuhold A, et al. MRI and magnetic resonance arthrography of the acetabular labrum: Comparison with surgical findings [in German]. *Roto Fortschr Ged Rontgenstr Neuen Bildgeb Verfahr.* 2001;173:702–707.
25. Allen WC, Cope R. Coxa saltans: The snapping hip revisited. *J Acad Orthop Surg.* 1995;3:303–308.
26. Tietz CC, Garrett WE, Miniaci A, et al. Tendon problems in athletic individuals. *J Bone Joint Surg.* 1997;79A:138–152.
27. Jacobsen T, Allen WC. Surgical correction of the snapping iliopsoas tendon. *Am J Sports Med.* 1990;18:470–474.
28. Lieberman J, Altchek D, Salvati E. Recurrent dislocation of a hip with a labral lesion. Treatment with a modified bankart repair. *J Bone Joint Surg.* 1993;75A:1524–1527.
29. Nunziata A, Blumenfeld I. Cadera a resort: A proposito de una variedad. *Prensa Med Argent.* 1951;38:1997–2001.
30. Schaberg JE, Harper MC, Allen WC. The snapping hip syndrome. *Am J Sports Med.* 1984;12:361–365.
31. Staple TW, Jung D, Mork A. Snapping tendon syndrome: Hip tenography with fluoroscopic monitoring. *Radiology.* 1988;166:873–874.
32. Binnie JF. The snapping hip. *Ann Surg.* 1913;58:59–66.
33. Mayer L. Snapping hip. *Surg Gynecol Obstet.* 1919;29:425–428.
34. Zoltan DJ, Clancy WG Jr, Keene JS. A new operative approach to snapping hip and refractory trochanteric bursitis in athletes. *Am J Sports Med.* 1986;14:201–204.
35. Altenberg AR. Acetabular labrum tears: A cause of hip pain and degenerative arthritis. *South Med J.* 1977;70:174–175.
36. Dorrell JH, Catterall A. The torn acetabular labrum. *J Bone Joint Surg.* 1986;68B:400–403.
37. Ikeda T, Awaya G, Suzuki S. Torn acetabular labrum in young patients: Arthroscopic diagnosis and management. *J Bone Joint Surg.* 1988;70B:13–16.
38. Sullivan CR, Bickel WH, Lipscomb PR. Recurrent dislocation of the hip. *J Bone Joint Surg.* 1955;37A:1256–1270.
39. Suzuki S, Awaya G, Okada Y. Arthroscopic diagnosis of ruptured acetabular labrum. *Acta Orthop Scand.* 1986;57:513–515.
40. Arvidsson I. The hip joint: Forces needed for distraction and appearance of the vacuum phenomenon. *Scand J Rehabil Med.* 1990;22:157–161.
41. Bombelli R, ed. *Structure and Function in Normal and Abnormal Hips.* 3rd Ed. New York: Springer-Verlag; 1993.
42. Crawford MJ, Dy CJ, Alexander JW, et al. The biomechanics of the hip labrum and the stability of the hip. *J Orthop Res.* 2007;465:16–22.
43. Shindle MK, Ranawat AS, Kelly BT. Diagnosis and management of traumatic and atraumatic hip instability in the athletic patient. *Clin Sports Med.* 2006;25:309–326.
44. Flory PJ, Garrett RR. Phase transition in collagen and gelatin systems. *J Am Chem Soc.* 1958;80:4836–4845.
45. Flory PJ, Weaver ES. Helix coil transition in dilute aqueous collagen solutions. *J Am Chem Soc.* 1959;82:4518–4525.
46. Hayashi K, Hecht P, Thabit G III, et al. The biologic response to laser thermal modification in an in vivo sheep model. *Clin Orthop Relat Res.* 2000;373:265–276.
47. Hecht P, Hayashi K, Cooley AJ, et al. The thermal effect of monopolar radiofrequency energy on the properties of joint capsule: An in vivo histologic study using a sheep model. *Am J Sports Med.* 1998;26:808–814.
48. Liao WL, Hedman TP, Vangsness CT Jr. Thermal profile of radiofrequency energy in the inferior glenohumeral ligament. *Arthroscopy.* 2004;20:603–608.
49. Medvecky MJ, Ong BC, Rokito AS, et al. Thermal capsular shrinkage: Basic science and clinical applications [review]. *Arthroscopy.* 2001;17:624–635.
50. Hecht P, Hayashi K, Lu Y, et al. Monopolar radiofrequency energy effects on joint capsular tissue: Potential treatment for joint instability. An in vivo mechanical and biomechanical, morphological and biochemical study using an ovine model. *Am J Sports Med.* 1999;27:761–771.
51. Miniaci A, Codsi MJ. Thermal capsulorrhaphy for the treatment of shoulder instability. *Am J Sports Med.* 2006;34(8):1356–1363.
52. Gartsman GM, Roddey TS, Hammerman SM. Arthroscopic treatment of bidirectional glenohumeral instability: 2–5 year follow-up. *J Shoulder Elbow Surg.* 2001;10:28–36.
53. Mishra DK, Fanton GS. Two-year outcome of arthroscopic bankart repair and electrothermal-assisted capsulorrhaphy for recurrent anterior shoulder instability. *Arthroscopy.* 2001;17:844–841.
54. Noonan TJ, Tokish JM, Briggs KK, et al. Laser assisted thermal capsulorrhaphy [review]. *Arthroscopy.* 2003;19:815–819.
55. D'Alessandro DF, Bradley JP, Fleischli JE, et al. Prospective evaluation of thermal capsulorrhaphy for shoulder instability: Indications and results, 2–5 year follow-up. *Am J Sports Med.* 2004;32:21–33.
56. Miniaci A, McBirnie J. Thermal capsular shrinkage for treatment of multidirectional instability of the shoulder. *J Bone Joint Surg Am.* 2003;85:2283–2287.
57. Levine WN, Clark AM Jr, D'Alessandro DF, et al. Chondrolysis following arthroscopic thermal capsulorrhaphy to treat shoulder instability: A report of 2 cases. *J Bone Joint Surg Am.* 2005;87:616–621.
58. Petty DH, Jazraxi LM, Estrada LS, et al. Glenohumeral chondrolysis after shoulder arthroscopy: Case reports and review of the literature. *Am J Sports Med.* 2004;32:509–515.
59. Rath E, Richmond JC. Capsular disruption as a complication of thermal alteration of the glenohumeral capsule. *Arthroscopy.* 2001;17:E10.
60. Wong KL, Williams GR. Complications of thermal capsulorrhaphy of the shoulder. *J Bone Joint Surg Am.* 2001;83(Suppl 2, pt 2):151–155.
61. Massie WK, Howorth MB. Congenital dislocation of the hip. Part 1. Methods of grading results. *J Bone Joint Surg Am.* 1950;32:519–531.
62. Tonnis D, Legal H, Graf R, eds. *Congenital Dysplasia and Dislocation of the Hip in Children and Adults.* Berlin, Germany: Springer-Verlag; 1987.
63. Good C, Shindle MK, Kelly BT, et al. Glenohumeral chondrolysis after shoulder arthroscopy with thermal capsulorrhaphy. *Arthroscopy.* 2007;23(7):797.e1–797.e5.
64. Lequesne M, de Seze. False profile of the pelvis. A new radiographic incidence for the study of the hip. Its use in dysplasias and different coxopathies. *Rev Rhum Mal Osteoartic.* 1961;28:643–652. [French].
65. Wiberg G. Studies on dysplastic acetabular and congenital subluxation of the hip joint. With special reference to the complication of osteoarthritis. Parts HV. *Acta Chir Scand Suppl.* 1939;58:7–38.
66. Matsui M, Masuhara K, Nakata K, et al. Early deterioration after modified rotational acetabular osteotomy for the dysplastic hip. *J Bone Joint Surg Br.* 1997;79:220–224.
67. Sanchez-Sotelo J, Trousdale RT, Berry DJ, et al. Surgical treatment of developmental dysplasia of the hip in adults: 1. Non-arthroplasty options. *J Am Acad Orthop Surg.* 2002;10:321–333.
68. Ganz R, Klaue K, Vinh TH, et al. A new periacetabular osteotomy for the treatment of hip dysplasias: Technique and preliminary results. *Clin Orthop.* 1988;232:26–36.
69. Crockarell J Jr, Trousdale RT, Cabanela ME, et al. Early experience and results with the periacetabular osteotomy: The Mayo clinic experience. *Clin Orthop.* 1999;363:64–72.
70. Siebenrock KA, Scholl E, Lottenbach M, et al. Bernese periacetabular osteotomy. *Clin Orthop.* 1999;363:9–20.
71. Trousdale RT, Ekkernkamp A, Ganz R, et al. Periacetabular and intertrochanteric osteotomy for the treatment of osteoarthrosis in dysplastic hips. *J Bone Joint Surg Am.* 1995;77:73–85.
72. Matta JM, Stover MD, Siebenrock K. Periacetabular osteotomy through the Smith-Petersen approach. *Clin Orthop.* 1999;363:21–32.
73. Trumble SJ, Mayo KA, Mast JW. The periacetabular osteotomy: Minimum 2 year follow-up in more than 100 hips. *Clin Orthop.* 1999;363:54–63.
74. Hussel JG, Mast JW, Mayo KA, et al. A comparison of different surgical approaches for the peri-acetabular osteotomy. *Clin Orthop.* 1999;363:64–72.
75. Hussel JG, Rodriguez JA, Ganz R. Technical complications of the Bernese periacetabular osteotomy. *Clin Orthop.* 1999;363:81–92.
76. Ping ME, Trousdale RT, Cabanela ME, et al. Intraoperative electromyographic monitoring during periacetabular osteotomy. *Clin Orthop.* 2002;400:158–164.
77. Myers SR, Eijer H, Ganz R. Anterior femoroacetabular impingement after periacetabular osteotomy. *Clin Orthop.* 1999;363:93–99.
78. Wong-Chung J, Ryan M, O'Brien TM. Movement of the femoral head after Salter osteotomy for acetabular dysplasia. *J Bone Joint Surg Br.* 1990;72:563–567.
79. Sutherland DH, Greenfield R. Double Innominate osteotomy. *J Bone Joint Surg Am.* 1977;59:1082–1091.
80. Le Coeur P. Corrections des defauts d'orientation de l'articulation coxofemorale par oteotomie de l'os iliaque. *Rev de Chir Orthop.* 1965;51:211–212.
81. Hopf A. Hip acetabular displacement by double pelvic osteotomy in the treatment of hip joint dysplasia and subluxation in young people and adults [German]. *Z Orthop Ihre Grenzgeb.* 1966;101:559–586.
82. Steel HH. Triple osteotomy of the innominate bone. *J Bone Joint Surg Am.* 1973;55:343–350.
83. Carlioz H, Khouri N, Hulin P. Osteotomie pelvienne triple juxtacotyloidienne. *Rev de Chir Orthop.* 1982;68:497–501.

84. Tonnis D, Behrens K, Tsharani F. A modified technique of triple pelvic osteotomy. *J Ped Orthop.* 1981;1:241–249.
85. Eppright RH. Abstract: Dial osteotomy of the acetabulum in the treatment of dysplasia of the hip. *J Bone Joint Surg Am.* 1975;57:1172.
86. Sanchez-Sotelo J, Berry DJ, Trousdale RT, et al. Surgical treatment of developmental dysplasia of the hip in adults: II. Arthroplasty Options. *J Am Acad Orthop Surg.* 2002;10:334–344.
87. Chudik S, Lopez V. Hip dislocations in athletes. *Sports Med Arthrosc Rev.* 2002;10:123–133.
88. Giza E, Mithofer K, Matthews H, et al. Hip fracture-dislocation in football: A report of two cases and review of the literature. *Br J Sports Med.* 2004;38:E17.
89. Lamke LO. Traumatic dislocations of the hip: Follow-up on cases from the Stockholm area. *Acta Orthop Scand.* 1970;41:188–198.
90. Mitchell JC, Giannoudis PV, Millner PA, et al. A rare fracture-dislocation of the hip in a gymnast and review of the literature. *Br J Sports Med.* 1999;33:283–284.
91. Stiris MG. Magnetic resonance arthrography of the hip joint in patients with suspected rupture of the labrum acetabulare. *Tidsskr Nor Laegeforen.* 2001;121:698–700.
92. Dameron T Jr. Bucket-handle tear of the acetabular labrum accompanying posterior dislocation of the hip. *J Bone Joint Surg Am.* 1959;41:131–134.
93. Nelson C. Traumatic recurrent dislocation of the hip: Report of a case. *J Bone Joint Surg Am.* 1970;52:128–130.
94. Rasleigh-Belcher H, Cannon S. Recurrent dislocation of the hip with a bankart-type lesion. *J Bone Joint Surg Br.* 1966;68:398–399.
95. Simmons R, Elder J. Recurrent post-traumatic dislocations of the hip in children. *South Med J.* 1972;65:1463–1466.
96. Slavic M, Dungl P, Spindrick J, et al. Recurrent traumatic dislocation of the hip in a child. Significance of early arthrography. *Arch Orthop Trauma Surg.* 1986;104:385–388.
97. Townsend R, Edwards G, Bazant F. Posttraumatic recurrent dislocation of the hip without fracture. *J Bone Joint Surg Br.* 1969;194.
98. Liebenberg F, Dommisse G. Recurrent posttraumatic dislocation of the hip. *J Bone Joint Surg Br.* 1969;51:632–637.
99. Dall D, MacNab I, Gross A. Recurrent anterior dislocation of the hip. *J Bone Joint Surg Am.* 1970;52:574–576.
100. Heinzelmann P, Nelson C. Recurrent traumatic dislocation of the hip: Report of a case. *J Bone Joint Surg Am.* 1976;58:895–896.
101. Yamamoto Y, Takatoshi I, Ono T, et al. Usefulness of arthroscopic surgery in hip trauma cases. *Arthroscopy.* 2003;19:269–273.
102. Mullis BH, Dahners LE. Hip Arthroscopy to remove loose bodies after traumatic dislocation. *J Orthop Trauma.* 2006;20:22–26.
103. Upadhyay SS, Moulton A, Srikrishnamurthy K. An Analysis of the late effects of traumatic posterior dislocation of the hip without fracture. *J Bone Joint Surg Br.* 1983;65:150–152.
104. DeLee JC. Fractures and dislocations of the hip. In: Rockwood CA, Green DP, eds. *Fractures in Adults.* 2nd Ed. Philadelphia, PA: J. B. Lippincott: 1984:1211–1356.
105. Letournel E. Acetabular fractures. *Clin Orthop.* 1980;151:81–106.
106. Matta JM, Anderson LM, Epstein HC. Fracture of the acetabulum. *Clin Orthop.* 1986;205:230–250.
107. Evans CH, Mazzocchi RA, Nelson DD, et al. Experimental arthritis induced by intra-articular injection of allogenic cartilaginous particles into rabbit knees. *Arthritis Rheum.* 1984;27:200–207.
108. Thompson VP, Epstein HC. Traumatic dislocation of the hip. *J Bone Joint Surg Am.* 1951;33:746–778.
109. Armstrong JR. Traumatic dislocation of the hip: Review of 101 dislocations. *J Bone Joint Surg Br.* 1948;30:430–445.
110. Stewart MJ, McCarroll HR, Mulhollan JS. Fracture dislocation of the hip. *Acta Orthop Scand.* 1975;46:507–525.
111. Brav CEA. Traumatic dislocation of the hip. *J Bone Joint Surg Am.* 1962;44:1115–1134.
112. Svoboda S, Williams DM, Murphy KP. Hip arthroscopy for osteochondral loose body removal after a posterior hip dislocation. *Arthroscopy.* 2003;19:777–781.
113. Epstein HC. Posterior fracture-dislocations of the hip: Long term follow-up. *J Bone Joint Surg Am.* 1974;56:1103–1127.
114. Epstein HC. Traumatic dislocations of the hip. *Clin Orthop.* 1973;92:116–142.

CHAPTER

10

Anil S. Ranawat
Jon K. Sekiya

Cartilage Injuries of the Hip

INTRODUCTION

As the field of joint preservation surgery has continued to grow, much of its attention has focused on the prearthritic hip. This burgeoning interest is related to the growing clinical literature, emerging basic science, improved imaging studies, development of hip-specific arthroscopic instrumentation, and new safe joint preserving surgical windows to the hip joint. As in knee, numerous procedures are available to treat hip cartilage injuries and mitigate symptoms and hopefully control progression of arthritic disease. These include, but are not limited to, chondroplasty, microfracture, autologous chondrocyte implantation, autograft and allograft osteochondral transfer, and metallic resurfacing.[1–3] Due to cartilage's intrinsic limited healing capacity,[4] cartilage injuries have been difficult to treat in all joints. Only recently have orthopedic surgeons developed treatment strategies and algorithms to treat hip cartilage injuries, which have been reported to be as high as 50% of all intra-articular hip derangements in a series of athletes.[5] This review addresses the pathoanatomy and physiology of cartilage injuries of the hip and focus on joint preserving techniques, including both arthroscopic and open surgery, used to treat them.

HISTORY AND PHYSICAL EXAMINATION

The onset of symptoms of hip chondral injuries can be either acute or chronic. Acute injuries are usually dramatic, while chronic injuries may only present after an innocuous trauma with minimal dysfunction and symptoms. Any persistent symptoms such as intermittent catching or pain elicited by provocative maneuvers should prompt a more extensive diagnostic workup. The history and physical examination is critical in the workup of hip pain. The clinician must determine the location, frequency, pattern, and radiation of symptoms, and separate intra-articular pathology from extra-articular pathology including pelvic and back pain.

Intra-articular hip symptoms can be mechanical in nature such as clicking and locking, which are commonly seen with acute chondro-labral injuries. Other intra-articular symptoms can be groin pain, "C-sign," stiffness, and decreased hip range of motion, the latter two being more suggestive of an effusion or synovitis. Other important historical information includes determining what factors exacerbate or relieve the symptoms and duration of symptoms. Intra-articular hip pain can commonly radiate to the medial knee due to irritation of the femoral nerve. Thigh or buttock pain radiating to below the knee is more likely to be related to a neurological disorder such as spinal stenosis or a herniated lumbar disc.[6,7]

Extra-articular sources of hip pain are extensive. The examiner must elicit if the pain is from the lateral or anterior thigh, groin/adductor region, sacral-iliac joint or lower back, true pelvis (intra-abdominal), reproductive organs, etc. Many times, these sources of hip pain can overlap so a detailed history is crucial.

Since the differential diagnosis of hip pain is so broad, the examiner must detail the patient's history based on three subjects: past medical history, any hip surgery/trauma or pediatric hip disease, and any social or occupational hazards that predispose the hip to early dysfunction. First, a past medical history is elicited such as a history of coagulopathy, collagen-vascular disorders, inflammatory diseases, or a history of malignancy. If any of these are positive, then appropriate bloodwork should be ordered. Second, the examiner asks the patient regarding any prior hip surgery or trauma and the treatment thereafter with specific attention to early pediatric diseases such as slipped femoral epiphysis, dysplasia, and Perthes.[6,7] Finally, it is essential to know the history of alcohol abuse, prolonged steroid therapy, use of nonsteroidal anti-inflammatory drugs (NSAIDs), and sporting activity. Activity in sports can clue the physician into a possible source of complaints. Patients who play soccer, rugby, martial arts, or who are long-distance runners have a higher incidence of sports hernia injuries as well as labral tears and chondral injuries.

The physical examination begins with first assessing the position of the hip at rest and then with weight bearing and motion. For instance, a hip that is abducted, flexed, and externally rotated provides the largest joint capsule volume, suggesting the presence of an effusion or synovitis. Next, with the patient standing, a Trendelenburg test should be performed to assess for abductor weakness.[6,7] Other postural tests include checking for pelvic obliquity, leg length discrepancies, scoliosis, foot and limb alignment, and muscle contractures.[8] The patient should then be asked to ambulate. If the gait is of a Trendelenburg type, an intra-articular disease process may be suggested. Finally, a complete lumbar spine examination to include motor, sensory, range of motion, reflexes, and straight-leg raises must be performed to rule out this area as the cause of symptoms.

The next phase of the examination is the palpation of bony prominences and soft tissue structures as well as an assessment of range of motion of both hips. Structures that should be palpated include the great trochanter and the course of the iliotibial band, pubic symphisis, and adductors, and a check for hernias should also be done. Next, both passive and active range of motion exam should be performed with the hip in both extension and flexion. Any side-to-side differences should be noted and could indicate potential areas of pathology, specifically loss of internal rotation, which suggests early arthritic process and excessive resting external rotation, which in turn suggests some capsular laxity.[9]

The final phase of the examination is specialty hip testing. Although there is no specific examination maneuver to assess for chondral injuries, the flexion internal rotation is highly sensitive for intra-articular pathology.[10] Other maneuvers include the scour sign, which elicits clicking, catching, or other mechanical symptoms associated with chondro-labral injuries. Lastly, other provocative maneuvers should be performed such as resisted straight leg raise, flexion abduction internal rotation (FABER) test, and Ober test.

IMAGING

Plain radiographs are the cornerstone of all diagnostic hip workups. Although not specific for chondral injuries, they supply invaluable information about the bony architecture and osseous environment of the hip. The standard series should include accurate anterior–posterior pelvis and the affected hip in orthogonal views. There are numerous choices for lateral radiographs: cross-table, frog-leg, extended long neck lateral, and false profile. All of these radiographs have specific advantages and disadvantages. If the patient had a recent trauma, then oblique acetabular views (obturator and iliac) and a fine cut computed tomography can help delineate bony abnormalities and fractures in more detail. Information gained from plain radiographs includes the degree of arthritic disease, fractures, dislocation/subluxations, or loose bodies. Ultrasound is useful mostly to check for effusions and has limited role in chondral injuries depending on the skill of the examiner. A bone scan should be obtained if malignancy or occult fractures are suspected.

Magnetic resonance imaging (MRI) is a valuable modality in diagnosing chondral injuries of the hip. It has the best sensitivity and specificity compared to other modalities.[11] MRI does have some limitations, as Sekiya et al.[12] showed that MRI is inadequate at measuring cartilage in avascular necrosis (AVN)and Byrd and Jones[10] have shown low sensitivity and specificity for diagnosing chondral injuries in general.

Improvements in imaging with MRI arthrograms (MRAs) and cartilage-specific sequences have significantly improved its effectiveness. The advent of the MRA allows for better evaluation of the cartilage surface, though some literature claims that there is a high false-negative rate, which may limit the extent of the true articular surface damage.[11,13] In an MRA, dilute gadolinium is injected into the joint capsule, which distends the capsule and allows better visualization of the articular cartilage. Labral tears will show an abnormal linear extension of solution into the labrum. Chondral lesions are defined by an outline of the cartilage defects from gadolinium (Fig. 10.1). Keeney et al.[13] compared MRA with arthroscopy of the hip and showed that the MRA detected 76% of the acetabular tears. Also, articular cartilage findings on MRA were confirmed using arthroscopy only 62.7% of the time. In Keeney's study, MRA had a sensitivity of 47%, specificity of 89%, a positive predictive value of 84%, and negative predictive value of 59%.[9] Another advantage of an arthrogram is that it is both a therapeutic and a diagnostic injection since both an anesthetic and a steroid can be injected with the gadolinium.[10,14]

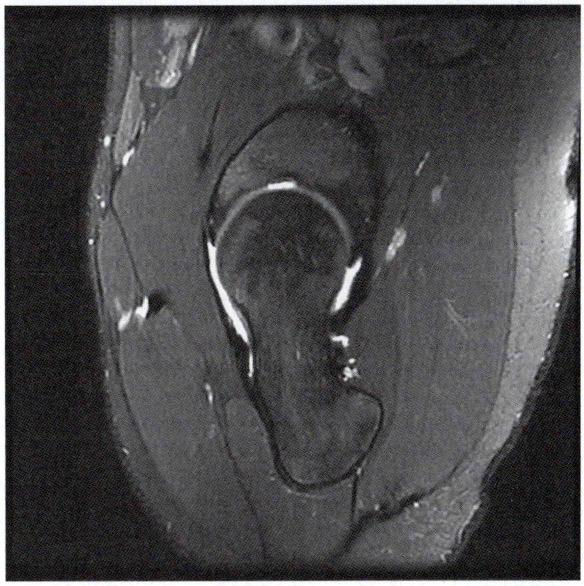

Figure 10.1. Axial fat saturated MRA of a right hip showing a traumatic full-thickness acetabular chondral lesion.

Although gadolinium-enhanced MR arthrography is currently the most promising imaging modality, it still has some limitations and requires an invasive injection. Potter et al.[15] have demonstrated the utility of cartilage sensitive MRI for the detection of these lesions which can be performed successfully without the use of gadolinium. In the work of Mintz et al., similar cartilage-specific sequence was correlated with arthroscopic findings. For articular cartilage defects of the femoral head and acetabulum, there was good concordance (92% and 86% within one grade) between MRI and surgical findings.[16]

PATHOPHYSIOLOGY AND ETIOLOGY OF CHONDRAL LESIONS

Chondral injury is an elusive source of hip pain.[17,18] Traditionally, chondral damage around the hip has been associated with either progressive joint deterioration (osteoarthritis or rheumatoid arthritis) or proximal femur and acetabular fractures. However, isolated traumatic hip articular injuries can occur from impact loading across the joint, the so called "lateral impact injury." Besides trauma and degenerative conditions, other etiologies of chondral injuries include loose bodies/synovial chondramatosis, sequelae of pediatric disease, focal osteonecrosis, osteochondritis dissecans, capsular laxity, and femoroacetabular impingement (FAI).

Chondral injuries can be either acute or chronic and either partial or full thickness. They can also be either primarily femoral or acetabular. Femoral lesions usually fail from shear forces near the tidemark with deep lesions, while acetabular lesions are more commonly due to compressive forces and range from osteomalacia to full-thickness lesions.[19] They can be related to conditions that primarily affect cartilage, the subchondral bone or both. They are commonly associated with labral tears but this depends on the underlying etiology of the chondral injury.[20] Location of the injuries also depends on underlying pathology. In one series of 457 hips over a 6-year period, the anterior acetabulum was affected in 59% of the hips. Other locations included the superior acetabulum in 24%, and the posterior acetabulum in 25%. Deeper lesions, Outerbridge grade III and IV lesions,[21] were found primarily in the anterior acetabulum in 70% of cases, while only 36% and 27%, respectively, in the posterior and superior acetabulum.[20]

PROXIMAL FEMUR AND ACETABULAR FRACTURES

Traditionally, most chondral damage in the hip was secondary to high velocity injuries leading to hip trauma. It has been shown the anatomic reduction is a favorable prognostic sign for long-term function of the joint.[22] Other injury patterns include hip subluxations and dislocations with associated femoral head or acetabular fractures. The mainstay of treatment by traumatologists is anatomic reduction on both the acetabular and femoral side. Arthroscopic assisted approaches have also been attempted to assess reduction as well debride malreductions.[23]

DEGENERATIVE JOINT DISEASE/ARTHRITIS

As in the knee, chondral injuries are most often the natural sequelae of arthritic conditions. The etiology can be primary osteoarthritis or secondary conditions such as an inflammatory disorder, prior trauma, pediatric disease, etc. Although there is a limited role for joint lavage and debridement in any arthritic joint, a definitive procedure is usually preferable.[20,24–26]

ISOLATED CHONDRAL INJURIES

The "lateral impact injury" is a common injury pattern in young, fit adult males who sustain a direct blow over the greater trochanter in contact sports and activities.[27] Due to the subcutaneous nature and high bone density properties of the greater trochanter, energy and load are transferred from the trochanter intra-articularly into the hip joint surface resulting in chondral lesions of the femoral head or acetabulum without associated osseous injury (Fig. 10.2). Arthroscopic findings in this clinical scenario will commonly support this lateral impact mechanism and these areas can be appropriately debrided or microfractured.[18]

LOOSE BODIES/SYNOVIAL CHONDROMATOSIS

Loose bodies are free floating cartilage fragments usually originating from traumatic injury, degenerative conditions, or synovial proliferative disorders.[14,28–31] The history typically reveals mechanical symptoms, such as locking and clicking. Bony fragments can be seen on radiographs, while both cartilage and bony fragments may be seen on MRI (Fig. 10.3). Loose bodies are commonly found in the posterior region of the central compartment or in the peripheral compartment, especially in the posterior and medial femoral neck region; thus, arthroscopic removal of loose bodies has been a classic indication for hip arthroscopy. Synovial chondromatosis can be quite extensive and usually requires an extensive arthroscopic procedure with numerous working and viewing portals.

SEQUELAE OF PEDIATRIC HIP DISEASE

A common etiology of chondral injury is the sequelae of pediatric hip disease, which include but are not limited to hip dysplasia, Legg–Calves–Perthes disease, slipped capital femoral epiphysis, and coax vara. These various conditions create unfavorable biomechanical environment which may develop into chondral injuries and in certain cases advanced arthrosis. These conditions are best treated with early diagnosis and prevention. If early chondral injuries develop, then these lesions are usually case specific and can be handled either open or arthroscopic.[32]

OSTEONECROSIS

Focal osteonecrosis of the femoral head represents a subchondral disorder with articular manifestations. If the lesion is identified prior to collapse, it can be used to remove associated loose bodies, evaluate the articular cartilage covering the defect, and

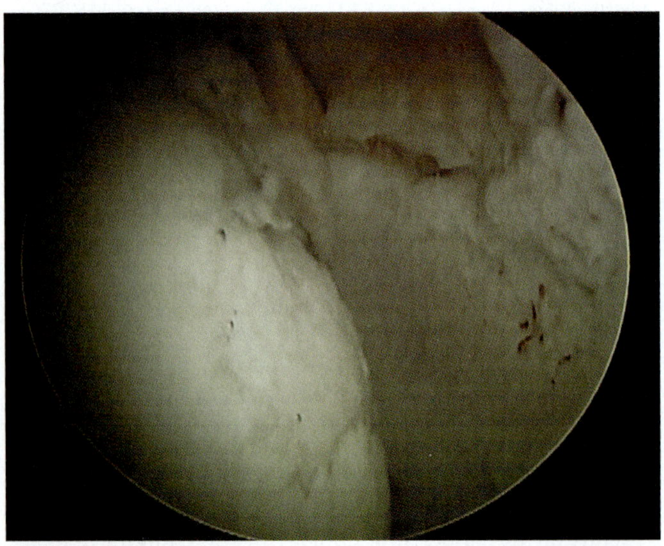

Figure 10.2. Arthroscopic view of left hip in central compartment showing a full-thickness traumatic femoral head lesion.

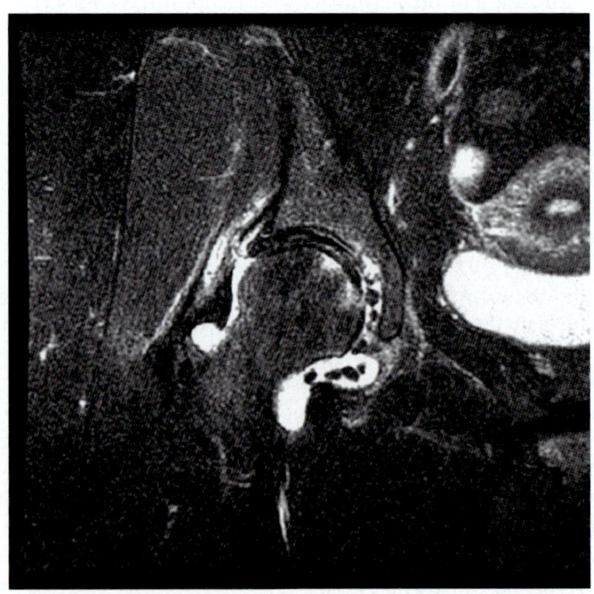

Figure 10.3. Coronal fat saturated MRA of a right hip showing multiple osteochondral lesions consistent with synovial chondromatosis.

debride the defective portions (Fig. 10.4).[33] If the articular cartilage segment is intact, joint preservation surgery such as free vascularized fibular grafting may be attempted, potentially with better success, given the intact articular cartilage.[12] Furthermore, it is possible to drill the necrotic zone under direct visualization thereby protecting surrounding articular cartilage. In these cases, arthroscopically assisted core drilling and bone grafting can be performed to revascularize the necrotic region. Arthroscopic evaluation of the core tract can also be done to assess the presence of bleeding bone. Byrd and Jones[29] treated four patients with osteonecrosis of the femoral head and reported the worst results in the three patients with the most advanced necrosis.

OSTEOCHONDRITIS DISSECANS

Like focal osteonecrosis, osteochondritis dissecans is actually a subchondral disorder with chondral manifestations. It almost exclusively affects the femoral head versus the acetabulum. Hip arthroscopy can be utilized to remove the osteochondral fragment and debride the resultant lesion. This disease is rare and the successful treatment with hip arthroscopy was only reported in few case reports.[32,34]

CAPSULAR LAXITY

Excessive capsular laxity whether primary or secondary in nature is a recognizable etiology of chondro-labral damage. The laxity of the anterior hip structures due to either an inherent collagen problem (primary) or repetitive loading (secondary) causes repetitive impingement of the proximal femur and acetabulum leading to chondral injuries. This can usually be treated conservatively with physical therapy but can also be treated arthroscopically where both the chondro-labral injury as well as underlying laxity can be addressed.[35]

FEMOROACETABULAR IMPINGEMENT

FAI has recently been recognized as one of the most common etiologies of chondro-labral injuries.[20] The two types of FAI can be from abnormalities in the proximal femur, cam type, or abnormalities in the acetabulum, pincer lesions. However, most commonly, both abnormalities exist. The underlying type of impingement results in unique chondral injury patterns. In cam impingement, the proximal femur abuts the acetabulum during flexion resulting in shear forces causing anterior–superior acetabular cartilage damage with separation and delamination of the cartilage but with preservation of the labrum (Fig. 10.5A).[36] In pincer impingement, the cartilage damage is more circumferential around the acetabulum and does not penetrate as deep as it does in cam impingement but with more labral pathology and ossification (Fig. 10.5B). In Pincer impingement, repeated abutment of the anterior femoral head on the acetabulum results in a moment arm on the postero-inferior acetabulum and creates the "so-called" contre-coup-cartilage injury of the postero-inferior acetabulum. Most commonly, however, there is some combination of both pathologies (Fig. 10.6).

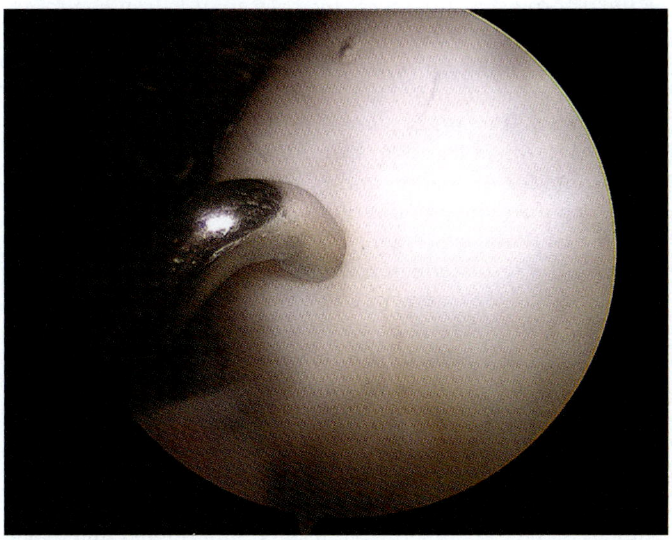

Figure 10.4. Arthroscopic view of AVN with soft cartilage and loss of subchondral support with "ballotable" cartilage.

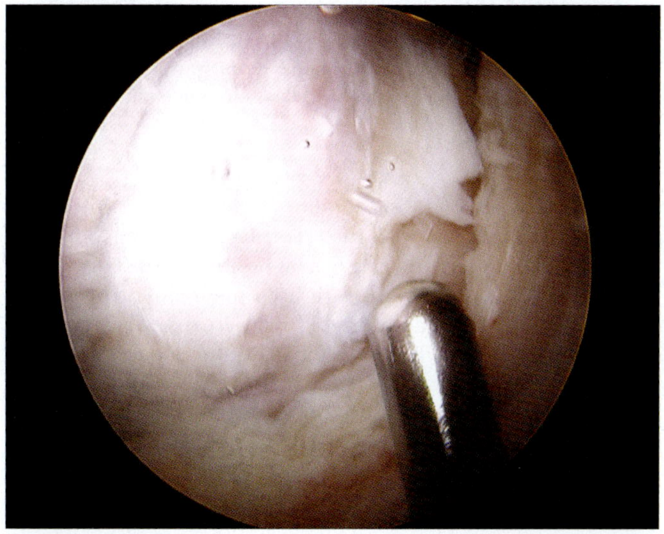

A

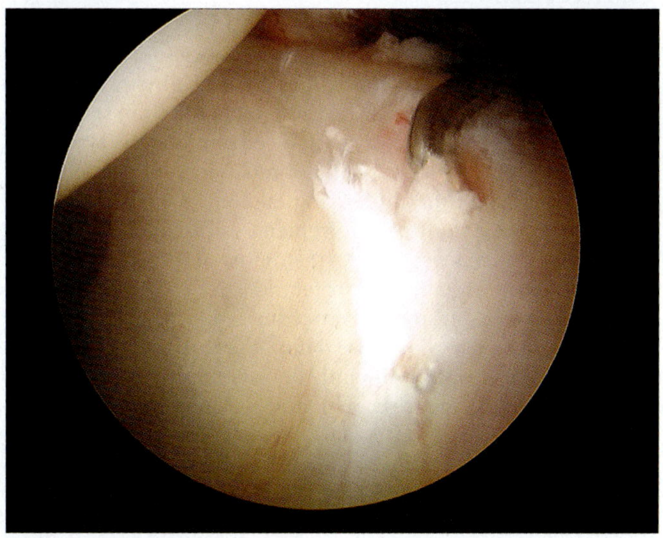

B

Figure 10.5. Arthroscopic view of **(A)** Peripheral compartment showing a cam-type lesion at the osteochondral junction and **(B)** Central compartment showing the sequelae of a pincer-type lesion with labral tearing ossification and circumferential chondral damage.

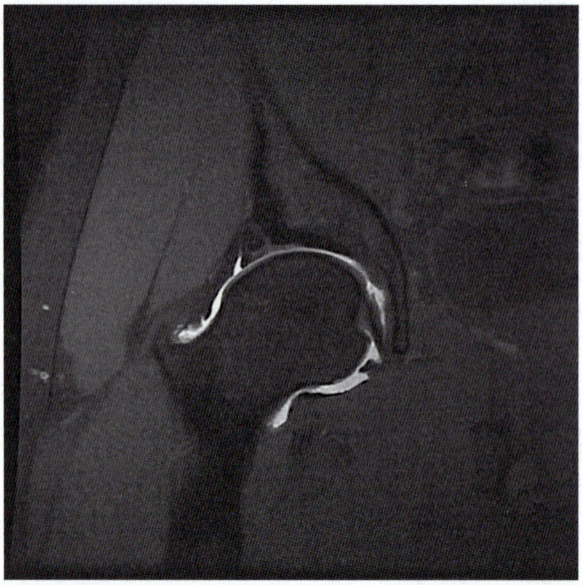

Figure 10.6. Coronal fat saturated MRA of a right hip showing the classic pattern of chondro-labral acetabular injury associated with both cam and pincer features of femoroacetabular impingement.

The treatment of these conditions depends on the severity of involvement. As with most cartilages injuries, both the injury and the underlying cause must be addressed. This can be performed with good results with both open and arthroscopic procedures.[37–40] The mainstay of open treatment is surgical dislocation of the hip but anterior procedures have also been described in arthroscopy.[41–44] Although arthroscopic tools and procedures are constantly developing, many authors still argue that hip arthroscopy limit the ability to successfully address all lesions.[37,45]

TREATMENT

The mainstay of treatment for cartilage injuries of hip consists of prompt diagnosis and modalities such as physical therapy, NSAIDs, or steroid injections. If these modalities fail to control symptoms, then surgical treatment is recommended. There are numerous accepted surgical options and as in the knee, the procedure depends on the underlying etiology, overall alignment of the joint, the extent of involvement, and size of the lesion. For more advanced processes, treatment options include procedures such as acetabular and femoral osteoplasties, redirectional osteotomies, trap door procedures, hip resurfacing, and total hip arthroplasty. For more defined lesions in a prearthritic well-aligned joint, options include debridement, microfracture, and isolated cartilage restoring and resurfacing procedures (allograft/autograft/autologous chondrocyte implantation [ACI] and metallic arthrosurface implants). Although open surgery is still the gold standard, these procedures are increasingly being treated by new arthroscopic techniques.[46,47]

ARTHROSCOPIC TECHNIQUES

Although new reconstructive procedures are emerging, arthroscopic debridement of cartilage injuries is still the most common hip arthroscopic procedure. This is most commonly performed for patients with mechanical symptoms for loose bodies, impingement, or after trauma. The technique is highly effective usually using hip-specific instruments such as straight and curved shavers and flexible heat probes.[14] This procedure can be done in either the supine or lateral position, and usually only two arthroscopic portals are necessary depending on the size and location of the lesion.

Since microfracture of the knee has been shown a safe and effective procedure,[1,48–50] many arthroscopists have applied the same principles to the hip.[47,51–54] Microfracture provides an enriched environment for tissue regeneration by taking advantage of the body's own healing abilities. After the procedure, a marrow clot is established within the affected area. This clot provides an environment for pluripotential marrow cells and mesenchymal stem cells to differentiate into stable tissue within the lesion. Fibrocartilaginous tissue is the final product covering the previous lesion.

The indications for microfracture of the hip are similar to that of the knee. These include focal and contained lesions, typically less than 2 to 4 cm in size. Some authors have empirically noted that lesions less than 400 mm^2 tend to respond better to microfracture than lesions 400 mm^2 or greater.[48] Intact subchondral bone is critical. The cartilage loss can either be full thickness in weight-bearing areas or unstable partial lesions. Indications for microfracture include impingement, trauma, pediatric hip disease, or early degenerative hip disease. Other considerations for performing the procedure include patient age, activity level, and the ability to comply with postoperative rehabilitation.

Contraindications to the procedure include stable partial thickness defects, subchondral bony disease, large subchondral defects associated with cartilage defects, significant arthritis, and a patient's inability to comply with a post-operative rehabilitation regiment.

The technique of microfracture begins with positioning of the patient, which can be either supine or lateral decubitus. Meticulous attention needs to be paid to proper positioning and portal placement to avoid neurological complications. We prefer the supine position as it allows for ease of distraction of the affected hip for access into the joint.[47] It also permits easier use of image intensification and more straightforward instrument handling. The patient is placed on a fracture table with a well-padded perineal post to protect against pudendal nerve injury. Traction is placed on the affected limb using a foot stirrup with at least 7 to 15 mm of joint distraction for adequate room for evaluation and instrumentation. The C-arm is used to confirm the amount of traction needed and for portal placement. Portal placement includes anterior, anterolateral, and rarely posterolateral portals.[55–57] Portals for hip arthroscopy are standard anterolateral and anterior portals. We rarely need to use the posterolateral portal. Once the arthroscope is introduced, the joint is evaluated in standard fashion from the anterolateral portal, a thorough intra-articular hip inspection is performed. Care is taken to also inspect the entire anterior portion of the hip joint including the entire anterior labrum, acetabular fossa, ligamentum teres, and fovea capitus. In acetabular fossa, two normal variants may exist and appear like cartilage lesions. They are stellate crease, which is located superior and has a star-like appearance and the physeal scar, a remnant of the triradiate cartilage and can be anterior or posterior in the fossa. The arthroscope is then moved from the anterolateral portal to the anterior portal to visualize the posterior portion of the hip joint as well as the posterior recess, while any instruments are placed in the anterolateral portal.[58] If necessary, accessory posterior or anterior portals are made at this point. Next, attention is turned to the defect.

Once the chondral defect is identified, the extent of the lesion is documented (Fig. 10.7A). Debridement of all

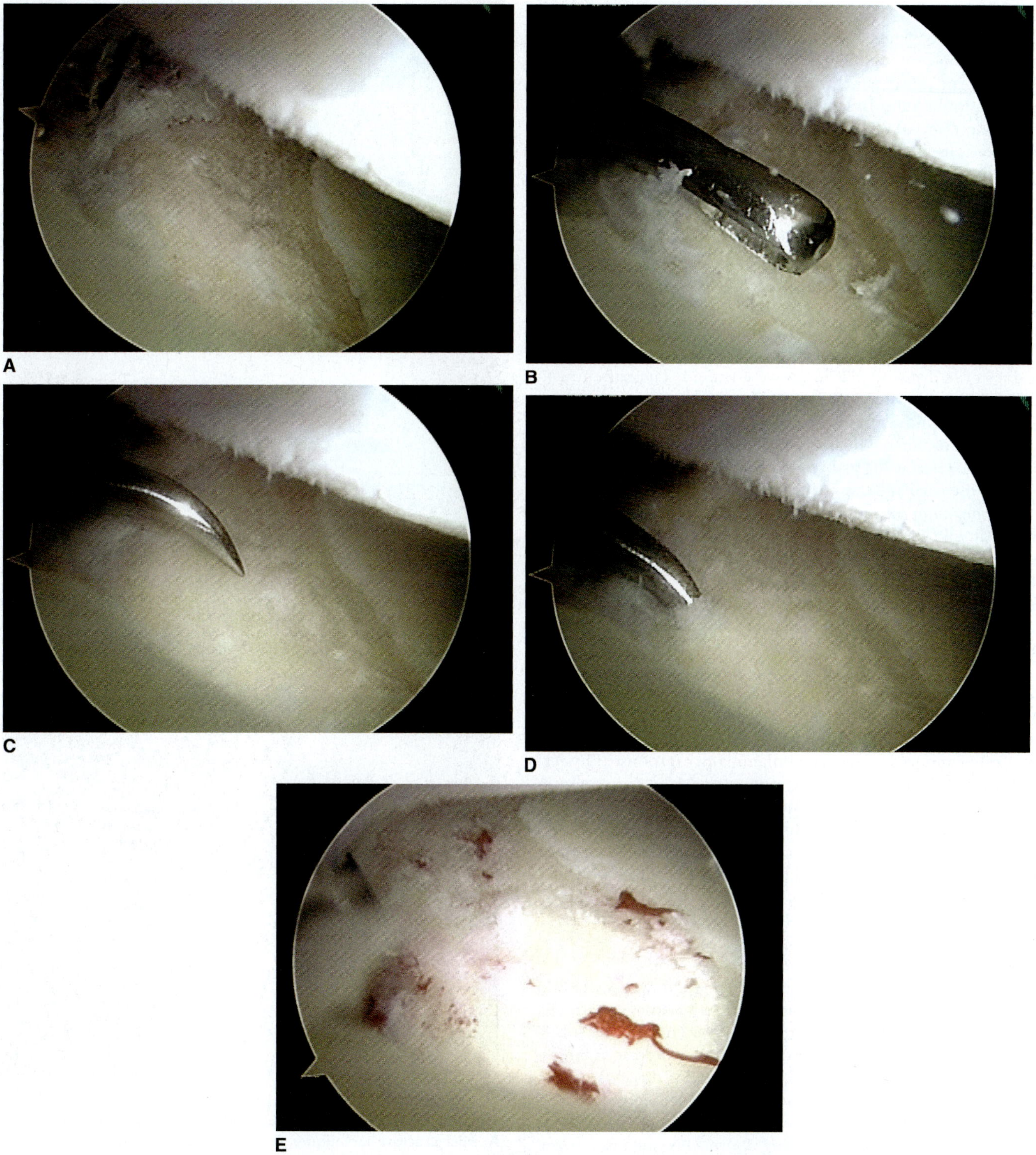

Figure 10.7. Microfracture of a grade IV superolateral acetabular chondral lesion in a patient with chronic femoroacetabular impingement. **A:** Grade IV chondral lesion of the superolateral acetabulum. **B:** Ring curette is used to remove the calcified cartilage layer from the planned microfracture bed. **C:** A microfracture awl is positioned for impaction. **D:** The awl is impacted. **E:** After the arthroscopic fluid is turned off, bleeding is visualized signaling an appropriate microfracture technique.

remaining unstable cartilage from the exposed bone is completed using a full radius resector and curettes. A ring curette is particularly useful for preparation of the defect and creating a smooth, perpendicular border (Fig. 10.7B). Particular attention must be paid while debriding the surrounding rim of the defect. Debridement should be deep enough to remove the calcified cartilage layer while maintaining the integrity of the subchondral plate.[1] The edges of the lesion should be perpendicular to the adjacent, unaffected cartilage to allow for the marrow clot to form more effectively. Arthroscopic awls are used to make multiple holes (microfractures) in the exposed subchondral plate (Fig. 10.7C & D). As many holes as possible should be placed, leaving about 3 to 4mm between each. A depth of approximately 2 to 4mm is enough to visualize fat droplets/bleeding from the holes once the arthroscopic fluid pressure is released (Fig. 10.7E). After bleeding is confirmed, the fluid pressure is re-established and any associated procedures are performed. If there is any concern for loose bodies or need for visualization of the femoral head–neck junction, the peripheral compartment is entered with the hip in 45° of flexion and 30° of external rotation with arthroscope in the anterior portal. The portals and/or incisions are closed in standard fashion, and a sterile dressing placed over the wound. The patient usually is discharged the same day.[1,6,47,48]

Other techniques have also been attempted in order to repair cartilage flaps. First, a microfracture is performed as previously described. Then using arthroscopic techniques and absorbable sutures, the cartilage flap is repaired (Fig. 10.8A–C).

The most important principle in postoperative management is to maintain the marrow clot and thus the ideal environment for healing while regaining range of motion and strength. Crutch-assisted 30lb flat-foot weight bearing is allowed for 4 weeks with advancement to full weight bearing to 6 weeks. A continuous passive motion machine is utilized throughout the 4-week period. Initial physical therapy consists of passive motion progressing to active-assisted motion and eventually active motion with particular emphasis on regaining hip internal rotation. Specific limitations also depend on associated procedures performed. Cold therapy is a good initial modality for pain relief and to decrease the inflammatory response. Physical therapy should focus early on motion and later on strength. Stationary bicycle exercises without resistance are useful and can be started immediately. Impact sports are delayed until at least 4 to 6 months postoperatively, and resumed only after range of motion, strength, and functional agility have returned to normal.[6,47,48]

OPEN TECHNIQUES

There are numerous described surgical windows to the hip joint. Each has unique advantages and disadvantages with different indications for different procedures. They can be subdivided into traditional approaches such as the anterior or Smith-Peterson,[59,60] anterolateral or Watson-Jones,[61–63] direct lateral or transgluteal Hardinge,[64] posterior or "Southern approach,"[65–67] and the posterolateral or Kocher–Langenbeck approach[68–70] or the more modern joint preserving approaches such as a surgical dislocation[71] or mini-open anterior approach.

The technique of a surgical dislocation has been well described.[71] Its purpose is to preserve the blood supply of the femoral head while obtaining a 360° view of both the femoral head and acetabulum if possible. It takes advantage of the anatomy of the medial femoral circumflex vessels and its relationship

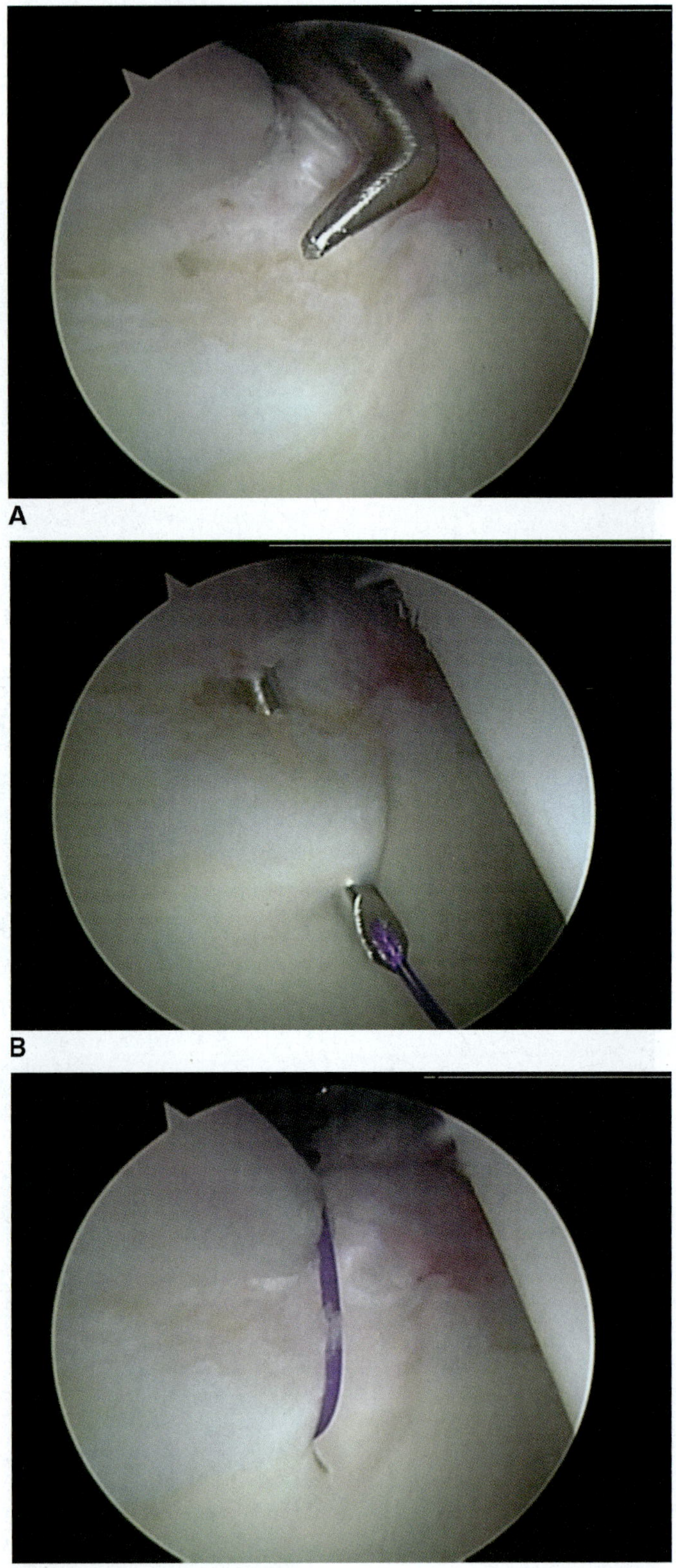

Figure 10.8. Microfracture and cartilage repair of a grade IV lesion. **A:** Microfracture techniques with awl. **B,C:** Absorbable suture passed and arthroscopic knot tied to stabilize cartilage flap.

to the obturator externus. Unlike traditional approaches, a surgical dislocation affords a much more expansive view of the hip but with more surgical morbidity due to a large dissection, complications from a trochanteric osteotomy, and possible AVN. An alternative technique is the mini-open anterior approach which may or may not be supplemented with arthroscopy.[43,44]

This mini-open approach is a less extensile modification of the Smith-Peterson and was initially described by Sekiya et al.[43,44] The incision is approximately 4 cm in length, 1 cm below the anterior inferior iliac spine. The approach uses the plane between the sartorius and tensor fascia latae superficially and then the rectus femoris and gluteus medius. If the procedure is supplemented with arthroscopy, the hip capsule is distended with saline and then the arthroscopic portals are placed via direct visualization of the capsule. It is technically less difficult than traditional hip arthroscopy and may reduce the risk of neurovascular damage and labral or cartilage damage that might occur during the placement of instruments with traditional arthroscopy. It may also have less morbidity than an open dislocation but has an inferior view and access to the hip joint.

Both joint-preserving approaches afford the operative surgeon an opportunity to reconstruct an osteochondral defect. As in the knee, there are various reconstructive options which include but are not limited to osteochondral autograft, allograft, arthrosurface implant, and ACI. The approach and technique chosen are dependent on the size and nature of the lesion. As in the knee, attention is focused on reconstructing the primary weight-bearing portions. Autografts from the proximal femur or ipsilateral knee can be used[72] (Fig. 10.9).

RESULTS

There is an emerging literature on the treatment of hip chondral injuries. Farjo et al.[73] evaluated 28 hips that underwent arthroscopy for acetabular labral tears with a minimum follow-up of 13 months. They found that patients with degenerative changes noted radiographically or arthroscopically on either the femoral or acetabular chondral surfaces were significantly associated with a poorer outcome. Byrd and Jones[29] prospectively evaluated 38 hip arthroscopies with a modified Harris hip score at 2 years postoperatively. There was a median score improvement of 28 points from preoperative to latest follow-up. Their cohort included a subset of 15 patients with a diagnosis of chondral injury, and this subset had a median improvement of 18 points. No specific mention was made in the article on the type of treatment to the chondral injury that was performed during arthroscopy. In an even smaller cohort, Byrd and Jones[74] also treated three patients with grade IV lesions with the microfracture technique who at 2 years returned to high level sporting activities. McCarthy et al.[54] described a cohort of ten elite athletes that underwent hip arthroscopy for a variety of diagnoses. Of these, four patients had evidence of chondral injury on the acetabular side that underwent an unspecified treatment. All ten athletes returned to compete in their sport. Kelly et al.[14] described in their review of hip arthroscopy the use of microfracture for full-thickness cartilage defects.

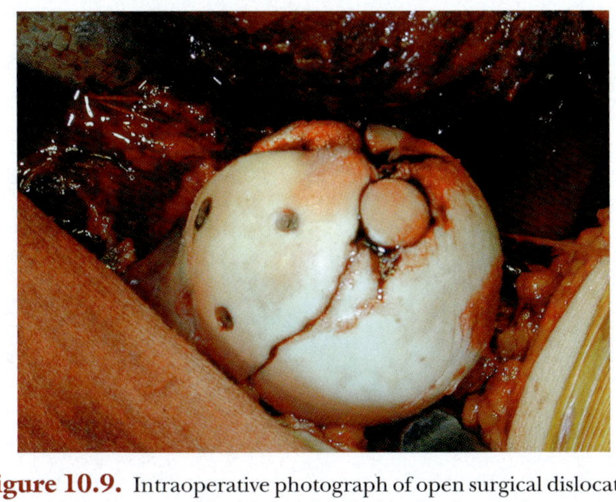

Figure 10.9. Intraoperative photograph of open surgical dislocation of a Pipkin injury treated with bioabsorbable fixation and an autograft plug taken from the non-weight-bearing portion of the proximal femur. (Courtesy of Dr RL Buly.)

CONCLUSIONS

Cartilage injuries in the hip joint are becoming increasingly recognized as a source of hip pain. The etiologies are quite variable including degenerative conditions, traumatic lesions, lesions from FAI, and capsular laxity. As our diagnostic and imaging modalities improve, numerous methods of treatment for these conditions are constantly growing and evolving. As in the knee, the procedure is dictated by numerous factors including the size of the lesion, the condition of remaining aspect of the joint, the overall alignment of the joint, and the underlying etiology of the defect. These lesions can be addressed both arthroscopically and through open surgery. The most common and reproducible arthroscopic technique is the microfracture technique for full-thickness chondral lesions. However, long-term outcome needs yet to be reported as the indications for microfracture are expanded and the experience grows with the use of microfracture technique utilizing hip arthroscopy. Prospective, long-term clinical studies with validated outcome measures are necessary to determine the indications and efficacy of all joint preserving techniques.

REFERENCES

1. Steadman JR, Rodkey WG, Rodrigo JJ. Microfracture: Surgical technique and rehabilitation to treat chondral defects. *Clin Orthop Relat Res.* 2001;391(Suppl.):S362–S369.
2. Sledge SL. Microfracture techniques in the treatment of osteochondral injuries. *Clin Sports Med.* 2001;20(2):365–377.
3. Gross AE. Repair of cartilage defects in the knee. *J Knee Surg.* 2002;15(3):167–169.
4. Buckwalter JA. Articular cartilage: Injuries and potential for healing. *J Orthop Sports Phys Ther.* 1998;28(4):192–202.
5. Byrd JW, Jones KS. Hip arthroscopy in athletes. *Clin Sports Med.* 2001;20(4):749–761.
6. McCarthy JC. The diagnosis and treatment of labral and chondral injuries. *Instr Course Lect.* 2004;53:573–577.
7. DeAngelis NA, Busconi BD. Assessment and differential diagnosis of the painful hip. *Clin Orthop Relat Res.* 2003;406:11–18.
8. Shindle MK, Voos JE, Heyworth BE, et al. Hip arthroscopy in the athletic patient: Current techniques and spectrum of disease. *J Bone Joint Surg Am.* 2007;89(Suppl. 3):29–43.
9. Braly BA, Beall DP, Martin HD. Clinical examination of the athletic hip. *Clin Sports Med.* 2006;25(2):199–210, vii.
10. Byrd JW, Jones KS. Diagnostic accuracy of clinical assessment, magnetic resonance imaging, magnetic resonance arthrography, and intra-articular injection in hip arthroscopy patients. *Am J Sports Med.* 2004;32(7):1668–1674.
11. Newberg AH, Newman JS. Imaging the painful hip. *Clin Orthop Relat Res.* 2003;406:19–28.
12. Sekiya JK, et al. Hip arthroscopy in staging avascular necrosis of the femoral head. *J South Orthop Assoc.* 2000;9(4):254–261.
13. Keeney JA, Peelle MW, Jackson J, et al. Magnetic resonance arthrography versus arthroscopy in the evaluation of articular hip pathology. *Clin Orthop Relat Res.* 2004; 429:163–169.
14. Kelly BT, Williams RJ III, Philippon MJ. Hip arthroscopy: Current indications, treatment options, and management issues. *Am J Sports Med.* 2003;31(6):1020–1037.
15. Potter HG, Linklater JM, Allen AA, et al. Magnetic resonance imaging of articular cartilage in the knee: An evaluation with use of fast-spin-echo imaging. *J Bone Joint Surg.* 1998;80A(9):1276–1284.
16. Mintz DN, Hooper T, Connell D, et al. Magnetic resonance imaging of the hip: Detection of labral and chondral abnormalities using noncontrast imaging. *Arthroscopy.* 2005;21(4):385–393.

17. Byrd JW. Hip arthroscopy: The supine position. *Clin Sports Med.* 2001;20(4):703–731.
18. Byrd JW. Lateral impact injury: A source of occult hip pathology. *Clin Sports Med.* 2001;20(4):801–815.
19. Byrd JW. Intraarticular hip injuries. In: *AOSSM.* Calgary, 2007.
20. McCarthy JC, Lee JA. Arthroscopic intervention in early hip disease. *Clin Orthop Relat Res.* 2004;429:157–162.
21. Outerbridge RE. The etiology of chondromalacia patellae. *J Bone Joint Surg Br.* 1961;43-B:752–757.
22. Mears DC, Velyvis JH, Chang CP. Displaced acetabular fractures managed operatively: Indicators of outcome. *Clin Orthop Relat Res.* 2003;407:173–186.
23. Yamamoto Y, Ide T, Ono T, et al. Usefulness of arthroscopic surgery in hip trauma cases. *Arthroscopy.* 2003;19(3):269–273.
24. McCarthy JC. Hip arthroscopy: When it is and when it is not indicated. *Instr Course Lect.* 2004;53:615–621.
25. McCarthy JC, Lee JA. The role of hip arthroscopy: Useful adjunct or devil's tool? *Orthopedics.* 2002;25(9):947–948.
26. McCarthy JC, Day B, Busconi B. Hip arthroscopy: Applications and technique. *J Am Acad Orthop Surg.* 1995;3:115–122.
27. Byrd JW. Lateral impact injury: A source of occult hip pathology. *Clin Sports Med.* 2001; 20(4):801–815.
28. Byrd JW. Hip arthroscopy for posttraumatic loose fragments in the young active adult: Three case reports. *Clin J Sport Med.* 1996;6(2):129–134.
29. Byrd JW, Jones KS. Prospective analysis of hip arthroscopy with 2-year follow-up. *Arthroscopy.* 2000;16(6):578–587.
30. Svoboda SJ, Williams DM, Murphy KP. Hip arthroscopy for osteochondral loose body removal after a posterior hip dislocation. *Arthroscopy.* 2003;19(7):777–781.
31. Elmali N, Esenkaya I, Alkan A. Synovial chondromatosis: A report of four cases with three diverse localizations. *Acta Orthop Traumatol Turc.* 2003;37(2):173–177.
32. Roy DR. Arthroscopic findings of the hip in new onset hip pain in adolescents with previous Legg-Calve-Perthes disease. *J Pediatr Orthop B.* 2005;14(3):151–155.
33. McCarthy J, Puri L, Barsoum W, et al. Articular cartilage changes in avascular necrosis: An arthroscopic evaluation. *Clin Orthop Relat Res.* 2003;406:64–70.
34. Hardy P, Hinojosa JF, Coudane H, et al. Osteochondritis dissecans of the acetabulum: Apropos of a case. *Rev Chir Orthop Reparatrice Appar Mot.* 1992;78(2):134–137.
35. Shindle MK, Ranawat AS, Kelly BT. Diagnosis and management of traumatic and atraumatic hip instability in the athletic patient. *Clin Sports Med.* 2006;25(2):309–326, ix–x.
36. Beck M, Kalhor M, Leunig M, et al., Hip morphology influences the pattern of damage to the acetabular cartilage: Femoroacetabular impingement as a cause of early osteoarthritis of the hip. *J Bone Joint Surg Br.* 2005;87(7):1012–1018.
37. Parvizi J, Leunig M, Ganz R. Femoroacetabular impingement. *J Am Acad Orthop Surg.* 2007;15(9):561–570.
38. Philippon MJ, Stubbs AJ, Schenker ML, et al. Arthroscopic management of femoroacetabular impingement: Osteoplasty technique and literature review. *Am J Sports Med.* 2007;35(9):1571–1580.
39. Espinosa N, Beck M, Rothenfluh DA, et al. Treatment of femoroacetabular impingement: Preliminary results of labral refixation. Surgical technique. *J Bone Joint Surg Am.* 2007;89(Suppl. 2 Pt 1):36–53.
40. Espinosa N, Rothenfluh DA, Beck M, et al. Treatment of femoroacetabular impingement: Preliminary results of labral refixation. *J Bone Joint Surg Am.* 2006;88(5):925–935.
41. Beck M, Leunig M, Parvizi J, et al. Anterior femoroacetabular impingement: Part II. Midterm results of surgical treatment. *Clin Orthop Relat Res.* 2004;418:67–73.
42. Ganz R, Parvizi J, Beck M, et al. Femoroacetabular impingement: A cause for osteoarthritis of the hip. *Clin Orthop Relat Res.* 2003;417:112–120.
43. Clohisy JC, McClure JT. Treatment of anterior femoroacetabular impingement with combined hip arthroscopy and limited anterior decompression. *Iowa Orthop J.* 2005;25:164–171.
44. Sekiya JK, Wojtys EM, Loder RT, et al. Hip arthroscopy using a limited anterior exposure: An alternative approach for arthroscopic access. *Arthroscopy.* 2000;16(1):16–20.
45. Sussman PS, Ranawat AS, Lorich DG, et al. Arthroscopic versus open osteoplasty of the head-neck junction a cadaveric investigation. *Arthrosc.* 2007;23(12):1257–1264. Epub 2007 Oct 29.
46. Beaule PE, Clohisy JC, Schoenecker P, et al. Hip arthroscopy: An emerging gold standard. *Arthroscopy.* 2007;23(6):682.
47. Crawford K, Philippon MJ, Sekiya JK, et al. Microfracture of the hip in athletes. *Clin Sports Med.* 2006;25(2):327–335.
48. Steadman JR, Briggs KK, Rodrigo JJ, et al. Outcomes of microfracture for traumatic chondral defects of the knee: Average 11-year follow-up. *Arthroscopy.* 2003;19(5):477–484.
49. Steadman JR, Miller BS, Karas SG, et al. The microfracture technique in the treatment of full-thickness chondral lesions of the knee in National Football League players. *J Knee Surg.* 2003;16(2):83–86.
50. Steadman JR, Rodkey WG, Briggs KK. Microfracture to treat full-thickness chondral defects: Surgical technique, rehabilitation, and outcomes. *J Knee Surg.* 2002;15(3):170–176.
51. Byrd JW. Hip arthroscopy in the supine position. *Operat Tech Sports Med.* 2002;10(4): 184–195.
52. Byrd JW. Hip arthroscopy in athletes. *Instr Course Lect.* 2003;52:701–709.
53. Byrd JW. Hip arthroscopy: Patient assessment and indications. *Instr Course Lect.* 2003;52:711–719.
54. McCarthy J, Barsoum W, Puri L, et al. The role of hip arthroscopy in the elite athlete. *Clin Orthop Relat Res.* 2003;406:71–74.
55. Mason JB, McCarthy JC, O'Donnell J, et al. Hip arthroscopy: Surgical approach, positioning, and distraction. *Clin Orthop Relat Res.* 2003;406:29–37.
56. Monllau JC, Solano A, Leon A, et al. Tomographic study of the arthroscopic approaches to the hip joint. *Arthroscopy.* 2003;19(4):368–372.
57. Clarke MT, Arora A, Villar RN. Hip arthroscopy: Complications in 1054 cases. *Clin Orthop Relat Res.* 2003;406:84–88.
58. Ranawat AS, Kelly BT. Anatomy of the hip: Open and arthroscopic structure and function. *Operat Tech Orthop.* 2005;15(3):160–174.
59. Smith-Peterson M. A new supra-articular subperiosteal approach to the hip joint. *Am J Orthop Surg.* 1917;15:592.
60. Smith-Peterson M. Approach to and exposure of the hip joint for mold arthroplasty. *J Bone Joint Surg.* 1949;31A:40.
61. Charnley J. *Low Friction Arthroplasty of the Hip: Theory and Practice.* New York: Springer-Verlag; 1979.
62. Harris W. A new lateral approach to the hip. *J Bone Joint Surg.* 1967;49A:891.
63. Hirsch D. Personal Communication Re: Antero-Lateral Exposure of Hip. Watson-Jones, 1981.
64. Hardinge K. The direct lateral approach to the hip. *J Bone Joint Surg.* 1982;64B:17–19.
65. Hoppenfeld S, DeBoer P. *Surgical Exposures in Orthopaedics: The Anatomic Approach.* 3rd Ed. Philadelphia, PA: Lippincott Williams & Wilkins; 2003.
66. Moore AT. The self-locking metal hip prosthesis. *J Bone Joint Surg.* 1957;39A:811.
67. Moore AT. The Moore self-locking vitallium prosthesis in fresh femoral neck fractures: A new low posterior approach (the southern exposure). *Instructional Course Lecture of the American Academy of Orthopedic Surgeons.* 1959;16.
68. Kocher T. *Operative Surgery.* In: Siles HJ, Paul CB, eds. London: Black; 1911.
69. Langenbeck B. Ueber die Schussfracturen der Gelenke und ihre Behandlung, 1868.
70. Mehlman CT, Meiss L, DiPasquale TG. Hyphenated-history: The Kocher–Langenneck surgical approach. *J Orthop Trauma.* 2000;14(1):60–64.
71. Ganz R, Gill TJ, Gautier E, et al. Surgical dislocation of the adult hip a technique with full access to the femoral head and acetabulum without the risk of avascular necrosis. *J Bone Joint Surg.* 2001;83B(8):1119–1124.
72. Gardner MJ, Suk M, Pearle A, et al. Surgical dislocation of the hip for fractures of the femoral head. *J Orthop Trauma.* 2005;19(5):334–342.
73. Farjo LA, Glick JM, Sampson TG. Hip arthroscopy for acetabular labral tears. *Arthroscopy.* 1999;15(2):132–137.
74. Byrd JW, Jones KS. Osteoarthritis caused by an inverted acetabular labrum: Radiographic diagnosis and arthroscopic treatment. *Arthroscopy.* 2002;18(7):741–747.

CHAPTER

11

Marc J. Philippon
Connor J. Hay
David A. Kuppersmith
Karen K. Briggs

Hip Injuries in the High-Level Athlete

INTRODUCTION

Hip injuries can cause significant disability in the elite athletes, resulting in an inability to participate in their sport due to debilitating pain, mechanical symptoms, instability, or a decline in their performance due to their hip. With jogging, the hip joint is forced to withstand loads of up to eight times body weight and likely encounters higher forces during vigorous athletic competition, potentially causing acute or chronic injury.[1,2] Many types of injuries can occur about the hip in the athlete, including muscle strains, contusions, avulsion injuries, labral tears, and hip dislocations and subluxations.[3]

Hip injuries in the elite athlete result from both acute, traumatic episodes, and repetitive stress and strain. Forceful dislocation of the hip must be treated emergently by means of expert closed reduction (to avoid femoral neck fracture) or open surgical reduction. More subtle hip subluxation injuries may often go unrecognized and undertreated. When witnessed or reported, traumatic hip subluxations warrant a careful exam and consideration for an urgent MRI to evaluate the extent of injury and resultant intracapsular bleeding, which may require surgical evacuation.

Repetitive stress to the hip occurs across a wide variety of athletic pursuits. Athletes involved in dancing, hockey, soccer, football, baseball, and basketball frequently place supraphysiologic demands on their hips. The repetitive nature of these stresses over the course of time at the elite level of play may contribute to the wide spectrum of hip injuries seen in these athletes. Hip injuries requiring arthroscopic treatment occur in a wide range of sport. Athletes present with an inability to participate in their sport due to pain and have failed conservative treatment for 6 to 12 weeks. Commonly, on preoperative physical examination and diagnostic imaging, there is evidence of femoroacetabular impingement (FAI) and associated labral tears, requiring surgical intervention to correct these abnormalities.

CLINICAL DIAGNOSIS

Potential generators of hip pain and dysfunction can be broadly classified as intra-articular and extra-articular (Table 11.1). Careful consideration must be made for the bony anatomy and alignment of the athlete's hip. Developmental dysplasia of the hip (DDH), deformity from slipped capital femoral epiphysis or Legg–Calve–Perthes disease, and FAI strongly influence both intra-articular and extra-articular injury patterns in the hip.

With FAI, the patient has bony morphologic abnormalities that alter the force distribution within the joint, triggering damage to the acetabular labrum, and articular cartilage of the hip. Cam, pincer, and mixed-type impingement is common among the athletic population presenting with hip pain, loss of range of motion, and disability in athletics. Furthermore, these structural abnormalities oftentimes place athletes at a higher risk for labral pathology, as the labrum is the first structure encountered during contact with both types of impingement. Labral tears are commonly the result of repetitive sports-related injury as opposed to an isolated traumatic event[4] and symptoms may be exacerbated with rigorous athletic activity (Fig. 11.1). Crawford et al.[5] recently explored the mechanical factors leading to the formation of labral tears and their effect on hip kinematics. Using a 3D motion analysis system, the stability of six cadaveric hips was measured during loading maneuvers.[5] They found that a breach of integrity of labral function is shown to lead to a decreased femoral stability relative to the acetabulum during extreme ranges of motion.[5]

Additionally, instability within the hip joint may be seen among athletes who have experienced traumatic dislocation or subluxation of the femoral head, with most athletic hip dislocations occurring in contact sports such as football or hockey. Atraumatic instability also exists among patients presenting with global ligamentous laxity or disorders such as Ehlers–Danlos syndrome, Down syndrome, Marfan syndrome, or DDH.[6] Recurring athletic activities may cause increased tension in the hip joint capsule and surrounding ligaments, leading to capsular elongation and it is often seen in conjunction with a labral tear.[2]

Athletes with unrecognized intra-articular hip pathologies often endure prolonged, frustrating, and confusing interactions with their trainers, therapists, and physicians. Many athletes are diagnosed with groin injuries, sports hernia, piriformis syndrome, coxa sultans, and/or various lumbar spine pathologies.

The sports hernia is commonly seen in the elite athlete. The inguinal hernia is caused by overuse. Shearing forces across the symphysis pubis cause stress on inguinal wall musculature. There can also be an abnormal insertion of the rectus abdominus. The internal oblique is torn at the pubic tubercle or the external oblique is torn. Entrapment of the ilioinguinal nerve has also been documented. Athletes present with a lump in the groin, a positive cough impulse, and pain. Accurate diagnosis of

TABLE 11.1 Common Causes of Hip Pain

Primary Labrum	*Primary Chondral*	*Primary Capsule*	*Systemic*	*Extra-articular*
Trauma	Lateral impact	Laxity	Hormonal	Snapping hip
Laxity	Subluxation	Adhesive capsulitis	Rheumatoid	Trochanteric bursitis
Bony impingement	Dislocation	Synovitis/Inflammation	Poly-articular	Ischial bursitis
	AVN		Autoimmune	Psoas bursitis
Dysplasia	Loose bodies		RSD	Osteitis pubis
Degenerative	Synovial		Regional pain syndrome	Sports hernia
	Chromotosis			Piriformis syndrome
	Chondrocalcinosis			Adductor muscles strain or tendinopathy
	Degeneration			Stress fractures
				Infection

Courtesy of Marc J. Philippon, MD.

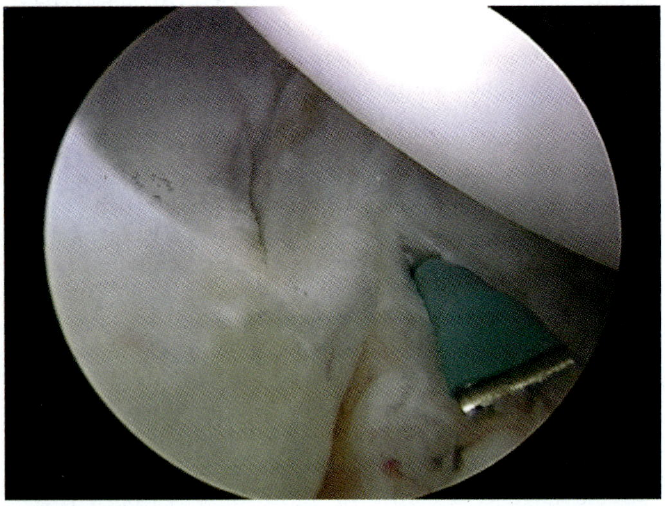

Figure 11.1. Labral tear demonstrated with radiofrequency probe. (Courtesy of Marc J. Philippon, MD.)

the sports hernia remains challenging. A recent study reported a 10-fold increase in the number of patients seen with sports hernia over a 20-year period.[7] A diagnostic algorithm is currently being developed to assist with the diagnosis of the common pathology seen in elite athletes (Fig. 11.2).

Intra-articular pathology may require surgical intervention. The physical exam is extremely important for determining the source of the patient's symptoms. First, an evaluation of the patients' lumbar spine and a focused neurologic evaluation should be performed. This allows the surgeon to rule out any nonhip pathologies that could be causing their pain. We then like to perform a series of tests for range of motion and strength of the perihip musculature. It is common to see a reduction of internal rotation and pain during testing of patients with impingement.[8] Furthermore, we will perform anterior and posterior impingement tests to further stress the labrum and reproduce symptoms of pain (Fig. 11.3). Finally, we will perform a hip dial test to determine the integrity of the anterior capsule and iliofemoral ligament. With the patient in a supine position, we will evaluate the position of the lower extremity with respect to the long axis of the body. By pressing on the inside of the patient's foot and watching for rebound, we can determine how tight or lax this capsular tissue has become.

It is very important with any of these provocative tests to determine if the pain the patients are experiencing is the same pain that has brought them to your clinic. One effective way in which this can be accomplished is to perform a lidocaine and kenalog injection in the office. After sterile prep, an 18-gauge spinal needle is placed within the hip capsule and the steroid/lidocaine mixture administered. After approximately 5 min, we can repeat the same physical exam tests and quantify the improvement in the patient's symptoms. This is typically diagnostic and can be therapeutic during the time the patient is awaiting surgical intervention.

Advances in arthroscopic techniques and instrumentation have made hip arthroscopy an increasingly attractive alternative to longer, more invasive open approaches to address pathology within the hip joint. The classic open technique required the patient to endure traumatic intraoperative episodes combined with lengthy long-term rehabilitation. In the athletic population, arthroscopic approaches to the hip may facilitate a more rapid return to play.

INDICATIONS

Proper patient selection is the key to excellent outcomes for both the surgeon and the patient alike. The ideal candidate for the procedure has a history and physical exam that correlates well with radiographic and advanced imaging studies demonstrating intra-articular hip pathology. The patient must have predominantly healthy cartilage in the hip and a minimum joint space of 2 mm, measured in a weight-bearing AP radiograph (Fig. 11.4). They must also have failed to respond to a minimum 3-month regimen of targeted physical therapy and NSAIDs. Finally, they must be well-informed of the procedure and the intensive postoperative treatment plan and demonstrate commitment to the process from start to finish. Relative contraindications would include morbid obesity (given positioning and instrumentation difficulties), advanced arthritis,

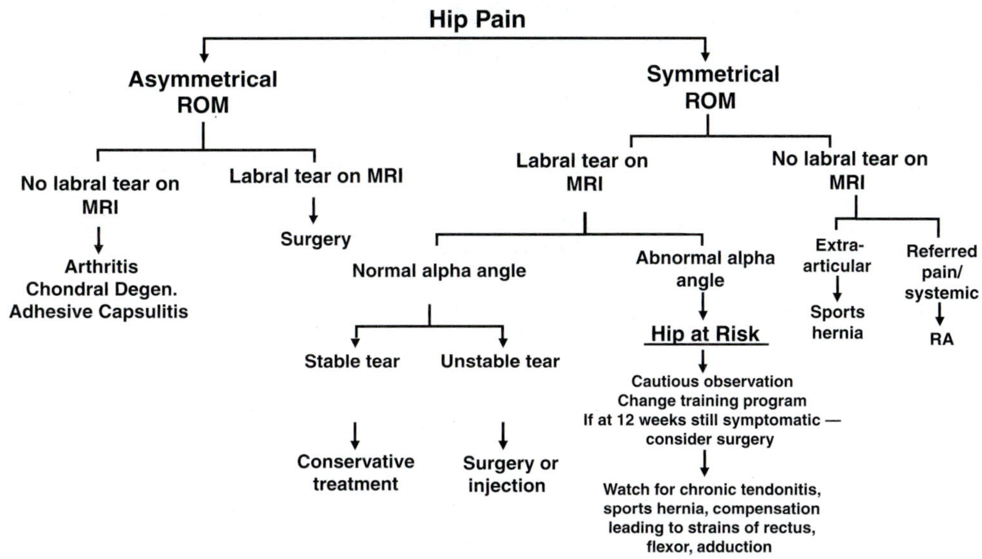

Figure 11.2. Current treatment algorithm for hip pain. (Courtesy of Marc J. Philippon, MD.)

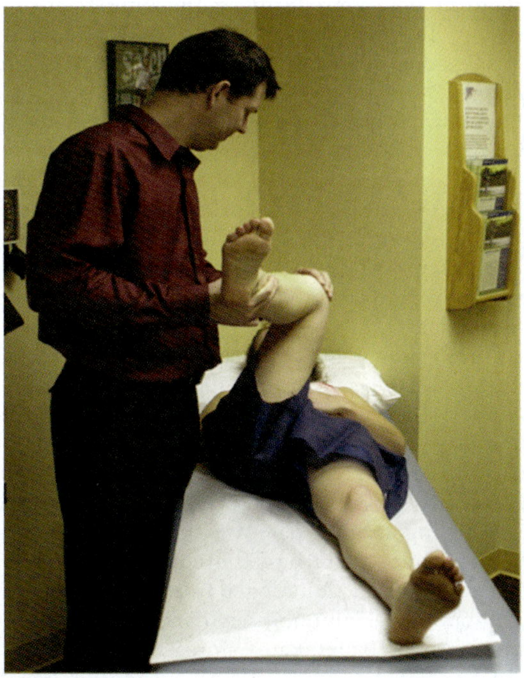

Figure 11.3. Demonstration of impingement test. (Courtesy of Marc J. Philippon, MD.)

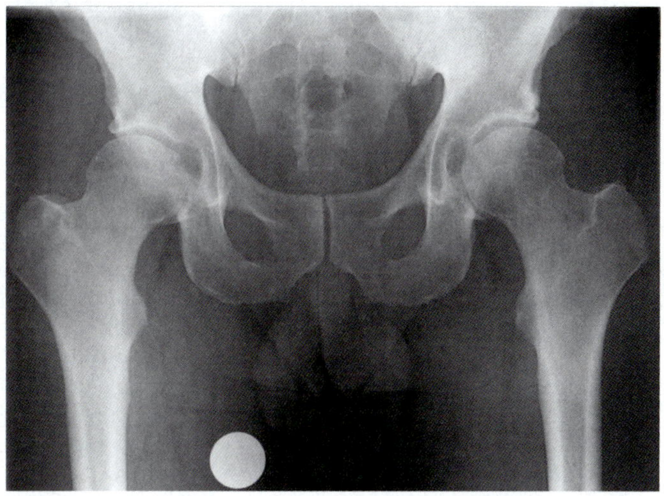

Figure 11.4. AP lateral radiograph. (Courtesy of Marc J. Philippon, MD.)

avascular necrosis (AVN) and joint collapse, severely dysplastic hips, chronic intra-articular infection, and patient's unwillingness to comply with strict rehabilitation protocol.

SURGICAL FINDINGS IN THE ELITE ATHLETE

Injury patterns in the hip may vary by the sport the athlete plays. In professional football players, athletes are subjected to high-impact trauma as well as axial loading with rotational forces.[9] The senior author recently focused on the surgical treatment of ten football players who presented with hip pain. This group of patients had labral tears, but the common finding was associated with significant chondral injuries.[9] Similarly, Feeley et al.[10] monitored hip-related injuries in the National Football League (NFL) from 1997 to 2006. The authors found 738 hip injuries, which accounted for 3.1% of all injuries seen in the NFL within this time period. They found that the most common type of injury was hip flexor strain, followed by contusion, intra-articular injury, and a sprain. This pattern is similar to other contact sports such as soccer, basketball, and lacrosse.

In hockey, athletes are subjected to significant, high-impact forces on their hip as well as significant abduction/external rotation movements.[9] Strains are very common, as is hip flexor tendonitis, and it is not unreasonable to speculate that these injuries work in conjunction with underlying, intra-articular pathologies such as a labral tear, chondral injuries, or loose bodies.[9] Emery et al.[11] analyzed groin and abdominal strain injuries retrospectively among elite male hockey players in the

National Hockey League (NHL) over six seasons of play. They found that the majority of the injuries reported were adductor groin muscle strains and that the incidence of groin/abdominal strain injuries increased from 12.99 injuries/100 players/year in the 1991/1992 season to 19.87 injuries/100 players/year in the 1996/1997 season.

Hip-related injuries are also common among baseball players due to significant axial loading forces with rotational components common to baseball-related movements.[9] Specifically, baseball pitchers transfer weight at the end of the throw on their landing leg or have extra load on winding up during their early phase of throwing, subjecting their hip joint to increased loads.[9] Furthermore, baseball catchers are subjected to extra load on their hip joint due to their squatted position for extended periods of time.[9]

Professional dancers frequently encounter hip-related injuries involving capsular laxity and instability. Ballet dancers subject their hip to significant extremes of motion, especially rotation, leading to significant instability due to capsular stretching.[9] Repetitive external rotation of the hip and axial loading may cause capsular laxity, resulting in excess stress being placed on the ligamentum teres and tears may result.[2] Furthermore, a labral tear in conjunction with capsular elongation can lead to rotational instability and eventually to significant discomfort.[9] These dancers are commonly treated with thermal capsulorrhaphy and capsular plication to correct ligamentous elongation and capsular laxity.

POSTOPERATIVE REHABILITATION

The initial treatment following hip arthroscopy is to protect the repaired tissue while starting early passive range of motion within a restricted range. The athlete must adhere to weight-bearing restrictions to help mitigate pain. Hip circumduction, flexion, and internal rotation are emphasized in the early stages of rehabilitation. Circumduction at 70° and neutral is also stressed to prevent adhesions between the circular fibers of the zona obicularis and the femoral neck. Internal rotation is stressed due to the removal of the impingement; however, a "pinching" sensation is avoided to prevent stress and inflammation on the surgical repair.

Patients advance to the next level of rehabilitation based on pain reduction, range of motion, motor control, and weight-bearing status. The next phase of rehabilitation usually begins at postoperative week 2 to 3, with progressive resistive exercise in addition to continued passive range of motion (PROM) and gait training. Hip flexion is progressed as tolerated by the patient. The treadmill (including underwater treadmills) should never be used by the patient from this point forward due to the secondary shearing forces across the anterior hip joint as a result of the moving tread. The criteria to progress to the next rehabilitation phase are full range of motion, normal gait, and greater than 70% hip adduction, abduction, extension, internal rotation, and external rotation in comparison to uninvolved limb.[12]

The advanced phases of rehabilitation consist of muscular endurance and cardiovascular conditioning. Advanced plyometric activities are started to prepare the patient for the general sport test. The sport test is a functional test comprised of four exercises with a 20-point scoring system. It is meant to test the patient's ability to demonstrate endurance and functional strength in the lower extremity, good explosion of and absorption onto the involved lower extremity in a lateral and rotational direction, and the ability to flex and extend into a lunge position without pain, fatigue, or compensation. The four tests are the single knee bends, side-to-side lateral movement, diagonal side-to-side movement, and forward box lunges. The sport test is used as a presurgery functional exam as well as a return to training/play functional test. Athletes must achieve a passing score on the sport test prior to returning to training and eventual return to athletic competition.

The sport-specific rehabilitation phase is intended to integrate the athlete into team practice in preparation for competitive return to high-level sport. The importance of this phase is full return-to-competition without limitations in elite sport function other than restrictions on full contact training.

OUTCOMES

Between October 2000 and September 2005, the senior author treated 45 professional athletes with arthroscopic hip surgery for FAI. Forty-two athletes (93%) returned to professional sport following hip arthroscopy and the three players who did not return had diffuse osteoarthritis at the time of arthroscopy.[2] Thirty-five of the forty-five athletes (78%) remained active at the professional level at an average of 1.6 years after hip arthroscopy.[12]

Additionally, 30 professional football players were recently treated because of an inability to participate in their sport due to persistent hip pain. Thirteen of the fourteen players who were minimum 1 year post-op returned to full competitive play during the season of or the season following surgery. Seven of the thirteen players who have returned are currently active and playing at an average of 2.2 years after surgery (Philippon et al., unpublished data).

Thirty professional hockey players also presented to the senior author for unremitting and debilitating hip pain. These players underwent arthroscopic labral repair and treatment for FAI. All of these patients returned to sport at an average of 3.8 months (range 1 to 11 months) after surgery. Follow-up was obtained on 24 (80%) of the 30 players at an average of 18.2 months following surgery. The average Modified Harris Hip score (MHHS) improved from 69 preoperatively to 95 postoperatively. Patient satisfaction ranged from 7 to 10 with a median of 10 (Philippon et al., unpublished data).

Furthermore, 31 ballet dancers presented between January 2002 and December 2004 for anterior superior labral tears. Twenty-four dancers had associated partial ligamentum teres tear, 20 underwent partial iliopsoas release, and three underwent acetabular microfracture. All patients improved on MHHS and 91% of the patients were symptom free following arthroscopy. Twenty-eight patients returned to athletic performance at an average of 16 weeks following treatment (Philippon et al., unpublished data).

Between August 2000 and September 2006, 14 professional athletes were treated for traumatic hip dislocation. All patients were found to have some form of either labral or chondral pathology. All 14 athletes returned to full competition following arthroscopic intervention for hip pain after traumatic hip dislocation (Philippon et al., unpublished data).

Finally, a group of professional or Olympic-level athletes were monitored to determine the outcomes following hip arthroscopy. A group of 22 athletes underwent surgery between August 1999 and August 2001 and their respective sports included ballet, baseball, figure skating, football, golf, taekwondo, tennis, and soccer. At a minimum of 48 months, all patients had improvement in their MHHS and 92% of the players returned to sport following surgery. All of the athletes who returned to play remained active in their sport at 2-year follow-up (Philippon et al., unpublished data).

CONCLUSIONS

Hip arthroscopy has provided the orthopaedic surgeon with the ability to address pathology in the hip and return the elite athlete to competition. With proper patient selection and patient compliance, this procedure reports a very high success rate. In addition to this success rate, relatively low complication rates with this operative approach are the impetus behind the recent focus in orthopedic literature and at national meetings across the globe. Continued innovation, led by the pioneering orthopedic surgeons, will further advance the successes we have seen in the last 5 to 7 years.

REFERENCES

1. Crowninshield RD, Johnston RC, Andrews JG, et al. A biomechanical investigation of the human hip. *J Biomech.* 1978;11:75–85.
2. Philippon MJ, Schenker ML. Athletic hip injuries and capsular laxity. *Oper Tech Orthop.* 2005;15:261–266.
3. Anderson K, Strickland SM, Warren R. Hip and groin injuries in athletes. *Am J Sports Med.* 2001;29:521–533.
4. Bharam S. Labral tears, extra-articular injuries and hip arthroscopy in the athlete. *Clin Sports Med.* 2006;25(2):279–291.
5. Crawford MJ, Dy CJ, Alexander JW, et al. The 2007 Frank Stinchfield Award: The biomechanics of the hip labrum and the stability of the hip. *Clin Orthop Relat Res.* 2007;465:16–22.
6. Philippon MJ. The role of arthroscopic thermal capsulorrhaphy in the hip. *Clin Sports Med.* 2001;20:817–829.
7. Meyers WC, McKechnie A, Philippon MJ, et al. Experience with "sports hernia" spanning two decades. *Ann Surg.* 2008;248(4):656–665.
8. Philippon MJ, Maxwell RB, Johnston TL, et al. Clinical presentation of femoroacetabular impingement. *Knee Surg Sports Traumatol Arthrosc.* 2007;15:1041–1047.
9. Philippon MJ. Arthroscopy of the hip in the management of the athlete. In: McGinty JB, ed. *Operative Arthroscopy.* Philadelphia, PA: Lippincott Williams & Wilkins; 2003, p. 60.
10. Feeley BT, Powell JW, Muller MS, et al. Hip injuries and labral tears in the national football league. *Am J Sports Med.* 2008;36:2187–2195.
11. Emery CA, Meeuwisse WH, Powell JW. Groin and abdominal strain injuries in the national hockey league. *Clin J Sports Med.* 1999;9(3):151–156.
12. Philippon MJ, Schenker ML, Briggs KK, et al. Femoroacetabular impingement in 45 professional athletes: Associated pathologies and return to sport following arthroscopic decompression. *Knee Surg Sports Traumatol Arthrosc.* 2007;15:908–914.

CHAPTER

12

Michael Leunig
Mark R. Williams
Reinhold Ganz

Treatment of Femoroacetabular Impingement—Open

INTRODUCTION

Hip osteoarthritis is now recognized as a more complex process than purely a biomechanical mismatch leading to concentric or eccentric joint overload and subsequent wear of the articular cartilage.[1,2] The presence of a subgroup of patients who develop osteoarthritis in joints with normal articular structure and alignment suggests that alternative mechanisms are responsible. In most cases of idiopathic and in all cases of secondary osteoarthritis, the cause may be due to femoroacetabular impingement (FAI).[3]

CONCEPT OF FEMOROACETABULAR IMPINGEMENT

Some radiological signs of FAI have been reported previously with description of the "pistol grip" deformity seen on AP radiographs in patients with this phenomenon.[4] However, the effects of this abnormal anatomical relationship on the biomechanics of the hip joint were only described in more recent times.[5] In a subgroup of patients, it is apparent that there is reduced joint clearance at the extremes of movement, typically flexion of the hip joint, combined with a degree of internal rotation. The physical abutment of the abnormally shaped femoral neck on the acetabular rim over time may be responsible for injury to the acetabular labrum and rim and, subsequently, damage to the acetabular articular cartilage. This mechanism may be responsible for the development of osteoarthritis in these patients.

TYPES OF FEMOROACETABULAR IMPINGEMENT

Assessment of the pattern of labral and chondral injuries in this group of patients has led to the identification of two distinct types of FAI (Fig. 12.1).[5] In cases where there is a loss of anterior offset of the femoral neck, there are high shear stresses on the cartilage of the acetabulum and repetitive damage. This is known as cam impingement. The chronic effect of this process is initially acetabular cartilage injury, subsequently followed by acetabular labral injury, seen as chondral avulsion and labral detachment.[6,7]

Where increased acetabular coverage leads to the femoral neck abutting against the acetabular rim in extremes of motion, this is known as pincer impingement. The acetabular labrum appears to be the first structure to fail, with subsequent intrasubstance degeneration and cyst formation and further deepening of the acetabular socket due to bone apposition at the involved rim, which exacerbates the problem.[8] Pincer FAI can lead to a "contrecoup" injury at the postero-inferior cartilage as the femoral head is levered against the anterior acetabular rim.

TREATMENT OPTIONS

Conservative treatment may be considered initially as activity modification, rest, and NSAIDS may alleviate the symptoms to a degree that is acceptable for the patient to tolerate. However, in the younger patients with high physical demands, this is not always acceptable and may not be complied with. Furthermore, these management strategies may have been attempted without alleviation of symptoms to a satisfactory level. In this instance, surgery can be considered if the specific morphological and pathological abnormalities are detected on magnetic resonance arthrography.

Surgical treatment can be approached in a variety of ways, but the type of underlying abnormality and pathology should be considered in selecting the technique. Arthroscopy is an emerging technique in patients suffering from localized anterior FAI, but while the secondary effects of the morphological abnormality can be easily treated (labral pathology), it is technically more challenging to address the underlying cause. Surgical dislocation of the hip via an open approach provides complete visualization of the acetabular and femoral surfaces, allowing identification of lesions of the chondral surface and labrum. In addition, the structural morphological changes such as lack of anterior femoral neck offset and acetabular overcoverage can be addressed with relative ease.[9,10] Surgical dislocation is the approch of choice for the complex impingement situations. The open treatment of FAI will now be discussed in detail.

BLOOD SUPPLY OF THE FEMORAL HEAD

One of the key issues and difficulties with using an open approach in the treatment of intracapsular procedures such as

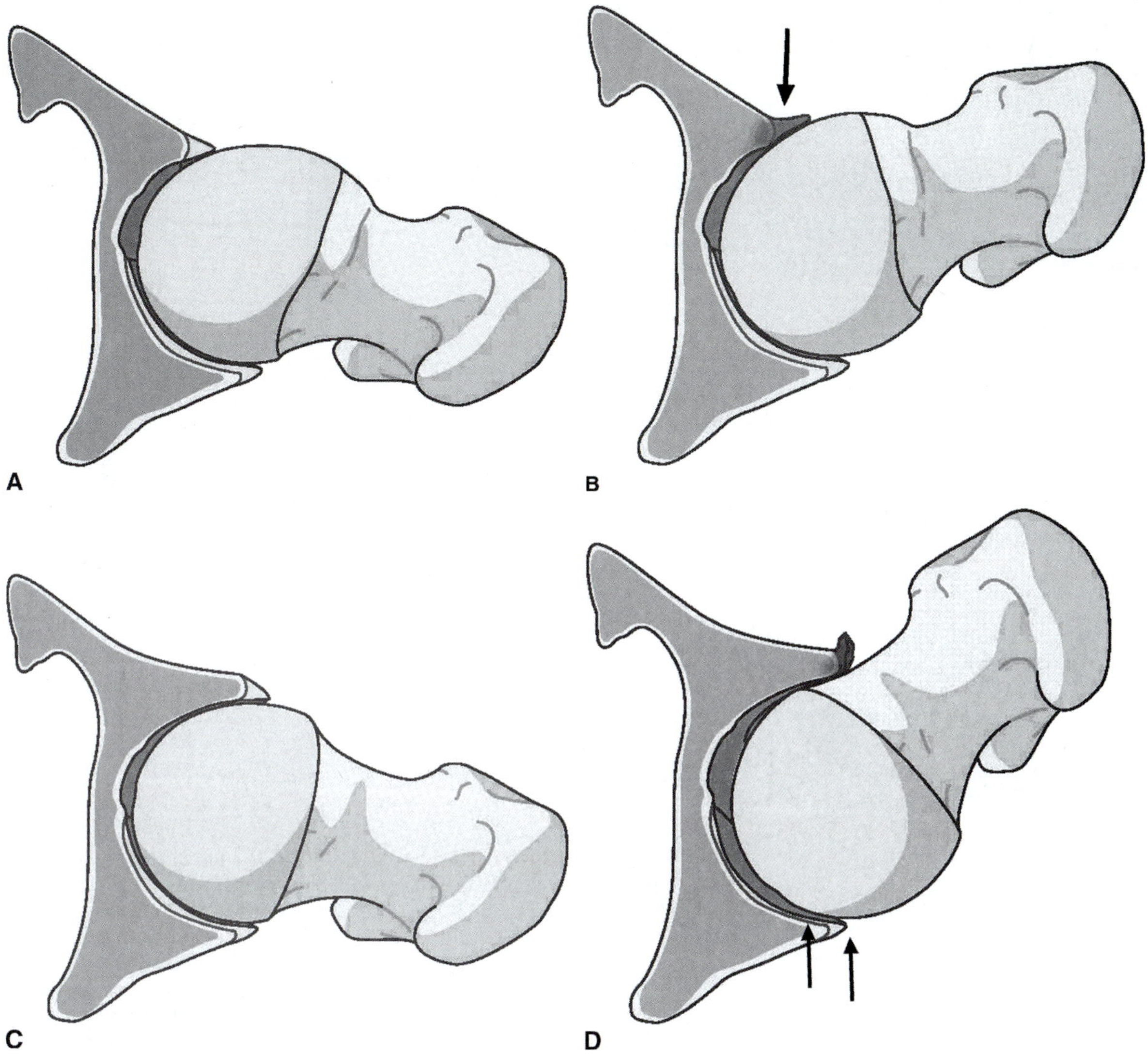

Figure 12.1. The two forms of FAI are shown. Cam FAI occurs when the lack of offset on the femoral neck **(A)** leads to mainly anterior damage (*arrow*) through repetitive trauma between the femoral neck and acetabulum during hip flexion **(B)**. Pincer FAI occurs secondary to acetabular overcoverage **(C)** causing anterior abutment and subsequent "contrecoup" injury to the cartilage of the postero-inferior acetabulum (*arrows*) during hip flexion **(D)**. (From Leunig M, Robertson W, Ganz R. Femoroacetabular impingement: Diagnosis and management including open surgical technique. *Tech Sports Med.* 2007;15:178–88, with permission.)

FAI relates to the blood supply of the hip and how to preserve this during surgery. Studies dating back more than 40 years have shown that the primary supply to the head of the femur is the deep branch of the medial femoral circumflex artery (MFCA). A previous series of 24 cadaveric hips injected with neoprene latex into the femoral or internal iliac vessels demonstrated that the MFCA is the main blood supply to the femoral head.[11] The vessel was surgically dissected out in the cadaveric specimens and found to cross obturator externus posteriorly, thereafter passing anteriorly to the short external rotators before perforating the joint capsule at the level of superior gemellus. The study also demonstrated that the vessel remained intact without excessive tension in hip dislocation, providing the external rotators and obturator externus remained intact.[11]

Unfortunately, the commonly utilized posterior approach requires division of the short external rotators, and in doing so, the artery is severely endangered. As a result of this, a new technique allowing operative exposure and dislocation of the femoral head was developed.

SURGICAL DISLOCATION OF THE HIP

The basis for a surgical approach in the treatment of FAI was preservation of the blood supply to the hip. The approach combined and utilized features from several previously described approaches, with the general principle of an anterior dislocation of the femoral head from a postero (-lateral) approach. However, in order to protect the MFCA, the external rotators are left intact, and the joint capsule is obtained from the anteriorly exposed part using a trochanteric flip osteotomy. The surgical technique is explained in detail below.

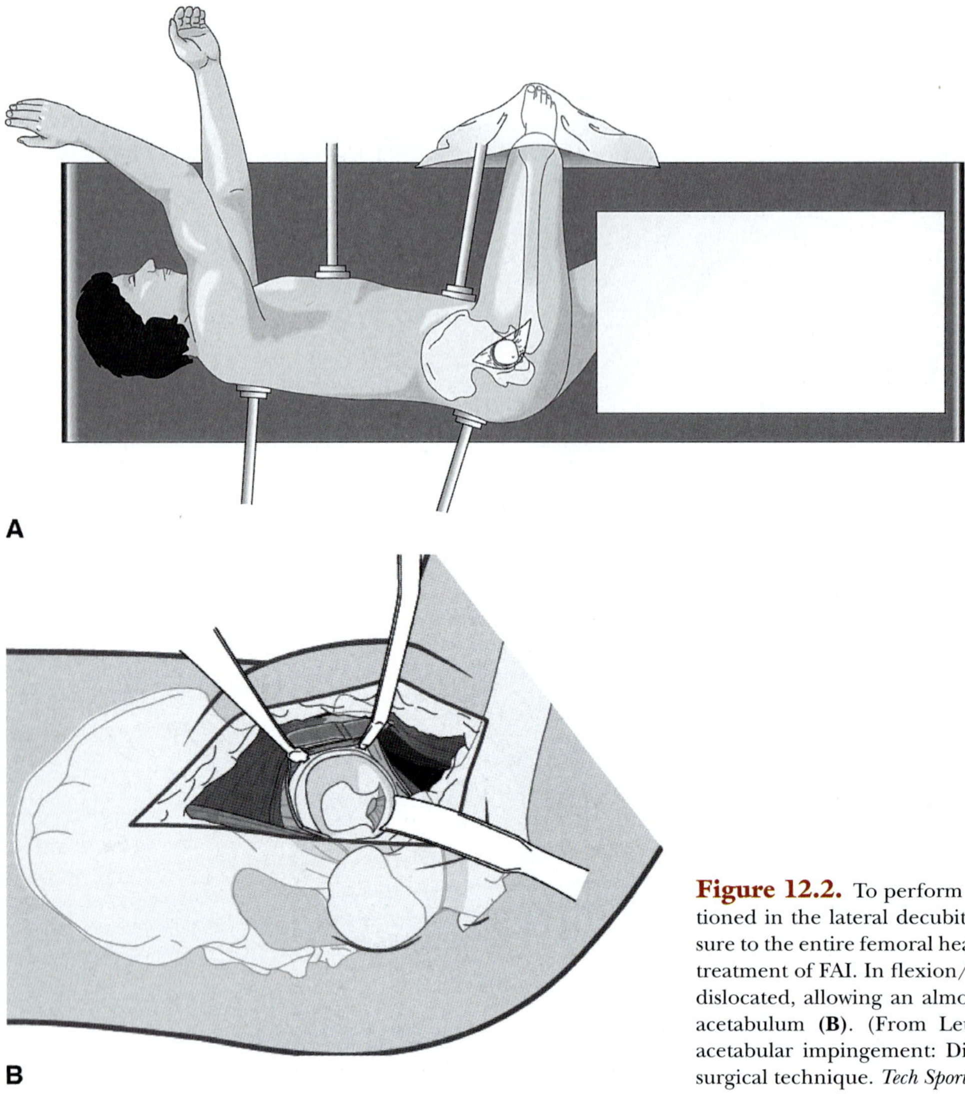

Figure 12.2. To perform surgical hip dislocation, the patient is positioned in the lateral decubitus position **(A)**. This technique with exposure to the entire femoral head and acetabulum allows identification and treatment of FAI. In flexion/external rotation, the femoral head can be dislocated, allowing an almost circumferential inspection of the entire acetabulum **(B)**. (From Leunig M, Robertson W, Ganz R. Femoroacetabular impingement: Diagnosis and management including open surgical technique. *Tech Sports Med.* 2007;15:178–88, with permission.)

POSITIONING

The patient is positioned in a standard lateral decubitus position (Fig. 12.2A).[5] Correct orientation is important to allow accurate assessment of acetabular orientation during the procedure, and the use of three or four specific holding devices is recommended. The use of a bolster to protect the lower limb is recommended.

SKIN PREPARATION/DRAPING

The entire lower extremity is disinfected up to the level of the rib cage, followed by draping from the level of the iliac crest to the mid thigh, with sterile enclosure of the calf and foot. A sterile leg pouch should be attached to the assistant's side of the table to protect the sterile field during dislocation of the hip.

INCISION

A Gibson approach is recommended rather than a Kocher–Langenbeck approach, with a 15 to 25 cm incision along the anterior border of greater trochanter being usually sufficient. The advantage of this approach to the superficial structures is that the gluteus maximus muscle is not split, avoiding damage to the muscle and its neurovascular supply.

DISSECTION

Following the incision to the skin, the subcutaneous tissue is sharply dissected with thorough hemostasis to the level of the fascia lata. The anterior border of the gluteus maximus is identified by branches from the inferior gluteal artery which pass within the fascia before running superficially into the subcutaneous fat layer. The fascia lata is incised anterior to the curved border of gluteus maximus and then parallel in line with the femur. The muscle and these perforating vessels are preserved, and in doing so, branches of the inferior gluteal nerve supplying the anterior gluteus maximus are also protected. The greater trochanter is exposed and the bursa is reflected anteriorly. A small trochanteric branch of the medial circumflex artery can be identified running anteriorly from the posterior border of the trochanteric crest and hemocauterized. The trochanteric flip osteotomy can now be performed.

TROCHANTERIC OSTEOTOMY

Internal rotation of the leg of about 20° to 30° should be performed to expose the posterior border of gluteus medius prior to making the osteotomy. The osteotomy fragment should provide continuity between the gluteus medius and minimus superiorly and the vastus lateralis via the osteotomy fragment. Conversely, the piriformis and short external rotators should remain attached to the nonosteotomized femur.

The osteotomy should run from the posterosuperior border of the greater trochanter distally toward the posterior border of the vastus lateralis muscle and remain parallel with the long axis of the femoral shaft. Although the osteotomy was originally described as a single cut made with an oscillating saw, we would now recommend the use of a "triplanar" osteotomy to increase the mechanical stability of the osteotomy fragment. The osteotomy should commence at the posterosuperior border of the greater trochanter, with two broad chevron type cuts leaving a step of 5 mm between both. The distal cut should end medially to the proximal. Moreover, it is recommended that the osteotomy cuts do not perforate the anterior cortex of the trochanter, but instead, an osteotome is used to lever the fragment forward anteriorly until the cortex is controlled fractured. This process creates a third plane to the osteotomy as the anterior cortex typically detaches leaving an anterior ridge of cortex attached to the stable bone. This creates a triplanar osteotomy fragment that when reattached has the advantage of increased stability in both anterior/posterior and superior/inferior directions. It also allows a greater ease of anatomical refixation of the fragment at the end of the procedure. The resulting fragment should have an approximate thickness of 10 to 15 mm.

The osteotomy fragment is retracted anteriorly using a Hohmann retractor, and any remaining soft tissue attachments are sharply detached. These may include a small portion of the posterior gluteus medius tendon and the piriformis tendon. This process is aided by external rotation and flexion of the leg to mobilize the osteotomy fragment anteriorly. Care must be taken during the procedure to avoid damage to the MCFA—both during the initial stages of the osteotomy cut and in releasing the fragment.

After anterior retraction of the fragment in continuity with the gluteus medius and vastus lateralis, the underlying piriformis and gluteus minimus muscles are exposed. Access to the capsule is achieved by developing the interval strictly between these muscles, to avoid injury to the constant anaostomosis between the deep branch of the MCFA and the inferior gluteal artery. Careful dissection of the gluteus minimus from its capsular attachment is performed to expose the capsule.

CAPSULOTOMY

The capsulotomy should now be performed, with a linear incision along the line of the femoral neck, with a posterosuperior extension along the acetabular rim and an inferomedial extension over the front of the capsule towards the anteroinferior border of the acetabulum. It is important to avoid extending the capsulotomy cut past the lesser trochanter to protect the MFCA while the posterosuperior extension should not extend past the piriformis tendon as the vessel may be injured at this point also. The labrum must also be preserved. This creates a z-shaped capsulotomy for the right hip or a mirrored z for the left hip. The hip can now be inspected for signs of FAI and secondary injury.

OPEN INSPECTION

The initial appearance of the capsule and femoral head can now be made, with attention given to the degree of synovial effusion and synovitis, and observation of the posterosuperior retinaculum and vessels can be done. The sphericity of the femoral head can be assessed, and any FAI can be demonstrated by flexing and internally rotating the hip on table. Labral and chondral injuries may also be observed during this maneuver although a more thorough assessment should be made after dislocation of the femoral head. Not infrequently the anteroinferior, the posterosuperior and/or the posteroinferior is the area of additional impingement.

The anterior dislocation (Fig. 12.2B)[5] of the femoral head is made with the leg flexed and externally rotated (protected in a sterile leg bag) combined with traction on the calcar using a bone hook to produce enough subluxation to expose the ligamentum teres. This can be carefully cut with curved scissors, taking care not to damage the chondral surfaces of the acetabulum or femoral head. Following release, the femoral head can be comfortably dislocated anteriorly and complete inspection of the femoral head, acetabular cartilage, bony rim, and labrum can be made by altering the position of the leg in flexion to expose the articular surfaces. A blunt probe can be used to examine the labrum for detachments or tears and assess the cartilage for softening or delamination.

INTRAOPERATIVE TREATMENT

One of the main advantages of open surgery in the treatment of FAI is following the inspection of the hip, several procedures can be performed to the acetabulum, labrum, and femoral neck under direct vision, with high precision and without the risk od collateral damage to the cartilage.[12] Furthermore, the effectiveness of these techniques can be assessed on table by flexing and internally rotating the hip at the end of the procedure, demonstrating any residual impingement.

ACETABULAR IMPINGEMENT

If acetabular retroversion is noted preoperatively and confirmed intraoperatively, resection of the anterior rim can be performed (Fig. 12.3).[5] However, to perform this procedure, the labrum must be first detached from the acetabular rim by sharp dissection. The typical location for acetabular rim lesions is the anterosuperior margin, but as mentioned earlier, other localisations are possible.

Thereafter, the excessive rim segment can be removed with a curved osteotome. The amount of rim resected should be assessed preoperatively from plain radiographs. The use of the lateral center edge angle to measure the degree of overcoverage and plan the degree of surgical resection is useful. Ultimately however, intraoperative assessment is used to assess the degree of overcoverage causing impingement, with excision of the rim until no impingement is likely to occur on the acetabular side.

Following resection of the acetabular bone, the labrum should be reattached using two to four small bone anchors to a bed of bleeding cancellous bone, with nonabsorbable sutures employed to avoid an inflammatory response. With the bone anchor in situ in the cancellous acetabular bone, the suture

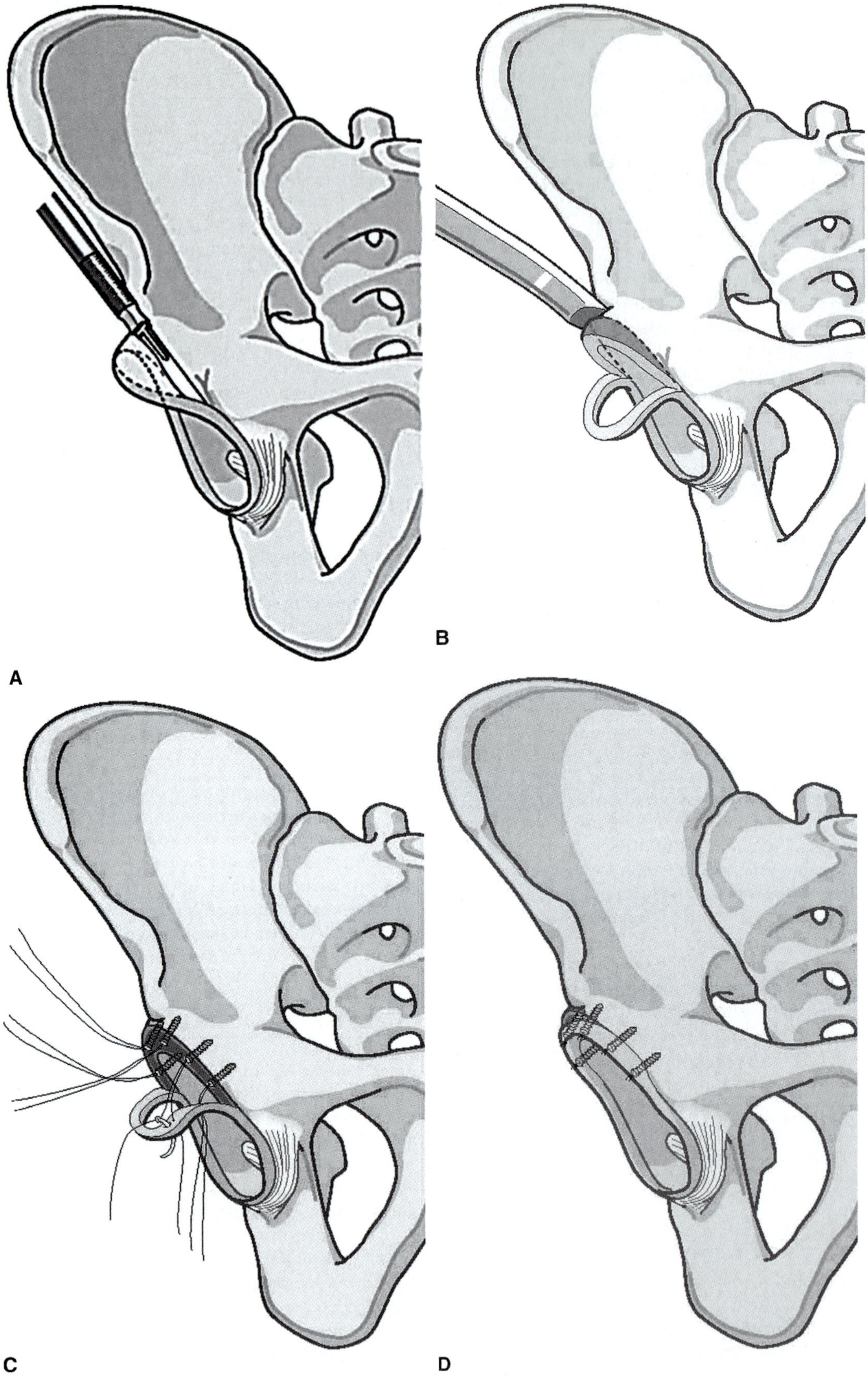

Figure 12.3. Resection of excessive anterior rim **(A)** in acetabular retroversion with a curved osteotome **(B)** can be performed after labral detachment as part of the approach to the acetabular rim. After sufficient rim resection **(C)**, labral refixation is performed by the use of bone anchors **(D)**. (From Leunig M, Robertson W, Ganz R. Femoroacetabular impingement: Diagnosis and management including open surgical technique. *Tech Sports Med.* 2007;15:178–88, with permission.)

should be passed through the base of the labrum, however tidening of the sutures should be postponed after definitive reduction of the head. The suture should be tied on the non-articular surface of the labrum.

FEMORAL IMPINGEMENT

The femoral head should be assessed for nonsphericity using transparent spherical templates. The commonest location for this pathology is the anterosuperior head/neck junction, with the abnormal cartilage having a slightly hypervascular, pink appearance (Fig. 12.4).[5] The presence of a cyst near the peripheral border of the nonspherical segment is sometimes noted which indicates the point of maximum impingement.

The abnormal bone can be removed carefully using curved chisels until a normal head/neck offset is recreated, taking great care not to injure the terminal branches of the MFCA that run along the posterosuperior aspect of the femoral neck. Unfortunately, this area may also be nonspherical, in which case, the debridement should start proximally on the head and reach the point where the vessels enter their intraosseous course.

Careful removal of the bone with regular reassessment using the spherical templates should be performed to avoid overresection, which may increase the risk of neck fracture and lead to the loss of a labral seal against the femoral head. The risk of fracture is a possibility with excessive resection, although studies have shown that even large neck resections do not adversely affect the femoral neck mechanically.

Prior to relocation, perfusion from the foveal artery should be confirmed by assessing the foveal artery for bleeding, and observing any bleeding from the raw cancellous surface created following the neck debridement. Bone wax can be applied to this surface prior to relocation.

Hip relocation can be achieved with simple traction and controlled internal rotation. Following relocation and tidening of the labral sutures, the range of movement can be assessed to look for residual impingement prior to closure.

CLOSURE

Capsular closure without excessive tension is recommended to avoid compression of the retinacular vessels. The trochanteric fragment should be reduced according to the triplanar osteotomy steps and reattached using 3.5 or 4.5 mm screws. With the triplanar trochanteric osteotomy, 3.5 mm screws are usually sufficient and produce less soft tissue irritation. As a result, late removal of these smaller headed screws is less likely to be required. The fascia lata, fat, and cutaneous layers can be carefully closed with running or single sutures. Drains are rarely indicated.

POSTOPERATIVE RECOVERY

Depending on the type of trochanteric osteotomy and intra-articular pathology, the patient should be mobilized postoperatively to touch weight bearing for 4 to 6 weeks with limited abduction and flexion until there is radiographic evidence of trochanteric osteotomy union (Fig.12.5). The patient can usually be discharged after 5 to 7 days but is continued on low molecular weight heparin until full mobilization can occur.

SUMMARY

The open treatment of FAI via a trochanteric flip approach provides excellent surgical access for evaluation of pathology affecting the acetabulum, labrum, and femur. The morbitity of this approach is minimal. Furthermore, the surgical treatment of the impingement can be performed readily using the technique described in this chapter. By eliminating FAI, osteoarthritic change in the hip secondary to this pathology can be prevented or delayed, with good mid-term results seen in patients with early osteoarthritis.[13]

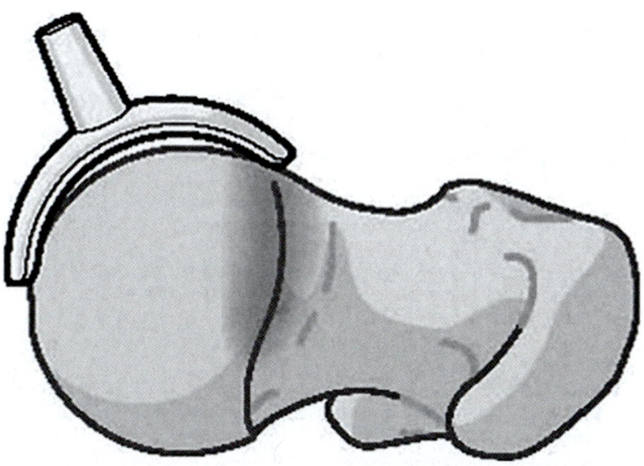

A

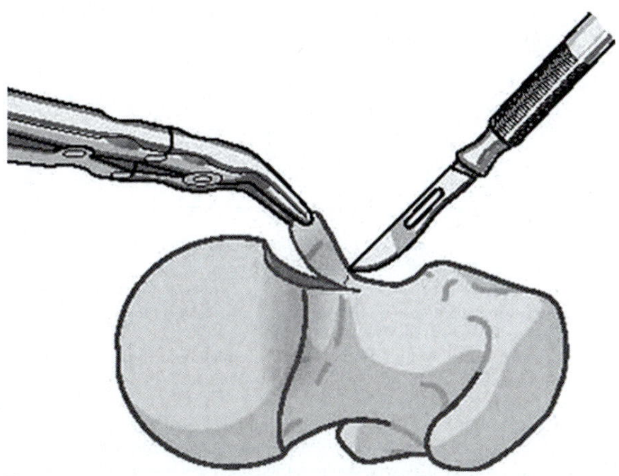

B

Figure 12.4. Resection osteoplasty from the femoral head/neck junction can be used to recreate the normal concave contour of the femoral neck. **A:** Transparent templates are used to determine femoral head sphericity. **B:** Femoral osteochondroplasty is performed to restore the insufficient offset. (From Leunig M, Robertson W, Ganz R. Femoroacetabular impingement: Diagnosis and management including open surgical technique. *Tech Sports Med.* 2007;15:178–88, with permission.)

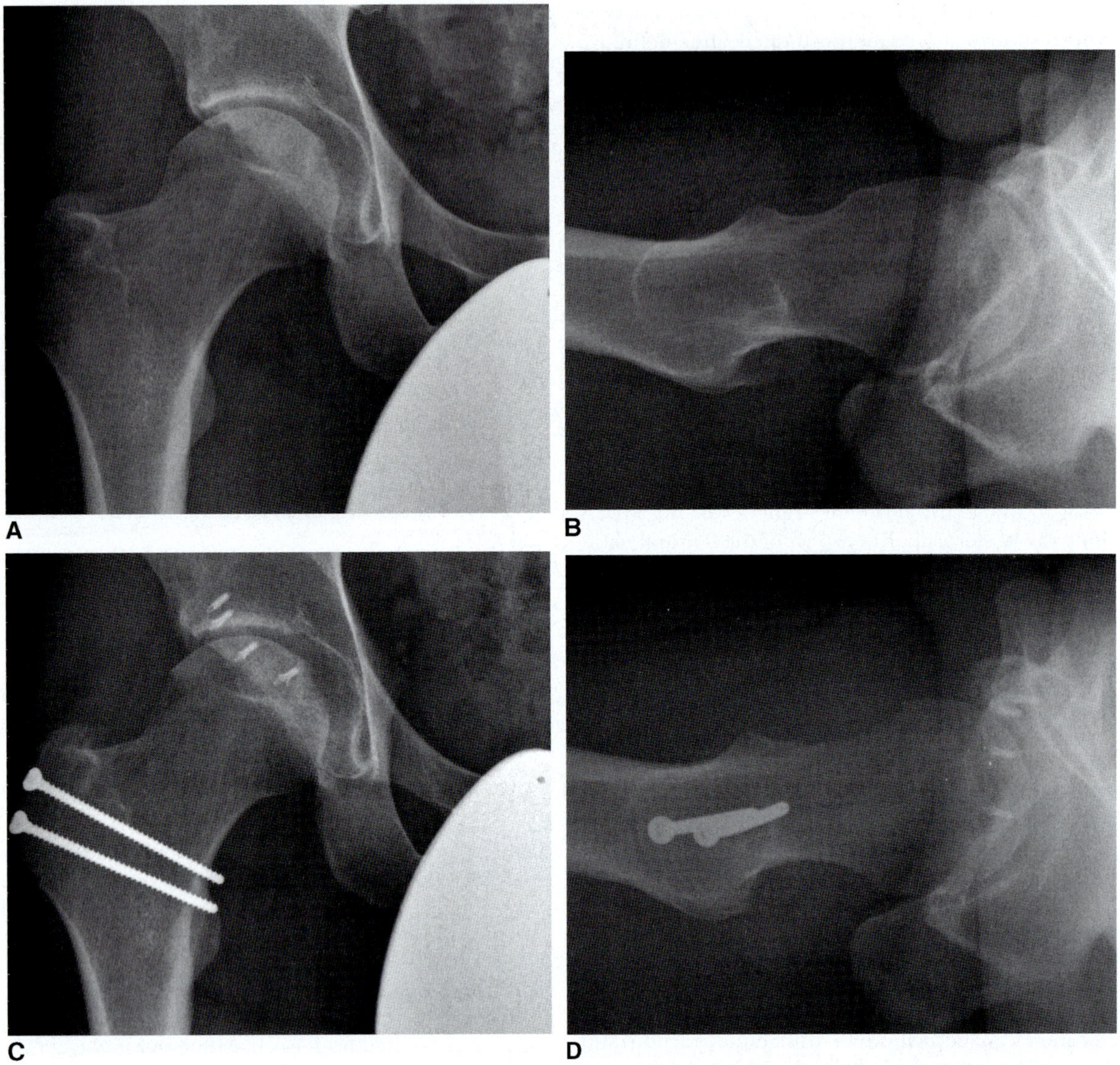

Figure 12.5. **A:** AP hip taken from a correctly oriented pelvic radiograph. **B:** Cross-table lateral radiograph in a patient with combined (cam and pincer) FAI. Addressing of acetabular retroversion using rim trimming and labral refixation **(C)** and improvement of femoral offset **(D)** using surgical dislocation through a transtrochanteric approach.

REFERENCES

1. Pauwels F, ed. *Biomechanics of the Normal and Diseased Hip: Theoretical Foundation, Technique and Results of Treatment. An Atlas.* Berlin, Germany: Springer-Verlag; 1976.
2. Murray RO. The aetiology of primary osteoarthritis of the hip. *Br J Radiol.* 1965;38:810–824.
3. Ganz R, Parvizi J, Beck M, et al. Femoro-acetabular impingement: An important cause of early osteoarthritis of the hip. *Clin Orthop Relat Res.* 2003;417:112–120.
4. Stulberg SD, Cordell LD, Harris WH, et al. Unrecognised childhood disease: A major cause of idiopathic osteoarthritis of the hip. *Proceedings of the Third Meeting of the Hip Society.* St Louis, MO: Mosby; 1975:212–228.
5. Leunig M, Robertson W, Ganz R. Femoroacetabular impingement: Diagnosis and management including open surgical technique. *Tech Sports Med.* 2007;15:178–88.
6. Ito K, Minka MA II, Leunig M, et al. Femoroacetabular impingement and the cam effect: A MRI based quantitative anatomical study of the femoral head-neck offset. *J Bone Joint Surg Br.* 2001;83:171–176.
7. Eijer H, Myers SR, Ganz R. Anterior femoroacetabular impingement after femoral neck fracture. *J Orthop Trauma.* 2001;15:475–481.
8. Siebenrock SA, Schoeniger R, Ganz R. Anterior femoro-acetabular impingement due to acetabular retroversion: Treatment with periacetabular osteotomy. *J Bone Joint Surg Am.* 2003;85:278–286.
9. Mercati E, Guary A, Myquel C, et al. A postero-external approach to the hip joint. Value of the formation of a digastric muscle. *J Chir (Paris).* 1988;103:223–231.
10. Ganz R, Gill TJ, Gautier E, et al. Surgical dislocation of the adult hip: A technique with full access to femoral head and acetabulum without the risk of avascular necrosis. *J Bone Joint Surg Br.* 2001;82:679–683.
11. Gautier E, Ganz K, Krugel N, et al. Anatomy of the medial femoral circumflex artery and its surgical implications. *J Bone Joint Surg Br.* 2000;82:679–683.
12. Lavigne M, Parvici J, Beck M, et al. Anterior femoroacetabular impingement Part I: Technique of joint preserving surgery. *Clin Orthop.* 2004;418:61–66.
13. Beck M, Leunig M, Parvici J, et al. Anterior femoroacetabular impingement Part II: Clinical midterm results. *Clin Orthop.* 2004;418:67–73.

CHAPTER

13

Aaron A. Bare
Carlos A. Guanche

Femoroacetabular Impingement

INTRODUCTION

Understanding the etiology of hip osteoarthritis in the middle-aged patient population has been challenging. Femoroacetabular impingement (FAI) has offered an explanation for a subset of these patients since the dysfunction and pain secondary to the altered morphology of the femoral neck and acetabulum have now been made known. These congenital or development deviations of the anatomy may alter load-bearing mechanics, leading to joint degeneration. Structural alterations of the femoral neck or acetabulum may cause impingement at terminal degrees of motion, especially flexion and internal rotation. Lack of normal head–neck offset (cam impingement) or increased acetabular retroversion (pincer impingement) may change the load-bearing properties of the labrum and bone interface, resulting in labral tears and chondral delaminations. Repetitive contact between the femoral neck and acetabular labrum can lead to chronic groin pain and may serve as a catalyst for hip arthritis.

Stulberg described the "pistol grip" femoral neck deformity as an abnormally shaped femoral neck with a decreased head–neck offset. This type of deformity has been shown to be a risk factor in the development of degenerative arthritis. A large percentage of these patients, especially younger ones, had degenerative labral tears at the time of hip arthroplasty. While there is currently no established causal relationship between FAI and arthritis, one can extrapolate from our current understanding that an impinging lesion may begin or contribute to the degenerative cascade.[1,2]

FAI may result in activity limiting hip pain in the young, athletic patient often in the presence of subtle radiographic abnormalities. Symptoms often develop in the middle-aged patient without trauma or a history of childhood abnormalities. Repetitive micro trauma to the peripheral labrum can lead to chondral injuries and degenerative labral tears. The common development of symptoms in middle age suggests pathology surfaces after many years of impingement. Now recognized as a source of hip pain in the athletic population, treatment offers pain relief and restoration of more normal femoral neck and/or acetabular morphology. Whether this can abate the degenerative process has yet to be proven.

HISTORY/BACKGROUND

A nonspherical femoral head has been associated with early development of osteoarthritis.[1] Also, a degenerative acetabular labrum has been linked to arthritic hips in young patients.[3–5] The presence of underlying acetabular chondral defects approximately doubles in the presence of labral tears at the time of hip arthroplasty.

The concept of hip impingement was introduced by Murray in 1965 using the term "head tilt."[6] Stulberg et al. introduced "pistol grip" deformity to describe the radiographic abnormality of the dysplastic femoral neck and suggested this abnormal relationship as a possible cause of osteoarthritis. The etiology of the decreased head–neck junction is yet to be fully understood, but it has been attributed to mild or subclinical slipped capital femoral epiphysis.[7]

A revival of interest surfaced early this century as Ganz popularized the concept of FAI in the presence of spherical femoral heads.[2] The impingement occurs in an area known as the peripheral compartment, which is intracapsular but outside of the central weight-bearing area of the joint. Either an abnormally shaped femoral neck with decreased head–neck offset or excessive anterior acetabular over coverage from excessive retroversion will create femoral neck and acetabular labral contact in positions of end range of flexion. Other conditions that may lead to abnormal stress or contact include slipped capital femoral epiphysis or previous femoral neck fractures.[6] A congenital anatomical variant of the proximal lateral femoral physis may develop into an abnormal head–neck offset (Fig. 13.1). An increase in the lateral epiphyseal extension into the cranial hemisphere of the femoral head has been correlated with decreased head–neck offset.[7] Therefore, developmental variants such as subclinical capital epiphyseal slips or lateral physeal variants are believed to contribute to the altered bone structures of the hip joint.

Beck et al. noted that all patients treated operatively for FAI had labral lesions in the anterosuperior quadrant.[1] The presence of labral and cartilaginous injuries correlated with an absent anterolateral offset of the head–neck junction. Therefore, impingement tends to take place in the anterosuperior quadrant.

TYPES OF IMPINGEMENT

Abnormal contact between the proximal femur and acetabulum may result from a variety of conditions. A developmental lack of normal femoral head–neck offset from a slipped capital femoral epiphysis or abnormal lateral physeal extension,

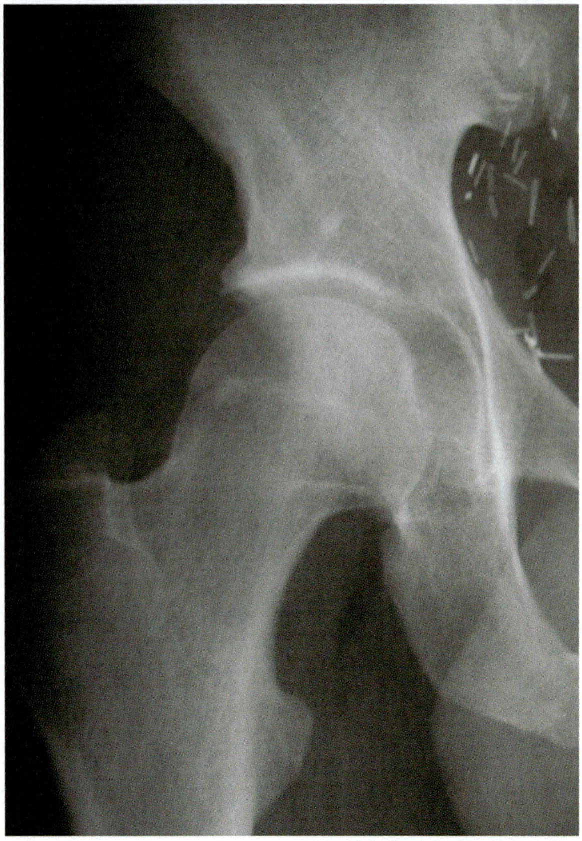

Figure 13.1. Abnormal extension of the proximal femoral epiphysis in a lateral direction can lead to a proximal femoral offset that is deficient and lead to labral tearing.

excessive acetabular retroversion, previous femoral neck fractures, or previous periacetabular osteotomies all can result in pain in the groin region with subtle radiographic abnormalities. Chronic impingement may overload the articular cartilage causing chondral injury or delamination defects of the anterior acetabular labrum with separation and tearing of the adjacent labrum.

Ganz et al.[2] described two distinct patterns of FAI based on the pattern of chondral and labral lesions during direct observation, these were termed cam and pincer impingement. Cam impingement occurs when a nonspherical femoral head–neck rotates in the acetabulum. This mechanism defines a mismatch between the anterolateral femoral neck and acetabular radius, presenting as a lack of normal head–neck offset. There is often a bone lesion or subtle prominence on the superior femoral neck on plain radiographs (Fig. 13.2). During flexion (and often exacerbated with internal rotation), the compressive and shear forces on the acetabulum overload the articular cartilage. This shearing force at the anterosuperior acetabulum can cause acetabular chondral delaminations and articular sided labral detachments. Occasionally, the forces will avulse the articular cartilage from the labral rim, creating a cleft seen on MRI. This condition is encountered more commonly in young, active males.[8]

Pincer impingement occurs from direct contact on the acetabular rim at the femoral neck. Excessive anterior acetabular coverage, seen more often with coxa profunda or acetabular retroversion, is the primary culprit (Fig. 13.3). The femo-

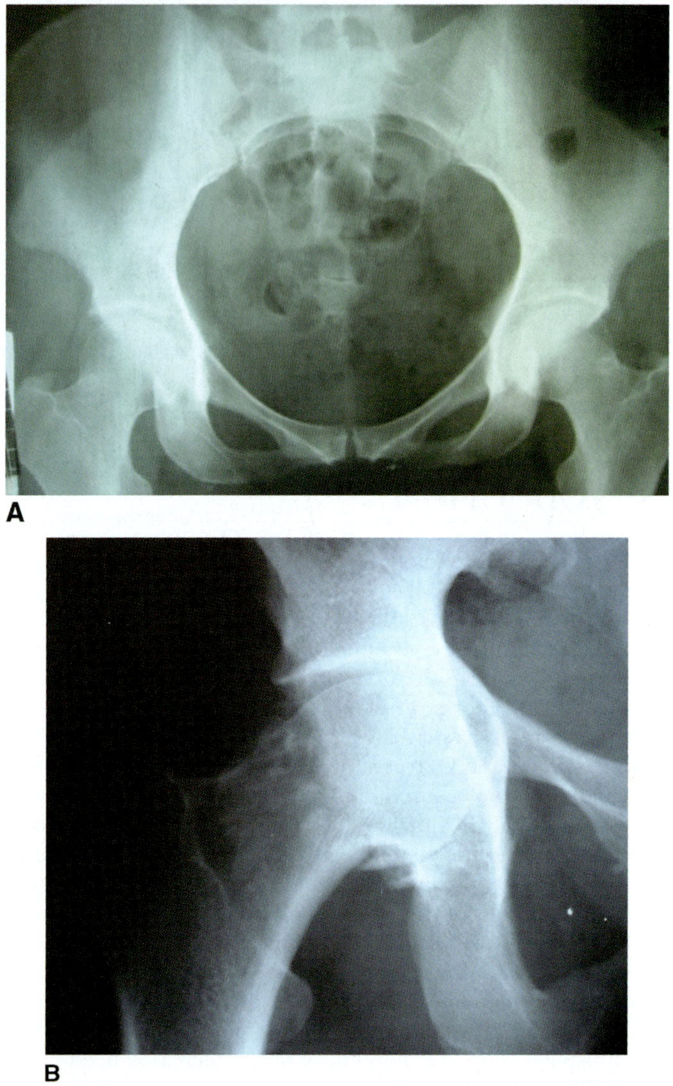

Figure 13.2. **A:** AP pelvis radiograph depicting a normal hip joint on the right side and an abnormal retroversion on the left. **B:** AP view of a right hip with profunda acetabulae leading to pincer impingement and subsequent degenerative changes.

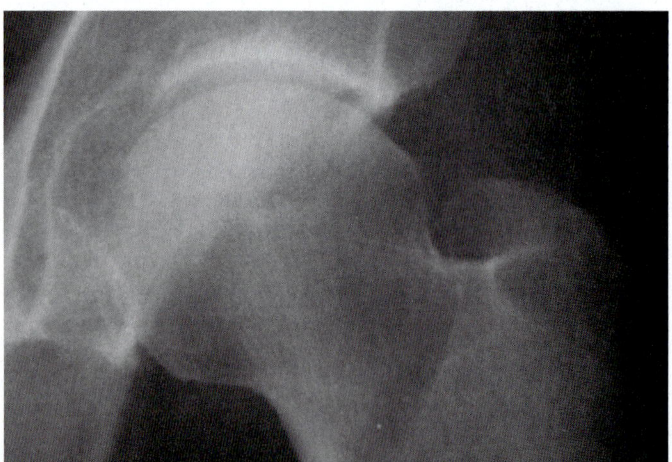

Figure 13.3. AP view of cam impingement secondary to abnormal offset.

ral head may be of normal appearance. Pincer impingement causes a compression or crushing of the labrum between the femoral neck and acetabulum. The first structure to fail appears to be a small area of the labrum causing labral degeneration, intrasubstance ganglions, or labral ossification (Fig. 13.4). Continued abutment against an ossified labrum can lever the femoral head out of the socket, creating head contact on the posteroinferior acetabulum with resultant chondral lesion or reactive osteophytes in that quadrant. Pincer impingement has been suggested to be more prevalent in women, mostly in those who engage in athletic activities.[2]

In many instances, the pathologies overlap. A significant proportion of patients will have a combination of pincer and cam impingement as an etiology for their clinical symptomatology (Fig. 13.5). It is important to address both of these pathologies at the time of surgery or further degeneration of the labrum and joint may occur.

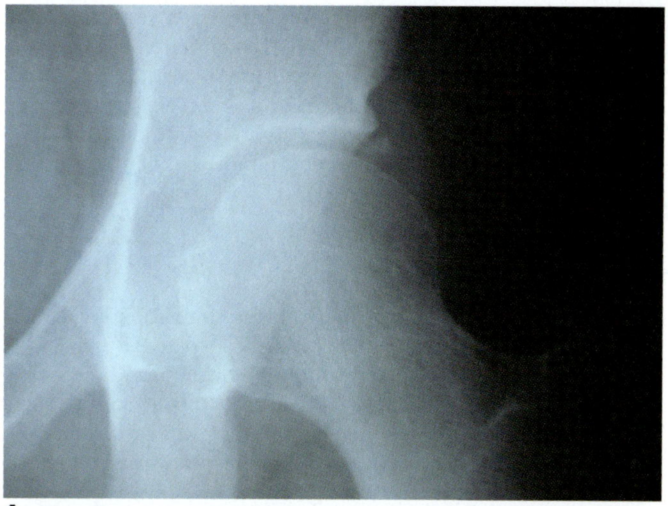

A

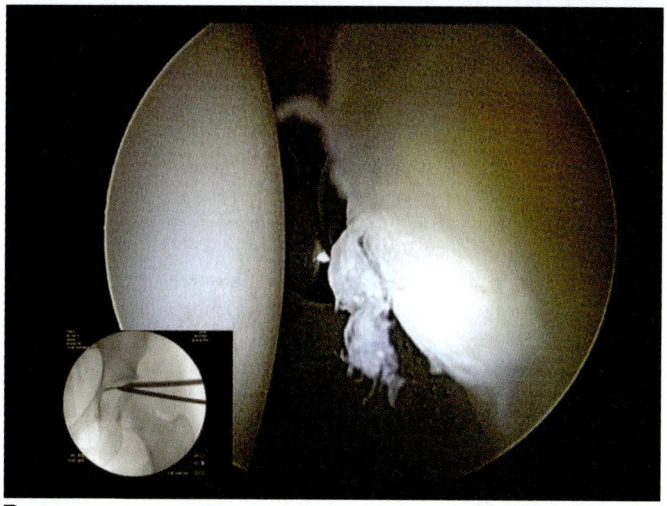

B

Figure 13.4. Perilabral ossification secondary to chronic pincer impingement. **A:** AP radiograph depicting lateral calcification. **B:** Intraoperative image showing decompression of calcific lesion (labral tissue is on the right).

CLINICAL PRESENTATION

HISTORY

Patients with excessive acetabular retroversion or decreased femoral head–neck offset have less clearance between the superior femoral neck and the acetabular labrum. Therefore, during activities that require more flexion than flat ground walking, groin pain develops. Groin pain during sports, climbing stairs, and during or after prolonged sitting are hallmark complaints. Symptoms range from mild to severe and are often intermittent and insidious in presentation. Many patients will report a history of mild symptoms for several years, which have slowly progressed without a history of trauma. Excessive demands such as athletic activities will tend to exacerbate the complaints. Occasionally, pain may be referred to the knee. Often, given a diagnosis of a hip strain in the presence of presumed normal radiographs without degenerative changes, athletes may receive extraordinary workups or may be given incorrect diagnoses such as sports hernia and chronic groin strain. This occurs with radiographs that show FAI changes but are presumed to be normal by the examining physician.[8]

PHYSICAL EXAMINATION

Patients with hip impingement often exhibit decreased internal rotation in adduction. These maneuvers are often accompanied by pain. The impingement test, done by passively internally rotating the adducted hip and flexed hip, will often elicit groin pain. Motion may be limited secondary to pain or from the mechanical impingement at end ranges of motion and this is often measured as decreased internal rotation. However, the lesion may be present bilaterally, so radiographs help confirm the presence or absence of a contralateral lesion. The symptoms are usually localized anteriorly and depending on the locations of the lesions, lateral or posterior pain may also be present. Athletes may report difficulty with squatting, lateral movements, as well as starting and stopping.[8] The presence of clicking and/or locking may represent a delaminated chondral lesion or labral tear. Stability and strength are usually normal, as is gait.

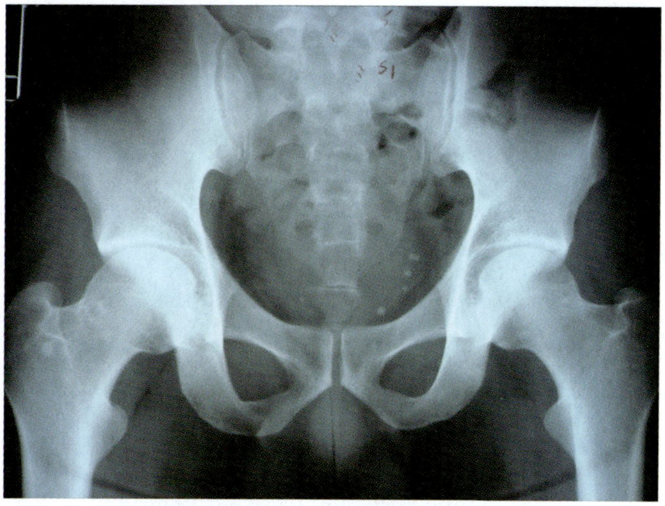

Figure 13.5. Combined pincer and cam impingement in a 45-year-old male patient with mechanical symptomatology.

A thorough examination should be performed to rule out other causes of groin pain such as sports hernia, lateral femoral cutaneous neuropathy, bursitis, snapping hip syndrome, and lumbar radiculopathy. In addition to the impingement test, the FABER (flexion, abduction, and external rotation) test should be performed. The nonspecific test has been shown to correlate with FAI. An increased vertical distance between the lateral edge of the knee and the examination table has been observed in FAI.[8]

IMAGING

Standard radiographs often illustrate the morphological relationships of the femoral head and neck. A true AP pelvis, AP and lateral of the affected hip highlight structural landmarks allowing assessment of head–neck offset and acetabular version. Either a frog or cross-table lateral view will confirm a cam lesion. The lateral radiograph illustrates the anterior neck and offers an offset comparison to the posterior neck for cam lesions. Meyer et al.[9] suggested that a cross-table lateral in internal rotation or a Dunn view in 45° of hip flexion offer the best analysis of femoral head–neck asphericity.

Several radiographic measures evaluate the femoral neck for dysplasia. The lateral center edge angle (CE angle of Wiberg) is measured on the AP view from the center of the femoral head vertically and an angle measured from the lateral rim. An angle less than 20° is consistent with dysplasia. Greater than 25° is considered normal, with an angle between 20° and 25° considered borderline. The femoral head extrusion index is the percentage of the femoral head outside of the acetabular roof. Greater than 25% is consistent with dysplasia.[10]

The alpha angle specifically analyzes the femoral head–neck offset and is an indicator of cam impingement.[9] This is measured as a concentric circle drawn around the femoral head. This angle is formed between a line that begins at the center of the femoral head and runs perpendicular to a line through the center of the femoral neck and a second line from the center of the femoral head to the point where the head–neck junction falls outside of the concentric circle. Cam impingement exists with an alpha angle >55° on any radiographic projection (Fig. 13.6).

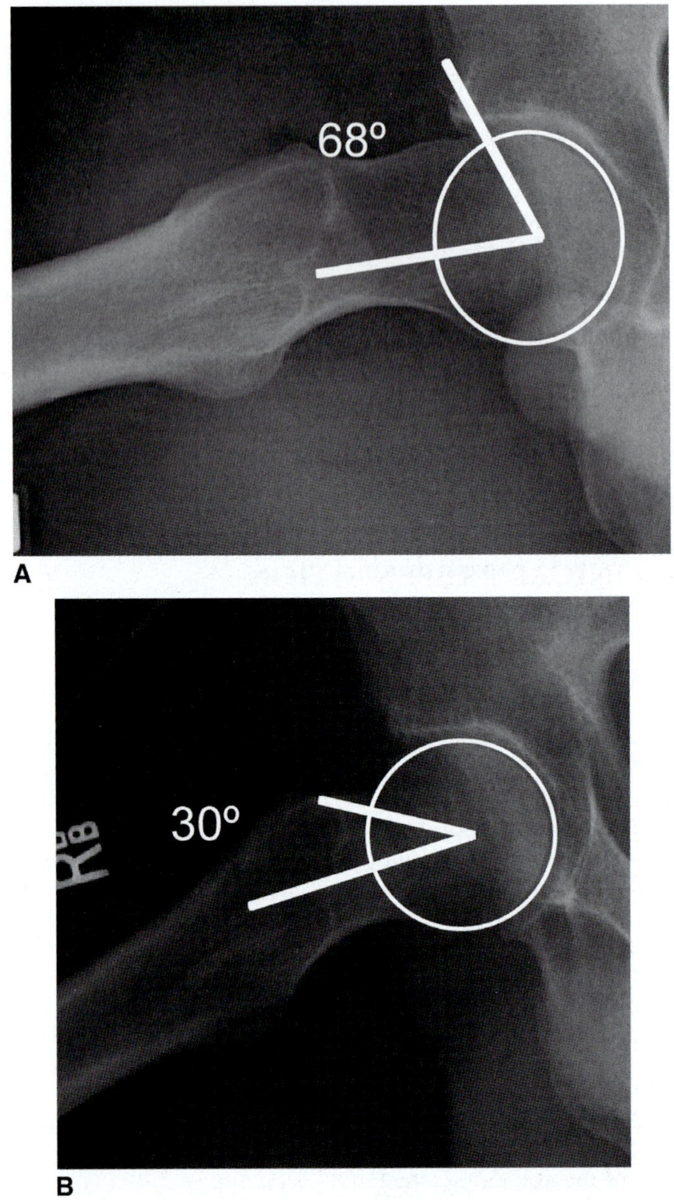

Figure 13.6. The alpha angle. This angle is formed between a line that begins at the center of the femoral head and runs perpendicular to a line through the center of the femoral neck and a second line from the center of the femoral head to the point where the head neck junction falls outside of the concentric circle. An angle greater than 55° is diagnostic of decreased offset.

Measuring acetabular version requires a true AP pelvis radiograph.[9] The film should align the coccyx and symphysis pubis with a separation distance of 1 to 2 cm (Fig. 13.7). Lines are then traced from the anterolateral edge of the acetabulum along the anterior and posterior projections of the rim. With normal version, the lines should not cross. If the anterior wall is traced more laterally than the posterior wall, the acetabulum is retroverted. This creates a "figure-of-eight" tracing as the anterior wall crosses the posterior wall. In converse, if the posterior line is traced more laterally than the anterior wall, the acetabulum is anteverted (Fig. 13.8). If the tracings do not cross, then the acetabulum is felt to be in neutral version. In the early stages of FAI, the joint space is rarely affected.

Further diagnostic imaging can document intra-articular pathology and assist in preoperative planning. MRI arthrograms are capable of detecting labral and, less reliably, chondral injuries. Marcaine should be combined with the gadolinium-DPTA for diagnostic measures. Asymmetric fluid presence surrounding the femoral neck on T2 images suggests inflammation in the peripheral compartment. The arthrogram will also define the three-dimensional (3D) anatomy of the femoral head–neck offset, herniation pits, paralabral cysts, and ossification of the acetabular rim. While MRI arthrograms have very good sensitivity and specificity for detecting labral and chondral lesions, they are limited in their ability to reliably detect chondral delaminations.[11] A CT scan with 3D image reconstructions is an excellent preoperative planning adjunct, especially if treating the lesion arthroscopically. The 3D CT scan offers a thorough analysis of a cam or pincer lesion, especially for those that are believed to extend posteriorly on plain radiographs.

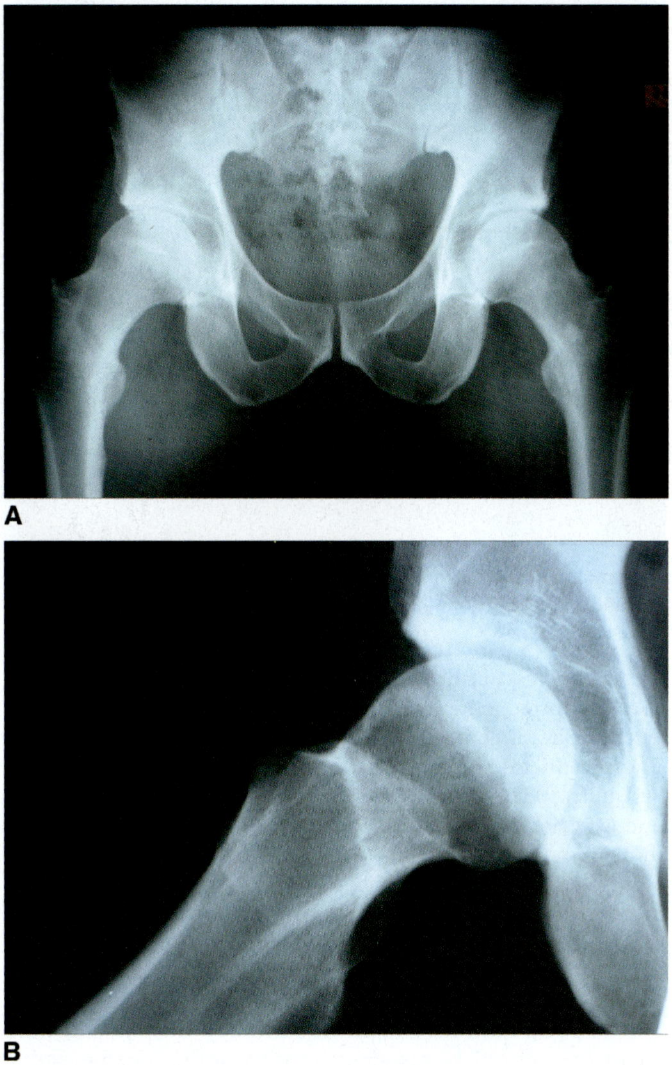

Figure 13.7. Normal AP pelvic radiograph (**A**) and frog lateral views (**B**).

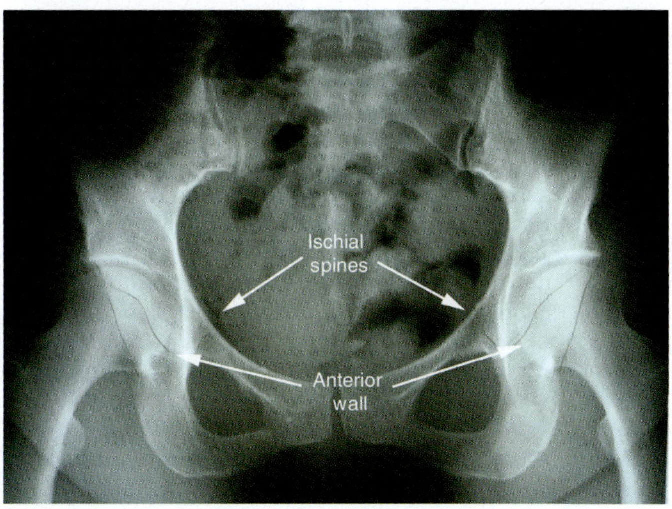

Figure 13.8. Radiographic depiction of retroversion of the acetabulum.

TREATMENT

Activity modification, anti-inflammatories, and physical therapy with emphasis on hip and core strengthening exercises will often minimize symptoms to a tolerable level. These modalities, however, will not alter the anatomical problem. Those who improve with conservative care and no longer require treatment should be educated that this condition may lead to future joint deterioration. Exacerbation of, or worsening of, symptoms in the future should warrant repeat radiographs and possibly surgical intervention. At this time, no data exists to support prophylactic treatment of femoral neck or acetabular lesions in order to decrease the risk of future development of degenerative joint disease.

Open and arthroscopic treatment of both cam and pincer lesions have been reported with good results. Traditionally, operative management of hip dysplasia has been performed with a variety of open osteotomies. Ganz et al. have popularized a periacetabular osteotomy for young patients with dysplastic hips.[2] The osteotomy is performed through one incision, allowing a multidirectional correction, thus preserving the blood supply to the acetabulum. Their results showed 72% good to excellent results with patients with labral tears having less favorable results.[12] Some patients with persistent pain were found to have an anterior overcorrection of their osteotomy, creating a relative over coverage or retroversion of the acetabulum. They concluded that impingement was the source of the patients' pain. These patients, with new onset of pincer impingement, were treated with surgical hip dislocation and resection osteoplasty of the acetabular rim and femoral neck.

For anterior FAI, Ganz et al.[13] developed a joint preserving surgical approach to address the offending acetabular and/or femoral neck lesion while protecting the femoral head blood supply. They found that protecting the lateral epiphyseal branch of the medial femoral circumflex artery allows sacrificing the capsular arteries without risking avascular necrosis.[14] An average follow-up of 19 patients over 5 years produced good or excellent results in 14 patients with no evidence of osteonecrosis. They concluded that this procedure produced overall good results in most patients with anterior FAI as long as there were limited degenerative hip changes.[13]

Hip arthroscopy has become an accepted treatment for labral tears, loose bodies, and several other intra-articular problems. More recently, FAI has been addressed with this modality. Assessing the central compartment of the hip has become less technically challenging as we have gained a better understanding of hip traction and developed hip-specific arthroscopic instrumentation. Previously thought too technically demanding,[15] several authors have reported techniques outlining an arthroscopic equivalent procedure to treat FAI.[8,16,17,18,19] This technique minimizes the morbidity of an open hip dislocation and trochanteric osteotomy while lessening the recovery and rehabilitation process. Short-term results have also been encouraging.[17,18,19,20]

Dienst et al.[21] outlined a systematic approach to the peripheral compartment, without the use of traction. Arthroscopic treatment of FAI hinges on access to the central (weight-bearing) compartment for chondral and labral lesions as well as the peripheral (intra-articular, non-weight-bearing cartilage) compartment for femoral neck and acetabular dysplasia.

The concept of separating the hip into two compartments is an important principle in the management of FAI. The central compartment includes the weight-bearing head, articular cartilage, acetabular fossa, and the ligamentum teres. The peripheral compartment contains the non-weight-bearing head, the femoral neck, hip capsule, synovial folds, and intrinsic ligaments. Hip arthroscopy can be performed in either the supine[22] or lateral[18] position. The order of treating the central or peripheral compartment pathology is left up to the surgeon. Sufficient traction and portal placement are important for entry and manipulation within the central compartment. Anterior, anterolateral, and posterolateral portals are utilized. C-arm fluoroscopy should be used periodically throughout the procedure to document the appropriate position of instrumentation, especially as portals are established. Thirty and seventy degree arthroscopes visualize most of the central compartment through the anterolateral portal with far medial and posterior visualization through the posterolateral portal. Many patients with pathology in the central compartment will have chondral or labral lesions and they are typically located in the anterosuperior quadrant. Chondral delamination lesions may be hidden to arthroscopic visualization, so the articular surfaces should be thoroughly probed. At the end range of flexion, acetabular, and femoral head–neck impingement may lever the head posterolaterally, creating degenerative lesions of posterior acetabulum known as contrecoup lesions (Fig. 13.9).

Chronic impingement against the peripheral labrum in pincer impingement often creates a degenerative labral lesion not amenable to repair (Fig. 13.10). However, with cam lesions, the shear stress may create articular sided labral detachments amenable to repair. These labral lesions may be associated with chondral delaminations that are best treated with debridement or microfracture (Fig. 13.11). Microfracture can be utilized for exposed bone following chondral lesion debridement and is best suited for Outerbridge grade 3 or 4 lesions. Limiting traction time to 2h is important to lessen the risk of traction neuropraxias of the sciatic and pudendal nerves. Following the treatment of central compartment pathology, traction should be immediately released.

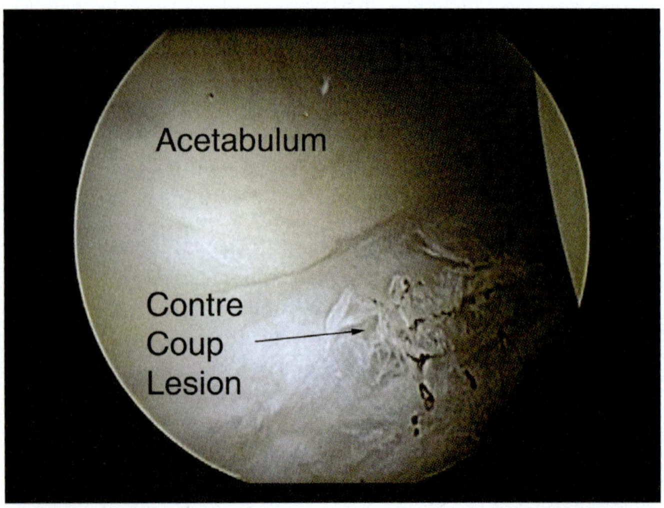

Figure 13.9. Contrecoup lesion in the posterior acetabular labrum in a patient with significant anterior labral tearing secondary to acetabular retroversion.

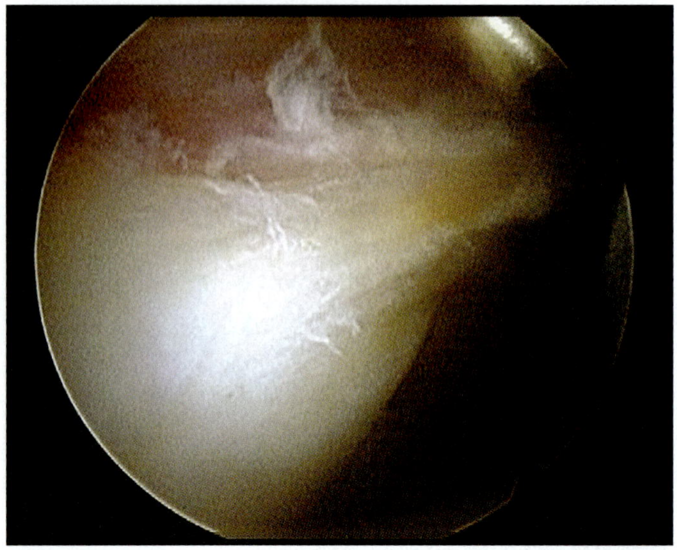

Figure 13.10. Pincer type of labral tear in a patient with significant acetabular retroversion.

While the central compartment contains the products of chronic impingement (labral tears and chondral injuries), the peripheral compartment houses the offending pathology. The peripheral compartment has been defined systematically by Dienst.[21] The hip capsule attaches to the intertrochanteric line anteriorly while superiorly it is bounded by the capsular reflection onto the hip labrum. Visualization of the peripheral compartment is best performed without traction with the hip in 20° to 30° of flexion, which relaxes the anterior hip capsule. Capsular relaxation offers a more predictable access to the anterior and lateral neck as well as the peripheral labrum and acetabulum.[17,21,23]

The peripheral compartment is entered in a manner similar to the central compartment with a spinal needle, guide wire, and dilators through the anterolateral portal under fluoroscopic guidance. The spinal needle should meet resistance as it skives off the anterior neck, through the anterior capsule (Fig. 13.12). The guide wire should meet resistance as it is advanced against the medial capsule. Advancement of the guide wire beyond the acetabulum under fluoroscopic guidance suggests that the wire is not contained in the peripheral compartment. A diagnostic, systematic examination is performed from the anterolateral portal.[21] An anterior, limited capsulectomy is performed using the anterior portal for instrumentation.[17,18] The limited anterior capsulectomy increases space and working area without affecting hip stability. The arthroscopic peripheral compartment examination proceeds in a counter-clockwise direction beginning with the anterior neck and proceeding through the medial neck, medial head, anterior head, lateral head, and posterior area.[21] The traction-free, flexed hip can be rotated to visualize far lateral or medial structures. In addition, the impingement process, whether due to femoral or acetabular lesions (or both), is now visualized.

Based on preoperative planning, the femoral neck, acetabulum, or both are addressed. Synovitis at the capsular reflection on the labrum is often seen as well as corresponding soft tissue

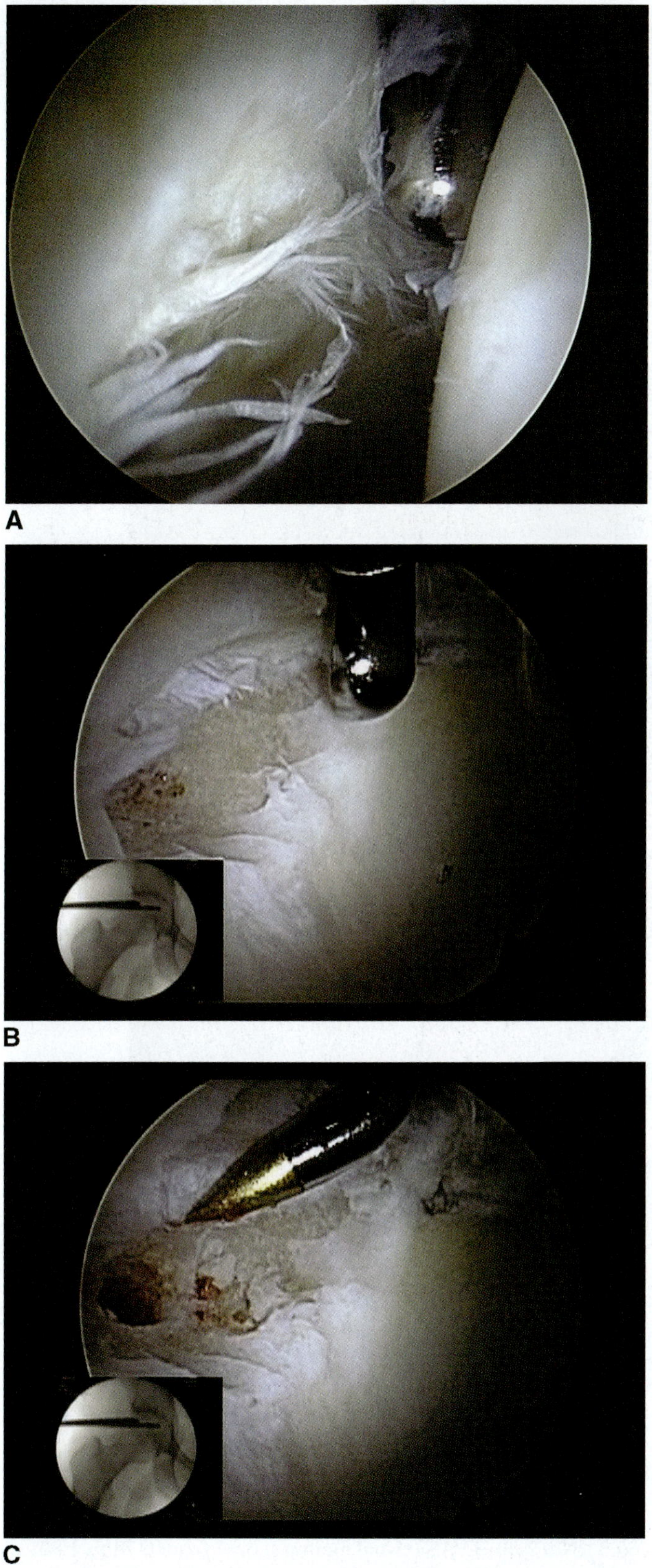

Figure 13.11. **A:** Labral tear seen in a patient with significant cam impingement. **B:** Area of chondral delamination following debridement. **C:** Chondroplasty awl creating channel for chondral regenerative process.

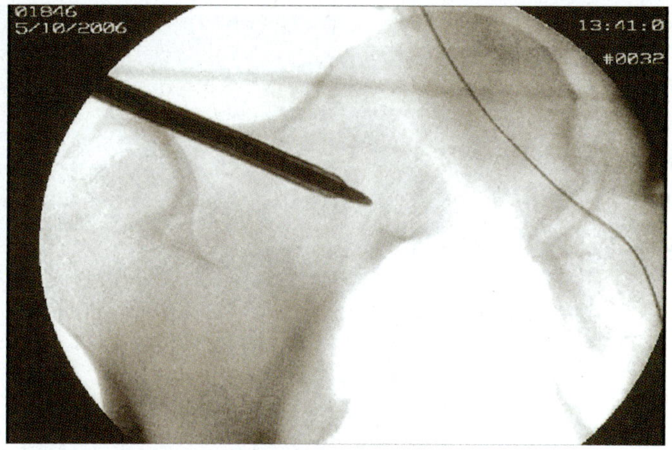

Figure 13.12. Position of arthroscope to begin diagnostic arthroscopy of the peripheral compartment. The point of entry on the skin is the anterolateral portal. Radiographically, the entry should be about 2 cm above the greater trochanter and aim toward the medial physeal scar.

disruption over the anterolateral neck. For the treatment of cam impingement, the anterior accessory lateral portal is established using fluoroscopy as necessary. This portal is developed approximately 4 to 5 cm distal to the anterolateral portal along the same coronal plane and offers good visualization of the femoral neck for cam impingement. The arthroscope is then switched from the anterolateral to the accessory portal and the anterolateral portal becomes the working portal. A burr is utilized to shape the femoral neck with the assistance of fluoroscopy. Internally rotating the leg to access the far lateral neck is an important principle since anterolateral cam lesions often extend posteriorly (Fig. 13.13). Hip arthroscopy specific traction tables allow leg manipulation in space without traction. Mardones has shown that up to 30% of the femoral neck can be safely resected without compromising the structural integrity of the femoral neck. The amount of resection, however, should be individualized since the degree of offset and anatomical impingement vary greatly from patient to patient.[24]

Treating pincer lesions from acetabular retroversion is addressed from the central compartment. Anterior overhang is often the culprit with an associated ossified anterosuperior labrum secondary to chronic impingement. The procedure known as "rim trimming" often necessitates the labral detachment and repair following resection of the overhang.[25] Establishing the junction between the labrum and bone with an arthroscopic osteotome or a fine tip radiofrequency device allows a clean detachment. The diseased labrum will often lend information regarding the location of the offending acetabular lesion. After the margins have been identified, a motorized shaver clears the soft tissue from the overhanging acetabulum followed by a motorized burr to resect the bony acetabular prominence (typically 5 to 7 mm). Avoiding excessive acetabular resection is important to protect it from iatrogenic hip instability. Reattachment of the labrum following bone resection is performed with suture anchors (Fig. 13.14). This procedure is also performed under fluoroscopic guidance and with a true AP pelvis, the crossover sign should be routinely checked, stopping when neutral version has been achieved. Following resection of

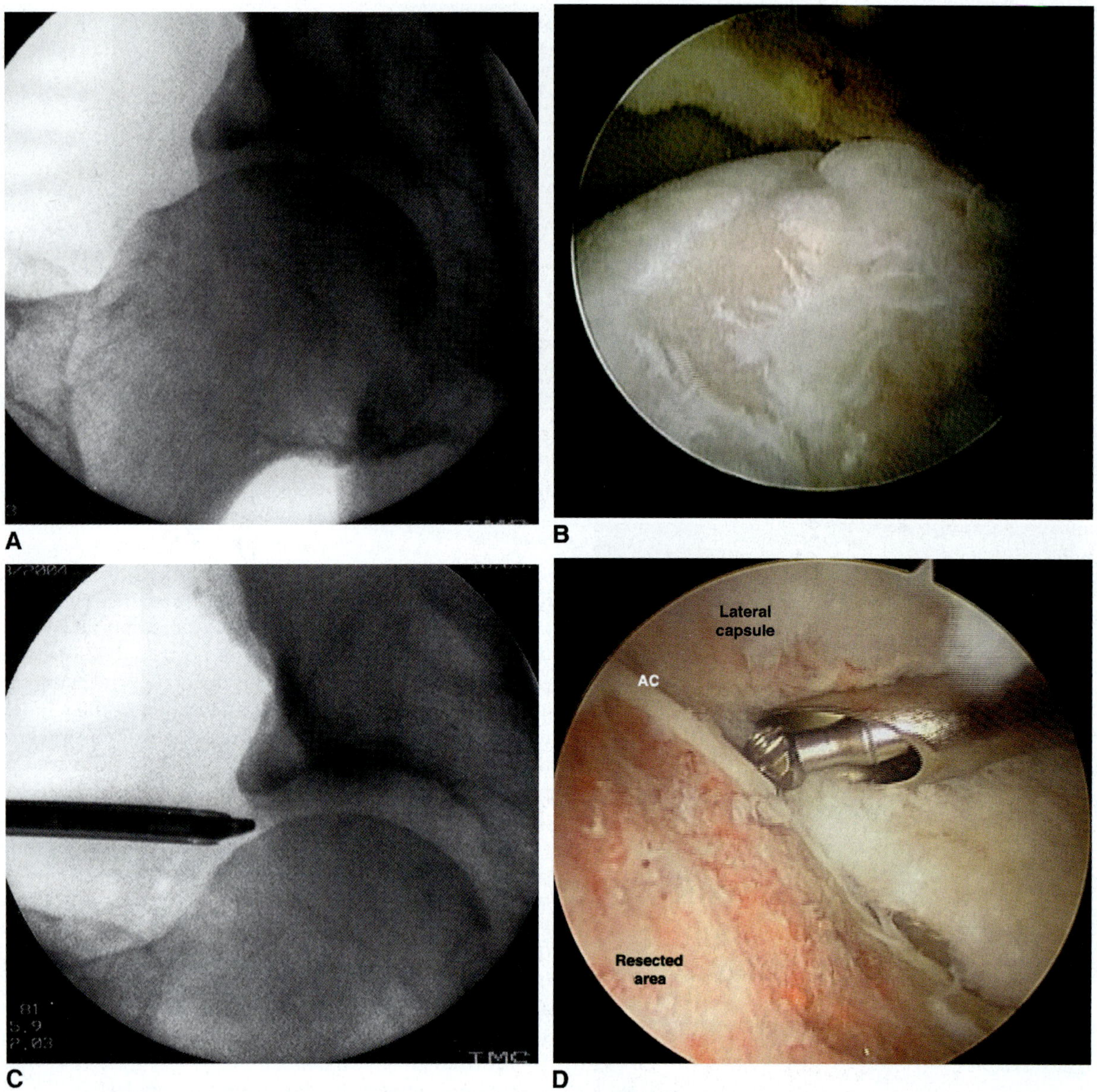

Figure 13.13. Treatment of a cam lesion. **A:** Radiograph of impingement lesion. **B:** Intraoperative view of impingement lesion. **C:** Radiograph following resection of the lesion. **D:** Intraoperative view of resected lesion.

the pincer impingement, the arthroscope should be placed in the peripheral compartment to visualize the head–neck junction during range of motion. Mixed lesions are common and treatment of both pincer and cam lesions is often necessary to eliminate the impingement.[26]

Early results of arthroscopic treatment of FAI are encouraging and have paralleled the results of the open approach. In a review of 45 elite athletes with FAI treated arthroscopically, all patients had symptomatic relief and were able to return to sport.[19] In a larger series of 320 patients treated arthroscopically, 90% had resolution of the preoperative impingement sign and were satisfied with their outcome.[20] Guanche presented 24 consecutive patients with an average of 16 months follow-up and showed significant improvement in pain and function.[17] The average NAH score (nonarthritic hip score) improved from 64.7 to 97 while WOMAC scores improved from 74.9 to 93 at last follow-up. Seventeen patients had anterosuperior cartilage delaminations lesions. Nineteen patients with Tonnis grade I radiographic changes did significantly better than those with more advanced arthritis.[27] Larson et al. reported 100 consecutive patients with a mean age of 35 years at an average of 9 month follow-up.[20] Isolated cam lesions were identified in 17, pincer in 28, and combined lesions were noted in 55 patients. Thirty required labral repair or labral refixation. Harris hip scores improved on an average from 60.5 to 81.5, SF-12 from 60.3 to 75.7, and VAS (visual analog score) from 6.74 to 1.85, all statistically significant. Of note, six patients developed heterotopic ossification, none symptomatic. Three patients required total hip arthroplasty with all three having Outerbridge 4 chondral delamination injuries to the acetabulum greater than 2 cm at the time of surgery (preoperative Tonnis grade I, two patients, and grade II, one patient).

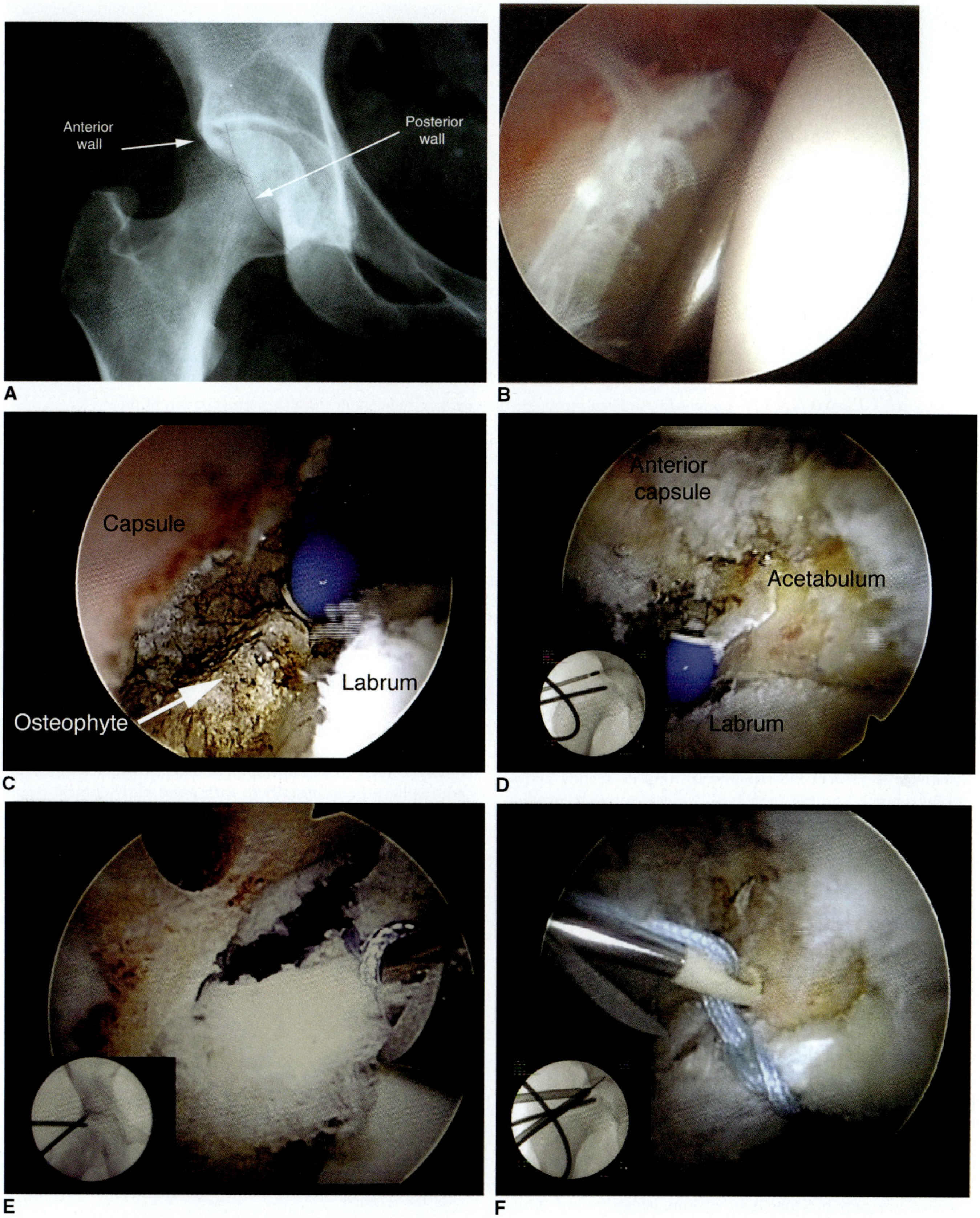

Figure 13.14. Treatment of pincer lesion in a right hip. **A:** Preoperative radiograph of lateral and anterior overhang. **B:** Labral tearing extending over the anterior acetabulum. **C:** Area of bony prominence following labral takedown. **D:** Final bony resection. **E:** Labral tissue prepared with circumferential suture. **F:** Suture anchor insertion into superior acetabulum.

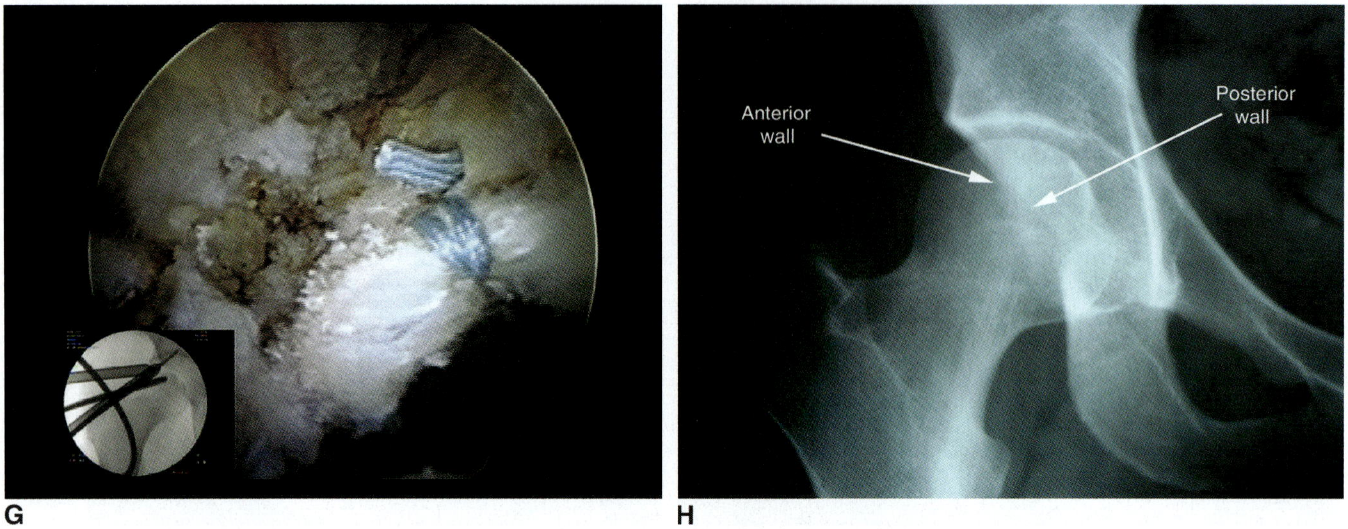

Figure 13.14. (Continued) **G:** Final repair. **H:** Postoperative radiograph revealing normalization of the center edge angle.

POSTOPERATIVE REHABILITATION

Following arthroscopic management of FAI, treatment focuses on protection of the osteoplasty and labrum as well as prevention of heterotopic ossification. The use of a strong nonsteroidal anti-inflammatory is recommended for 2 weeks postoperatively. The postoperative activity restrictions fluctuate depending on the amount of resection as well as the presence of labral debridement or repair. For a typical cam impingement resection including femoral neck osteoplasty with labral debridement, 4 weeks of protected weight bearing is recommended. For pincer lesions that are treated with labral takedown and repair with acetabular rim trimming, restrictions include weight bearing and motion to protect the repaired labrum. Protecting active external rotation and hip flexion for 4 weeks serves to protect the repaired labrum. Physical therapy is begun at 2 weeks to restore full passive motion prior to institution of full active motion at 4 weeks.

DISCUSSION

The recent interest in FAI and its potential long-term effect on the hip joint have increased awareness of both identification and management. FAI should be screened in young- and middle-aged athletes with activity related hip pain. The subcategories of cam and pincer impingement offer valuable information regarding the cause of the abnormal contact. Properly taken radiographs usually allow determination of both femoral head–neck offset as well as acetabular version. Abnormal version or offset in addition to positive clinical findings guide initial conservative treatment for FAI.

Exercises, medications, and therapy will not eliminate the abnormal anatomy but may help to diminish symptoms to an acceptable level. For failed conservative measures, arthroscopic management of both cam and pincer impingement has shown successful early clinical results. A more complete understanding of the mechanisms and origin of the impinging lesions has led to techniques that restore abnormal head–neck offset and acetabular version to more normal values. A better understanding of the anatomy of the peripheral compartment and the safety of peripheral compartment osteoplasties has lead to widespread acceptance and utilization of arthroscopic management of femoroacetabular lesions.

CONCLUSION

Hip pain in the athletic population secondary to FAI may lead to chronic pain and sport-specific limitations. In the absence of severe hip dysplasia, coxa vara or degenerative joint disease, treatment of femoroacetabular lesions has led to promising clinical results. While both open and arthroscopic surgical procedures have been described, with good early clinical results, arthroscopy offers less morbidity and recovery time, with potentially an earlier return to sport.

Chronic impingement is believed to lead to, or at least contribute to, the early degenerative cascade. The role of operative treatment of impinging lesions and hip dysplasia to halt the degenerative process is theoretical at this time. Long-term outcome and future prospective studies are needed to further our understanding of FAI and guide treatment algorithms.

REFERENCES

1. Beck M, Leunig, Parvizi J, et al. Anterior femoroacetabular impingement: II. Clinical midterm results. *Clin Orthop Relat Res.* 2004;418:67–73.
2. Ganz R, Parvizi J, Beck M, et al. Femoroacetabular impingement: A cause for early osteoarthritis of the hip. *Clin Orthop Relat Res.* 2003;417:112–120.
3. Leunig M, Beck M, Woo A, et al. Acetabular rim degeneration: A constant finding in the aged hip. *Clin Orthop.* 2003;413:201–207.
4. McCarthy JC, Noble PC, Schuck MR, et al. The role of labral lesions to development of early degenerative hip disease. *Clin Orthop Relat Res.* 2001;393:25–37.
5. Santori N, Villar R. Arthroscopic findings in the initial stages of hip osteoarthritis. *Orthopedics.* 1999;22:405–409.
6. Stulberg SD, Cordell LD, Harris WH, et al. Unrecognized childhood hip disease: A major cause of idiopathic osteoarthritis of the hip, In: *The Hip: Proceedings of the Third Meeting of the Hip Society.* St Louis, MO: CV Mosby;1975, pp. 212–228.
7. Goodman DA, Feighan JE, Smith AD, et al. Subclinical slipped capital femoral epiphysis. Relationship to osteoarthritis of the hip. *J Bone Joint Surg Am.* 1997;79:1489–1497.
8. Philippon MJ, Schenkere ML. Arthroscopic treatment of femoroacetabular impingement in the athlete. *Clin Sports Med.* 2006;25:299–308.

9. Meyer DC, Beck M, Ellis T, et al. Comparison of six radiographic projections to assess femoral head/neck asphericity. *Clin Orthop.* 2006;445:181–185.
10. Mast JW, Brunnerr RL, Zebrack J. Recognizing acetabular version in the radiographic presentation of hip dysplasia. *Clin Orthop.* 2004;418:48–53.
11. Leunig M, Podeszwa D, Beck M, et al. Magnetic resonance arthrography of labral disorders in hips with dysplasia and impingement. *Clin Orthop Relat Res.* 2004;418:74–80.
12. Siebenrock KA, Schoeniger R, Ganz R. Anterior femoro-acetabular impingement due to acetabular retroversion: Treatment with periacetabular osteotomy. *J Bone Joint Surg Am.* 2003;85:278–286.
13. Ganz R, Gill TJ, Gautier E, et al. Surgical dislocation of the adult hip: A technique with full access to the femoral head and acetabulum without the risk of avascular necrosis. *J Bone Joint Surg Br.* 2001;83:1119–1124.
14. Gautier E, Ganz K, Krugel N, et al. Anatomy of the medial femoral circumflex artery and its surgical implications. *J Bone Joint Surg Br.* 2000;82:679–683.
15. Lavigne M, Parvizi J, Beck M, et al. Anterior femoro-acetabular impingement: I. Technique of joint preserving surgery. *Clin Orthop Relat Res.* 2004;418:61–66.
16. Clohisy JC, McClure JT. Treatment of anterior femoroacetabular impingement with combined hip arthroscopy and limited anterior decompression. *Iowa Orthop.* 2005;25:164–171.
17. Guanche CA, Bare AA. Arthroscopic treatment of femoroacetabular impingement. *Arthroscopy.* 2006;22:95–106.
18. Guanche CA, Bare AA. Arthroscopic treatment of femoroacetabular impingement. *Arthroscopy.* 2006;22:95–106.
19. Philippon MJ, Schenker M, et al. Femoroacetabular impingement in 45 professional athletes: Associated pathologies and return to sport following arthroscopic decompression. *Knee Surg Sports Traumatol Arthrosc.* 2007;15(7):908–914.
20. Larson CM, Giveans MR. Arthroscopic debridement versus refixation of the acetabular labrum associated with femoroacetabular impingement. *Arthroscopy.* 2009;25: 369–375.
21. Dienst M, Godde S, Seil R, et al. Hip arthroscopy without traction: In vivo anatomy of the peripheral hip joint cavity. *Arthroscopy.* 2001;17:924–931.
22. Byrd JW. Hip arthroscopy utilizing the supine position. *Arthroscopy.* 1994;10:275–280.
23. Bare AA, Guanche CA. Hip impingement: The role of arthroscopy. *Orthopedics.* 2005;28: 266–273.
24. Mardones RM, Gonzalez C, Chen Q, et al. Surgical treatment of femoroacetabular impingement: Evaluation of the effect of the size of resection. *J Bone Joint Surg Am.* 2005;87: 273–279.
25. Philippon MJ, Schenker, et al. A new method for acetabular rim trimming and labral repair. *Clin Sports Med.* 2006;25(2):293–297.
26. Beck M, Kalhor M, Leunig M, et al. Hip morphology influences the pattern of damage to the acetabular cartilage: femoroacetabular impingement as a cause of early osteoarthritis of the hip. *J Bone Joint Surg Br.* 2005;87:1012–1018.
27. Tonnis D, Heinecke A. Acetabular and femoral anteversion: Relationship with osteoarthritis of the hip. *J Bone Joint Surg Am.* 1999;81:1747–1770.

CHAPTER

14

Aaron A. Bare
Carlos A. Guanche

Intra-articular Hip: Miscellaneous Disorders

Approximately 2.5% of all sports related injuries could be linked to the hip region. Up to 10% of reported high school athletic injuries involve the hip.[1] While extra-articular musculotendinous and intra-articular labral injuries dominate the injury spectrum, several less common, intra-articular lesions also present as hip pain. These lesions are often challenging to diagnose and treat. However, with improved imaging modalities and arthroscopic techniques, minimally invasive treatment of less common intra-articular lesions is now possible. An understanding of the full spectrum of intra-articular diseases of the hip offers patients definitive answers regarding both diagnosis and treatment.

Normally, the hip joint functions flawlessly under normal physiologic loads, which may reach up to five times the body weight. When a pathologic process alters the function of the homeostatic chemical and mechanical forces within the joint, articular cartilage breakdown can occur and joint deterioration may follow. Detecting and treating these pathological processes before joint breakdown occurs may preserve the integrity of the hip joint. Once bony changes have occurred, the process of joint deterioration often becomes irreversible. Young patients with acute and rate-limiting pain, believed to be originating from the hip joint, necessitate further workup.

The majority of intra-articular pathology does not respond well to conservative measures. Diagnostic imaging tools, such as MRI arthrograms, not only allow the discovery of the intra-articular lesions but also offer evaluation of the articular cartilage. The status of the articular cartilage will offer information regarding prognosis following surgical intervention. Intra-articular lesions often respond well to surgical debridement and removal of the offending lesion. Treatment of intra-articular lesions can be performed either arthroscopically or open. Arthroscopy offers a minimally invasive procedure with excellent visualization of the femoroacetabular joint to treat intra-articular pathology. It spares extensive surgical dissection and violation of the hip capsule. While the range of pathology amenable to arthroscopic treatment in the hip continues to expand, open exposure of the joint remains an option for conditions not amenable to arthroscopic technique, such as management of large osteochondral lesions. The goal of management of intra-articular pathology is to restore normal intra-articular anatomy and biomechanical forces. Inferior results should not be accepted as a consequence of an inexperienced hip arthroscopist.

Burman[2] introduced hip arthroscopy in 1931. Shoulder and knee arthroscopic procedures flourished in the 1980s. The 21st century has seen an increase in both the number of arthroscopic procedures performed and the number of arthroscopists treating hip disorders. Current indications for treating intra-articular hip disorders include removal of loose bodies, labral tears debridement or repair, avascular necrosis, synovial and connective tissue disorders, chondral lesions, and a select population of degenerative arthroses.

LOOSE BODIES

Loose bodies within the joint can cause pain and may mimic a snapping hip. These mobile, intra-articular lesions may occur as an isolated entity following trauma or present with multiple lesions such as in synovial chondromatosis. Anterior groin pain, episodes of clicking or locking, buckling, giving way, and persistent pain during activity suggest an intra-articular loose body. McCarthy and Busconi[3] showed that loose bodies within the hip, whether ossified or not, correlate with locking episodes and inguinal pain.

In cases of traumatic injury or dislocation, suspicion should be high for loose bodies to explain hip symptoms. Besides hip trauma, other diseases known to be associated with loose bodies include Perthes disease, osteochondritis dissecans (OCD), avascular necrosis (AVN), synovial chondromatosis, and osteoarthrosis. Computed tomography (CT) imaging can assist in evaluation of suspected osseous loose bodies, such as after dislocation. Keene and Villar[4] advocate early arthroscopic retrieval of loose bone fragments from the joint to eliminate additional insult to the articular surface. Whether or not the loose body is ossified, CT imaging is more sensitive in detecting loose bodies than MRI.[5]

Although arthrotomy remains the traditional, gold standard for direct joint observation and loose body removal, the morbidity of the open approach is significant as it requires hip dislocation. Hip arthroscopy eliminates the vast majority of the associated morbidity from soft tissue dissection, capsular incision, and hip dislocation. With the appropriate hip distraction and portal placement, the hip can be fully visualized, loose bodies removed, and additional intra-articular pathology such as labral and chondral lesions treated at the same time.

McCarthy and Busconi[3] reported that radiographs did not visualize 67% of loose bodies in the hip. When persistent symptoms of locking or catching are present, further workup for loose bodies should be performed with a CT scan if trauma was the precipitating injury. If labral pathology is suspected, an MRI arthrogram offers the best imaging modality. With documentation of intra-articular loose bodies and corresponding symptoms, surgical arthroscopy offers the most ideal treatment solution (Fig. 14.1).

Osteoarthritis changes in the hip can be caused by intra-articular bone and chondral fragments or from incongruity at the articular surface. Osteoarthrosis has been shown to develop at a rate of approximately 25% to 55% at 10 years following native hip dislocation, with simple dislocations having the most favorable outcome.[6] Yamamoto et al. evaluated 11 consecutive hip dislocations arthroscopically. In seven patients, small osteochondral fragments or treatable chondral lesions were not seen on radiographs or CT scans. Although the series was small, the results suggest a broadening indication for hip arthroscopy following dislocation, especially in the setting of mechanical symptoms without radiographic findings.

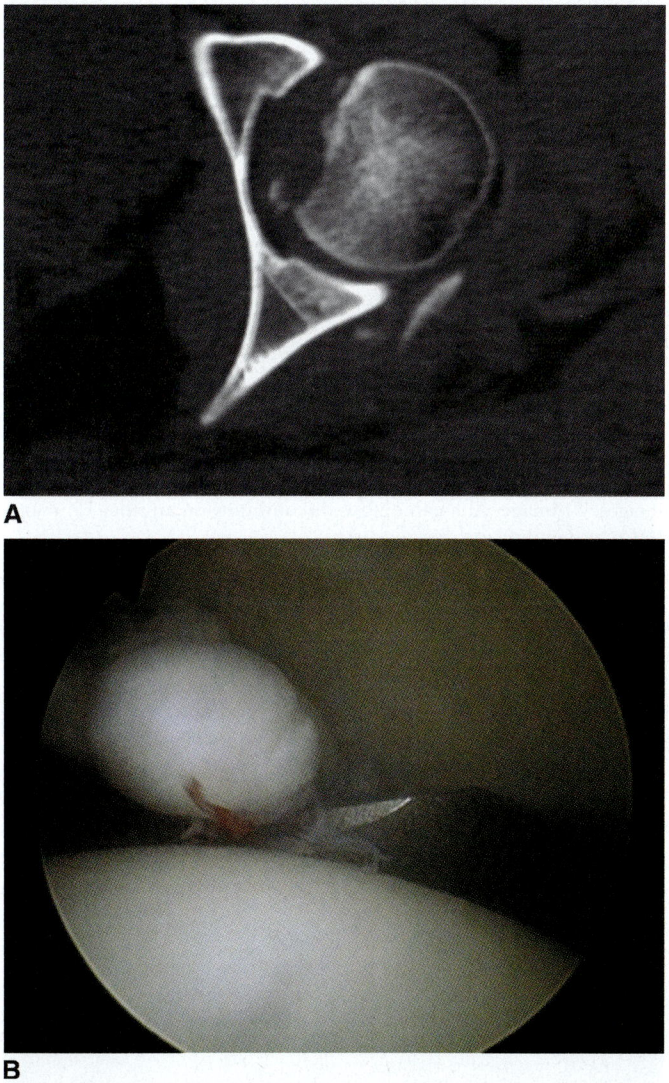

Figure 14.1. Loose bodies in the hip following trauma. **A:** Axial CT illustrates loose bodies within the hip joint along with a femoral head defect following a posterior hip dislocation. **B:** Arthroscopy of the joint allows for loose body removal.

The presence of a loose body within the articulating surface of any joint theoretically will result in destruction of articular hyaline cartilage and ultimately premature arthritic joint destruction. The significance of a symptomatic loose body in the hip joint should not be underestimated and treatment should not be delayed. When hip disease or a pathological condition results in loose body formation, symptomatic improvement can be expected after surgical removal, but the future of the joint remains dependent on the natural history of the underlying condition. The minimally invasive nature of hip arthroscopy makes the procedure ideal for establishing an early preventive strategy to treat symptomatic patients.

CHONDRAL LESIONS

Articular surface lesions create an irregular contour of the joint surface and lead to abnormal intra-articular forces with motion and weight bearing, predisposing the patient to the development of progressive degenerative disease. Chondral injuries are found following trauma and have been associated with degenerative labral lesions as well with early arthritic hips. One study reported that 74% of patients with a torn labrum had some degree of articular surface damage.[7] In 80% of those patients, the labral and articular lesion occurred in the same quadrant. They also found a correlation among the patient's age, labral tear, and severity of the articular cartilage injury. The frequency and severity of cartilage lesions increased with age, and 24% of chondral injuries were observed arthroscopically in patients less than 30 years of age compared to 81% of patients with chondral lesions in those older than 60 years of age.

Arthroscopic debridement of chondral flaps can be performed through a standard arthroscopic approach. Chondral flaps are debrided and associated labral pathology is treated as well. Full-thickness chondral defects, more often associated with trauma, can be treated with microfracture or acute repair of large full-thickness acute lesions. Arthroscopic microfracture as well as drilling or internal fixation of osteochondral lesions, especially large defects, can be challenging and an open approach should be considered if an arthroscopic technique would compromise the result.

LIGAMENTUM TERES

A triangular-shaped ligament, the ligamentum teres, arises from the posteroinferior region of the cotyloid fossa and inserts into the base of the femoral head. It provides blood supply to the femoral head in children while its function in adults remains unclear. Gray and Villar[8] suggest that a ligamentum teres injury causing symptoms without a history of a dislocation may be more common than previously reported. Byrd and Jones[9] reported that a ruptured ligamentum was the third most commonly encountered intra-articular pathology during arthroscopy. The ligament becomes taut in flexion, adduction, and external rotation, suggesting a plausible mechanism for injury.[8]

Gray and Villar[8] noted 20 ligamentum teres injuries in 472 consecutive hip arthroscopies. They discovered three distinct patterns of injury: complete rupture, partial tears, and degenerative ligaments associated with degenerative arthrosis (Fig. 14.2).

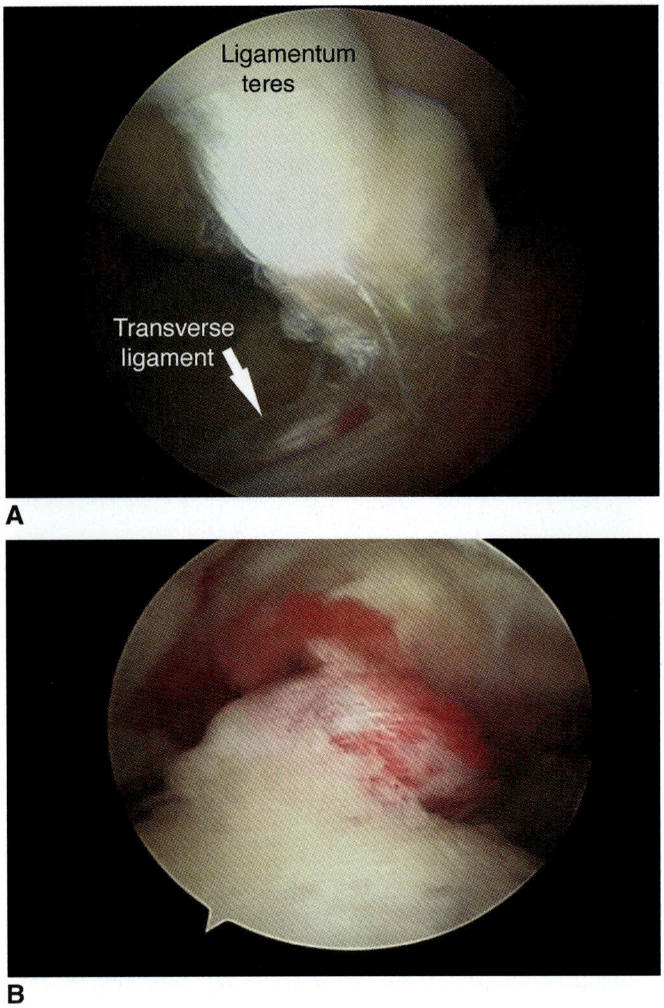

Figure 14.2. Ligamentum teres tear. **A:** Arthroscopy confirms a complete ligamentum rupture. **B:** A partial ligamentum tear with surrounding synovial inflammation.

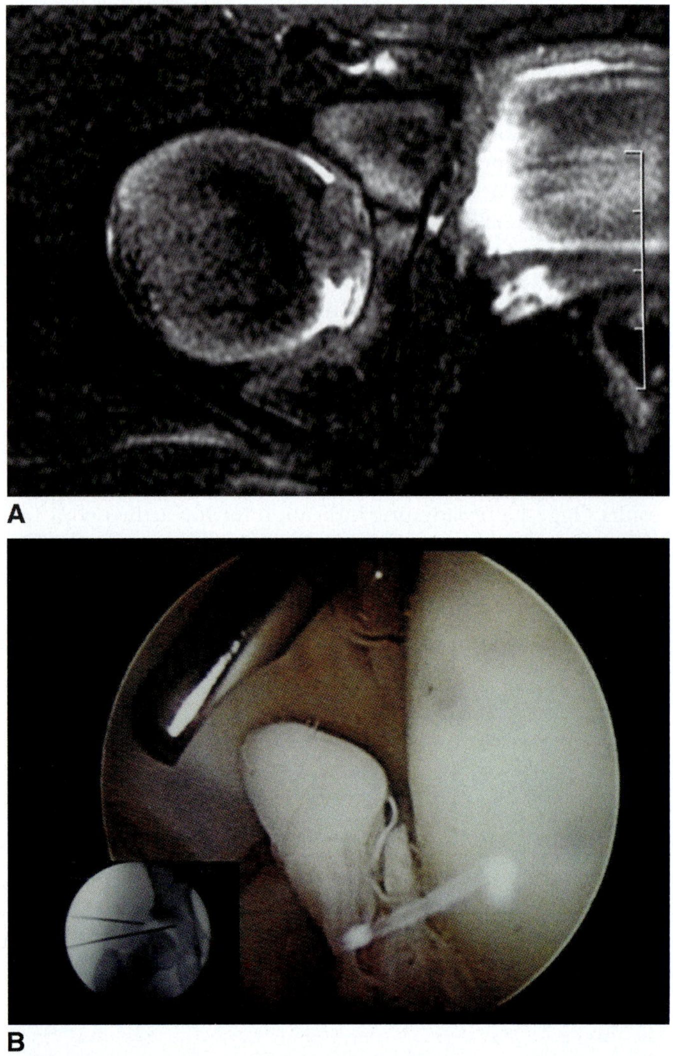

Figure 14.3. Ligamentum tears are best visualized on axial MRI images. T1 image. **A:** Ligamentous discontinuity on an axial T2 image. **B:** Corresponding arthroscopic view.

Complete ruptures were associated with trauma, and labral or chondral injuries were often present. Partial tears often occurred without associated pathology and presented as hip pain of unknown etiology. The degenerative ligaments all had articular degenerative changes on both the femoral and acetabular surfaces. All patients presented with groin or thigh pain and most complained of a limp or clicking sensation with weight bearing. They were unable to elicit any specific exam finding pathognomonic symptom for ligament tears and reported that the imaging studies did not aid in the diagnosis (Fig. 14.3). Byrd and Jones reported 41 lesions of the ligamentum teres among 271 consecutive hip arthroscopies. In 23, the injury was traumatic, with 12 complete and 11 partial ruptures; 18 were hypertrophic or degenerative. In patients with traumatic injuries, 80% complained of mechanical symptoms.[9] Of the 23, 15 were from high velocity trauma and eight from twisting injuries. Preoperative diagnosis of ligamentum injuries was made on two of 23 cases. Eight lesions were isolated findings at the time of arthroscopy and 15 patients had additional pathology requiring treatment. All patients improved with arthroscopic debridement, with an average preoperative hip score of 47 and postoperative score of 90 and more than 1 year of follow-up (Fig. 14.4).

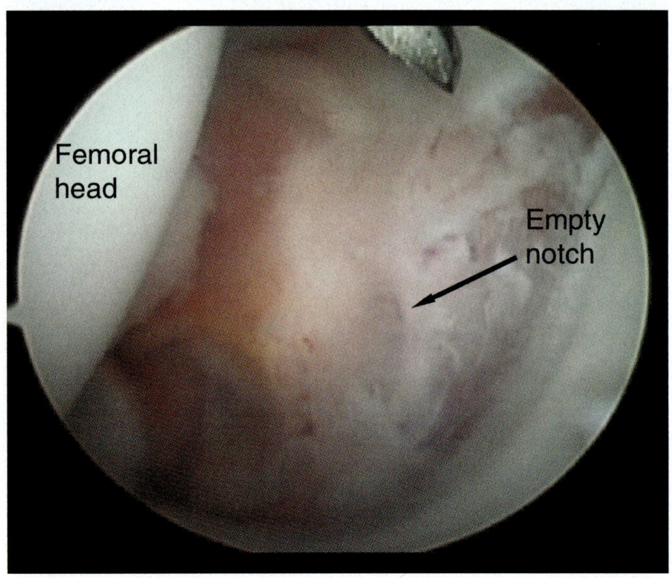

Figure 14.4. Base of the acetabular notch following debridement of the ligamentum.

Overall, ligamentum teres ruptures respond well to arthroscopic debridement. One should consider a ligamentum teres injury for patients with complaints of mechanical symptoms following trauma or a twisting injury. Radiographic and MRI studies will often be interpreted as normal. We suggest routinely looking for the ligament on axial and coronal images to become more comfortable with its presence on MRI. Debridement of a complete or partial rupture has not been shown to produce detrimental effects on hip stability; however, the complete function of the ligament has not been fully elucidated.

OSTEONECROSIS

Osteonecrosis can cause severe pain and disability in young patients, occurring most commonly between the third and fifth decades of life.[10] Approximately 10,000 to 20,000 new cases of hip osteonecrosis are reported each year in the United States.[11] It has been estimated that up to 10% of total hip arthroplasties are performed because of avascular necrosis.[12] Osteonecrosis can result from trauma that disrupts the blood supply of the femoral head. Other nontraumatic risk factors include corticosteroid use, heavy alcohol consumption, sickle cell disease, Gaucher and Caisson disease as well as hypercoaguable states. However, the etiology of a large percentage of patients remains idiopathic. Without treatment, avascular necrosis often progresses to articular collapse and degenerative joint disease. Prior to femoral head collapse, joint preserving procedures such as core decompression, vascularized fibular grafts, and osteotomies attempt to obviate the problem by stimulating the vascular supply to the involved area of the femoral head.

While the traditional joint preserving procedures attempt to alter the intrinsic composition of the diseased subchondral bone, intra-articular changes do occur, most often in the form of chondromalacia, chondral flaps, and loose bodies. Arthroscopic evaluation of the joint offers the ability to treat intra-articular pathology and improve mechanical symptoms. Prior to subchondral collapse, some patients complain of mechanical symptoms such as locking, buckling, and clicking.[10] O'Leary et al.[13] reported the results of hip arthroscopy for the treatment of 37 cases of hip AVN. They found that outcomes were most favorable for patients with mechanical symptoms without articular collapse. As would be expected, patients with degenerative changes and no mechanical symptoms had the worst outcomes. Of patients with stage III or IV Ficat, only 34% had significant pain relief following arthroscopy.

Patients with stage III (crescent sign without collapse) or stage IV (joint space collapse) are likely best treated with a total hip arthroplasty, hemiarthroplasty, or femoral head resurfacing. However, there exists a small subset of patients who present primarily with mechanical symptoms and who may benefit from arthroscopy. Resurfacing arthroplasty (Fig. 14.5) of the femoral head preserves bone stock and only removes the diseased portion of the head while not compromising future conversion to a total hip arthroplasty. This procedure is indicated for Ficat stage III or early stage IV disease with no acetabular changes. Mont et al.[12] showed that resurfacing arthroplasty had a survival rate of 90% at 10 years, nearly identical to the total hip arthroplasty population. While survival rates appear promising, patient outcomes tend to be less predictable with good or excellent results at an early follow-up between 60% and 80%. Stage IV Ficat disease is best treated with total hip arthroplasty.

In general, the goal in treating AVN of the hip is to improve patients' symptoms and give them the best opportunity to prevent subchondral collapse and degeneration, which often occurs at a young age. Patients without subchondral collapse and those complaining of pain associated with mechanical symptoms will often improve following arthroscopy. The degree of improvement often hinges on the amount of articular disease present at the time of the procedure. Arthroscopy may also be preformed in conjunction with patients undergoing joint preservation procedure and is best suited for osteonecrosis patients before the femoral head begins to collapse.

Arthroscopy may also have a role in the evaluation and treatment of OCD and Perthes disease.[14] Treatment parameters parallel those for osteonecrosis and the prevalence is estimated to be significantly less than in the knee.[15] Sporadic case reports have reported OCD in the hip in young patients.[16] Perthes, often more common than OCD of the hip in children, is often monitored conservatively, focusing attention on preserving range of motion with frequent follow-up evaluations and radiographs. Conservative treatment is often successful.

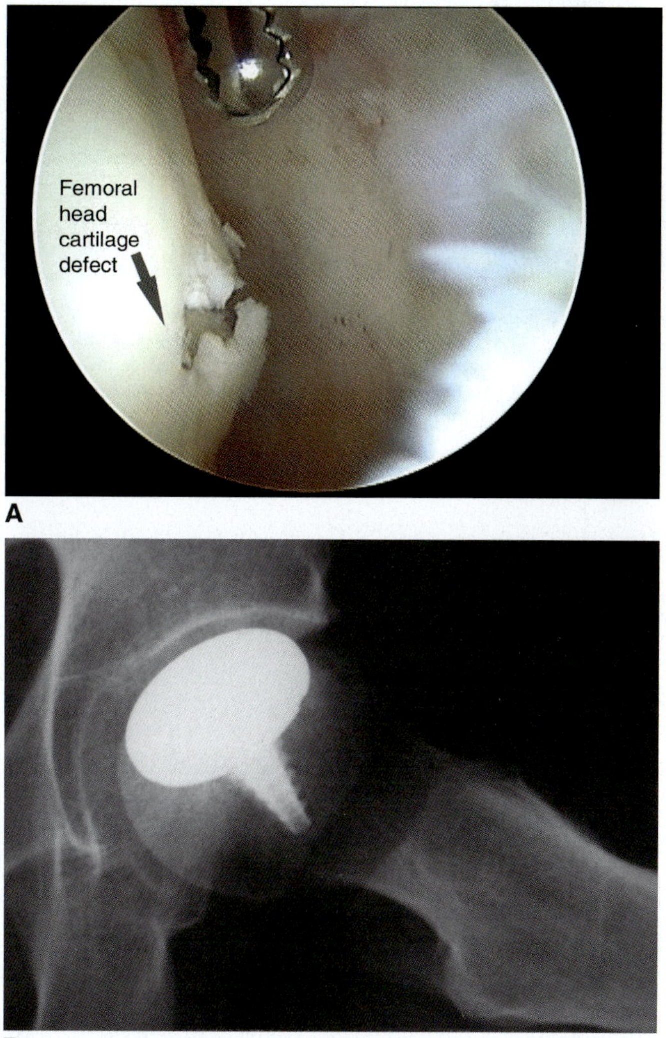

Figure 14.5. Avascular necrosis of the femoral head. **A:** Femoral head AVN with involvement of a large portion of the femoral head. **B:** Resurfacing arthroplasty of the femoral head.

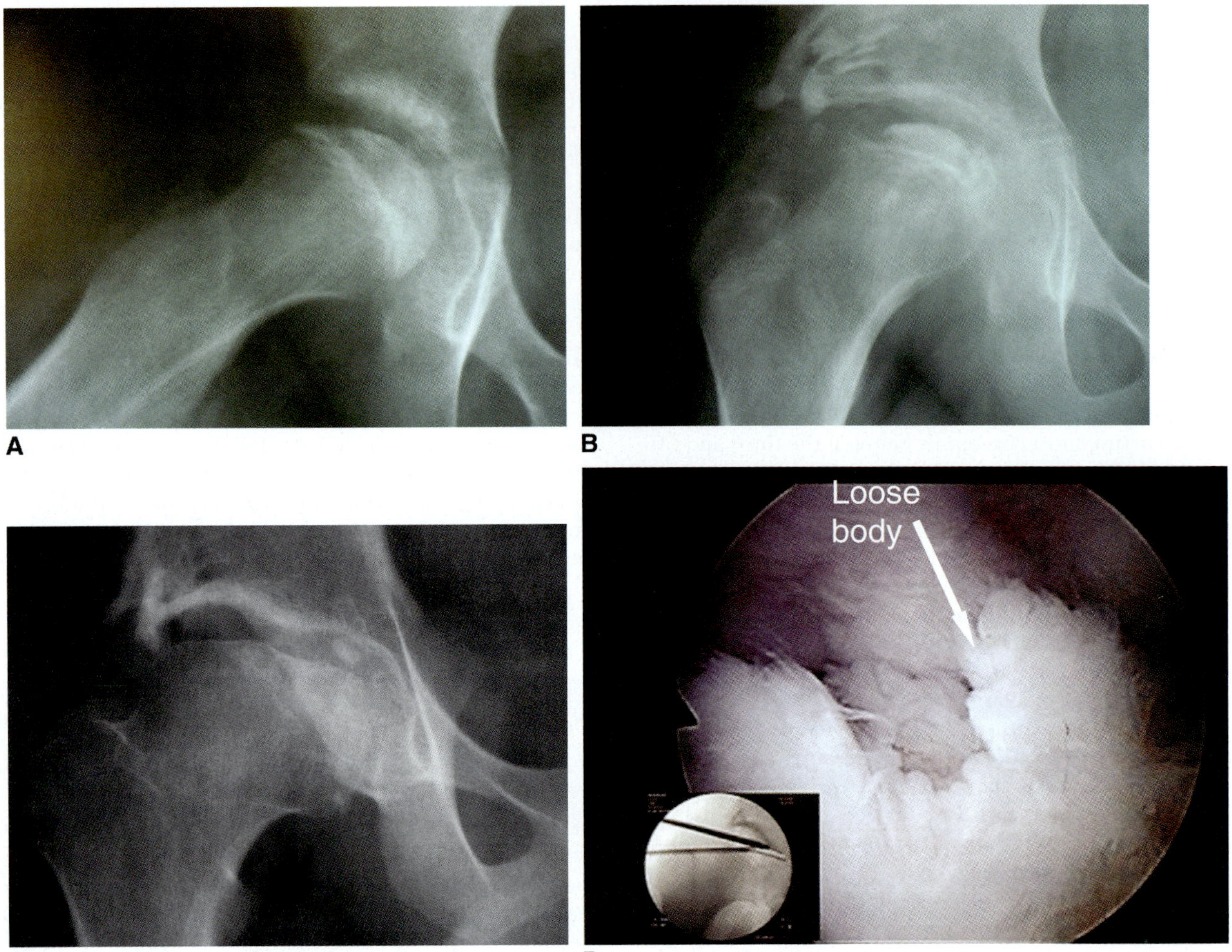

Figure 14.6. Legg–Perthes disease in an 18-year-old patient. **A:** Initial radiograph at age 10. **B:** AP radiograph at age 16 following shelf procedure. **C:** AP radiograph at age 18 with mechanical symptomatology. **D:** Intraoperative view of loose body in acetabular notch.

However, if young patients with either OCD or Perthes develop symptomatic mechanical symptoms, consideration should be given to arthroscopic evaluation of joint surfaces. Chondral flaps or loose bodies can be treated with limited morbidity to the patient (Fig. 14.6).

DEGENERATIVE JOINT DISEASE

Hip arthroscopy has a limited role in treating the symptoms of osteoarthrosis. Similar to knee and shoulder osteoarthrosis, arthroscopy may offer no benefit and, in some cases, may exacerbate symptoms. The best indications for arthroscopy include those patients who are with mechanical symptoms and minimal joint space collapse (Fig. 14.7).

Santori and Villar[17] reported a series of 234 consecutive hip arthroscopies of which 66% had normal radiographs. More than 30% had evidence of early degenerative changes documented at the time of arthroscopy. Therefore, osteoarthritis of the hip can present clinically prior to the development of radio-

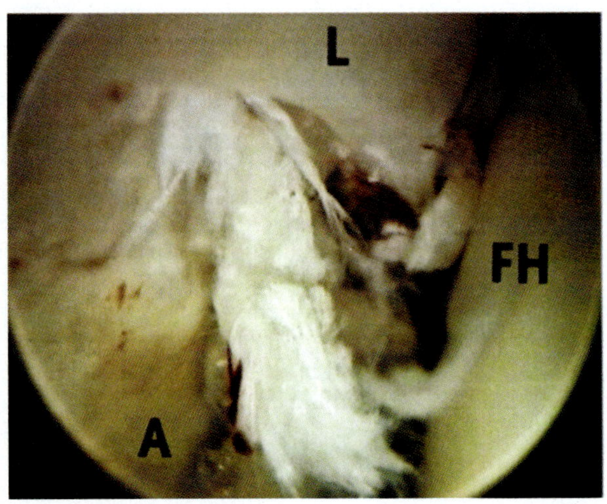

Figure 14.7. Arthroscopic view of a 65-year-old patient with mechanical symptomatology. Note the loose labral tissue and areas of chondral delamination immediately behind the frayed labrum. A, acetabulum; L, labrum; FH, femoral head.

graphic changes, with those complaining of mechanical symptoms responding most favorably to arthroscopic debridement.

SYNOVIAL DISORDERS

SYNOVIAL CHONDROMATOSIS

The most common synovial-based proliferative disorders include synovial chondromatosis, pigmented villonodular synovitis (PVNS), and inflammatory arthropathies such as rheumatoid arthritis. Also, other conditions that result in acute and chronic synovitis of the hip such as hemosideric deposits from hemophilia as well as deposits from chondrocalcinosis may benefit from arthroscopic treatment. Early treatment of progressive synovial diseases may curb the progression of articular destruction.

Synovial chondromatosis or intrasynovial cartilage metaplasia can produce multiple intra-articular or extra-articular loose bodies. Although it is more commonly reported in the knee, shoulder, and elbow, hip involvement is not uncommon.[18] Typically, symptoms include the onset of dull, aching pain, catching or locking, and often restrictions in range of motion. Periarticular loose bodies are seen on radiographs less than 50% of the time as they are often not calcified.[19]

The best imaging modality for intra-articular synovial disease is a gadolinium enhanced MRI (arthrogram). Multiple filling defects suggest synovial chondromatosis. Conservative management of multiple intra-articular lesions can lead to articular erosions and hip subluxation. Hip arthroscopy will offer removal of the offending lesions, often with immediate symptom relief (Fig. 14.8). Consideration should be given to performing a con-

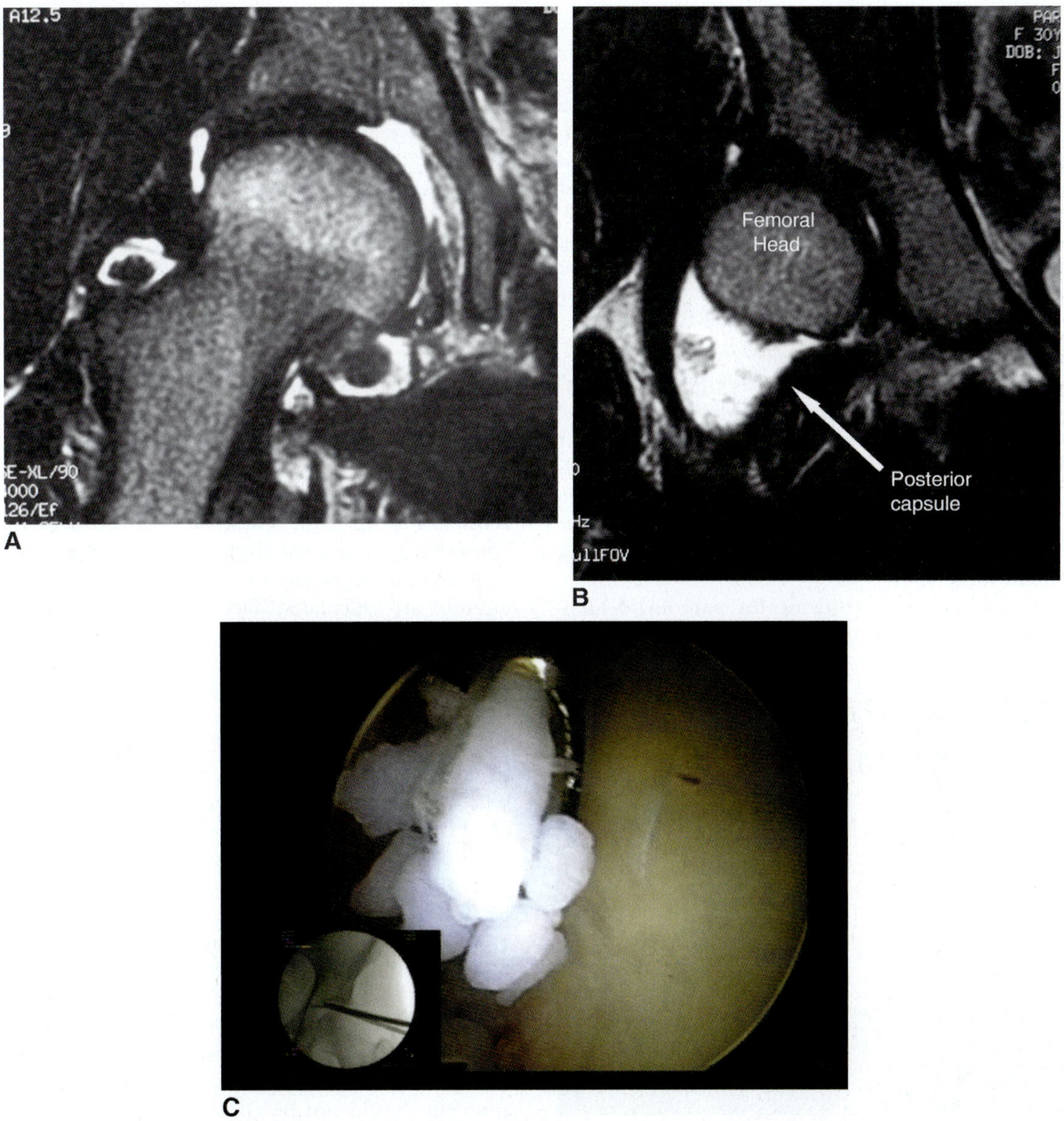

Figure 14.8. Synovial chondromatosis. **A:** Coronal MRI view depicting multiple chondral loose bodies (T2 weighted). **B:** Coronal MRI (close-up view) depicting multiple small loose bodies inferiorly. Note the multiple small, relatively gray loose bodies within the posterior recess. **C:** Arthroscopic visualization of the central portion of the joint with multiple chondral loose bodies.

comitant synovectomy. The role of synovectomy has not been fully elucidated or completely embraced as some authors have recommended loose body removal only[20–22] and others loose body removal and extensive synovectomy.[18,23] Realistically, a complete synovectomy will not be performed due to technical limitations.

The open approach is an option in intra-articular lesions and may be the best option in extensive disease. With either approach, it is critical to perform a thorough hip arthroscopy to include the peripheral compartment in these cases as the bulk of the pathology is often in this area. Recurrence rates have not been published but can be extrapolated from synovial chondromatosis in the knee and shoulder. Recurrence rates have been published between 7% and 23%.[18,24] We recommend arthroscopic loose body removal and synovectomy for all lesions amenable to arthroscopic treatment and formal open debridement and synovectomy for recurrences, paying particular attention to the peripheral compartment.

PIGMENTED VILLONODULAR SYNOVITIS

PVNS is a nonneoplastic disorder that most commonly occurs in the knee, but hip involvement has been reported.[25,26] It can affect any synovial lined structures including bursa, tendons, and intra-articular compartments. It typically presents in younger patients, with an average age within the fourth or fifth decade, without gender predilection. It should be considered in the differential diagnosis of this age group in patients with hip pain.

Similar to chondrocalcinosis, the pathogenesis remains unknown. It has been attributed to a chronic inflammatory response or a benign but locally aggressive growth of fibrohistiocytic origin. Long-standing PVNS of the hip often results in hip degeneration.[25] Treatment includes debulking of the lesion, synovectomy, and possible chemical or radio nuclear adjunctive therapy (Fig. 14.9). Hips with superimposed degenerative arthrosis are treated with total hip arthroplasty. As these lesions present in the middle-age population, early diagnosis and treatment may prevent a younger patient from requiring joint replacement surgery.

Hip arthroscopy can produce tissue for pathologic identification, can allow evaluation of the joint surfaces, and has the ability to perform a partial synovectomy. As a complete synovectomy is technically challenging, adjunctive chemical synoviothesis in addition to partial synovectomy offers the most minimally invasive treatment option. This treatment regimen is most successful for patients with no or very limited degenerative joint disease. If the lesion recurs, as is common for PVNS,[25] a more aggressive open complete synovectomy can be attempted. Total hip arthroplasty will offer pain relief if joint deterioration occurs, yet this modality in the young patient population is not desirable.

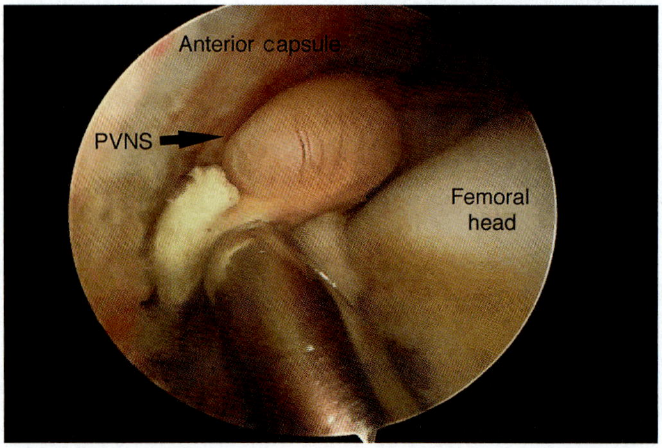

Figure 14.9. PVNS in a 28-year-old patient with significant pain and mechanical symptomatology. View is of left hip; viewed in peripheral compartment from the anterolateral portal. PVNS, pigmented villonodular synovitis.

SYNOVIAL PLICAE

In the knee, diagnosis and treatment of plicae is well described.[27,28] There have been sporadic case reports of symptomatic plicae in other joints such as the elbow, ankle, and hip. Six cases of symptomatic hip plicae have been published.[29–31] Hip plicae have been described in cadavers[32] and are often discovered during routine hip arthroscopy or arthrography.[31] Plicae are present as unusually large folds that are vulnerable to impingement between the articular surfaces.

Patients may have a palpable click during the examination with passive motion. One case report by the senior author noted that flexion, abduction, and external rotation created pain as well as a click and this corresponded to a plica along the anteromedial aspect of the femoral neck.[29] Plain films and nonenhanced MRI are often normal. Gadolinium enhanced MRI arthrography is obtained with the suspicion of a labral tear (Fig. 14.10). MRI arthrogram may reveal an elongated ligamentous appearing structure extending from the region of the femoral head–neck to a region of the hip capsule. Chondromalacia, if present, suggests repetitive impingement from the plica on the articular surface.

Although plica syndrome of the hip is reportedly rare, its true incidence may be underappreciated. The presence of plicae should be considered in the differential diagnosis of recalcitrant hip pain. Suspicion of a hip plica that has failed conservative treatment should be treated with diagnostic hip arthroscopy, debridement of the plicae, and thorough evaluation of the articular surfaces, looking in particular for associated chondromalacia.

CAPSULAR LAXITY

Instability of the hip is much less common than shoulder instability, but its presence can cause a significant amount of disability.[14] The hip joint relies less on the surrounding soft tissue structures for stability because of the constrained osseous stability. The labrum provides a great deal of stability at extremes of motion, especially flexion. With a torn of absent labrum, a great deal of force is transmitted through the capsule.[14]

Hip instability can be difficult to diagnose. Patients are often performing a motion of pelvic rotation and external rotation to elicit symptoms.[33] Motions such as swinging a golf club or throwing a football often precipitate symptoms in active patients.[14] The cause of instability may be traumatic or atraumatic and the clinician should not be confused with the voluntary external snapping hip syndrome as a result of a subluxing iliotibial band across the greater trochanter. Connective tissue disorders such as Ehlers–Danlos, Marfan, or Down syndrome may contribute to ligamentous laxity.

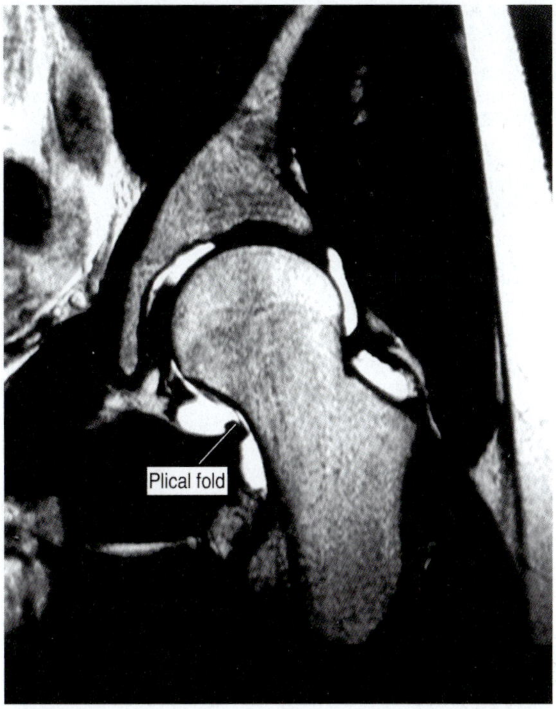

A

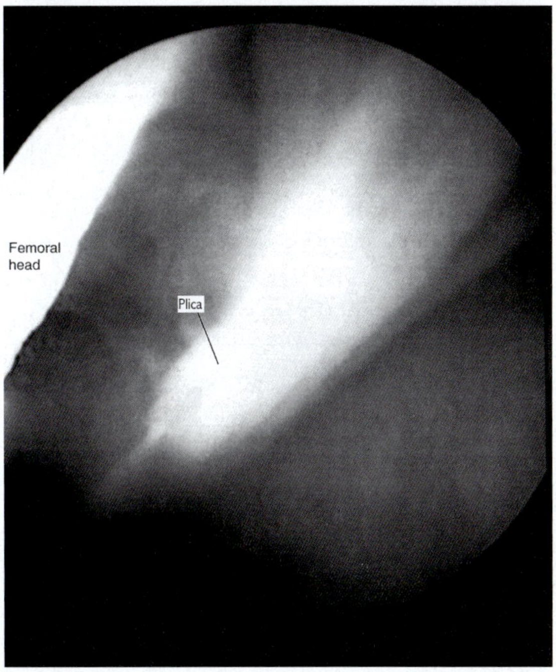

B

Figure 14.10. Synovial plica of the hip. **A:** A sagittal MRI reveals a synovial plica along the inferior neck. **B:** Arthroscopic image of plica. View is of the inferior neck in a right hip visualized from the posterolateral portal.

Bellabarba et al.[34] linked a group of patients with hip instability without trauma to acetabular dysplasia. Iatrogenic instability secondary to pincer impingement resection of the acetabulum may result from excessive bone resection from the anterior overhang. Adequate reattachment of the labrum following bone resection of the acetabulum is critical for maintaining stability.

Traumatic dislocations can lead to capsular redundancy and clinical laxity. Liebenberg and Dommisse[35] described the development of capsular redundancy after recurrent posterior dislocation of the hip. They suggest that the presence of hip instability in these patients likely results from a damaged capsulolabral complex. The labrum may be torn and may not function as it did prior to the injury. Thus, with a deficient labral contribution to stability, the hip relies more on a redundant capsule. Repetitive capsular stress creates further laxity and instability.

SUMMARY

There are many types of intra-articular pathologies that can cause significant pain and mechanical symptomatology. A thorough evaluation of all patients is warranted to ensure that the proper diagnosis is made in all patients. Although hip labral tears are, by far, the most common problem, it is important to know that a certain percentage of patients will not fall into this category. The treating physician should be comfortable in diagnosing these uncommon problems and treating them effectively, either arthroscopically or in an open fashion.

REFERENCES

1. DeAngelis NA, Busconi BD. Assessment and differential diagnosis of the painful hip. *Clin Orthop.* 2003;406(1):11–18.
2. Burman M. Arthroscopy or the direct visualization of joints. *J Bone Joint Surg.* 1931;4:669–695.
3. McCarthy JC, Busconi BD. The role of hip arthroscopy in the diagnosis and treatment of hip disease. *Orthopedics.* 1995;18:753–756.
4. Keene GS, Villar RN. Arthroscopic anatomy of the hip: An in vivo study. *Arthroscopy.* 1994;10:392–399.
5. Potter HG, Linklater JM, Allen AA, et al. Magnetic resonance imaging of articular cartilage of the knee. *J Bone Joint Surg.* 1998;80A:1276–1288.
6. Yamamoto Y, Ide T, Ono T, et al. Usefulness of arthroscopic surgery in hip trauma cases. *Arthroscopy.* 2003;19(3):269–273.
7. McCarthy JC, Noble PC, Schuck MR, et al. The role of labral lesions to the development of hip disease. *Clin Orthop.* 2001;393:25–37.
8. Gray AJR, Villar RN. The ligamentum teres of the hip: An arthroscopic classification of its pathology. *Arthroscopy.* 1997;13:575–578.
9. Byrd JWT, Jones KS. Traumatic rupture of the ligamentum teres as a source of hip pain. *Arthroscopy.* 2004;20(4):385–391.
10. McCarthy J, Barsoum W, Puri L, et al. The role of hip arthroscopy in the elite athlete. *Clin Orthop.* 2003;406:71–74.
11. Etienne G, Mont MA, Ragland PS. The diagnosis and treatment of nontraumatic osteonecrosis of the femoral head. *Instr Course Lect.* 2004;53:67–85.
12. Mont M, Rajadyaksha AD, Hungerford DS. Outcomes of limited femoral resurfacing arthroplasty compared with total hip arthroplasty for osteonecrosis of the femoral head. *Clin Orthop.* 2001;386:85–92.
13. O'Leary JA, Berend K, Vail TP. The relationship between diagnosis and outcome in arthroscopy of the hip. *Arthroscopy.* 2001;17(2):181–188.
14. Kelly BT, Williams RJ, Philippon MJ. Hip arthroscopy: Current indications, treatment options, and management issues. *Am J Sports Med.* 2003;31(6):1020–1037.
15. Linden B, Jonsson K, Redlund-Johnell I. Osteochondritis dissecans of the hip. *Acta Radiol.* 2003;44(1):67–71.
16. Rowe SM, Yoon TR, Jung ST, et al. Free osteochondral fragment caught in the acetabular fossa in the osteochondritis dissecans after Legg-Calve-Perthes' disease–reports of 2 cases. *Acta Orthop Scand.* 2003;74(1):107–110.
17. Santori N, Villar RN. Arthroscopic findings in the initial stages of hip osteoarthritis. *Orthopedics.* 1999;22:405–409.
18. Maurice H, Crone M, Watt I. Synovial chondromatosis. *J Bone Joint Surg.* 1988;70B:807–811.
19. Wilson WJ, Parr TJ. Synovial chondromatosis. *Orthopedics.* 1988:1179–1183.
20. Dorfmann H, Boyer T. Arthroscopy of the hip: 12 years of experience. *Arthroscopy.* 1999;15:67–72.
21. Shpitzer T, Ganel A, Engelberg S. Surgery for synovial chondromatosis: 26 cases followed up for 6 years. *Acta Orthop Scand.* 1990;61:567–569.
22. Okada Y, Awaya G, Ikeda T, et al. Arthroscopic surgery for synovial chondromatosis. *J Bone Joint Surg.* 1989;71B:198–199.
23. Murphy F, Dahlin D, Sullivan C. Articular synovial chondromatosis. J Bone *Joint Surg.* 1962;44A:77–86.
24. Ogilvie-Harris DJ, Weisleder L. Arthroscopic synovectomy of the knee: Is it helpful? *Arthroscopy.* 1995;11:91–95.
25. Goldman AB, DiCarlo EF. Pigmented villonodular synovitis: Diagnosis and differential diagnosis. *Radiol Clin North Am.* 1988;26:1327–1347.

26. Cotton A, Flipo RM, Chastanet P, et al. Pigmented villonodular synovitis of the hip: Review of radiographic features in 58 patients. *Skeletal Radiol.* 1995;24:1–6.
27. Dorchak JD, Barrack RL, Kneisl JS, et al. Arthroscopic treatment of symptomatic synovial plicae of the knee: Long-term follow-up. *Am J Sports Med.* 1991;19:503–507.
28. Johnson DP, Eastwood DM, Witherow PJ. Symptomatic synovial plicae of the knee. *J Bone Joint Surg.* 1993;75A:1485–1496.
29. Atlihan D, Jones DC, Guanche CA. Arthroscopic treatment of a symptomatic hip plicae. *Clin Orthop.* 2003;411:174–177.
30. Frich LH, Lauritzen J, Juhl M. Arthroscopy in the diagnosis and treatment of hip disorders. *Orthopedics.* 1989;12:389–392.
31. Helenon CH, Bergevin H, Aubert JD, et al. Plication of hip synovia at the upper border of femoral neck. *J Radiol.* 1896;67:737–740.
32. Fu Z, Peng M, Peng Q. Anatomical study of the synovial plicae of the hip joint. *Clin Orthop.* 1997;10:235–238.
33. Philippon MJ. The role of arthroscopic thermal capsulorrhaphy in the hip. *Clin Sports Med.* 2001;20:817–819.
34. Bellabarba C, Sheinkop KB, Kuo KN. Idiopathic hip instability. An unrecognized cause of coxa saltans in the adult. *Clin Orthop.* 1998;355:261–271.
35. Liebenberg F, Dommissee GF. Recurrent post-traumatic dislocation of the hip. *J Bone Joint Surg.* 1969;51B:632–637.

CHAPTER

15

Victor M. Ilizaliturri Jr.
Javier Camacho-Galindo

Snapping Hip Syndrome

INTRODUCTION

The snapping hip or *coxa saltans* is characterized by a snapping phenomenon that occurs in association with hip motion. It has been classified into three different types[1]: (i) External snapping hip syndrome was the earliest type described.[2] It is caused by the iliotibial band sliding over the greater trochanter. (ii) The internal snapping hip syndrome, which was first reported in Argentina,[3] is caused by the iliopsoas tendon snapping over the iliopectineal eminence or the femoral head. (iii) A third type, the so-called intra-articular snapping hip, refers to intra-articular pathology causing mechanical hip symptoms (locking, catching, and giving away). Because we are now more precise in the diagnosis and description of intra-articular hip pathology, we no longer use the term intra-articular snapping hip.[4]

EXTERNAL SNAPPING HIP SYNDROME

The external snapping hip syndrome is produced by a posterior thickening of the iliotibial band and an anterior thickening of fibers of the gluteus maximus. These fibers lie posterior to the greater trochanter. The thickened fibers snap on the greater trochanter with flexion and extension of the hip (Fig. 15.1). In some cases, the snapping phenomenon may be visible under the skin, and in some other cases, it may be palpated. This phenomenon is always voluntary and the patient often volunteers to demonstrate it.[1] Asymptomatic snapping must always be considered a normal occurrence.[5] Diagnosis is evident; the snapping will occur when flexing the hip and when extending from flexion. In cases that present severe snapping, this phenomenon may also be detected with internal and external rotation. The snapping phenomenon is also described by some patients as the ability to "dislocate the hip." This is often demonstrated by rotating the affected hip while tilting the pelvis in standing position. The voluntary "dislocators" are more frequently painless and should only be treated with stretching exercises of the iliotibial band. Symptomatic external snapping hip syndrome is always accompanied with pain in the trochanteric region. The pain is secondary to greater trochanteric bursitis. When Trendelenburg gait is also found, an associated abductor muscle tear must be suspected; this is an indication for surgical treatment. Anteroposterior pelvis X-rays should always be done to identify bony abnormalities, calcifications, or other pathology. The snapping phenomenon can be documented with dynamic ultrasonography and associated pathology such as tendonitis, bursitis, or muscle tears detected.[6,7] Iliopsoas bursitis and abductor muscle tears can be diagnosed using magnetic resonance imaging.[8,9]

Most of the symptomatic cases improve with stretching physical therapy, nonsteroidal anti-inflammatory therapy, and corticosteroid infiltration of the greater trochanter bursa.[1] When conservative treatment fails, surgical release is indicated. Open iliotibial band release or lengthening has been the traditional surgical option to treat the external snapping hip syndrome.[5,10–13] Recently, we have described a technique for endoscopic iliotibial band release for the treatment of external snapping hip syndrome.[14] Surgical release of the iliotibial band should always be combined with greater trochanteric bursectomy and a careful inspection of the abductor tendons.

ENDOSCOPIC ILIOTIBIAL BAND RELEASE

We position the patient lateral, similar to the setup for total hip replacement.[14] Surgical drapes most allow for free range of motion of the lower extremity to reproduce the snapping phenomenon during surgery. No traction is necessary to access the greater trochanteric bursa and the iliotibial band. The greater trochanter is marked on the skin using a skin marker. The greater trochanter is the main landmark for portal establishment. We utilize two portals, a proximal trochanteric and distal trochanteric. The area of snapping should be between the two portals and is also marked on the skin (Fig. 15.2). We start by infiltrating the space under the iliotibial band with 40 to 50 mL of saline (Fig. 15.3). Next, the inferior trochanteric portal is established using a standard arthroscopic cannula that is introduced under the skin and directed proximally to the site of the superior trochanteric portal using the blunt obturator to develop a working space above the iliotibial band. The site of the proximal trochanteric portal is identified arthroscopically using a needle inserted at the portal landmark, the skin incision is made and a shaver is introduced to dissect subcutaneous tissue from the iliotibial band situated between the portals. Hemostasia is performed in this step to allow clear visualization of the iliotibial band. Then, a radiofrequency hook probe is introduced from the proximal trochanteric portal and a 4 to 5 cm vertical retrograde cut is performed on the iliotibial band starting at the level of the inferior trochanteric portal, which

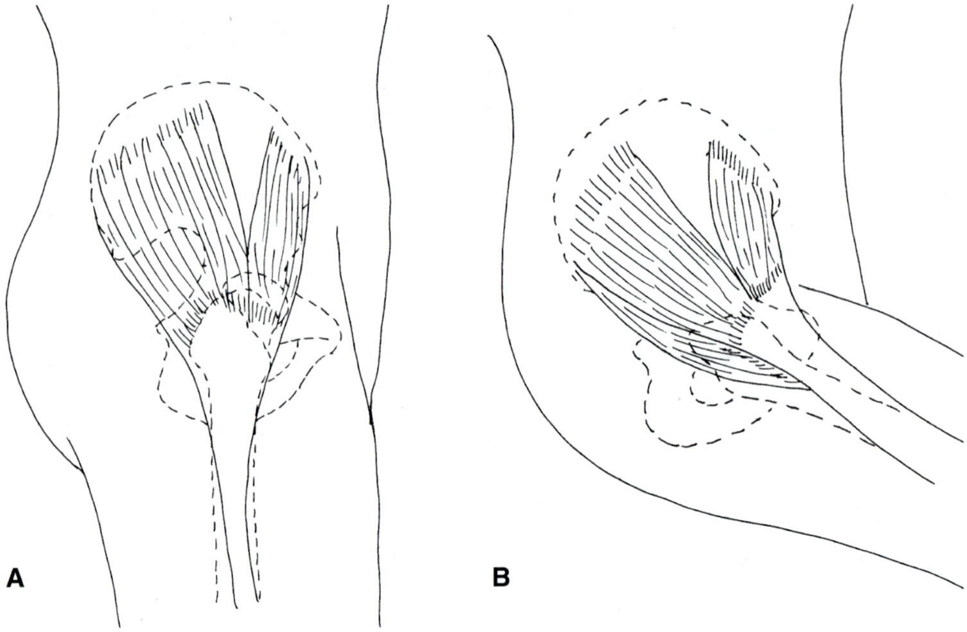

Figure 15.1. Schematic drawing that represents the snapping phenomenon of the posterior iliotibial band over the greater trochanter. **A:** The hip is in extension. **B:** The snapping phenomenon occurs as the hip is flexed. The phenomenon will occur again as the hip is brought back to extension.

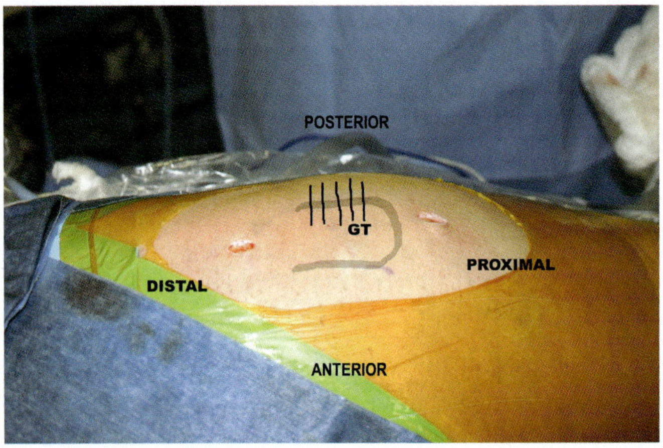

Figure 15.2. This photograph demonstrates portal sites for endoscopic iliotibial band release (The photograph was taken from the front). The patient is positioned in left lateral decubitus. The patient's head is to the right. Setup is similar to that of total hip replacement. The greater trochanter (GT) has been outlined. Proximal to the tip of the GT, the proximal trochanteric portal is observed. Distal to the tip of the greater trochanter, the distal trochanteric portal is observed. The black lines indicate the area of snapping (Note how the area of snapping is between the portals).

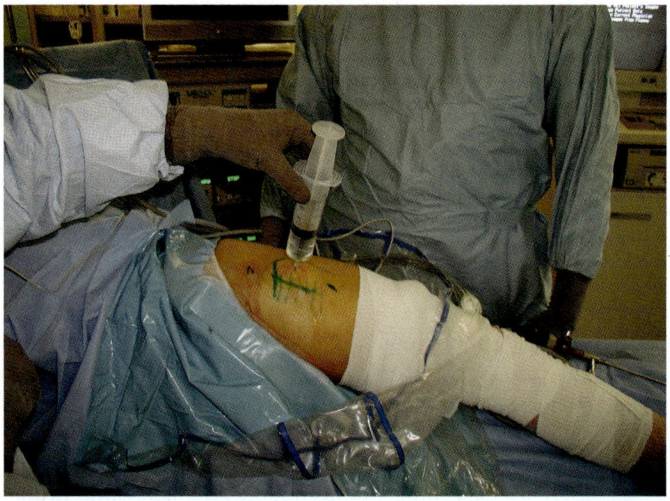

Figure 15.3. This photograph demonstrates a patient in left lateral decubitus prepared for endoscopic release of the iliotibial band (Note how the setup is similar to total hip replacement. To the right, the leg is draped for free range of motion. The photograph was taken from the back). The greater trochanter and the proximal and distal trochanteric portals have been outlined. The lines indicate the area of snapping. The space under the iliotibial band is being infiltrated with saline.

is the viewing portal (Fig. 15.4). The pump pressure should be kept low while working on the subcutaneous space to avoid complications with the skin. Once the vertical cut on the iliotibial band is complete, the pump pressure can be increased and a transverse anterior cut of 2 cm length is performed starting at the middle of the vertical cut (Fig. 15.5). The resulting superior and inferior anterior flaps are resected using a shaver, developing a triangular defect on the anterior iliotibial band that will provide access to the posterior iliotibial band. Next, a transverse posterior cut is started at the same level of the transverse anterior cut. This is the most important release and should be carried out until the snapping phenomenon is solved. Finally, the superior and inferior posterior flaps are resected, which results in a diamond-shaped defect on the iliotibial band (Fig. 15.6A & B). The greater trochanter will rotate freely within the defect without snapping. The greater trochanteric bursa should be removed through the defect on the iliotibial band and the abductor tendons inspected for tears.

When hip arthroscopy is also necessary, we start with the patient positioned lateral. We perform arthroscopy of the central and peripheral compartment of the hip; after hip arthroscopy is complete, the foot is released from the traction device and the endoscopic iliotibial band release performed as described.

RESULTS

Most of the reported results in the literature of external snapping hip syndrome are with open techniques. Recently, short term results of endoscopic release have been reported.[14] These results compare well with the results reported with open technique (Table 15.1).

INTERNAL SNAPPING HIP SYNDROME

The internal snapping hip syndrome is produced by the iliopsoas tendon over the iliopectineal eminence or the femoral head. The iliopsoas tendon is located lateral to the iliopectineal eminence when the hip is in full flexion; with hip extension, the tendon is displaced medially until it positions medial to the iliopectineal eminence producing a snap[1] (Fig. 15.7). The snapping phenomenon can occur without pain in up to 10% of the general population and should be considered a normal occurrence.[4]

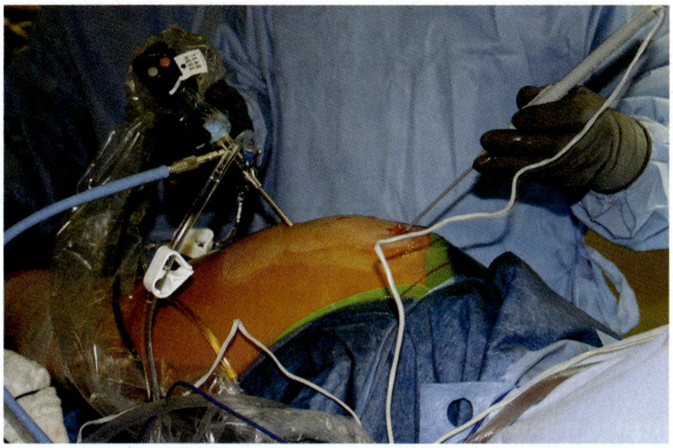

Figure 15.4. This photograph demonstrates instruments inside the portals for endoscopic release of the iliotibial band. The patient is in left lateral decubitus (The photograph was taken from the front). The arthroscope is inside the inferior trochanteric portal; a radiofrequency hook probe is inside the proximal trochanteric portal.

The symptomatic internal snapping hip syndrome always presents pain in the groin associated with the snapping phenomenon. The snapping phenomenon is reproduced when bringing the hip to extension from a flexed position. The patients report snapping while stair climbing or standing from a chair. The snapping phenomenon is always voluntary and reproducible.[1,4,15]

Physical examination of the internal snapping phenomenon is done with the patient supine by flexing the affected hip more than 90° and extending to neutral position. This may be accentuated with abduction and external rotation in flexion and adducting and internally rotating while extending. The snapping phenomenon is not visible at the groin. It may be audible or may be palpated by placing the hand over the affected groin. There is always an apprehension response from the patient when the snapping occurs.

Plain radiographs are usually normal; in some cases, a cam femoroacetabular impingement deformity may be documented[16,17]; psoas bursography may outline the tendon and, if combined with fluoroscopy, may document the snapping phenomenon dynamically. The main problem is that it depends on the ability of the technician to reproduce the snapping while examining hip motion within the range of view of the C-arm.[18] Ultrasonography of the iliopsoas tendon is a dynamic noninvasive study that may document the snapping phenomenon as well as pathologic changes of the iliopsoas tendon and its bursa. Psoas ultrasonography also depends on the ability and experience of the examiner.[19] Because almost half of the patients with

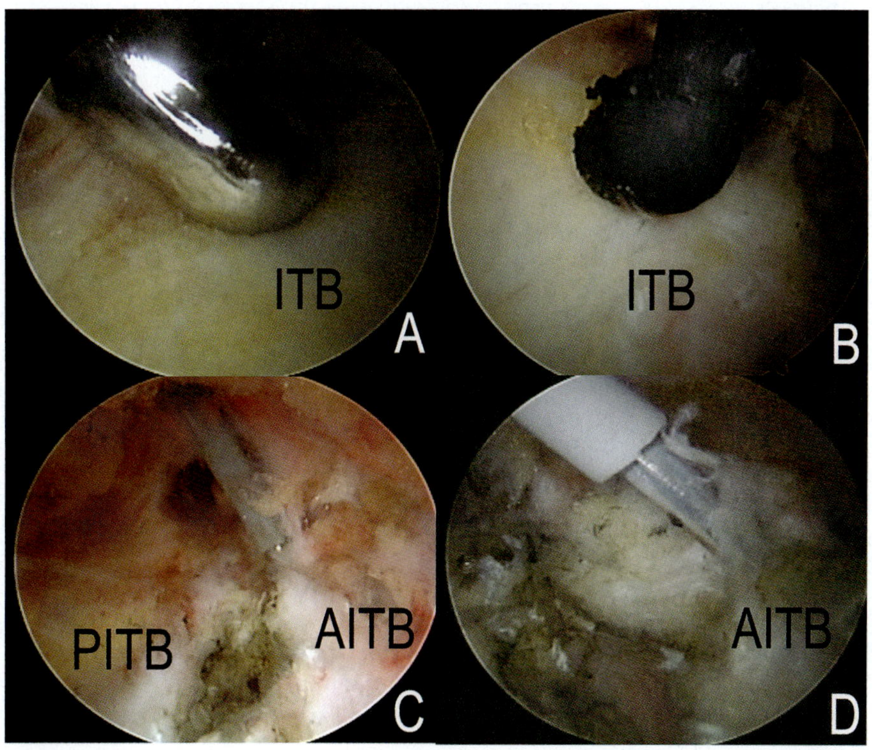

Figure 15.5. Series of arthroscopic photographs of endoscopic iliotibial band release in a right hip. **A:** A shaver is used to dissect subcutaneous tissue above the iliotibial band (ITB). **B:** Hemostasia is necessary for clear visualization of the ITB. A radiofrequency device is being used for hemostasia on the ITB. **C:** A hook radiofrequency probe is used to perform the initial retrograde vertical cut. The ITB is divided into two: anterior iliotibial band (AITB) and posterior iliotibial band (PITB). **D:** A transverse anterior cut is performed starting at the mid-portion of the AITB.

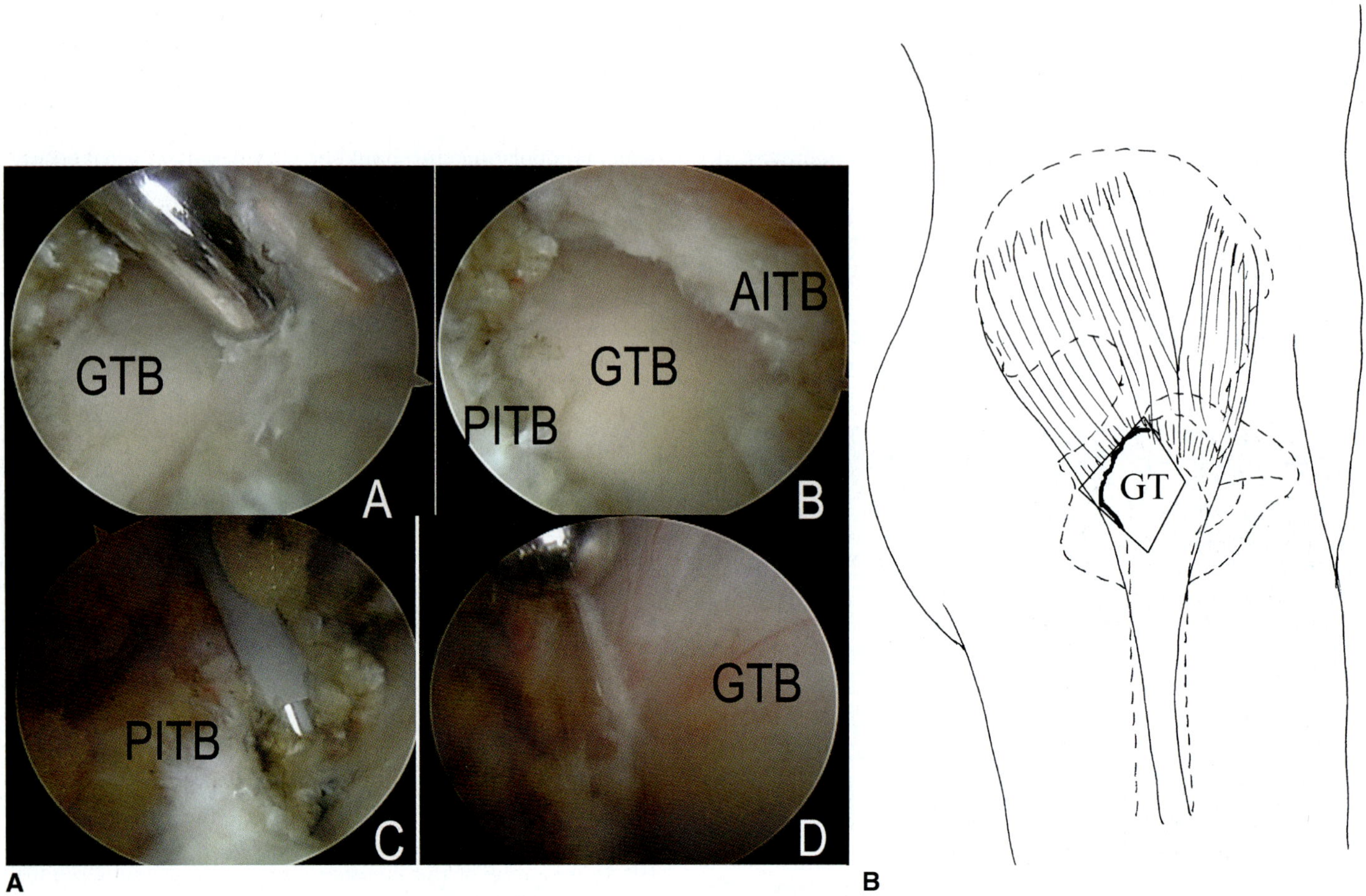

Figure 15.6. **A:** Series of arthroscopic photographs of endoscopic iliotibial band release in a right hip. *(A)* A shaver is used to resect the superior and inferior flaps of the transverse cut on the anterior iliotibial band (AITB). The greater trochanteric bursa (GTB) is visible through the defect. *(B)* When the superior and inferior flaps of the transverse cut on the AITB are complete, a triangular-shaped defect is obtained. The GTB is observed through the defect. The posterior iliotibial band (PITB) is to the left of the photograph. *(C)* A posterior transverse cut is started at the mid-portion of the PITB using a hook radiofrequency probe. *(D)* The superior and inferior flaps of the PITB are resected using a shaver. This results in a diamond-shaped defect. The GTB is observed through the defect. **B:** Schematic representation of a diamond-shaped defect on the iliotibial band.

TABLE 15.1 **Results of Surgical Treatment of External Snapping Hip Syndrome (Open and Endoscopic)**

Author	*Number of Hips*	*Technique*	*Follow-up*	*Pain*	*Resnapping*
Fery and Sommelet[13]	35	Open, crosscut and inverted flap suture	7 years	21 cases	10 cases
Faraj et al.[11]	11	Open, Z-plasty	12 months	3 cases	0
Provencher et al.[5]	9	Open Z-plasty	22 months	1	0
White et al.[10]	17	Open vertical incision and multiple transverse cuts	32.5 months	0	2 cases (reoperated)
Ilizaliturri et al.[14]	11	Diamond-shaped defect	25 months	0	1 case, improved with physical therapy

internal snapping hip syndrome have associated intra-articular hip pathology,[4,15] magnetic resonance arthrography is the diagnostic study we prefer. It may demonstrate intra-articular pathology and report changes related to the iliopsoas tendon and bursa. The snapping phenomenon cannot be documented using magnetic resonance arthrography.

Treatment is initially conservative with physical therapy, nonsteroidal anti-inflammatory therapy, and corticosteroid injec-

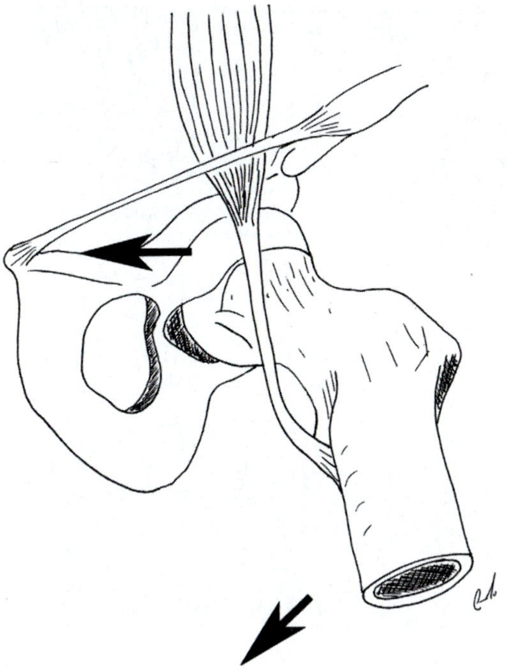

Figure 15.7. Schematic representation of a snapping iliopsoas tendon. The hip is in flexion and the tendon is positioned lateral to the iliopectineal eminence. As the hip is extended, the tendon is displaced medially producing a snap.

tions. If there is no positive response to conservative treatment, surgical treatment is indicated.[1]

Traditionally, open surgical treatment has been the standard procedure for the symptomatic internal snapping hip syndrome. Recently, endoscopic iliopsoas tendon release has been reported in the literature.[4,15,20,21]

Hip arthroscopy is always performed before endoscopic iliopsoas release; almost half of the patients with internal snapping hip syndrome present associated intra-articular pathology.[4,15,21] The patient can be positioned supine or lateral and the procedure can be performed successfully.

ENDOSCOPIC ILIOPSOAS TENDON RELEASE AT THE LESSER TROCHANTER

We position the patient in lateral decubitus for hip arthroscopy.[15] Arthroscopy of the central compartment is performed first using traction. Three portals are usually established for arthroscopy of the central compartment: anterolateral, posterolateral, and direct anterior.[22,23] Traction is released to access the peripheral compartment. Accessory portals are usually needed to access the hip periphery.[24,25]

After hip arthroscopy of the central and peripheral compartments is complete, instruments are taken out of the joint. The hip is positioned at 20° of flexion and external rotation to expose the lesser trochanter at the image intensifier (Fig. 15.8). A spinal needle is introduced through an accessory portal (superior accessory portal) established about 2 cm distal to a horizontal line directed anteriorly from the tip of the greater trochanter and 2 cm anterior of the anterior femur. The needle is directed to the lesser trochanter navigated by the image intensifier (Fig. 15.9). Orientation in the coronal plane is provided by the image intensifier. Orientation in the sagittal plane is provided by palpating the anterior aspect of the femur until the needle is positioned on the lesser trochanter. This will position the needle inside the iliopsoas bursa. After the spinal needle has been successfully positioned in the iliopsoas bursa, the stylus is removed and a flexible guidewire (nitinol) is introduced; the needle is removed and a cannulated switching stick from the Hip Access System (Smith & Nephew, Andover, MA) is passed into the iliopsoas bursa using the flexible guidewire as a monorail. A 4.5-mm double valve rotatable arthroscopic cannula is passed over the switching stick, which is then removed

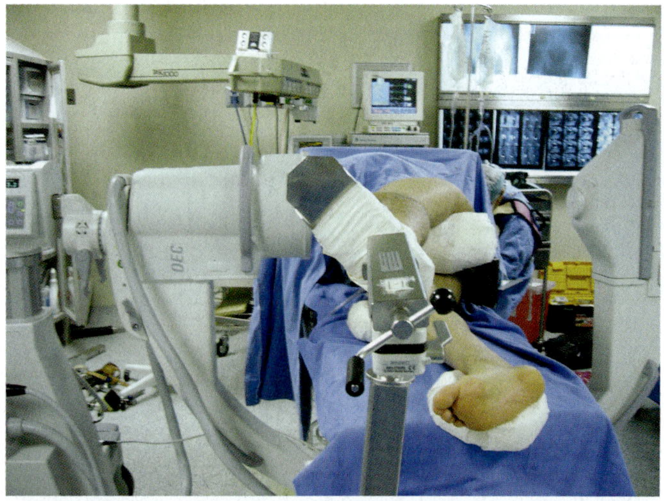

Figure 15.8. The patient is positioned in right lateral decubitus for arthroscopy of the left hip. Only the left foot is fixed to the traction device. Note how the left foot is externally rotated to allow visualization of the lesser trochanter at the image intensifier. The hip is flexed 20°. The C-arm is positioned horizontally under the operating table.

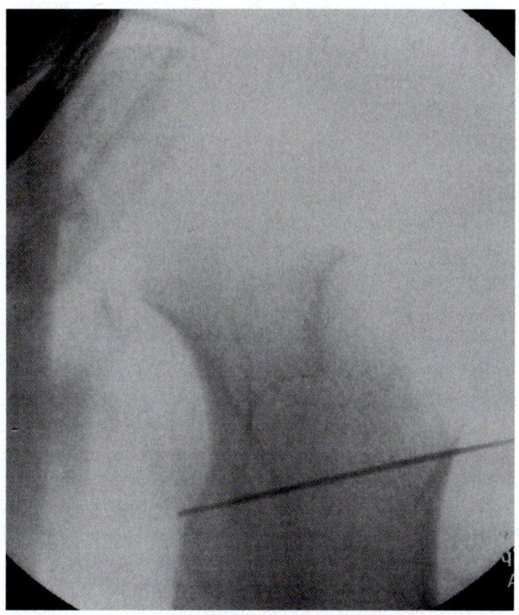

Figure 15.9. Fluoroscopy photograph that demonstrates a left hip in external rotation; the lesser trochanter is clearly visible. A needle is in position at the lesser trochanter.

and a 4.0mm 30° arthroscope introduced. The fluid pump is started and the iliopsoas tendon identified. A second accessory portal 3 to 4cm distal to the first one is established (inferior accessory portal) (Fig. 15.10A & B). A spinal needle is triangulated toward the tip of the arthroscope inside the iliopsoas bursa. The image intensifier can be utilized to assist navigating the needle (Fig. 15.11). The tip of the needle is identified endoscopically inside the iliopsoas bursa and a working portal is established using a flexible guidewire, a cannulated switching stick with a dilator, and finally a slotted cannula (Hip Access System; Smith & Nephew). A shaver is introduced through the

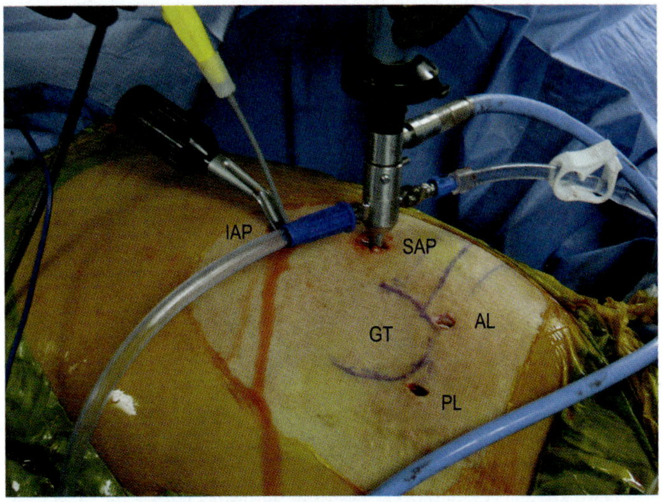

A

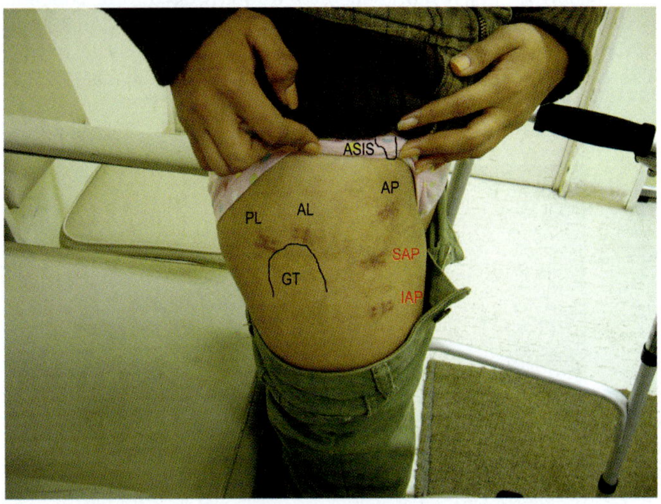

B

Figure 15.10. **A:** Photograph of a patient positioned in right lateral decubitus for arthroscopy of the left hip (the photograph was taken from behind the patient). The anterolateral (AL) and posterolateral (PL) portals for the central compartment are to the right of the photograph. The GT has been outlined. The arthroscope is inside the superior accessory portal (SAP). A slotted cannula is inside the inferior accessory portal (IAP) a radiofrequency hook probe is being introduced through the slotted cannula. **B:** Postoperative photograph. The GT and the anterior superior iliac spine are outlined. Initials for the AL, PL, and direct anterior portal (AP) are in black. Initials for the SAP and IAP are in red.

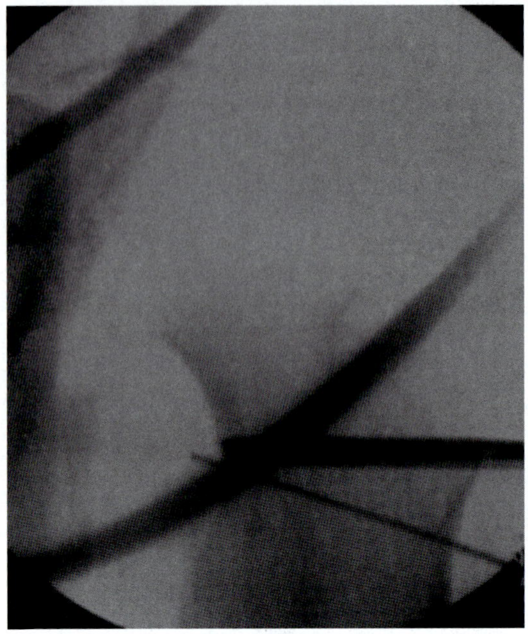

Figure 15.11. Fluoroscopy photograph that shows triangulation of the arthroscope and a spinal needle on the lesser trochanter in a left hip.

slotted cannula, which is then removed. The shaver is used to resect synovial tissue from the iliopsoas bursa and dissect the iliopsoas tendon. The slotted cannula is reinserted using the shaver as a guide. The shaver is removed and a radiofrequency hook probe inserted, the slotted cannula is removed and the radiofrequency probe utilized to release the iliopsoas tendon close to its insertion on the lesser trochanter (Fig. 15.12). The image intensifier can be utilized to verify the position of the radiofrequency hook probe before releasing the iliopsoas tendon (Fig. 15.13A & B).

TRANSCAPSULAR ILIOPSOAS TENDON RELEASE

The iliopsoas tendon can also be released endoscopically at the level of the femoral head–neck junction through an anterior hip capsulectomy.[20] We perform this procedure with the patient in lateral decubitus but it can also be performed with the patient in supine position. After arthroscopy of the central compartment is complete, instruments are taken out of the joint and traction is released. The hip is flexed 30° and externally rotated (Fig. 15.8). The hip periphery is accessed through an accessory portal as described for the iliopsoas tendon release at the lesser trochanter. The spinal needle is directed to the hip capsule at the level of the anterior femoral neck in an almost perpendicular angle to the femoral neck, cannulated instruments are utilized to establish a viewing portal. A second accessory portal (working portal) is established using a spinal needle guidewire technique and cannulated instruments by triangulating toward the tip of the arthroscope inside the hip periphery. The iliopsoas tendon is located immediately anterior to the hip capsule. It is always found in the space between the anterior zona orbicularis and anterior labrum proximal and anterior to the medial

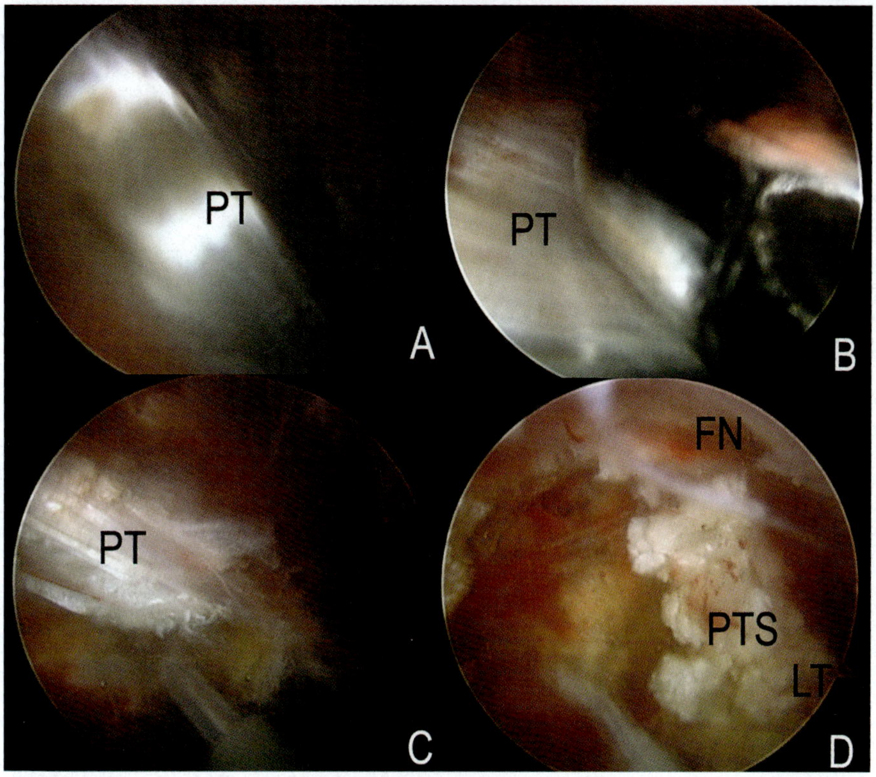

Figure 15.12. Series of arthroscopic photographs demonstrating an endoscopic iliopsoas tendon release on the lesser trochanter in a left hip. **A:** Arthroscopic view of the iliopsoas tendon (PT) in the iliopsoas bursa. **B:** A shaver is in use to remove synovial tissue from around the PT. **C:** A hook radiofrequency probe in use. The PT release is being performed in a retrograde fashion to cut away from the femoral nerve. **D:** After the release is complete the distal iliopsoas tendon stump (PTS) is on the lesser trochanter (LT). The femoral neck (FN) is at the top of the photograph.

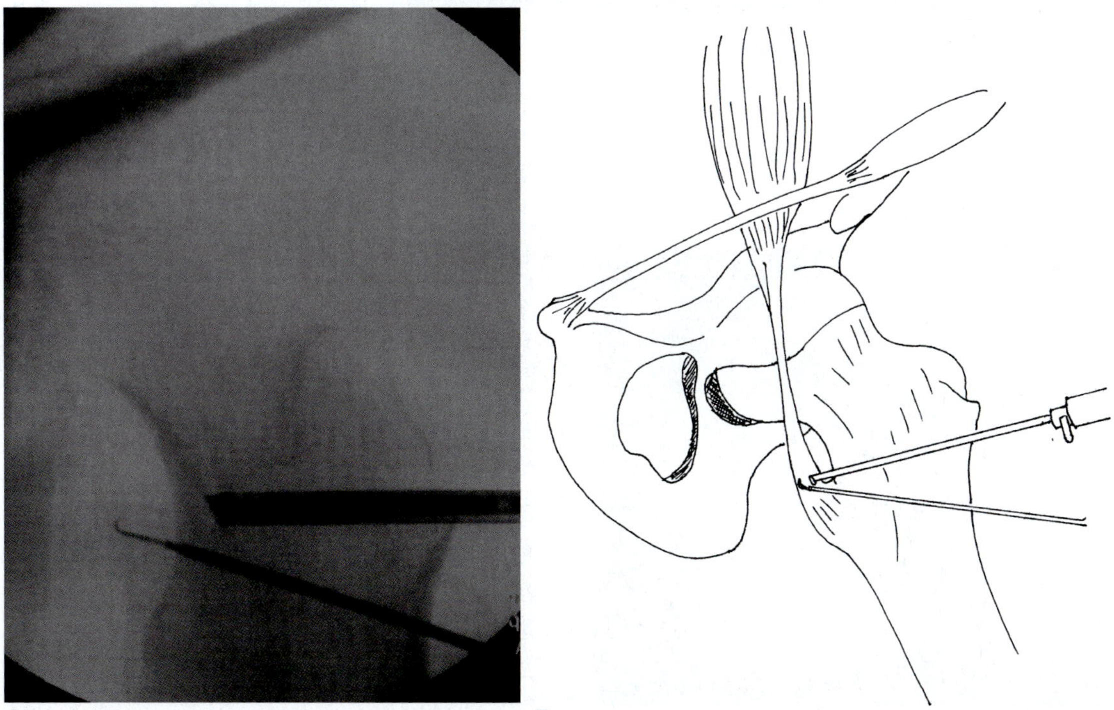

A **B**

Figure 15.13. **A:** Fluoroscopy photograph that demonstrates the position of the tip of the hook radiofrequency device before releasing the iliopsoas tendon. The position of the arthroscope is also demonstrated. **B:** Schematic representation of iliopsoas tendon release at the lesser trochanter. The arthroscope and the radiofrequency device are directed to the lesser trochanter.

synovial fold. A communication may exist at this level between the hip capsule and the iliopsoas bursa. In most cases, the hip capsule is thinner at this region and the iliopsoas tendon can be visualized through the thin portion of the hip capsule. A capsulectomy is performed at this level to gain accesss to the psoas tendon, we use a radiofrequency hook probe for this purpose through a slotted cannula. After the capsulectomy is done, synovial tissue from around the tendon is resected using a shaver. The tendon is released with a radiofrequency hook probe. A slotted cannula is also used to introduce and interchange instruments in the iliopsoas bursa through the defect on the anterior hip capsule (Figs. 15.14 and 15.15A & B). After

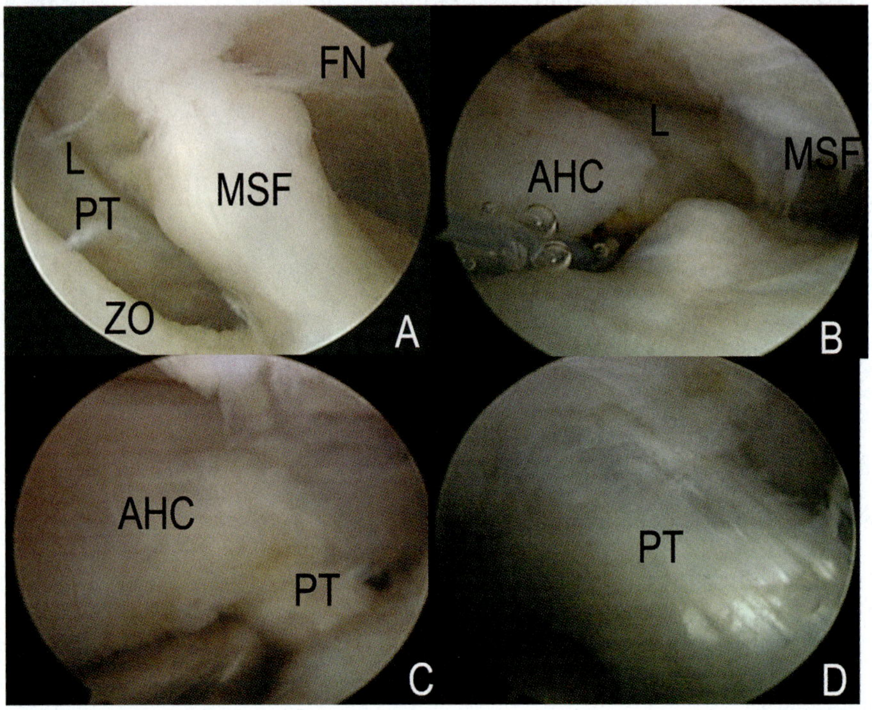

Figure 15.14. Series of arthroscopic photographs demonstrating a transcapsular iliopsoas tendon release in a left hip. **A:** The medial synovial fold (MSF) is to the center of the photograph, to the right, the femoral neck. To the left and bottom of the photograph, the anterior labrum (L) and the anterior zona orbicularis (ZO), respectively. Between the L and the ZO, there is a thin portion of the anterior hip capsule. Behind this thin portion is the PT. In some cases, there is a communication between the iliopsoas bursa and the hip capsule in this area. **B:** In this photograph, a defect on the anterior hip capsule (AHC) is being created using a radiofrequency hook probe to communicate the hip capsule and the iliopsoas bursa. The L is behind the capsulectomy. Part of the MSF is to the right of the photograph. **C:** A shaver is in use through the defect on the AHC to resect synovial tissue from around the PT. **D:** The PT as seen from the defect on the anterior hip capsule. Synovial tissue has been resected and the tendon is ready for release.

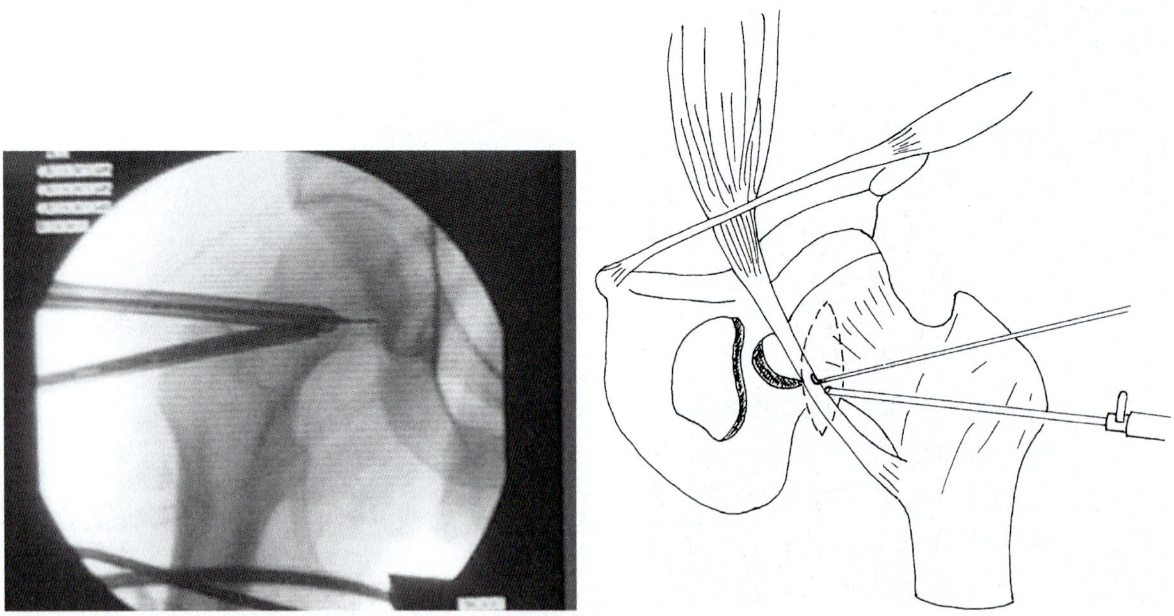

A B

Figure 15.15. **A:** Fluoroscopy photograph that demonstrates the position of the arthroscope and a radiofrequency hook probe (the radiofrequency device is observed through a slotted cannula) in a transcapsular iliopsoas tendon release. **B:** Schematic representation of a transcapsular iliopsoas tendon release. The arthroscope and the radiofrequency device are positioned inside the iliopsoas bursa through a window made on the anterior hip capsule.

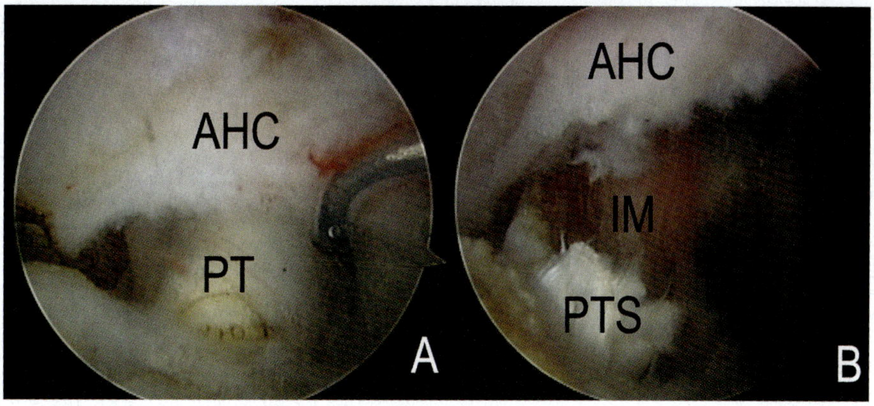

Figure 15.16. Arthroscopic photographs of a transcapsular iliopsoas tendon release in a right hip. **A:** The PT is observed inside the iliopsoas bursa through a defect created on the AHC. **B:** In the same view through the defect on the AHC, the iliopsoas tendon has been released and the distal PTS is at the bottom of the photograph. The intact fibers of the IM are observed behind the stump. AHC, anterior hip capsule; IM, iliacus muscle.

TABLE 15.2 Results of Surgical Treatment of Internal Snapping Hip Syndrome (Open and Endoscopic)

Author	*Number of Hips*	*Technique*	*Follow-up*	*Pain*	*Resnapping*
Taylor and Clarke[27]	17	Open release	17 months	0	5
Jacobson and Allen[28]	20	Open Z-plasty	20 months	2 (reoperated)	6
Dobbs et al.[29]	11	Open Z-plasty	4 years	0	1
Gruen et al.[30]	11	Open Z-plasty	3 years	0	0
Byrd[4]	9	Endoscopic release at the lesser trochanter	20 months	0	0
Ilizaliturri et al.[15]	7	Endoscopic release at the lesser trochanter	21 months	0	0
Dienst[20]	9	Endoscopic release (preserving iliacus muscle) transcapsular	3 months (technique report)	0	0
Flanum et al.[21]	6	Endoscopic release at the lesser trochanter	12 months	0	0

the tendinous portion of the iliopsoas has been released, the iliacus muscle is visible behind the retracted tendon stumps (Fig. 15.16). We do not release the iliacus muscle.

RESULTS

Endoscopic release of the iliopsoas tendon has been recently reported by different authors.[4,15,20,21] Results of endoscopic release of the iliopsoas tendon for internal snapping hip syndrome compare well with results reported for open release of lengthening techniques (Table 15.2).

DISCUSSION

Arthroscopy of the hip joint has evolved greatly in the last decade.[26] Technology to access the hip joint endoscopically has allowed the procedure to become standard in many centers around the world[23] and stimulated developments of new techniques and procedures. Endoscopic treatment of the snapping hip is safe and reproducible. Results of endoscopic techniques compare well with those of open techniques.

REFERENCES

1. Allen WC, Cope R. Coxa saltans: The snapping hip revisited. *J Am Acad Orthop Surg.* 1995;3:303–308.
2. Binnie JF. Snapping hip (Hanche a resort; Schnellend Hefte). *Ann Surg.* 1913;58:59–66.
3. Nunziata A, Blumenfeld I. Cadera a resorte: A propósito de una variedad. *Prensa Med Argent.* 1951;38:1997–2001.
4. Byrd JWT. Evaluation and management of the snapping iliopsoas tendon. *Tech Orthop.* 2005;20:45–51.
5. Provencher MT, Hofmeister EP, Muldoon MP. The surgical treatment of external coxa saltans (the snapping hip) by Z-plasty of the iliotibial band. *Am J Sports Med.* 2004;32:470–476.
6. Pelsser V, Cardinal E, Hobden R, et al. Extraarticular snapping hip: Sonographic findings. *AJR Am J Roentgenol.* 2001;176:67–73.
7. Choi YS, Lee SM, Song BY, et al. Dynamic sonography of external snapping hip syndrome. *J Ultrasound Med.* 2002;21:753–758.
8. Wunderbaldinger P, Bremer C, Schellenberger E, et al. Imaging features of iliopsoas bursitis. *Eur Radiol.* 2002;12:409–415.
9. Cvitanic O, Henzie G, Skezas N, et al. MRI diagnosis of tears of the hip abductor tendons (gluteus medius and gluteus minimus). *AJR Am J Roentgenol.* 2004;182:137–143.

10. White RA, Hughes MS, Burd T. A new operative approach in the correction of external coxa saltans. *Am J Sports Med.* 2004;32:1504–1508.
11. Faraj AA, Moulton A, Sirivastava VM. Snapping iliotibial band: Report of ten cases and review of the literature. *Acta Orthop Belg.* 2001;67:19–23.
12. Brignall CG, Stainsby GD. The snapping hip: Treatment by Z-plasty. *J Bone Joint Surg Br.* 1991;73:253–254.
13. Fery A, Sommelet J. The snapping hip: Late results of 24 surgical cases. *Int Orthop.* 1988;12:277–282.
14. Ilizaliturri VM Jr, Martinez-Escalante FA, Chaidez PA, et al. Endoscopic iliotibial band release for external snapping hip syndrome. *Arthroscopy.* 2006;22:505–510.
15. Ilizaliturri VM Jr, Villalobos FE, Chaidez PA, et al. External snapping hip syndrome: Treatment by endoscopic release of the iliopsoas tendon. *Arthroscopy.* 2005;21: 1375–1380.
16. Ganz R, Parvizi J, Beck M, et al. Femoroacetabular impingement: A cause for osteoarthritis of the hip. *Clin Orthop Relat Res.* 2003;417:112–120.
17. Ilizaliturri VM Jr, Nosa-Barrera JM, Acosta-Rodriguez E, et al. Arthroscopic treatment of femoroacetabular impingement secondary to paediatric hip disorders. *J Bone Joint Surg Br.* 2007;89-B:1025–1030.
18. Harper MC, Schaberg JE, Allen WC. Primary iliopsoas bursography in the diagnosis of disorders of the hip. *Clin Orthop Relat Res.* 1987;221:238–241.
19. Cardinal E, Buckwalter KA, Capello WN, et al. US of the snapping iliopsoas tendon. *Radiology.* 1996;198:521–522.
20. Wettstein M, Jung J, Dienst M. Arthroscopic psoas tenotomy. *Arthroscopy.* 2006;22:907,e1–e4.
21. Flanum ME, Keene JS, Blankenbaker DG, et al. Arthroscopic treatment of the painful "internal" snapping hip: Results of a new endoscopic technique and imaging protocol. *Am J Sports Med.* 2007;35:770–779.
22. Byrd JWT, Pappas JN, Pedley MJ. Hip arthroscopy: An anatomic study of portal placement and relationship to the extraarticular structures. *Arthroscopy.* 1995;11:418–423.
23. Ilizaliturri VM Jr, Mangino G, Valero FS, et al. Special instruments and technique for hip arthroscopy. *Tech Orthop.* 2005;20:9–16.
24. Dienst M, Godde S, Seil R, et al. Hip arthroscopy without traction: In vivo anatomy of the peripheral hip joint cavity. *Arthroscopy.* 2001;17:924–931.
25. Ilizaliturri VM Jr, Mangino G, Valero FS, et al. Hip arthroscopy of the central en peripheral compartments by the lateral approach. *Tech Orthop.* 2005;20:32–36.
26. Lubowitz JH, Poehling GG. Hip arthroscopy: An emerging gold standard. *Arthroscopy.* 2006;22:1257–1259.
27. Taylor GR, Clarke NM. Surgical release of the "snapping iliopsoas tendon." *J Bone Joint Surg Br.* 1995;77:881–883.
28. Jacobson T, Allen WC. Surgical correction of the snapping iliopsoas tendon. *Am J Sports Med.* 1990;18:470–474.
29. Dobbs MB, Gordon JE, Luhmann SJ, et al. Surgical correction of the snapping iliopsoas tendon in adolescents. *J Bone Joint Surg Am.* 2002;84:420–424.
30. Gruen GS, Scioscia TN, Lowenstein JE. The surgical treatment of internal snapping hip. *Am J Sports Med.* 2002;30:607–613.

CHAPTER

16

Travis G. Maak
James E. Voos
Bryan T. Kelly

The Peritrochanteric Compartment

INTRODUCTION

The advent of hip arthroscopy has led to an increased understanding of both intra-articular and extra-articular hip pathology. In 2006, Byrd[1,2] described the anatomic and surgical techniques involved in hip arthroscopy. Recent increasing enthusiasm for hip arthroscopy and minimally invasive surgery, combined with advances in magnetic resonance imaging (MRI) of the hip, have enabled orthopaedic surgeons to broaden the arthroscopic application. Arthroscopic treatment of intra-articular pathology including loose bodies, labral tears, ligamentum teres tears, chondral lesions, synovial chondromatosis, and femoroacetabular impingement have been previously described.[3]

Application of hip arthroscopy has since been expanded to allow visualization and treatment of extra-articular pathology—specifically in the peritrochanteric compartment.

Peritrochanteric compartment disorders including external coxa saltans or snapping hip, trochanteric bursitis, and gluteus medius and minimus tears, which were underappreciated prior to hip arthroscopy, have now been identified as significant causes of lateral hip pain. Some of these disorders were treated conservatively[4] or with open surgery[5,6]; however, these modalities have had varied efficacy and have been associated with significant postoperative morbidity. Conservative treatment is often the preferred treatment modality and includes corticosteroid and anesthetic injections[4] combined with a structured physical therapy regimen. Patients who fail the conservative treatment have previously required open surgery.[5–7]

Recent advances in hip arthroscopy have led to surgical treatment descriptions for many of the peritrochanteric compartment disorders. Recalcitrant trochanteric bursitis can be managed with arthroscopic trochanteric bursectomy.[4,8] Arthroscopic release of the external snapping iliotibial band can effectively treat external coxa saltans.[9] Debridement of gluteus medius and minimus tendonopathy secondary to calcific tendonitis has been described.[10] Repair of gluteus medius and minimus tears, which may cause much of the pain previously associated with refractory trochanteric bursitis, has also been reported.[11] These advances have increased the understanding of hip pain and have provided surgeons with more effective tools to address hip pathology.

This chapter describes the evaluation of the lateral aspect of the hip, the peripheral compartment of the hip anatomy, the associated pathologic entities, and the arthroscopic techniques used to effectively address them.

PATIENT EVALUATION

An in-depth patient history is one of the most effective tools for evaluating a complaint of hip pain. A historical description of hip pain can differentiate intra-articular versus extra-articular pathology. Extra-articular complaints can then be localized to lateral hip pain in the peritrochanteric compartment. When a description of extra-articular, lateral hip pain ismade, the diagnostic differential can be narrowed with descriptive characteristics specific to each peritrochanteric space disorder. These will be later described in each disorder section.

A thorough examination of the entire hip joint with a more focused evaluation of the lateral aspect of the hip should then be used to further define the offending peritrochanteric space disorder. A complete understanding of anatomic origins and insertions of the involved hip muscle groups is crucial to accurate diagnosis of these complex hip pathologies. This understanding is particularly important in the setting of concurrent intra-articular pathology.

Lateral hip pain can arise from direct pain from the peritrochanteric space or referred pain from intra-articular pathology. Palpation of the lateral hip aids in this differential as referred pain may be reproduced with passive and active joint motions, but should not produce tenderness with direct palpation. In this vein, palpation should begin with the origin of the gluteus maximus at the inferior–posterior aspect of the ileum and sacrum. The insertion can then be examined in two locations—the lateral base of the linea aspera on the proximal femur and the tensor fascia latae. Next, the gluteus medius should be palpated from its origin on the anterior and middle aspects of the ileum to its insertion on the middle facet of the greater trochanter. The gluteus minimus can be examined from its origin deep to the gluteus medius to its insertion at the greater trochanter anterior facet. The greater trochanteric bursa should also be appreciated overlying the greater trochanter at the mid-posterior proximal aspect of the femur.

Physical examination of muscle strength can be used to evaluate the abductor strength in the presence or absence of pain. This examination should be conducted with the hip in flexion to assess the tensor fascia latae, in neutral to evaluate the gluteus medius and in extension of the gluteus maximus. This examination should be performed with the knee both flexed and extended to allow tension and relaxation of the iliotibial band, respectively.

Ober test may be used during the physical examination to evaluate contractures of the abductor muscles. This test should also be conducted with the hip in flexion, neutral, and extension. Classically, Ober test is performed in hip extension to assess tension across the tensor fascia latae. The knee should then be flexed to relax the iliotibial band and to allow effective evaluation of the possible gluteus medius contracture. In this position, the knee should be able to internally rotate such that it can touch the table in the absence of pathologic tension.

PERITROCHANTERIC COMPARTMENT PATHOLOGY

EXTERNAL COXA SALTANS (SNAPPING HIP)

External Coxa Saltans, or "snapping hip," is characterized by a palpable or audible snapping as the hip is ranged from flexion to extension. This entity is most often seen during athletic activity but may occur with activities of daily life. Diagnosis of snapping hip is generally obtained with a combination of historical description and audible or palpable snapping on physical examination. However, dynamic sonography of the hip has been used as an adjuvant to confirming the diagnosis, especially when surgical treatment is indicated.[12]

While intra-articular, internal, and external categories of coxa saltans have been described, in most cases the snapping is external and has been attributed to an excessively thick, tense iliotibial band or gluteus maximus tendon moving over the greater trochanter.[13] Anatomically, with the hip extended, the iliotibial band lies posterior to the greater trochanter and slips anteriorly over the greater trochanter during hip flexion. The tight anterior attachments of the tensor fascia latae, the presence of the gluteus maximus posteriorly, and the association with gluteus medius aponeurosis restrict the iliotibial band over the greater trochanter throughout the hip range of motion.[14] The slipping motion termed external coxa saltans produces the perceived lateral hip pain. Additionally, inflammation or injury to the trochanteric bursa can further exacerbate the pain produced by iliotibial band snapping.

In most cases, external coxa saltans is either asymptomatic or can be treated conservatively with rest, activity modification, stretching, corticosteroid injections, and physical therapy.[13,14] While conservative treatment is often successful, some patients may remain symptomatic and require surgical treatment. Zoltan et al.[6] described an open surgical technique for the treatment of recalcitrant external coxa saltans, which involved excision of an ellipsoid-shaped portion of the iliotibial band overlying the greater trochanter and removal of the trochanteric bursa. Postoperative follow-up demonstrated 80% (4/5) of patients had significant improvement or relief of their symptoms, while 20% (1/5) failed the treatment. A minimally invasive technique using transverse step cuts in the fascia along a longitudinal facial incision has also been described.[15] Fourteen of sixteen hips remained asymptomatic postoperatively.

While these open techniques have shown positive results in treating external coxa saltans, peritrochanteric compartment arthroscopy is also a viable treatment modality. Treatment of external coxa saltans with endoscopic iliotibial band release has been described by multiple authors with promising results.[14,16] Ilizaliturri et al.[16] treated 11 patients with all patients experiencing no complaints and full return to previous activity level. Similarly, Jacobson et al.[14] treated 20 patients and reported that 19 of 20 experienced significant relief of symptoms.

TROCHANTERIC BURSITIS

Trochanteric bursitis and greater trochanteric pain syndrome are generally chronic entities prevalent in older females, and have been previously associated with long distance running, low back pain, coxa saltans, iliotibial band syndrome, and hip arthroplasty and osteotomy.[8,17–21] Diagnostic criteria are solely clinical and are characterized by chronic, intermittent aching pain over the lateral aspect of the hip. Conservative treatment in the form of one or two local corticosteroids and local anesthetic preparation injections combined with physical therapy is the mainstay of diagnosis and treatment.[4] The excellent diagnostic results produced by history, physical exam—including Little test,[22]—and relief with injection have obviated the need for routine MRI. This therapeutic regimen has demonstrated excellent responses in 66% of cases and improvement in the remaining 33%.[20] However, conservative therapy is not without drawbacks. Multiple or inappropriately placed corticosteroid injections have been associated with gluteus medius injury.[23] In this setting or if the patient fails conservative treatment, surgery may be required. MRI may be used to confirm potential gluteus medius and minimus tears and further guide surgical treatment. Open trochanteric bursectomy has been described for these refractory cases.[5,6] Trends toward arthroscopic treatment have also produced descriptions of endoscopic bursectomy in the literature.[7,8]

GLUTEUS MEDIUS AND MINIMUS TEARS

The insertions of the gluteus medius and minimus at the greater trochanter and tears at this insertion have been related to the insertion and tears of the rotator cuff tendons at the greater tuberosity.[24–26] As a result of this similarity, injuries to these abductor tendons have been termed "Rotator Cuff Tears of the Hip."[24–26] These tears have been identified during open debridement of recalcitrant trochanteric bursitis[25] and treatment of femoral neck fractures.[24] Descriptions of calcific tendonitis at the hip have also included relationships with gluteus medius and minimus tears, thus further substantiating the rotator cuff similarity.[27–29] The treatment has been described in an open fashion when encountered in the setting of refractory iliotibial band syndrome and total hip arthroplasty. The true incidence of gluteus medius and minimus tears is not known. A prospective study by Bunker et al.,[24] of 50 patients with fractures of the femoral neck revealed a 22% incidence of tears of the gluteus medius and minimus. In addition, Howell et al.[30] conducted another prospective study of 176 consecutive patients who underwent total hip arthroplasty for osteoarthritis and identified 20% with degenerative pathology.

As noted previously, suspected gluteus medius tendon tears in patients with trochanteric bursitis may be confirmed with MRI (Fig. 16.1). This modality aids to confirm the clinical suspicion in patients with refractory trochanteric bursitis, with lateral hip pain and an ambulatory limp likely related to hip abductor weakness.[23] Like trochanteric bursitis, open surgical techniques have been described for the treatment of these conditions. Arthroscopic treatment of trochanteric bursitis and calcific tendonitis of the gluteus medius and minimus has also been reported by Kandemir et al.[10] Voos et al.[11] recently

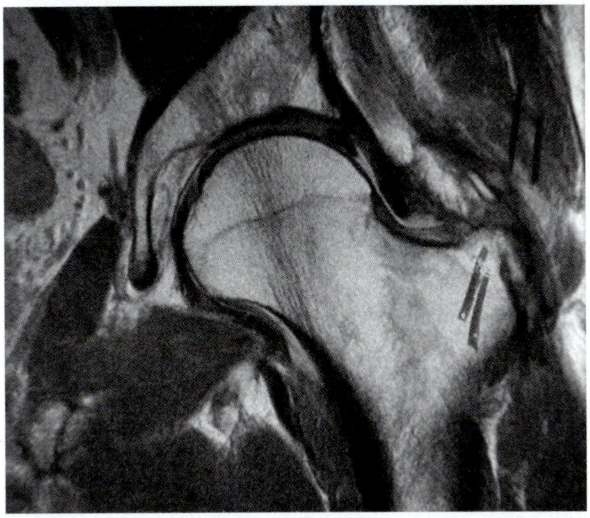

Figure 16.1. This coronal MRI of a left hip reveals a tear of the gluteus medius off of the greater trochanter.

reported an arthroscopic approach that provides access for the repair of gluteus medius and minimus tendon tears.

ARTHROSCOPIC ANATOMY AND TECHNIQUE

Improvements in radiographic imaging techniques including MRI have increased the surgeon's ability to predictably diagnose intra-articular and extra-articular disorders. Advancements in arthroscopic techniques and instrumentation have enabled better visualization and treatment of hip pathology. The increased visualization, both radiographically and arthroscopically, has subsequently improved the understanding of the intra-articular anatomy and the biomechanics of the hip—specifically from an arthroscopic perspective. Voos et al.[11] recently described the arthroscopic approach to and treatment of disorders in the peritrochanteric compartment, thus expanding this understanding to the extra-articular hip.

The central, intra-articular compartment is first inspected with the arthroscope to assess for concomitant hip pathology prior to examining the lateral compartment of the hip. With this done, complete attention is directed to the extra-articular spaces. The peritrochanteric compartment of the hip is a potential space which can be accessed easily with the use of an arthroscope. The borders consist of the iliotibial band and tensor fascia latae laterally, vastus lateralis inferomedially, abductor tendons superomedially, gluteus maximus muscle superiorly, and gluteus maximus tendon insertion on the linea aspera posteriorly. Within the space the trochanteric bursa can be found, and it is of variable thickness based on the degree of inflammation and duration of symptoms.

In evaluating the space endoscopically, a consistent, routine evaluation ensures that all pathologies are addressed. Examination of the space is performed through the placement of three portals.

The first portal is the anterior portal. It provides the best access to the peritrochanteric space. The portal is placed 1 cm lateral to the anterior superior iliac spine (ASIS) in the interval between the tensor fascia latae and sartorius. The cannula is directed into the peritrochanteric space with the leg in full extension, held in 0° of adduction, and 10° to 15° of internal rotation. The cannula is aimed posterior and swept back and forth between the iliotibial band overlying the greater trochanteric bursa and the greater trochanter. This technique is analogous to accessing the subacromial space in the shoulder where the iliotibial band is analogous to the undersurface of the acromion. When the portal is placed appropriately, a clear space between the iliotibial band and the greater trochanter can be easily identified. If in doubt, cannula placement can be confirmed under fluoroscopy. A second, distal posterior portal is placed midway between the tip of the greater trochanter and the vastus tubercle along the posterior one third of the greater trochanteric midline. This portal placement facilitates access distally and proximally for both diagnostic evaluation and operative intervention. A third portal is placed proximal to the tip of the greater trochanter in line with the distal posterior portal. This portal facilitates more proximal work, and can also be used for more distal visualization.

Proper portal placement is crucial to understanding the peritrochanteric space and should be first oriented at the gluteus maximus insertion into the linea aspera (Fig. 16.2). Inspection should proceed in a counterclockwise fashion starting distally and posterior at the gluteus maximus insertion. This is done using the 70° scope placed into the anterior portal, and both the light source and camera are positioned proximally and oriented distally. The peritrochanteric space is typically distended with approximately 50 mm Hg pressurization. Hemostasis can be obtained with either radiofrequency ablation or standard coagulation. Sometimes, fibrinous bands in this area will require excision.

The initial view includes the insertion of the gluteus maximus into the posterior border of the iliotibial band, which is the starting point to begin a stepwise inspection of the space. This insertion can be probed and the bursa cleaned from this area with a motorized shaver. Looking proximally with the camera, the longitudinal lines of the vastus lateralis are identified and can be traced up to the insertion at the vastus tubercle

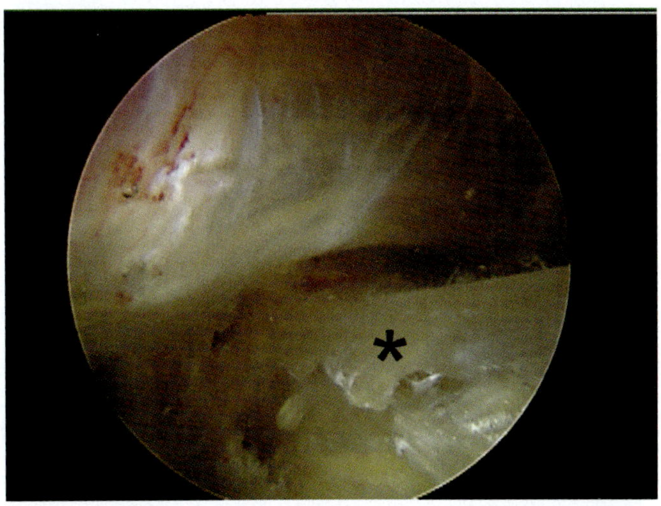

Figure 16.2. This arthroscopic image of the left hip demonstrates the insertion of the gluteus maximus (*) at the linea aspera. This image represents the initial view, which is the starting point to begin a stepwise inspection of the peritrochanteric compartment.

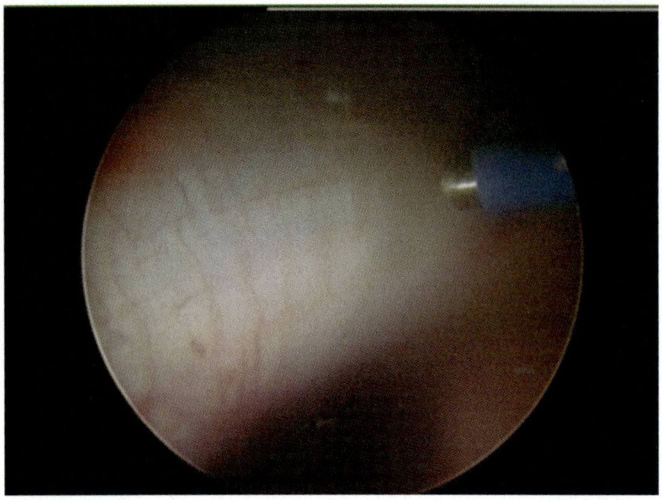

Figure 16.3. Arthroscopic probe identifying the vastus lateralis.

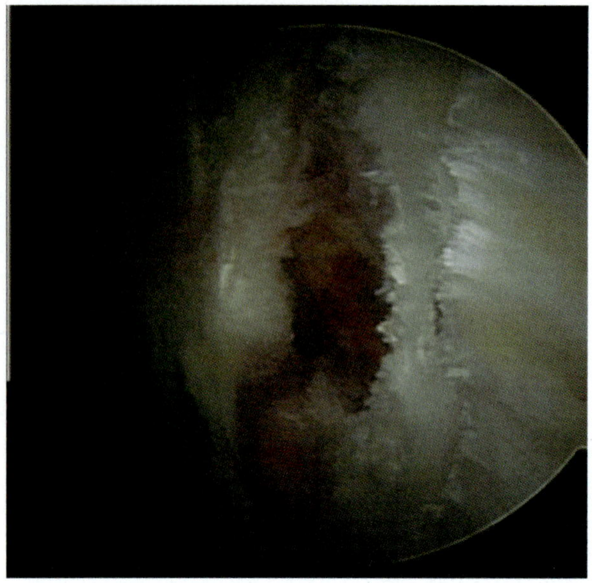

Figure 16.4. Arthroscopic image of the left hip demonstrating the iliotibial band following release for treatment of external snapping hip.

immediately anterior to the anterior facet (Fig. 16.3). The gluteus minimus tendon and muscle are visualized anteriorly with the scope source and camera placed laterally looking anterior and superior. As the scope is rotated superiorly, the gluteus medius will come into view with its insertion into the greater trochanter. It should be thoroughly probed and visualized to identify the presence of full-thickness tendon insertion tears. Further cleaning of the fibrinous bands of the trochanteric bursa overlying this area may be required for better access and visualization through the posterior portal. In cases of trochanteric bursitis, these fibrous bands are inflamed and can be fairly thick. Use of electrocautery or an arthroscopic 5.5 mm shaver is useful to remove this tissue. The gluteus maximus tendinous contribution to both the linea aspera and the tensor fascia can be visualized by looking laterally. Finally, the scope should be turned toward the iliotibial band. In particular, the posterior one third of the iliotibial band is implicated in coxa saltans externus and may be causing direct abrasive wear to the greater trochanter.

If the presence of coxa saltans externus is identified or snapping of the iliotibial band over this area has been refractory to nonoperative treatment, a release may be required with the use of an electrocautery device (Fig. 16.4). The release should be performed along the posterolateral portion of the greater trochanter beginning at the vastus tubercle insertion extending to the tip of the greater trochanter in a z-type release of 1 cm anterior, 3 cm distal, and 1 cm posterior with slight variations of this being required by digital and instrumented palpation in view of the particular fibers under the greatest amount of tension.

Surgery is indicated in patients who fail conservative treatment and have the evidence of abductor tendon tear on MRI. Prior to any surgical intervention, all patients should receive an injection of corticosteroid into the lateral compartment to assess for pain relief. The gluteus medius tendon should be examined in a manner similar to subacromial examination of the rotator cuff. All tears should have fibrinous, scarred bands released over the maximus or the medius. When a repairable tear is identified as in Fig. 16.5, the edges are debrided with a full-radius shaver and prepared for repair. The attachment site of the tendon at the greater trochanter is prepared with a full-radius shaver similar to the preparation of the footprint for rotator cuff tears (Fig. 16.6). Suture anchors can be placed into the

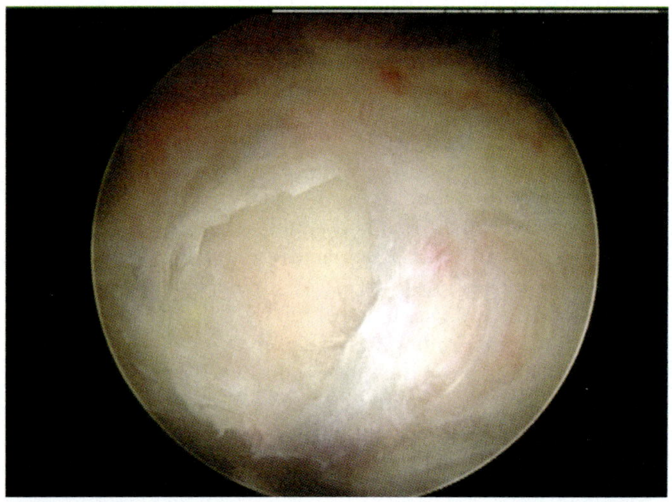

Figure 16.5. This image is an arthroscopic view of the left hip revealing a traumatic gluteus medius tear from the greater trochanter.

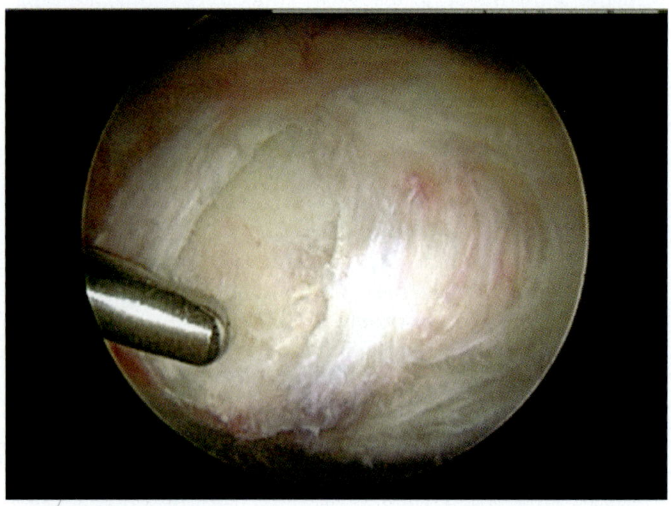

Figure 16.6. The attachment site of the tendon at the greater trochanter is prepared with a full-radius shaver similar to preparation of the footprint for rotator cuff tears.

footprint of the abductor tendons in a standard arthroscopic fashion (Fig. 16.7). We have used both metal and bioabsorbable sutures depending upon the bone quality. Fluoroscopic guidance may be helpful in directing the anchors in the appropriate direction and location (Fig. 16.8). Once the anchors are placed, the sutures are retrieved and passed sequentially through the edges of the prepared gluteus medius tendon with a suture passing device and tied under arthroscopic visualization with an arthroscopic knot pusher (Figs. 16.9 & 16.10).

REHABILITATION

Postoperative rehabilitation for patients undergoing bursectomy or iliotibial band release consists of weight bearing as tolerated with crutches for the first postoperative week. Full weight bearing is advanced without crutches, as the patients pain tolerates. Range of motion and hip strengthening without restrictions begins as soon as the patient's pain allows. It is important to avoid aggravating the lateral hip with too aggressive therapy immediately after surgery.

In patients undergoing repair of the gluteus medius and minimus tears, physical therapy consists of 6 weeks foot flat weight bearing with crutches. The patient is fitted with a hip abduction brace that blocks active abduction. No limitation of hip flexion or extension is required. Strengthening of the hip abductors should begin at 6 weeks. Running is not allowed until the patient displays equal abductor strength bilaterally to support the pelvis.

In the senior author's experience with short-term follow-up of patients at 1 to 2 years postoperative undergoing endoscopic repair of the gluteus medius, all patients have completely resolved lateral hip pain symptoms, returned to full activity and experienced no clinical failures of the repair.

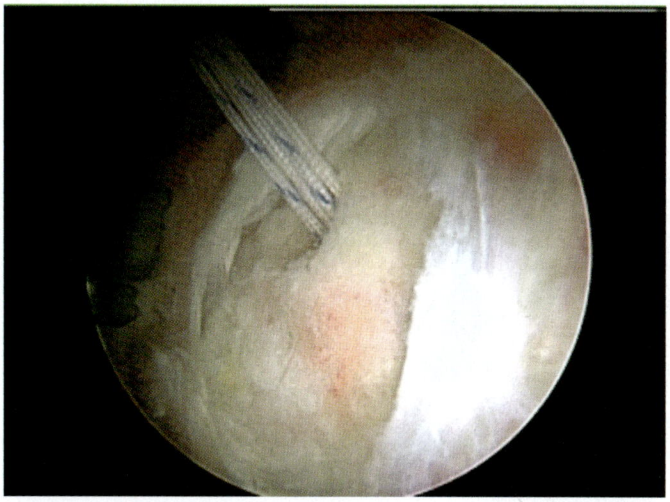

Figure 16.7. Arthroscopic view of the initial suture anchor placed in the prepared bed of the greater trochanter.

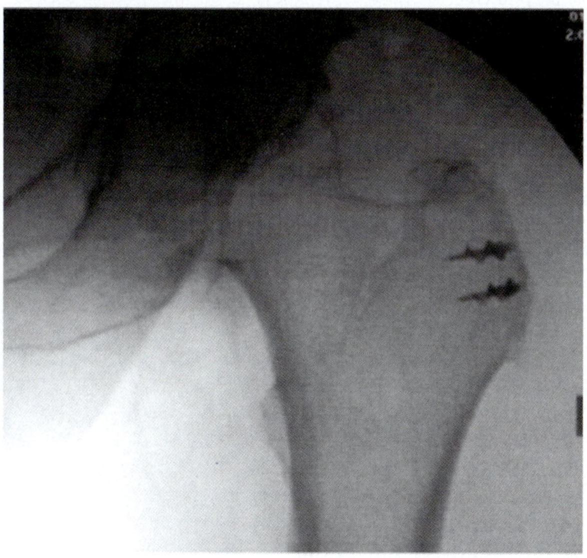

Figure 16.8. Intraoperative use of fluoroscopy to confirm adequate anchor placement in the greater trochanter of the left hip.

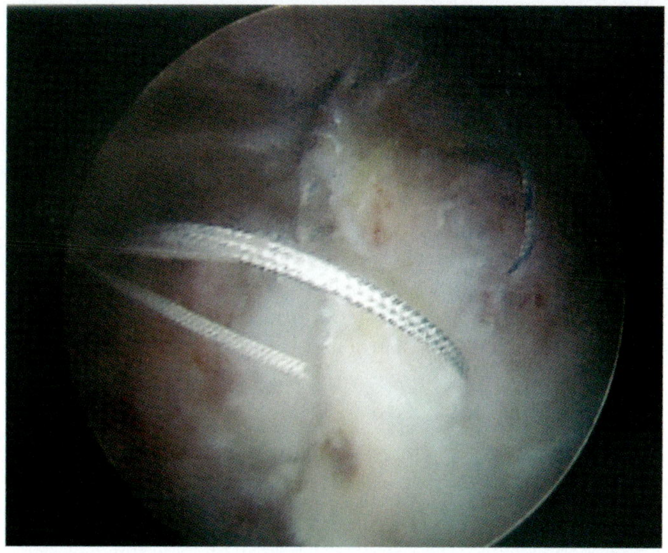

Figure 16.9. Retrieval and passage of sutures through the gluteus medius tendon are performed in a manner similar to that of the rotator cuff and tied under arthroscopic visualization.

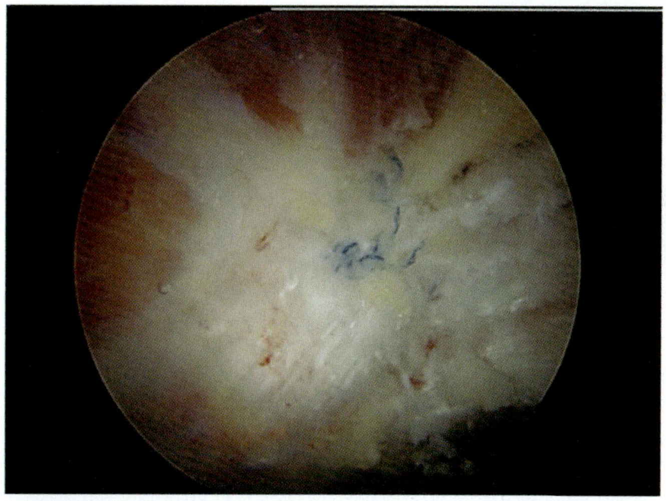

Figure 16.10. Arthroscopic image displaying the final repair of the gluteus medius after sutures have been tied with an arthroscopic knot pusher.

SUMMARY

Advancement in arthroscopic techniques has now enabled more effective identification and treatment of peritrochanteric compartment disorders, including external coxa saltans, trochanteric bursitis, and gluteus medius and minimus tears when conservative treatment has failed. A thorough understanding of arthroscopic anatomy of the hip and proper placement of portals is crucial for surgical ease and outcome success. Continued improvements through clinical studies and instrumentation will expand the viable treatment options and allow more effective management of extra-articular hip pain.

REFERENCES

1. Byrd JW. Hip arthroscopy. *J Am Acad Orthop Surg.* 2006;14(7):433–444.
2. Byrd JW. Hip arthroscopy: Surgical indications. *Arthroscopy.* 2006;22(12):1260–1262.
3. Kelly BT, Williams RJ III, Philippon MJ. Hip arthroscopy: Current indications, treatment options, and management issues. *Am J Sports Med.* 2003;31(6):1020–1037.
4. Fox JL. The role of arthroscopic bursectomy in the treatment of trochanteric bursitis. *Arthroscopy.* 2002;18(7):E34.
5. Govaert LH, van der Vis HM, Marti RK, et al. Trochanteric reduction osteotomy as a treatment for refractory trochanteric bursitis. *J Bone Joint Surg Br.* 2003;85(2):199–203.
6. Zoltan DJ, Clancy WG Jr, Keene JS. A new operative approach to snapping hip and refractory trochanteric bursitis in athletes. *Am J Sports Med.* 1986;14(3):201–204.
7. Brooker AF Jr. The surgical approach to refractory trochanteric bursitis. *Johns Hopkins Med J.* 1979;145(3):98–100.
8. Wiese M, Rubenthaler F, Willburger RE, et al. Early results of endoscopic trochanter bursectomy. *Int Orthop.* 2004;28(4):218–221.
9. Ilizaliturri VM Jr, Villalobos FE Jr, Chaidez PA, et al. Internal snapping hip syndrome: Treatment by endoscopic release of the iliopsoas tendon. *Arthroscopy.* 2005;21(11):1375–1380.
10. Kandemir U, Bharam S, Philippon MJ, et al. Endoscopic treatment of calcific tendinitis of gluteus medius and minimus. *Arthroscopy.* 2003;19(1):E4.
11. Voos JE, Rudzki JR, Shindle MK, et al. Arthroscopic anatomy and surgical techniques for peritrochanteric space disorders in the hip. *Arthroscopy.* 2007;23:1246.el–5.
12. Choi YS, Lee SM, Song BY, et al. Dynamic sonography of external snapping hip syndrome. *J Ultrasound Med.* 2002;21(7):753–758.
13. Allen WC, Cope R. Coxa saltans: The snapping hip revisited. *J Am Acad Orthop Surg.* 1995;3(5):303–308.
14. Jacobson T, Allen WC. Surgical correction of the snapping iliopsoas tendon. *Am J Sports Med.* 1990;18(5):470–474.
15. White RA, Hughes MS, Burd T, et al. A new operative approach in the correction of external coxa saltans: The snapping hip. *Am J Sports Med.* 2004;32(6):1504–1508.
16. Ilizaliturri VM Jr, Martinez-Escalante FA, Chaidez PA, et al. Endoscopic iliotibial band release for external snapping hip syndrome. *Arthroscopy.* 2006;22(5):505–510.
17. Clancy WG. Runners' injuries. Part two. Evaluation and treatment of specific injuries. *Am J Sports Med.* 1995;8(4):287–289.
18. Collee G, Dijkmans BA, Vandenbroucke JP, et al. Greater trochanteric pain syndrome (trochanteric bursitis) in low back pain. *Scand J Rheumatol.* 1991;20(4):262–266.
19. Collee G, Dijkmans BA, Vandenbroucke JP, et al. A clinical epidemiological study in low back pain: Description of two clinical syndromes. *Br J Rheumatol.* 1990;29(5):354–357.
20. Ege Rasmussen KJ, Fano N. Trochanteric bursitis: Treatment by corticosteroid injection. *Scand J Rheumatol.* 1985;14(4):417–420.
21. Tortolani PJ, Carbone JJ, Quartararo LG. Greater trochanteric pain syndrome in patients referred to orthopedic spine specialists. *Spine J.* 2002;2(4):251–254.
22. Little H. Trochanteric bursitis: A common cause of pelvic girdle pain. *Can Med Assoc J.* 1979;120(4):456–458.
23. LaBan MM, Weir SK, Taylor RS. "Bald trochanter" spontaneous rupture of the conjoined tendons of the gluteus medius and minimus presenting as a trochanteric bursitis. *Am J Phys Med Rehabil.* 2004;83(10):806–809.
24. Bunker TD, Esler CN, Leach WJ. Rotator-cuff tear of the hip. *J Bone Joint Surg Br.* 1997;79(4):618–620.
25. Kagan A II. Rotator cuff tears of the hip. *Clin Orthop Relat Res.* 1999;(368):135–140.
26. Kingzett-Taylor A, Tirman PF, Feller J, et al. Tendinosis and tears of gluteus medius and minimus muscles as a cause of hip pain: MR imaging findings. *Am J Roentgenol.* 1999;173(4):1123–1126.
27. Callaghan BD. Unusual calcification in the region of the gluteus medius and minimus muscles. *Australas Radiol.* 1977;21(4):362–366.
28. Gordon EJ. Trochanteric bursitis and tendinitis. *Clin Orthop.* 1961;20:193–202.
29. Leonard MH. Trochanteric syndrome; calcareous and noncalcareous tendonitis and bursitis about the trochanter major. *J Am Med Assoc.* 1958;168(2):175–177.
30. Howell GE, Biggs RE, Bourne RB. Prevalence of abductor mechanism tears of the hips in patients with osteoarthritis. *J Arthroplasty.* 2001;16(1):121–123.

CHAPTER

17

Victor M. Ilizaliturri Jr.
Alexander Tomic-Loftkjaer

The Role of Hip Arthroscopy in Pediatric Hip Disease

INTRODUCTION

Even though hip arthroscopy is an established and reproducible procedure,[1] its role in pediatric hip disease (PHD) is still developing and expanding. The pediatric hip can be subject to affections due to different etiologies: infectious, traumatic, or developmental. All of these etiologies may bring anatomical or clinical alterations on the short- and long-term. Hip arthroscopy offers a means to complete a diagnostic procedure, or to perform treatment in some cases, with the advantage of being minimally invasive in relation to open procedures. In the pediatric population, the ligamentum teres artery still supplies a significant portion of the blood flow to the femoral head. Open procedures with hip-controlled dislocation disrupt this blood supply increasing the risk of avascular necrosis, unlike the arthroscopic approach in which the ligament and its artery is usually preserved.[2]

Disorders that affect the pediatric hip may be intra-articular or extra-articular. Traumatic lesions may involve apophyseal injuries, labral injuries, chondral injuries, loose bodies formation, and/or hip dislocation.[3–6] Atraumatic affections of the hip which can induce childhood pain are septic arthritis (SAH), Legg–Calvé–Perthes (LCP) disease, slipped capital femoral epiphysis (SCFE), osteomyelitis, pyomyositis, transient synovitis, femoral neck stress fractures, tumors, juvenile rheumatoid arthritis (JRA), and developmental dysplasia (DDH). SAH, LCP disease, and DDH have been considered the most common affections that may lead to anatomic and functional alterations resulting in clinical disability despite treatment interventions.[7,8] These PHDs are susceptible to treatment through arthroscopic technique at different stages of their natural history or after treatment has been established.[2,9,10]

SEPTIC ARTHRITIS OF THE HIP

Atraumatic hip or knee pain in a young patient (0 to 6 years) requires ruling out a SAH due to potential damage to the joint if treatment is delayed.[11–13] SAH is usually diagnosed clinically and by employing laboratory studies including leukocyte count and erythrocyte sedimentation rate. Ultrasound guided hip aspiration is also routinely performed and may give a definitive diagnosis. Conventional radiographs may help rule out other hip affections with more evident anatomical alterations. The role of hip arthroscopy in this disease has been mostly as a means to perform joint lavage without the possible complications associated with a more classical open washout.[10,14,15] It also allows obtaining a culture sample and placing drainage.[2] Possible complications of an open procedure range from avascular necrosis to the esthetic implications of a scarring in a young patient. As an additional advantage, arthroscopy offers a less invasive way to obtain a biopsy to rule out JRA or transient synovitis (Fig. 17.1), which have been reported to present similarly to SAH. Chung et al.[14] present a series of patients as young as 2.4-year-old subject to hip arthroscopy due to SAH. They conclude that arthroscopic lavage and synovectomy may be performed safely in patients ranging from 2 to 7 years of age.

LEGG–CALVÉ–PERTHES DISEASE

LCP disease has been reported by some authors as the most common indication for hip arthroscopy in pediatric patients. The traditional indication for arthroscopy in this condition is to determine the severity of cartilage damage on the femoral head and the removal of loose bodies in more advanced cases (Fig. 17.2).[10,16,17] It may also be employed for debridement of labral and ligamentum teres tears.[18] Sequelae of LCP disease can be coxa magna, coxa brevis, coxa irregularis, and osteochondritis dissecans. Femoroacetabular impingement (FAI) may result after these deformities are established. This secondary anatomic alteration will lead to mechanical symptoms, diminished range of motion, and eventual degenerative osteoarthritis of the hip. Debridement of loose bodies and labral tears often results in improvement of mechanical symptoms of the hip.[13,19–21] More recent successful hip reshaping has been reported using arthroscopic techniques.[22] In the case of osteochondritis dissecans, it involves an incomplete healing of the necrotic epiphysis and the use of hip arthroscopy to determine the magnitude of the lesion and resection of necrotic tissue has been described.[17]

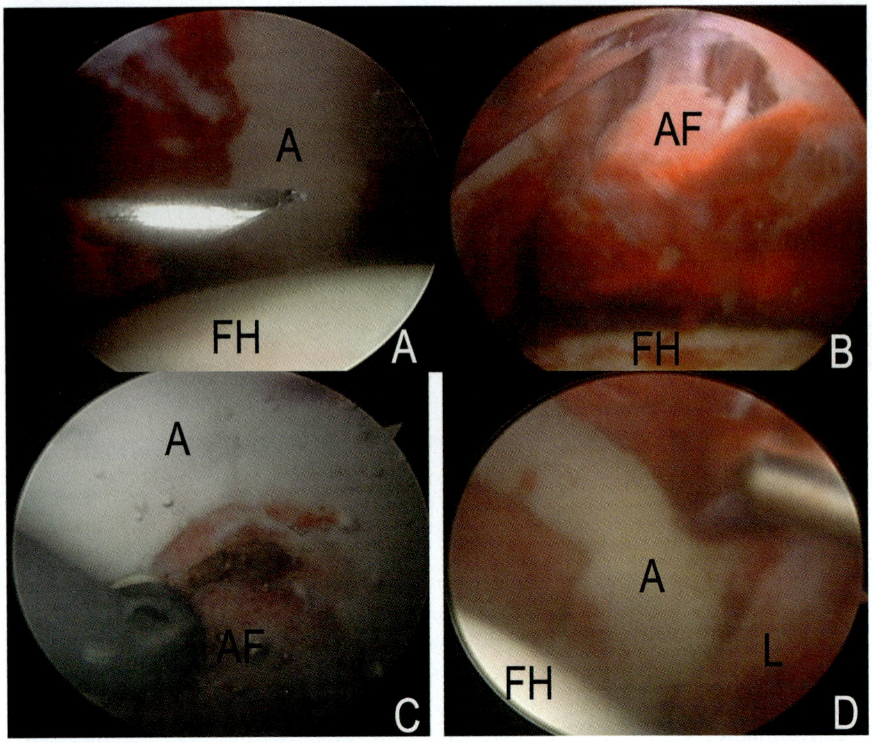

Figure 17.1. Series of arthroscopic photographs of a left hip with transient synovitis. **A:** The acetabulum (A) is at the top of the photograph and the femoral head (FH) is at the bottom. To the left, an arthroscopy needle is observed entering through the anterior hip capsule. Hypertrophic synovial tissue is around the needle. **B:** The acetabular fossa (AF) is occupied by hypertrophic synovium, the FH is at the bottom. **C:** The hypertrophic tissue presented in the prior photograph has been removed from the AF. The A is at the top. **D:** Hypertrophic synovium is observed infiltrating the sulcus between the posterior labrum (L) and the A. The FH is to the left. A shaver is used to resect the synovium.

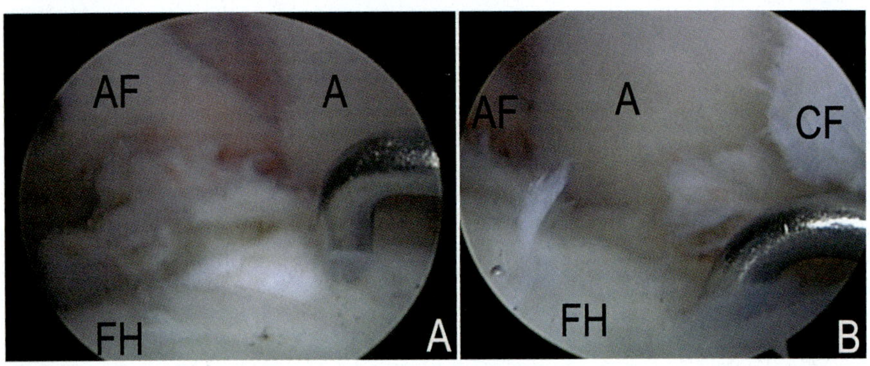

Figure 17.2. Series of arthroscopic photographs of a right hip with LCP disease. **A:** The acetabular fossa (AF) is to the left of the photograph. The ligamentum teres is hypertrophic. A probe is at the chondral defect on the femoral head (FH), which is secondary to Perthes disease. The acetabulum (A) is observed behind the probe. **B:** The defect on the FH is being depressed by the probe. The AF is to the left, the A is observed behind the FH, and a chondral flap (CF) is to the right of the photograph.

DEVELOPMENTAL DYSPLASIA OF THE HIP

Treatment for DDH in young patients implies obtaining a proper coverage of the femoral head by the acetabular rim. Multiple procedures are employed by pediatric orthopedists, ranging from external restraints to the maintenance of proper head position to femoral and pelvic osteotomies.

In older children or young adults, the indication and results of such procedures are less clear and predictable.[23] Even in those patients with satisfactory results, these procedures present themselves with anatomical alterations and may develop mechanical symptoms.[24] Labral tears and loose cartilage fragments can produce mechanical symptoms like catching and locking of the hip.[25] It has been reported on young adults suffering from DDH that labral lesions are the first cause of hip pain.[26] Dysplastic hips, if left untreated, will probably evolve to chondral lesions and eventually early hip osteoarthritis.[26]

The cases with indication of treatment employing the arthroscopic approach should be selected based on clinical history, understanding and correct examination, and interpretation of clinical studies.[22] The patient may present mechanical hip symptoms and reject an open approach. Traditional procedures such as augmentation, acetabular osteotomies, and reorientation have their own limitations.[27] Arthroscopic examination can determine the extent of the labral and ligamentum teres lesions and chondral involvement, which are predictors of the outcome.[24,28] It is an alternative in selected cases where the objective is to delay total hip replacement either because of medical indication or because of patient preferences, age, and expectations. This procedure is better in adults in the fourth or fifth decade of life with mild dysplasia and little degenerative changes.[24]

DDH cases in which closed reduction is unsuccessful may benefit from arthroscopic-assisted surgical treatment. Bulut et al.[29] present a small case series of children ranging from ages 11 to 14 months old. All children presented DDH, which did not respond to treatment with close reduction. The technique described includes a minimal anterior incision to perform tenotomy of the iliopsoas. The arthroscope is employed to visualize the acetabular space and remove the hypertrophic ligamentum teres, the transverse ligament, and the pulvinar. A short-term follow-up shows promising results; all cases improved their acetabular index, no leg length discrepancy or joint restriction was observed.

Patients previously treated for their DDH may present mechanical symptoms. Among the most common procedures are coverage osteotomies, proximal femoral osteotomies, and open reduction and tenotomies. In some of these cases, the presence of hardware may limit the information obtained in a complete workup. The presence of ligamentum teres ruptures and hypertrophy, labral entrapment, chondral lesions, and loose bodies in these cases has been reported. Excision of loose bodies and microfracture of osteochondral lesions has been done successfully (Fig. 17.3).[10,22,30–36,40] Hip arthroscopy may be an alternative to an open procedure in certain cases, but it may also be considered a complementary intervention to assess results and address some of its limitations.[24,49] Hip arthroscopy is no substitute for acetabular reorientation procedures in cases with moderate to severe acetabular dysplasia, especially in young patients that may benefit more from a procedure that normalizes the anatomy of the hip joint.[10,24]

SLIPPED CAPITAL FEMORAL EPIPHYSIS

SCFE results in an anatomic alteration of the femoral head–neck union. This shape has been described as a "pistol grip" deformity. Essentially, the head–neck anterior offset is diminished, resulting in a cam type FAI.[36,37] Arthroscopy has been employed with a diagnostic purpose determining the amount of cartilage injury and the presence of labral injury. The drainage of the hematoma and relief of intra-articular pressure reducing pain have also been reported.[38] It has also been described as an adjunct procedure to ensure the positioning of the pins in the treatment of SCFE. Finally, the resection of the anterolateral head–neck area in cases of FAI to reproduce a proper anterior offset in older patients has been reported.[49]

JUVENILE RHEUMATOID ARTHRITIS

Patients presenting with JRA may benefit from hip arthroscopy as a means to determine chondral lesions and amount of synovitis.[39,40] It offers a less invasive means to obtain a tissue biopsy to perform a definitive diagnosis. Finally, there have been reports of temporary relief with arthroscopic washout and synovectomy (Fig. 17.3).

TUMORS OF THE HIP

Benign tumors in the pediatric hip may be located intracapsularly. These may be managed with arthroscopic excision. A sample biopsy may be obtained through this technique with minimal morbidity and rapid functional recovery.[41] The use of arthroscopy has been reported in the treatment of osteoid osteoma,[41] chondroblastoma,[42] synovial chondromatosis,[43] and osteochondromas in multiple exostoses.[44] It can be used to address benign and pseudotumoral lesions.

FEMOROACETABULAR IMPINGEMENT

FAI is the result of overcoverage of the femoral head anterolaterally and/or an abnormal femoral head–neck union. It is usually diagnosed in adulthood, but it may be secondary to pediatric disorders already mentioned, such as LCP disease, SCFE, and

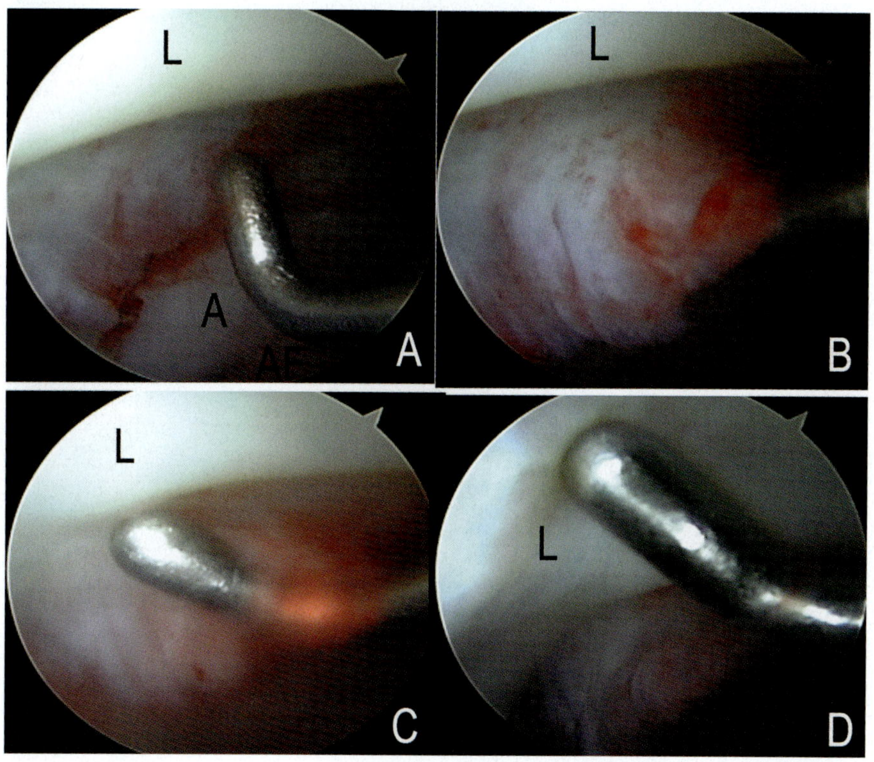

Figure 17.3. Series of arthroscopic photographs of a right hip with mild hip dysplasia. **A:** The labrum (L) is at the top. A probe is on a delamination cartilage flap medial to the anterior L. The acetabular fossa (AF) is at the bottom. **B:** A probe is used to manipulate the chondral flap (CF), the L is at the top. **C:** The CF is reduced to its original position using a probe, the L is lateral to the flap. **D:** The probe is used to verify the stability of L on the acetabular rim.

DDH. More subtle symptoms can be recognized in young athletes and have been positively correlated with findings in magnetic resonance image and radiographs.[49] Arthroscopic osteoplasty of the femoral head–neck union has been performed successfully in adult patients (Fig. 17.4). Acetabuloplasty to address anterolateral overcoverage in a pincer type FAI of the femoral head can be performed arthroscopically. Labral resection, detachment, and reattachment have been reported successfully as well by employing the arthroscopic technique.[10,22,30–36] In a recent study presented by Philippon et al.,[49] a small series (16 patients) of pediatric patients (13 to 16 years of age) in a short-term follow-up (average 10.6 months) presented results in the treatment of cam and/or pincer FAI. Femoral head–neck osteoplasty, acetabular trimming, labral debridement, or detachment–reattachment was performed as needed. Patient satisfaction was high and had favorable functional outcomes.

SURGICAL TECHNIQUE

The author's preferred technique and considerations for orthopedic patients have been previously published.[10]

We position the patient in the lateral decubitus as described by Glick and Sampson. A fracture table with special accessories for traction in lateral decubitus is used (Maquet, Rastatt, Germany). Basic portals for hip arthroscopy have been deeply discussed in the literature. We use three portals (anterolateral, posterolateral, and direct anterior) to access the central compartment (iliofemoral joint). The order in which these portals are established depends on the author. Accessory portals are useful for the hip periphery; we prefer inferior accessory portals that are usually positioned 2 to 4 cm below the level of the tip of the greater trochanter (GT) and between the anterior femur and a vertical line descending from the anterior superior iliac spine. Before an attempt to establish any portal is made, adequate separation of the joint space must be verified by applying traction and observing at least a 10-mm distance between the acetabulum and femoral head on the image intensifier. Access to the central compartment of the hip is only possible with effective traction. Our protocol for hip arthroscopy is described next: The anterolateral portal (AL) is located at the anterior–superior corner of the GT and is the first we establish because it lies in the middle of the "safe zone," which is limited anteriorly by a vertical line descending from the anterior–superior iliac spine; the femoral neurovascular bundle lies medial to this line. The posterior limit is the posterior aspect of the GT; the sciatic nerve lies at least 2 cm behind it. The AL is established by navigating an arthroscopy needle into the joint with fluoroscopic control and then the stylus of the needle is removed and a flexible guide wire (Nitinol) is passed through the needle and into the joint; the needle is then removed. With the guide wire in place, a cannulated switching stick from the Hip Access System (HAS) (Smith & Nephew, Andover, MA) is passed into the joint using the guide wire to direct it into the joint and then a standard 5.8 mm double-valve rotatable arthroscopic cannula (Dyonics/Smith & Nephew, Andover, MA) is passed over the

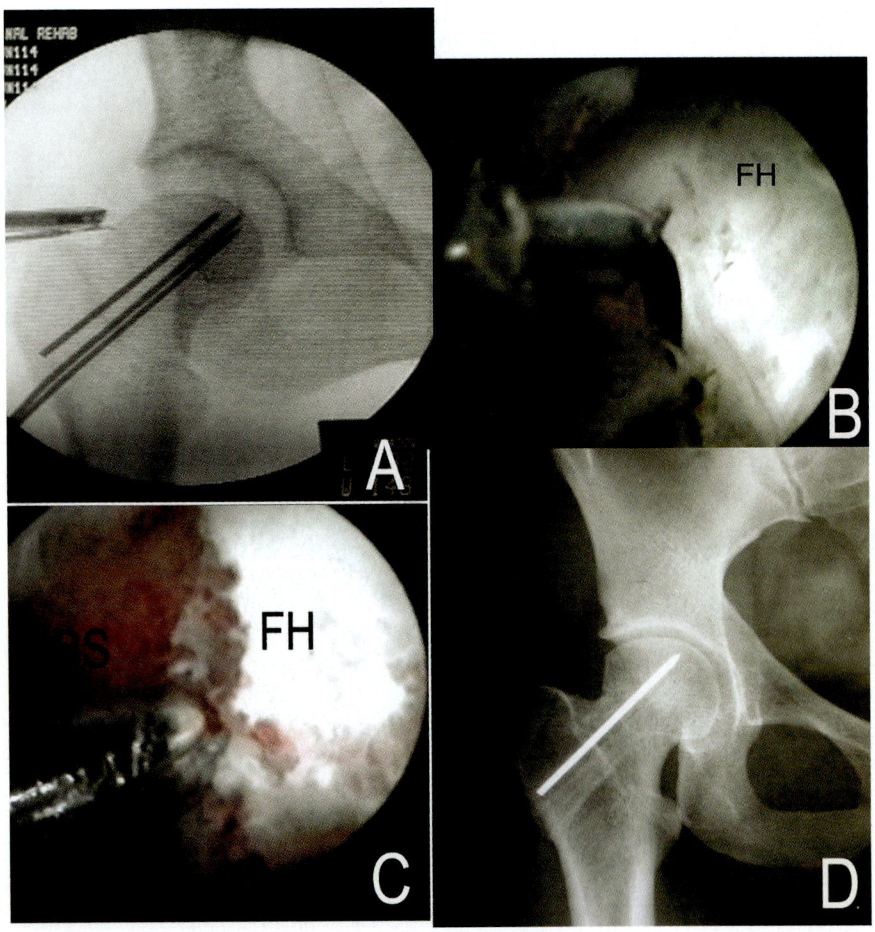

Figure 17.4. Series of photographs that illustrate a cam-type FAI decompression in a SCFE in a right hip. **A:** Fluoroscopy photograph of a capsulectomy. The arthroscope and a 90° radiofrequency probe are in position lateral to the hip labrum, the hip is still in traction. Note the pins that were used to fix the slipped capitelum. **B:** Arthroscopy photograph of a capsulectomy being performed on the anterior hip capsule (AC). The femoral head (FH) with the cam deformity is to the right. **C:** After the capsulectomy is completed, the cam deformity is reshaped. The burred surface (BS) is to the left and the FH to the right. A shaver is used to remove debris. **D:** Anteroposterior X-ray at 4 years postoperative. The reshaping was successful. Note the preservation of joint space. The ruptured pin is in the femoral neck and head.

cannulated switching stick, which is then removed with the guide wire and the 4.0-mm 30° arthroscope is placed in position. In the pediatric patient, fluoroscopic navigation is very important when femoral or acetabular deformities are present; adjustments to the point of entry at the anterior–superior corner of the GT may be necessary. A valgus deformity of the femoral neck will result in a higher position of the entry point for all the central compartment portals (anterolateral, posterolateral, and direct anterior). A varus deformity of the femoral neck requires portals that are closer to the tip of the GT and, in some cases, more separation between the femoral head and acetabulum. Distending the hip capsule by introducing 30 to 40 mL of saline solution will always result in an increment of the separation between the femoral head and the acetabulum without increasing the traction force. Distention will protect the intra-articular structures by increasing the available space to enter the joint. We always distend the capsule through the first needle that is passed into the joint. The posterolateral portal (PL) is the second we do, and it is located at the posterior–superior corner of the GT; a needle and a flexible guide wire are also used to start the PL, with or without fluoroscopic guidance. The needle is introduced parallel to the direction of the arthroscope at the AL and is visualized as it enters the joint with the arthroscope. When severe femoral or acetabular deformities are present, the use of fluoroscopy to navigate the establishment of this portal is advisable. It is important to confirm by direct arthroscopic visualization that the needle has not gone through the acetabular labrum or damages articular cartilage on the acetabulum or the femoral head. After the needle has been confirmed in a correct position, the stylus is removed and a guide wire is placed. The technique for establishing a working portal is then performed as follows: A cannulated switching stick and a portal enlarger (dilator) from the HAS (Smith & Nephew) are driven into the joint over the guide wire; when the position of the portal enlarger inside the joint is confirmed arthroscopically, the switching stick and guide wire are removed. A pistol-grip slotted cannula from the HAS (Smith & Nephew) is inserted into the joint using the portal enlarger as a guide; the enlarger is removed and the slotted cannula is ready for instrument introduction or portal shifting. In the case of the AP, the entry site is located at the crossing of a horizontal line directed medially from the GT and the vertical line descending from the anterior-superior iliac spine. This is the only portal located out of the plane of the image intensifier; therefore, it cannot be navigated like the AL and PL. When establishing the AP, the arthroscopy needle is directed 45° cephalad and 30° medially. The lateral femorocutaneous nerve lies at the AP site where it divides into three branches. Multiple puncture attempts increase the possibility of injuring this nerve. Acetabular deformity may further complicate the surgeon's orientation when establishing the AP; the use of aiming devices may help orient the needle in difficult cases.

COMPLICATIONS

The technique of hip arthroscopy has become more frequent. It is considered a relatively safe way to address many affections, either intra- or extra-articular of nature. The rate of complications reported ranges from 1% to 2%. Griffin and Villar[45] report a 1.6% of complications in a series of 640 consecutive procedures. The most common complication involves nerve palsies. These are associated to traction injuries and are reported to account for up to 0.8% of complications. Less frequent complications include damage to perineal structures, injury to the lateral femoral cutaneous nerve, extravasation of fluid with resulting abdominal pain, equipment failure, and inability to complete the procedure in obese patients. In a more recent follow-up, Clarke et al.[46] present complications recorded prospectively in 1,054 cases. About 1.4% of complications were recorded, neurapraxia being the most frequent, and one case of secondary SAH was the only major complication. The use of manual traction in patients ranging from 2.4 to 7.3 years of age, without reported complications, opens the possibility of this technique to such young patients.[14]

REFERENCES

1. Byrd JW. Hip arthroscopy. *J Am Acad Orthop Surg.* 2006;14:433–444.
2. DeAngelis NA, Busconi B. Hip arthroscopy in the pediatric population. *Clin Orthop Relat Res.* 2003;406:60–63.
3. Byrd JW. Hip arthroscopy for post-traumatic loose fragments in the young active adult: Three case reports. *Clin J Sports Med.* 1996;6:129–133.
4. Ikeda T, Awaya G, Suzuki S, et al. Torn acetabular labrum in young patients. *J Bone Joint Surg Br.* 1998;70:13–16.
5. Mehlmann CT, Hubbard GW, Crawford AH, et al. Traumatic hip dislocation in children: Long term follow-up of 42 patients. *Clin Orthop Relat Res.* 2000;376:68–79.
6. Quarrier NF, Wightman AB. A ballet dancer with chronic hip pain due to a lesser trochanter bony avulsion: The challenge of a differential diagnosis. *J Orthop Sports Phys Ther.* 1998;28:168–173.
7. Horn BD, Moseley CF. Current concepts in the management of pediatric hip disease. *Curr Opin Rheumatol.* 1992;4:180–190.
8. Weinstein SL. Natural history and outcomes of childhood hip disorders. *Clin Orthop Relat Res.* 1997;334:227–242.
9. Kocher MS, Lee B. Hip arthroscopy in children and adolescents. *Orthop Clin N Am.* 2006;37:233–240.
10. Ilizaliturri VM Jr, Martinez Escalante F, Camacho-Galindo J. Indications, surgical technique and findings of hip arthroscopy in pediatric hip disease (Arthroscopy of the pediatric hip). *Oper Tech Orthop.* 2005;15:231–238.
11. Blitzer CM. Arthroscopic management of septic arthritis of the hip. *Arthroscopy.* 1993;9:414–416.
12. Bould M. Arthroscopic diagnosis and treatment of septic hip arthritis of the hip joint. *Arthroscopy.* 1993;9:707–708.
13. Dorfmann H, Boyer T. Arthroscopy of the hip: 12 years of experience. *Arthroscopy.* 1999;15:67–72.
14. Chung WK, Slater GL, Bates EH. Treatment of septic arthritis of the hip by arthroscopic lavage. *J Pediatr Orthop.* 1993;13:444–446.
15. Kim SJ, Choi NH, Ko SH, et al. Arthroscopic treatment of septic arthritis of the hip. *Clin Orthop Relat Res.* 2003;407:211–214.
16. Kuklo TR, Mackenzie WG, Keeler KA. Hip arthroscopy in Legg–Calve–Perthes disease. *Arthroscopy.* 1999;15:88–92.
17. Bowen JR, Kumar VP, Joyce JJ III, et al. Osteochondritis dissecans following Perthes disease. *Clin Orthop Relat Res.* 1986;209:49–56.
18. Roy DR. Arthroscopic findings of the hip in new onset hip pain in adolescents with previous Legg–Calve–Perthes disease. *J Pediatr Orthop B.* 2005;15:151–155.
19. O'Leary AJ, Berend KR, Vail TP. The relationship between diagnosis and outcome in arthroscopy of the hip. *Arthroscopy.* 2001;24:339–343.
20. McCarthy JC, Busconi B. The role of the hip arthroscopy in the diagnosis and treatment of the hip disease. *Orthopedics.* 1995;18:753–756.
21. Farjo LA, Glick JM, Sampson TG. Hip arthroscopy for labral tears. *Arthroscopy.* 1999;15:132–137.
22. Ilizaliturri VM Jr, Nossa-Barrera M, Acosta-Rodriguez E, et al. Arthroscopic management of femoroacetabular impingement secondary to pediatric hip disorders. *J Bone and Joint Surg Br.* 2007;89-B:1025–1030.
23. Byrd JWT, Jones KS. Hip arthroscopy in the presence of dysplasia. *Arthroscopy.* 2003;10:1055–1060.
24. Ilizaliturri VM Jr, Chaidez PA, Valero FS, et al. Hip arthroscopy after previous acetabular osteotomy for development dysplasia of the hip. *Arthroscopy.* 2005;21:176–181.
25. McCarthy JC, Noble P, Schuck M, et al. The watershed labral lesion: Its relationship to early osteoarthritis of the hip. *J Arthroplasty.* 2001;16:81–87.
26. Klaue K, Durnin CW, Ganz R. The acetabular rim syndrome: A clinical presentation of dysplasia of the hip. *J Bone Joint Surg Br.* 1991;73:423–429.
27. Leunig M, Siebenrock KA, Ganz R. Rational of periacetabular osteotomy and background work. *Instr Course Lect.* 2001;50:229–238.
28. Noguchi Y, Hirosama M, Takasugi S, et al. Cartilage and labrum degeneration in the dysplastic hip generally originates in the anterosuperior weight-bearing area: An arthroscopic observation. *Arthroscopy.* 1999;15:496–506.
29. Bulut O, Öztürk H, Tezeren G, et al. Arthroscopic-assisted surgical treatment for developmental dislocation of the hip. *Arthroscopy.* 2005;21(5):574–579.

30. Brian T. Kelly, Daniel E. Weiland, Mara L. Schenker, et al. Arthroscopic labral repair in the hip: Surgical technique and review of the literature. *Arthroscopy.* 2005;21(12):1496–1504.
31. Mardones R, Tomic A, Vega R, et al. Tratamiento artroscópico del pellizcamiento femoro-acetabular combinado: Técnica quirurgica, Revista Chilena de Ortopedia y. *Traumatología.* 2006;47(2):53–108.
32. Philippon MJ, Schenker ML. A new method for acetabular rim trimming and labral repair. *Clin Sports Med.* 2006;25(2):293–297.
33. Ranawat AS, Kelly BT. Function of the labrum and management of labral pathology. *Oper Tech Orthop.* 2005;15(3):239–246.
34. Ide T, Akamatsu N, Nakajima I. Arthroscopic surgery of the hip joint. *Arthroscopy.* 1991;7:204–211.
35. Glick JM. Hip arthroscopy using the lateral approach. *Instr Course Lect.* 1988;37:223–231.
36. Snow SW, Keret D, Scarangella S, et al. Anterior impingement of the femoral head: A late phenomenon of Legg–Calve–Perthes' disease. *J Pediatr Orthop.* 1993;13:286–289.
37. Klaue K, Durnin CW, Ganz R. The acetabular rim syndrome. *J Bone Joint Surg Br.* 1991;73B:423–429.
38. Futami T, Kasahara Y, Suzuki S, et al. Arthroscopy for slipped capital femoral epiphysis. *J Pediatr Orthop.* 1992;12:592–597.
39. Holgersson S, Brattstrom H, Mogensen B, et al. Arthroscopy of the hip in juvenile chronic arthritis. *J Pediatric Orthop.* 1981;1:273–278.
40. Rydhold U, Wingstrand H, Egund N, et al. Sonography, arthroscopy, and intracapsular pressure in juvenile chronic arthritis of the hip. *Acta Orthop Scand.* 1986;57:295–298.
41. Khapchik V, O'Donell RJ, Glick JM. Arthroscopically assisted excision of osteoid osteoma involving the hip. *Arthroscopy.* 2001;17:56–61.
42. Thompson MS, Wooward JS. The use of the arthroscope as an adjunct in the resection of a chondroblastoma of the femoral head. *Arthroscopy.* 1995;11:106–111.
43. Byrd JW, Jones KS. Prospective analysis of hip arthroscopy with 2-year follow-up. *Arthroscopy.* 2000;16:578–587.
44. Bonnomet F, Clavert P, Abidine FZ, et al. Hip arthroscopy in hereditary multiple exostoses: A new perspective of treatment. *Arthroscopy.* 2001;17:E40.
45. Griffin DR, Villar RN. Complications in arthroscopy of the hip. *J Bone Joint Surg Br.* 1999;81:604–606.
46. Clarke MT, Arora A, Villar RN. Hip Arthroscopy: Complications in 1054 Cases. *Clin Orthop Relat Res.* 2003;406:84–88.

CHAPTER

18

Gary B. Fetzer
David A. Fischer

Hamstring Injuries

INTRODUCTION

Hamstring injuries are very common in athletic populations and can affect all levels, ranging from the recreational to the elite.[1–6] These represent a continuum of injuries, ranging from musculotendinous strains to avulsions. Fortunately, most of these injuries are strains that occur at the musculotendinous junction.[1,2] By definition, a strain is a partial or complete disruption of the musculotendinous unit.[3–5,7] Hamstring strains can result in significant pain and time lost to sport.[1,2] Avulsions of the proximal hamstring tendons from the ischium are much less common, although they can result in significant disability.[8–10] Diagnosis of proximal avulsions can be difficult and delay in diagnosis can complicate management of these injuries, especially when patients present months after injury.[2,9,11–13] While treatment of the common hamstring strain is typically uncomplicated, treatment of proximal hamstring avulsions has been controversial.[2,10,13,14]

In this chapter, we will discuss the clinical presentation, evaluation, management, and treatment of hamstring musculotendinous strain injuries and proximal hamstring avulsion injuries, with an emphasis on proximal avulsion injuries. We will also briefly review the pertinent anatomy and biomechanics of the hamstring complex. Special situations including ischial apophyseal avulsions and partial avulsions are discussed at the end of this chapter.

ANATOMY AND BIOMECHANICS

The anatomy and biomechanics of the hamstring complex is well described in the literature.[2,5,15–18] The hamstring muscle complex spans the posterior thigh and consists of three muscles: semitendinosus, semimembranosus (SM), and the biceps femoris (long head and short head). This muscle complex is unique because it crosses two joints and exerts forces and resultant mechanical effects at both the hip and knee.[1–4,15,18–20] With the exception of the short head of the biceps femoris, the hamstring complex originates from the ischial tuberosity and inserts distally below the knee on the proximal tibia. The short head of the biceps femoris originates from the linea aspera and the posterior femur. Muscle fibers of the biceps femoris are visible about 6 cm distal to the tuberosity and the proximal myotendinous junction encompasses nearly 60% of the total length of the muscle.[5] Furthermore, the same anatomical study revealed that the musculotendinous junction extends almost the entire length of the biceps femoris. The semitendinosus, SM, and the long head of biceps femoris are innervated by the tibial branch of the sciatic nerve, while the short head of the biceps femoris is innervated by the peroneal branch of the sciatic nerve.

The proximal hamstring complex has a strong bony insertion on the ischial tuberosity (Fig. 18.1). A recent cadaveric study has characterized the proximal hamstring footprint on the ischium.[18] They reported that the semitendinosus and the long head of biceps femoris have a common proximal tendon and footprint, while there is a distinct SM footprint (Fig. 18.2). The SM footprint is lateral to the crescent-shaped footprint of the common insertion of the semitendinosus and long head of the biceps femoris.

In skeletally immature individuals, the origin of the hamstring complex is from the ischial apophysis. This apophysis, along with the other pelvic apophyses, typically appears between ages 11 and 15 years.[19] Fusion of this secondary ossification center usually does not occur until ages 16 to 25 years.[19,21] This is relevant because the physis is typically the weakest structure of the growing skeleton, and injuries to the proximal hamstring tendon complex of skeletally immature individuals are typically apophyseal avulsions rather than tendinous avulsions off the ischium.

The sciatic nerve is one of the more important neurovascular structures of the posterior thigh. It typically lies lateral to the proximal hamstring tendon complex. Miller et al.[18] reported that the sciatic nerve lies about 1.2 cm from the most lateral aspect of the ischial tuberosity (Fig. 18.3). Injury to the sciatic nerve is possible from the trauma itself or iatrogenic during surgical repair. Sciatic nerve neurolysis is indicated during surgical treatment of chronic proximal avulsions. The posterior femoral cutaneous nerve, which supplies sensation to the posterior thigh, is located in the subcutaneous tissue. Careful dissection through the subcutaneous tissue will avoid injury to this nerve. Deep to the gluteus maximus muscle is the inferior gluteal nerve and artery. This neurovascular bundle is typically found deep to this muscle, and careful proximal retraction of the gluteus maximus must be performed to avoid injury.

The hamstring muscle complex is the main muscle group of the posterior thigh. As this complex crosses both the hip and knee joints, it is important in hip extension and knee flexion. As a result of being a "two-joint" muscle group, high forces are placed on the hamstring complex, which, many believe, predisposes it to injury.[2–5,7] Garrett et al.[4] reported a high proportion of Type II muscle fibers in cadaveric hamstrings

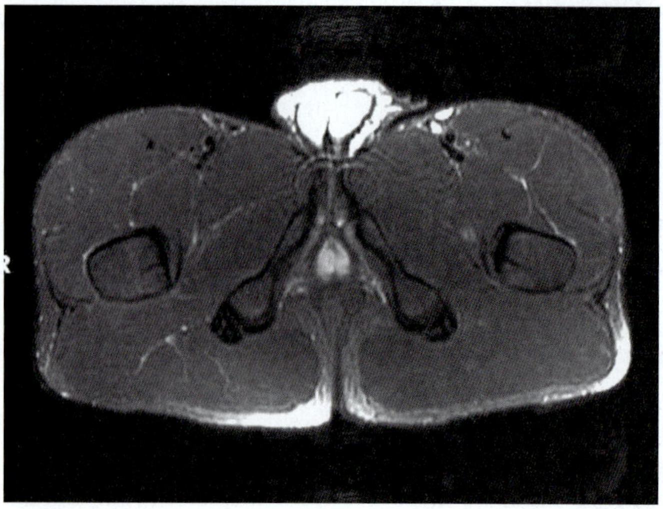

Figure 18.1. Axial MRI image demonstrating the normal hamstring complex insertion on the ischium.

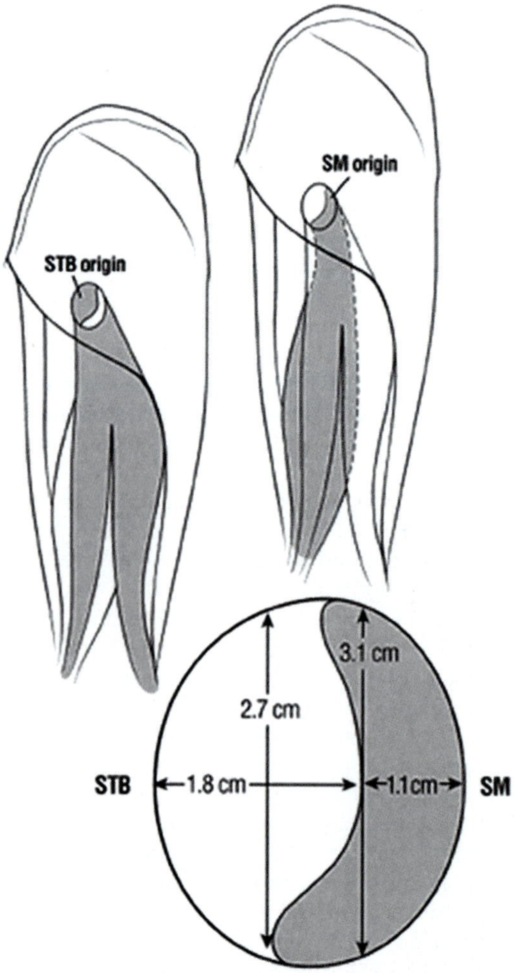

Figure 18.2. Illustration demonstrating the proximal hamstring footprint on the ischial tuberosity. The semimembranosus origin is lateral to the origin of the semitendinosus and long head of the biceps femoris. (Reprinted from Miller SL, Gill J, Webb GR. The proximal origin of the hamstrings and surrounding anatomy encountered during repair: A cadaveric study. *J Bone Joint Surg Am.* 2007;89(1):44–48.)

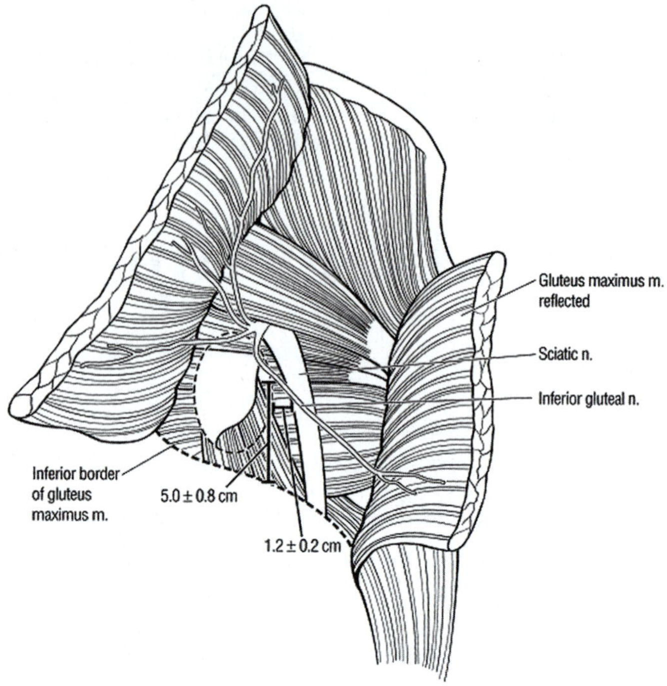

Figure 18.3. Illustration demonstrating the anatomical relationship of the proximal hamstring origin on the ischium and the sciatic nerve. (Reprinted from Miller SL, Gill J, Webb GR. The proximal origin of the hamstrings and surrounding anatomy encountered during repair: A cadaveric study. *J Bone Joint Surg Am.* 2007;89(1):44–48.)

compared to the quadriceps. These fast-twitch fibers indicate that strength and speed are important functions of the hamstring complex.[2–4] They further concluded that the muscle fiber composition, along with increased susceptibility of a "two-joint" muscle complex, results in an increased incidence of hamstring injuries.

During the gait cycle, the main function of the hamstring muscle group is to decelerate the knee at the end of the swing phase and provide push-off strength during the toe-off segment of the stance phase.[1,22] Electromyography (EMG) studies have implicated these two segments of the gait cycle most commonly in hamstring strains.[1,22,23]

MECHANISM OF INJURY/ CLASSIFICATION

Hamstring injuries are one of the most common injuries that sports medicine physicians encounter.[1,2,6] They commonly result from a wide variety of sporting activities, particularly those requiring rapid acceleration and deceleration.[1–3,6,24] Injuries can occur both in the early and late stages of athletic participation. Inadequate warm-up, inflexibility, fatigue during strenuous activity, previous injury and tendon degeneration, poor exercise technique and biomechanics, poor posture, leg-length inequality, and muscle strength imbalances are all risk factors reported in the literature for hamstring injuries.[2,6,7,10,24–27] The hamstring strain is a well recognized entity that results from excessive stretching of the musculotendinous unit.[2,3,24] Clinical and MRI studies have clearly identified that the biceps femoris is the most frequently injured muscle of the hamstring complex.[5,17,28–31] As its musculotendinous junction spans almost the length of the muscle, strains can occur even in the midthigh region. Hamstring strains are typically graded as mild (Grade I), moderate (Grade II), and severe (Grade III).[32] This is summarized in Table 18.1.

Avulsion injuries of the proximal hamstring complex are much less common. The typical mechanism of injury is an acute forced hip flexion with the knee in extension.[10,26] This is classically observed in water skiing (Fig. 18.4).[2,10,26] Similar to musculotendinous strains, proximal hamstring origin injuries commonly result from a wide variety of sporting activities that require rapid acceleration and deceleration.[9] Water skiing is by far the most common etiology of this injury. However, sprinting, soccer, rugby, weightlifting, ice skating, rollerblading, and snow skiing are also common etiologies reported in the literature.[2,10,26,33]

Proximal hamstring avulsion injuries can be classified as acute or chronic depending on the time frame from injury. Acute avulsions are typically defined as diagnosis and repair within 1 month of the injury.[9] Injuries can also be categorized as complete tendinous avulsions, partial tendinous avulsions, apophyseal avulsions, and degenerative (tendinosis) avulsions. Degenerative tears of the hamstring origin are more insidious in onset and are commonly seen as an overuse injury in middle- and long-distance runners.

TABLE 18.1 Hamstring Strain Classification

Grade	*Description*
I	Small disruption of the structural integrity of the musculotendinous unit
II	Partial tear, some musculotendinous fibers remain intact
IIIA	Complete tear of the musculotendinous unit
IIIB	Avulsion fracture at tendinous origin or insertion site

Reproduced from Brown TD, Brunet ME. Thigh. In: Delee JC, Drez DD, eds. *Orthopaedic Sports Medicine. Principles and Practice.* 2nd Ed. Philadelphia, PA: W.B. Saunders; 2003, p. 1487.

MUSCULOTENDINOUS INJURIES ("COMMON STRAIN")

CLINICAL EVALUATION

Clinical Examination

Diagnosis is usually made by clinical history and physical examination. Most hamstring strains are evaluated in the acute setting of athletic participation either by an athletic trainer or physician. Sudden onset of pain in the posterior thigh during strenuous activity is typical. A "tightness" or "pull" during exercise may be described by the athlete. An audible "pop" may also be appreciated by the athlete. Depending on the severity of the injury, pain may limit continuation of participation.

Physical examination is typically performed with the patient in the prone position. Examination with the knee slightly flexed will limit muscle spasms and make examination more comfortable. Inspection and palpation of the posterior thigh may reveal muscle spasm. Ecchymosis may only be observed if the fascial covering is also disrupted. Palpation of the entire posterior thigh is very important to localize the injury. Early after injury, focal tenderness and swelling will help localize the injury. However, with delayed examination, diffuse swelling and tenderness develop, which complicates localization. Low grade strains typically have limited swelling and tenderness, whereas with more severe strains, a palpable defect may be appreciated. However, some authors report that even in severe strains it is not uncommon to have difficulty palpating a defect.[27]

Radiographic Examination

Although the diagnosis of a common strain is usually made by history and physical examination, plain radiographs are occasionally indicated. If the athlete has proximal tenderness, is skeletally immature, has painful weight bearing, has pain out of proportion, or had an unusual mechanism of injury, radiographs are recommended. Typical radiographic views would be an anteroposterior view of the pelvis, as well as anteroposterior and lateral views of the femur. Prior to the advent of MRI, ultrasound and computed tomography were commonly used to confirm and characterize hamstring injuries.[5,29] Today, MRI examination is the most common imaging modality (Fig. 18.5).[17,29,31,34,35] Typical finding of hamstring strains is an increased signal on T2-weighted sequences, which represents edema and hemorrhage. Frank tears in the musculotendinous unit can also be seen. A considerable amount of objective

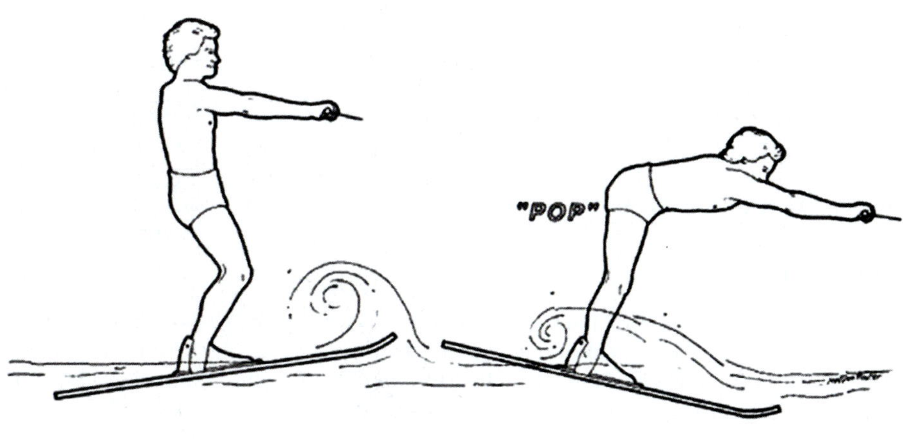

Figure 18.4. Illustration representing a common mechanism of injury for proximal hamstring avulsions. (Reprinted from Blasier RB, Morawa LG. Complete rupture of the hamstring origin from a water skiing injury. *Am J Sports Med.* 1990;18(4):435–437.)

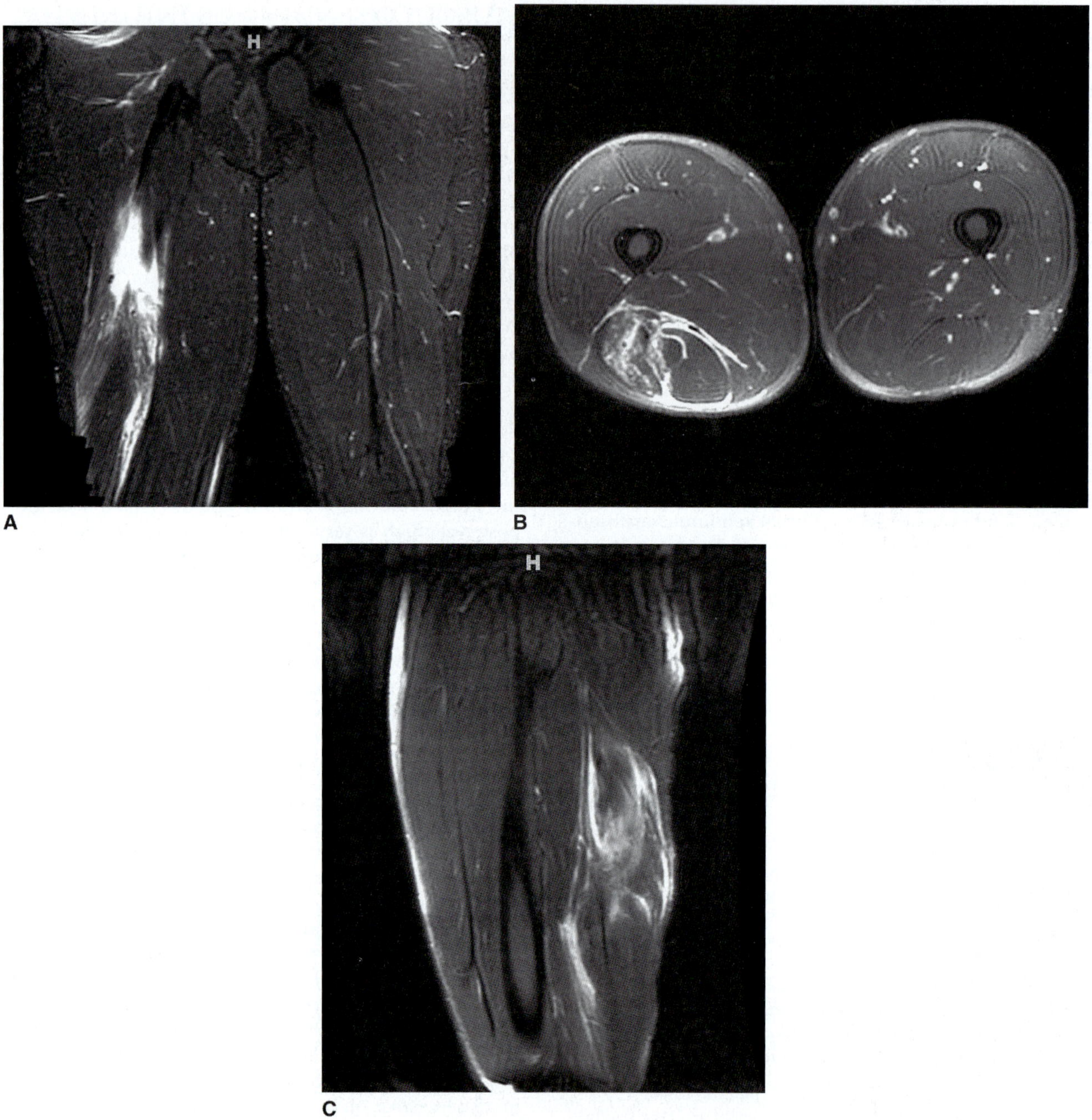

Figure 18.5. Coronal **(A)**, axial **(B)**, and sagittal **(C)** MRI sequences of a biceps femoris musculotendinous strain.

information can be obtained from an MR image of a hamstring strain (e.g., muscles involved, injury location, length of injury, cross-sectional area or volume of injury, etc.).[17,28,31,34–36] However, there is considerable debate in the literature whether MR is even necessary.[2,21,31,34–36] MRI examination is very expensive, and many question whether the information gained from the study outweighs the cost of the study.

TREATMENT

Treatment of common hamstring strains is typically straightforward.[1,2] The typical initial regimen consists of rest, ice, compression, and elevation. Acutely, pain control, as well as minimization of the swelling and hemorrhage, is the main focus. This is typically accomplished with ice, elevation, and compression. Although NSAIDs are also commonly given, there has been some controversy concerning the appropriate timing of administration.[37,38] Gentle stretching and range of motion exercises are begun within the parameters of pain, with strengthening added as tolerated by the athlete. Ultrasound and other modalities are also commonly used, but evidence to support this use is lacking.[39] Rehabilitation programs have been previously described and are best performed under the guidance of an athletic trainer or physical therapist to maximize outcome and prevent reinjury.[1–3,6,24,27,32]

Prevention and decreasing recurrence are also very important considerations. Important factors in preventing muscle strain injuries include improving flexibility, adequate warm-up, and pre-exercise stretching. Identifying weakness in hamstring muscles may allow prediction of risk for muscle strain and allow rehabilitation to correct the problem before injury.[7,40] Koulouris et al.[36] have suggested that longitudinal length of a strain is a risk factor for reinjury during the same season; however, this conclusion was not statistically supported. They also reported that players with recurrent hamstring strains in the same season had a longer rehabilitation period after the second injury.

Time until return to play is quite variable, ranging from days to weeks, and typically a function of the extent of the injury.[1,2] Minimizing the amount of time spent out of training and competition is critical not only for the professional athlete, but also for leisure and recreational athletes. There is debate in the literature concerning whether or not MRI can be used to predict return to play.[17,30,31,35,41,42] Verrall et al.[42] studied 83 Australian football players with posterior thigh injuries and reported that 82% were positive for hamstring injury using MRI. Hamstring muscle injury confirmed by MRI was associated with a longer absence from competition (27 vs. 16 days). Connell et al.[30] did MR assessments of acute and healing hamstring injuries and demonstrated that the longitudinal length of hamstring tears on MR had statistical correlation with recovery and was the best radiologic predictor for return to competition. Pomeranz and Heidt[31] used objective criterion regarding the extent and nature of injury to predict the convalescence interval. They reported that time lost from competition correlated with the percentage of abnormal muscle area and volume of muscle injury. Slavotinek et al.[35] found an association between rehabilitation time and volume of muscle injury and extent of cross-sectional area (>50% associated with longer recovery).

PROXIMAL HAMSTRING AVULSIONS

CLINICAL EVALUATION

Clinical Examination

Avulsion injuries of the proximal hamstring origin are much less common, and can be difficult to diagnose. Patients with acute injuries to the common hamstring origin typically present with acute pain in the proximal posterior thigh and buttock.[8–10,14,43] An audible or sensation of a "pop" is commonly reported. Painful weight bearing, weakness with knee flexion, and muscle spasms are also reported. With complete avulsions, rather significant swelling and ecchymosis develop over the next several days. The ecchymosis can be quite impressive and extend distally to the popliteal fossa. Sciatic nerve irritation is not an unusual complaint, and is likely a neurapraxia from a stretch injury to the nerve or a result of localized swelling and hematoma.[10]

In patients with delayed presentation, or chronic avulsions, common complaints are difficulty sitting for prolonged periods, difficulty "controlling" the leg, a sense of the leg "giving way," and a dull, aching pain in the gluteal and posterior thigh region.[9,11,14,26,43,44] These symptoms can be exacerbated by walking downhill, descending stairs, or with activities requiring rapid push-off. Degenerative tears of the hamstring origin are more insidious in onset and are difficult to diagnose. These particular patients report deep buttock pain or posterior thigh pain brought on during acceleration and at faster speeds.[2,8,13,45]

On physical examination, tenderness at the ischial tuberosity and along the proximal hamstring is common. A palpable defect in the posterior buttock region and ecchymosis spanning the entire posterior aspect of the leg may be appreciated. This defect may be difficult to appreciate secondary to localized swelling and hematoma. There may be hamstring asymmetry observed with attempted active knee flexion. A thorough neurovascular examination is important to identify any sciatic nerve deficits or irritation.

Radiographic Examination

Radiographic examination is an important component of the evaluation. Although plain radiographs are generally not diagnostic, avulsion fractures and other osseous abnormalities can be identified. In skeletally immature patients, comparison to the uninjured contralateral pelvis can be extremely useful if the diagnosis is uncertain. MRI examination is the most useful imaging modality to confirm diagnosis.[17,29,31,34,41] Sagittal and coronal T2-weighted sequences best delineate the injury and can estimate the retraction of the hamstring tendon (Fig. 18.6). In degenerative hamstring tendon avulsions, MRI often reveals tendon degeneration, associated thickening, and surrounding soft-tissue edema.

Ultrasound examination may be alternative imaging modality for patients unable to undergo MRI, especially if there is access to an experienced technologist familiar with musculoskeletal techniques.[3,5,17,31,34,46]

TREATMENT

Historically, management of proximal hamstring avulsions has been controversial.[8–11,14] Nonoperative treatment initially consists of rest, ice, and NSAIDs to decrease pain and control edema. Ambulatory aids (i.e., crutches) are usually needed to assist with gait. Gentle stretching and range of motion exercises are started as pain decreases. Normalization of gait, strengthening, and therapeutic exercises are started with a gradual return to athletic activity over a period of 4 to 6 weeks.[14] Complications of nonoperative treatment include weakness in hip extension and knee flexion, difficulty with prolonged sitting, difficulty controlling the leg, failure to return to sport, and development of symptoms similar to those of hamstring syndrome.[14,47] There is little information on the treatment of partial avulsions. Cohen and Bradley[14] have recommended nonoperative treatment for single tendon ruptures. Lempainen et al.[33] reported on a large series of patients with partial avulsions that failed conservation management, and ultimately underwent surgical management. Furthermore, nonoperative treatment of complete proximal hamstring avulsions has been shown to have unsatisfactory results in athletic populations.[10,14,43,48] Sallay et al.[10] clearly demonstrated a low rate of return to sports with any patient treated nonoperatively for complete tendinous avulsions. Other authors have also noted poor functional outcomes with nonoperative management.[43,48]

There is increasing literature demonstrating good to excellent outcomes with surgical management of acute complete avulsions (Table 18.2).[8,10,17,26,33,44,45] Blasier and Morawa[45] were one of the first to report surgical management of a complete tendinous avulsion in a water skier. Orava and Kujala[26] reported good outcomes in their series, which included four repairs, done within two months of injury. Klingele and Sallay[9] reported good to excellent outcomes in their series of 11 complete proximal tendinous avulsions (seven acute, four chronic). Ten of

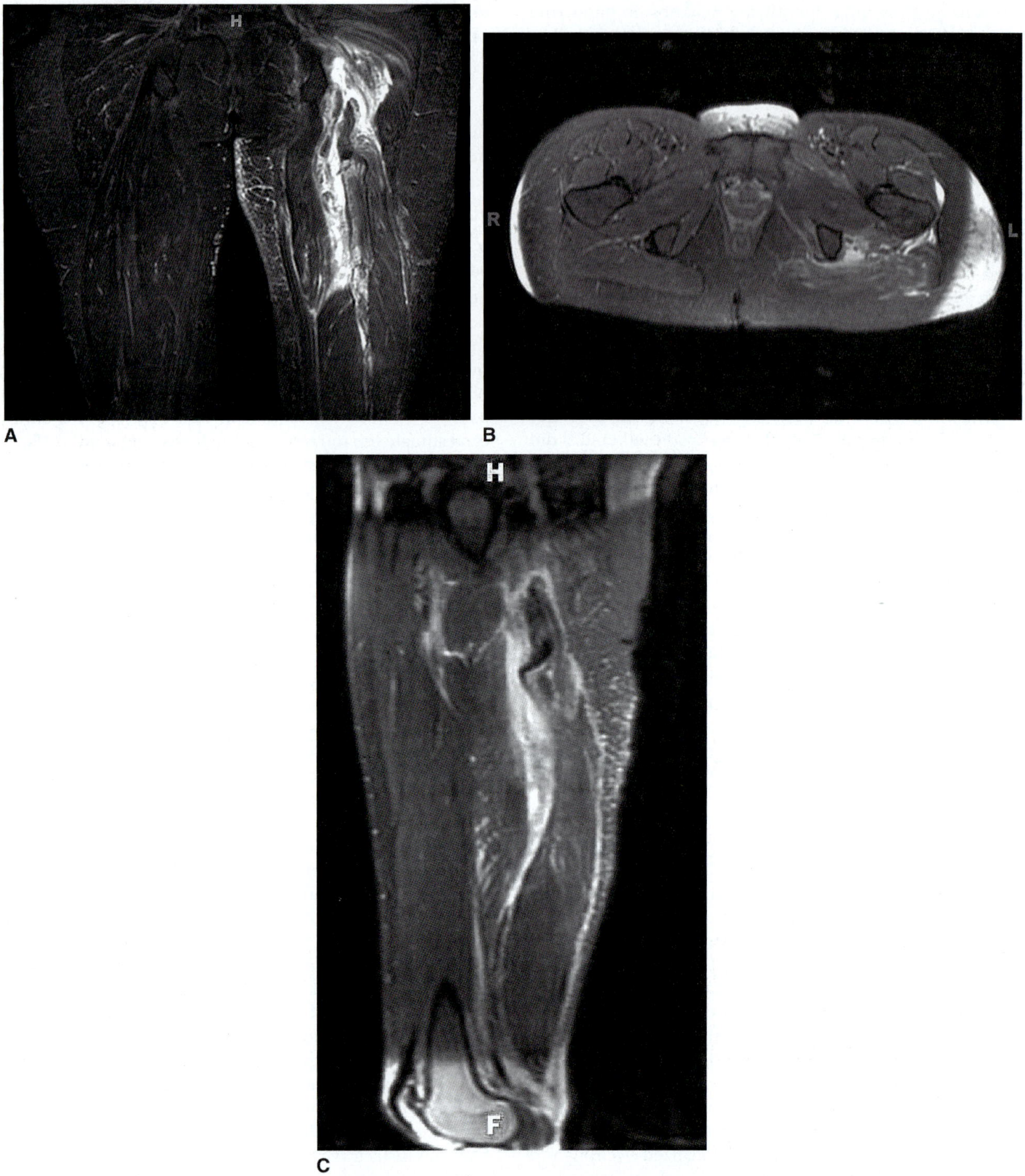

Figure 18.6. Coronal **(A)**, axial **(B)**, and sagittal **(C)** MRI sequences demonstrating an acute complete avulsion of the proximal hamstring tendon origin with retraction.

the eleven were satisfied with the outcome, and seven of the nine athletically active patients were able to return to sport at an average of 6 months. Isokinetic testing revealed an average of 91% return of hamstring function. Folsom and Larson[44] reported on 20 acute primary repairs in their series. At final follow-up, 75% were able to return to sport and 95% said they would have surgery again.

While surgical repair of acute avulsions have shown good to excellent results, the surgical outcomes of chronic avulsions have been more variable (Table 18.2).[9–11,16,26,44,49] Orava and Kujala[26] reported that surgical outcomes were not as good when surgery was performed later than 2 months from injury. Augmentation with fascia lata and plantaris tendon was needed in two patients and carbon fiber was also needed in one procedure. However,

TABLE 18.2 Acute and Chronic Complete Proximal Hamstring Avulsion Series

	Patients, N (Acute/ Chronic)	*Mean Follow-up (Months)*	*Mean Isokinetic Strength (%)*	*Comments*
Blasier and Morawa[45]	1 (1/0)	84	91	—
Sallay et al.[10]	2 (0/2)	18	—	Isokinetic testing at follow-up; 80% return of strength ($n = 1$)
Orava and Kujala[26]	8 (4/4)	5.7	—	Improved outcomes with acute repair
Cross et al.[11]	8 (0/8)	48	60.2	7/8 returned to recreational sports 91% satisfaction
Klingele and Sallay[9]	11 (7/4)	34	85.3	Distal fractional lengthening ($n = 2$)
Brucker et al.[16]	8 (6/2)	33.3	89	75% returned to sports
Chakravarty et al.[49]	4 (1/3)	14.6	90	75% returned to sports
Folsom and Larson[44]	25 (20/5)	20	83, 88[a]	15/20 acute repairs return to sports Three achilles tendon allograft recon.

[a]Acute repair group only; tested at both low speed (60°/s)/high speed (180°/s).

Klingele and Sallay[9] reported no difference between early (seven patients) and late repairs (four patients) with respect to functional outcome or return to sport. Two of their chronic cases required distal fractional lengthening of the hamstring muscles. They described a series of chevron incisions being made inferior to the distal myotendinous junction of the biceps and semitendinosus muscles. By applying firm traction, 2 to 3 cm of lengthening was obtained, which allowed anatomic repair. Cross et al.[11] demonstrated good functional outcomes even with delayed repair. Seven of their nine patients returned to preinjury sporting level. Folsom and Larson[44] reported good results with the use of an interpositional Achilles allograft for irreparable chronic ruptures. These authors utilized interference screw fixation of an Achilles allograft bone block into the pelvis. Thomsen and Jensen[50] published a case report of a chronic hamstring tendon rupture, which was repaired using a ligament augmentation device reinforced with a fascia lata graft. This fixation method led to good hamstring muscle strength and patient satisfaction at 8 months postoperatively. Lempainen et al.[51] reported good results on five repairs using fascia lata autograft. Four of the cases in this series were revision repairs, and one was a primary repair.

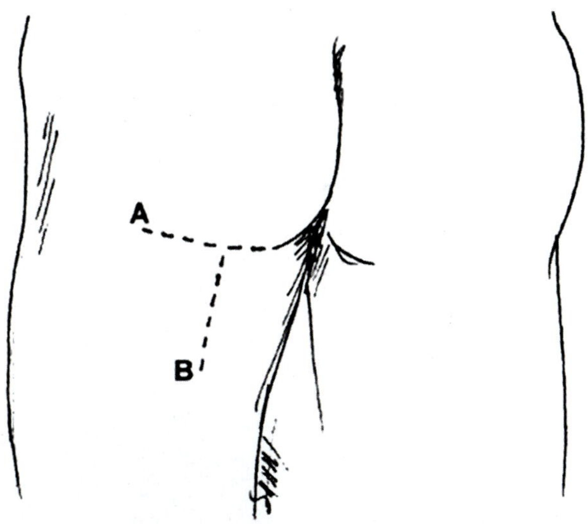

Figure 18.7. Illustration demonstrating surgical approaches for proximal hamstring repairs. (Reprinted from Klingele KE, Sallay PI. Surgical repair of complete proximal hamstring tendon rupture. *Am J Sports Med.* 2002;30(5):742–747.)

Surgical Technique for Direct Anatomic Repair (Acute)

The patient is typically positioned in the prone position with the knees slightly flexed. Surgical incision can be performed either with a longitudinal incision starting from the gluteal fold or a transverse incision in the gluteal fold (Fig. 18.7).[9] This decision is based on the amount of distal retraction and surgeon preference. Blunt dissection is performed through the subcutaneous tissue, with identification and protection of the posterior femoral cutaneous nerve. Identify the inferior border of the gluteus maximus muscle and retract it proximally. This exposes the fascia overlying the hamstring compartment and the injured tendon complex. The sciatic nerve is usually identified lateral to the common hamstring tendon and is followed proximally to the ischium. For acute repairs, neurolysis is usually not necessary, but identification of the nerve is useful to prevent iatrogenic injury. Sharp dissection through the fascial covering of the hamstring compartment is then performed. The injured proximal hamstring tendons are then identified and mobilized. The anatomic origin of the common hamstring tendons on the lateral, flat surface of the ischial tuberosity is identified. Fibrous tissue is debrided using an elevator and curette. Three or four 5 mm metallic suture anchors loaded with a large nonabsorbable suture are then inserted into the ischium. Repair of the hamstring tendon complex to the anatomic origin on the ischial tuberosity is then performed (Fig. 18.8). Hip extension and knee flexion can be used during the repair to help reduce the proximal tendon to the anatomic origin on the ischium.

Surgical Technique for Chronic Avulsions

In late repairs, primary direct repair should always be attempted. Late repairs usually require a more extensive mobilization of the proximal tendon complex from the surrounding scar tissue. In significantly retracted, chronic tears, or tears older than 3 months, the authors suggest having an allograft available. Sciatic nerve neurolysis is usually required in these cases, and should be done carefully. We routinely identify the nerve distally in normal tissue and then trace the nerve proximally. If direct anatomic repair is not possible, despite complete mobilization of the tendon, the authors feel that it is advisable to consider interpositional allograft if greater than 60° of knee flexion is required to achieve anatomic reattachment. We prefer an Achilles allograft. The calcaneal bone fragment of the thawed Achilles allograft was sharply removed. The allograft is then split longitudinally and each arm of the graft is tubularized with an

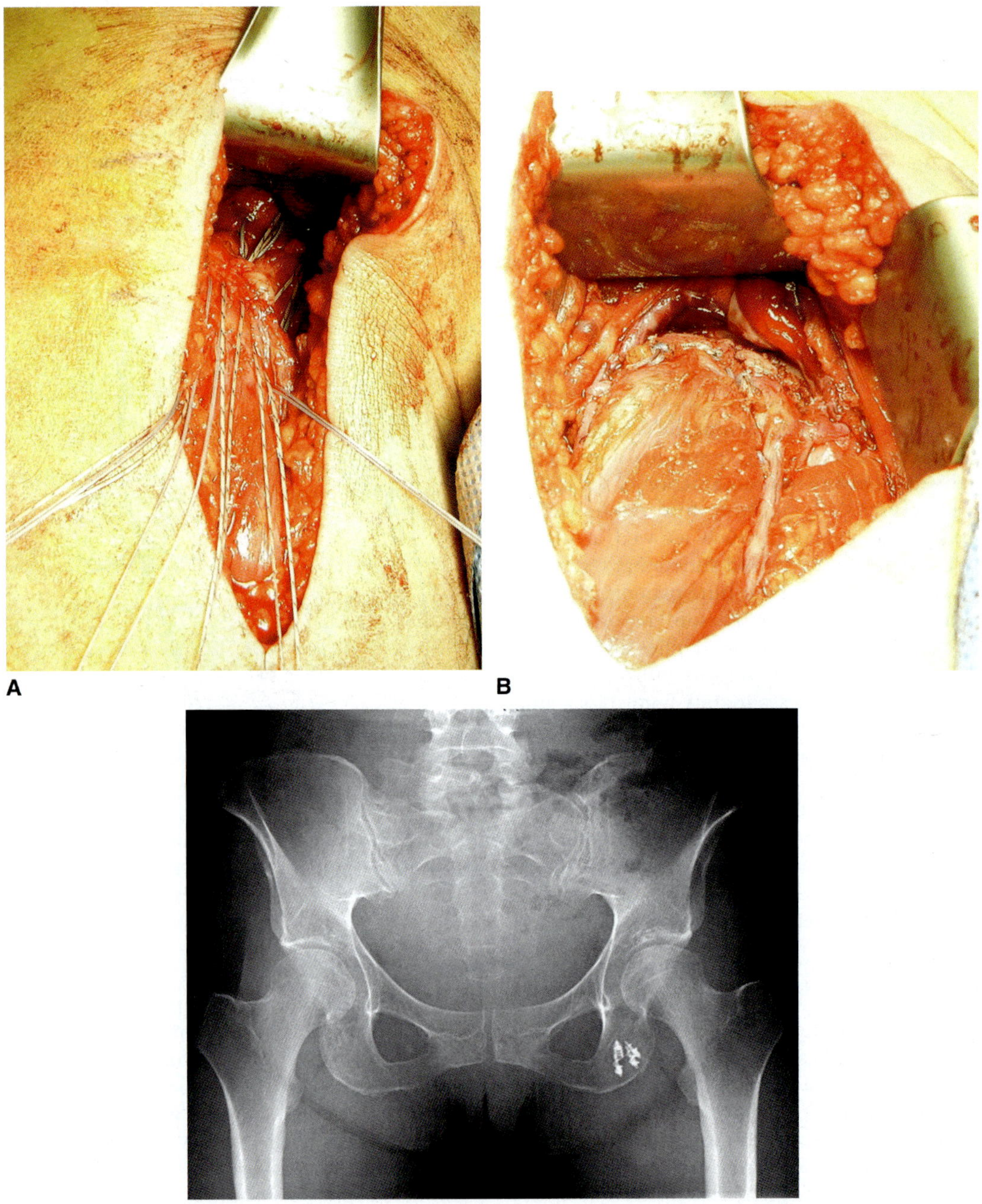

A B C

Figure 18.8. Intraoperative photographs of a direct anatomic repair of an acute complete proximal hamstring avulsion (**A,B**) and the postoperative radiograph (**C**).

absorbable suture (Fig. 18.9). The allograft is then interposed between the native common hamstring tendon and the ischial tuberosity. The calcaneal end of the Achilles tendon allograft was secured to the ischial origin utilizing three or four metallic bone anchors. Then, using a blunt hemostat, each limb of the allograft is weaved through the stump of the common hamstring in a figure-of-eight fashion. Each limb is then secured with a nonabsorbable synthetic braided suture both to the native hamstring tissue and onto itself. Tensioning of the interpositional graft is performed with the knee in approximately 45° to 50°of flexion.

POSTOPERATIVE CARE/REHABILITATION

There is little consensus in the literature on the postoperative management and rehabilitation of these injuries.[10,11,14,26,44,45] There are various recommendations concerning postoperative immobilization, length of protected weight-bearing, and when to begin physical therapy. The main goal in the early postoperative period (the "protection" phase) is to protect the repair to allow tendon-to-bone healing. During this phase, some authors use no immobilization,[26,51] while others recommend a hinged-knee brace,[11,44] a harness-suspension device,[9] a custom-fitted hip orthosis,[14] or even a hip spica cast.[45] Interestingly, there is no report on any difficulties or complications of regaining full extension even after this lengthy immobilization. The common theme in most of these series is to immobilize the extremity and protect the repair. With respect to weight bearing, most recommend a period of protected weight bearing, ranging from 4 to 8 weeks.[9–11,14,26,33,44,45,51] The second phase of the rehabilitation is the "mobilization" phase. During this phase, the main goal is normalization of gait with full weight bearing at about 4 to 6 weeks postoperatively. Active and active-assist range of motion can begin as tolerated. The third and final phase is the "strengthening" phase, and this is typically not instituted until about the 3-month mark.[11,33,44,51] Return to activity is as tolerated, as their strength allows. Isokinetic testing can be used to help guide rehabilitation and return to sport (Table 18.2).

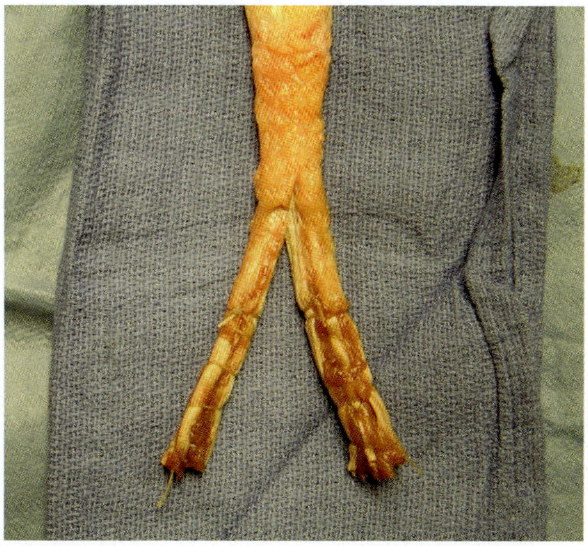

Figure 18.9. Preparation of the interpositional Achilles allograft for treatment of a chronic complete proximal hamstring origin avulsion.

The author's current postoperative protocol uses a standard hinged-knee brace locked in varying degrees of knee flexion based on the amount of tension at the time of repair (typically 30° to 60°). The brace is gradually extended over a period of about 4 weeks. Progressive weight bearing is allowed once the patient achieves full-knee extension. In the next phase of rehabilitation, the brace is discontinued, the patient is weaned from the crutches, and we emphasize normalization of gait and range of motion. Formal strengthening exercises are begun about 3 months postoperatively. We typically have patients undergo isokinetic testing at 6 and 12 months postoperatively to help guide rehabilitation and return to sport.

COMPLICATIONS

Complications following nonoperative and operative management of proximal hamstring avulsions are reported in the literature.[9,33,43,44,48,52] Sciatic nerve injury has been reported with both operative and nonoperative treatment of proximal hamstring avulsions.[9,43,48,52] There are three case reports of sciatic nerve entrapment following nonoperative management of proximal tendon avulsions or ischial apophyseal avulsion fractures.[43,48,52] Miller et al.[52] reported on a sensory deficit following nonoperative treatment of an avulsion fracture of the ischial tuberosity. Surgical exploration revealed the bony fragment impinging and piercing a portion of the sciatic nerve. Carmody and Prietto[48] reported on a water skier with a proximal hamstring tendinous avulsion who developed a progressive neurologic deficit that began as a sensory deficit and progressed to a foot drop. Street and Burks[43] reported a case of a sciatic nerve entrapment more than 15 years after initial injury presenting as a foot drop. EMG and MRI examination were performed in both of these cases to confirm diagnosis and localize the entrapment. Surgical exploration and neurolysis were performed without repair of the hamstring in both of these cases with good outcomes. Extensive scar tissue and fibrosis were found encasing the sciatic nerve in both cases.

Surgical complications reported in the literature include rerupture, hyperesthesia and hypoesthesia around the incision, superficial wound infections, hypertrophic scarring, deep infection requiring irrigation and debridement, development of complex regional pain syndrome.[9,33,44] Klingele and Sallay[9] reported one activity-related postoperative entrapment of the sciatic nerve in their series of 11 surgical repairs. Similarly, in the author's experience, we have noted one activity-related foot drop which ultimately required exploration and neurolysis. After neurolysis, the patient was able to return to recreational running and rock climbing without difficulty (unpublished data).

SPECIAL CIRCUMSTANCES

Ischial Apophyseal Avulsions

Avulsion fractures of the pelvic apophyses are commonly encountered.[12,19,20,53,54] The ischial apophysis is the site of origin of the hamstring muscle complex. The ischial apophysis appears between the ages of 11 and 15 years, and fuses to the pelvis between the ages of 16 and 25 years.[19,21,54] Until closure, this apophyseal growth plate is weaker than the tendinous insertion, thus injuries occur through the physis rather than the tendon. Ischial apophyseal avulsion injuries are rare and the management of these injuries is still debated.[12,14,19,20,52–57]

Historically, nonoperative treatment has been recommended as it was reported that these avulsion fractures did not lead to significant permanent disability.[19,58] Barnes and Hinds [55] reviewed 39 cases of ischial apophysis avulsions and reported that 68% did not heal by bony union. Nevertheless, it has been assumed that there would only be minimal disability even with a fibrous union. Metzmaker and Pappas[19] reported on six patients with ischial apophysis avulsions and noted five excellent and one good result with early, meticulous rehabilitation regardless of width of bony displacement. However, Miller et al.[52,56] and Hamada and Rada reported sciatic nerve entrapment following nonoperative management of an apophyseal avulsion. Additionally, other studies have suggested that significant pain, weakness, and limitations in functional performance are common, even after extensive rehabilitation.[20,54,56,57]

As a result, surgical management has also been offered as a treatment option. However, consensus of surgical indications is still lacking. Fragment displacement and fragment size as indicators for surgical management is debated in the literature.[12,53,56–58] Kujala et al.[12] recommended surgical intervention if displacement was greater than 2 cm, which was rare in their experience. Servant and Jones[57] reported an excellent outcome in the case of a sprinter with an ischial apophysis avulsion with 2.5 cm displacement treated with open reduction and internal fixation. They recommended open reduction and internal fixation if displacement was greater than 2 cm. Gill and Clark[58] recommended fixation if the fragment is displaced greater than 1.5 cm.

Surgical options include open reduction and internal fixation or fragment excision and reattachment of the tendon complex to the ischium. Supporters of open reduction and internal fixation suggest that nonoperative management of a displaced fragment or excision of the fragment will lead to loss of hamstring power.[12,20,53,56,57] However, support of this conclusion in the literature is lacking. Previous reports of decreased power following excision of the fragment are difficult to interpret because objective postoperative isokinetic data were not reported. In the author's experience, we have found that bony fragment excision and reattachment of the proximal hamstring complex can result in good functional outcome. It is the author's belief that even with minimal apophyseal displacement significant functional deficits can occur.

Partial Avulsions

There is limited data concerning the treatment of partial avulsions.[14,33] Cohen and Bradley[14] recommend consideration of nonoperative treatment for acute partial avulsions (one tendon ruptures). Lempainen et al.[33] reported on a series of 48 partial avulsions repairs, all of which failed initial nonoperative treatment. The conjoint tendon of the biceps femoris and semitendinosus was involved in the cases. They reported good and excellent results in 88% of the cases and 41 were able to return to their previous level of sports at an average of 5 months. They suggested that excellent outcomes are possible, even in delayed repair of partial avulsions. They further noted that the surgical procedure was technically less demanding in the acute phase as there was less need for sciatic nerve neurolysis. They recommended that surgical repair be considered even in partial avulsions.

SUMMARY

Hamstring injuries are common in athletic populations. Fortunately, most are musculotendinous strains, and treatment is generally straightforward. Proximal hamstring avulsion injuries can be debilitating, and a high index of suspicion is required. In athletic populations, nonoperative treatment may limit return to sport. Furthermore, direct anatomic repair of acute avulsions do result in good to excellent outcomes and return to sport. Chronic avulsions are more complicated, but good surgical results are supported in the literature. Direct anatomic repair of acute and chronic avulsions should be attempted in all cases. In cases where anatomic repair is not possible, alternative methods exist to allow repair to the ischium.

REFERENCES

1. Brown TD, Brunet ME. Thigh. In: DeLee JC DD, Miller MD, eds. *Orthopaedic Sports Medicine. Principles and Practice.* Vol. 2. Philadelphia, PA: WB Saunders; 2003, pp. 1481–1523.
2. Clanton TO, Coupe KJ. Hamstring strains in athletes: Diagnosis and treatment. *J Am Acad Orthop Surg.* 1998;6(4):237–248.
3. Garrett WE Jr. Muscle strain injuries. *Am J Sports Med.* 1996;24(Suppl. 6):S2–S8.
4. Garrett WE Jr, Califf JC, Bassett FH III. Histochemical correlates of hamstring injuries. *Am J Sports Med.* 1984;12(2):98–103.
5. Garrett WE Jr, Rich FR, Nikolaou PK, et al. Computed tomography of hamstring muscle strains. *Med Sci Sports Exerc.* 1989;21(5):506–514.
6. Worrell TW. Factors associated with hamstring injuries: An approach to treatment and preventative measures. *Sports Med.* 1994;17(5):338–345.
7. Burkett LN. Causative factors in hamstring strains. *Med Sci Sports.* 1970;2(1):39–42.
8. Ishikawa K, Kai K, Mizuta H. Avulsion of the hamstring muscles from the ischial tuberosity: A report of two cases. *Clin Orthop Relat Res.* 1988;232:153–155.
9. Klingele KE, Sallay PI. Surgical repair of complete proximal hamstring tendon rupture. *Am J Sports Med.* 2002;30(5):742–747.
10. Sallay PI, Friedman RL, Coogan PG, et al. Hamstring muscle injuries among water skiers: Functional outcome and prevention. *Am J Sports Med.* 1996;24(2):130–136.
11. Cross MJ, Vandersluis R, Wood D, et al. Surgical repair of chronic complete hamstring tendon rupture in the adult patient. *Am J Sports Med.* 1998;26(6):785–788.
12. Kujala UM, Orava S. Ischial apophysis injuries in athletes. *Sports Med.* 1993;16(4):290–294.
13. Kujala UM, Orava S, Jarvinen M. Hamstring injuries. Current trends in treatment and prevention. *Sports Med.* 1997;23(6):397–404.
14. Cohen S, Bradley J. Acute proximal hamstring rupture. *J Am Acad Orthop Surg.* 2007;15(6):350–355.
15. Agre JC. Hamstring injuries: Proposed aetiological factors, prevention, and treatment. *Sports Med.* 1985;2(1):21–33.
16. Brucker PU, Imhoff AB. Functional assessment after acute and chronic complete ruptures of the proximal hamstring tendons. *Knee Surg Sports Traumatol Arthrosc.* 2005;13(5):411–418.
17. Koulouris G, Connell D. Evaluation of the hamstring muscle complex following acute injury. *Skeletal Radiol.* 2003;32(10):582–589.
18. Miller SL, Gill J, Webb GR. The proximal origin of the hamstrings and surrounding anatomy encountered during repair: A cadaveric study. *J Bone Joint Surg Am.* 2007;89(1):44–48.
19. Metzmaker JN, Pappas AM. Avulsion fractures of the pelvis. *Am J Sports Med.* 1985;13(5):349–358.
20. Wootton JR, Cross MJ, Holt KW. Avulsion of the ischial apophysis: The case for open reduction and internal fixation. *J Bone Joint Surg Br.* 1990;72(4):625–627.
21. Anderson M, Hwang SC, Green WT. Growth of the normal trunk in boys and girls during the second decade of life; related to age, maturity, and ossification of the iliac epiphyses. *J Bone Joint Surg Am.* 1965;47(8):1554–1564.
22. Slocum DB, James SL. Biomechanics of running. *JAMA.* 1968;205(11):721–728.
23. Elliott BC, Blanksby BA. The synchronization of muscle activity and body segment movements during a running cycle. *Med Sci Sports.* 1979;11(4):322–327.
24. Liemohn W. Factors related to hamstring strains. *J Sports Med Phys Fitness.* 1978;18(1):71–76.
25. Knapik JJ, Jones BH, Bauman CL, et al. Strength, flexibility and athletic injuries. *Sports Med.* 1992;14(5):277–288.
26. Orava S, Kujala UM. Rupture of the ischial origin of the hamstring muscles. *Am J Sports Med.* 1995;23(6):702–705.
27. Safran MR, Garrett WE Jr, Seaber AV, et al. The role of warmup in muscular injury prevention. *Am J Sports Med.* 1988;16(2):123–129.
28. Askling CM, Tengvar M, Saartok T, et al. Acute first-time hamstring strains during high-speed running: A longitudinal study including clinical and magnetic resonance imaging findings. *Am J Sports Med.* 2007;35(2):197–206.
29. Brandser EA, el-Khoury GY, Kathol MH, et al. Hamstring injuries: Radiographic, conventional tomographic, CT, and MR imaging characteristics. *Radiology.* 1995;197(1):257–262.
30. Connell DA, Schneider-Kolsky ME, Hoving JL, et al. Longitudinal study comparing sonographic and MRI assessments of acute and healing hamstring injuries. *Am J Roentgenol.* 2004;183(4):975–984.

31. Pomeranz SJ, Heidt RS Jr. MR imaging in the prognostication of hamstring injury: Work in progress. *Radiology.* 1993;189(3):897–900.
32. Zarins B, Ciullo JV. Acute muscle and tendon injuries in athletes. *Clin Sports Med.* 1983;2(1):167–182.
33. Lempainen L, Sarimo J, Heikkila J, et al. Surgical treatment of partial tears of the proximal origin of the hamstring muscles. *Br J Sports Med.* 2006;40(8):688–691.
34. Koulouris G, Connell D. Hamstring muscle complex: An imaging review. *Radiographics.* 2005;25(3):571–586.
35. Slavotinek JP, Verrall GM, Fon GT. Hamstring injury in athletes: Using MR imaging measurements to compare extent of muscle injury with amount of time lost from competition. *Am J Roentgenol.* 2002;179(6):1621–1628.
36. Koulouris G, Connell DA, Brukner P, et al. Magnetic resonance imaging parameters for assessing risk of recurrent hamstring injuries in elite athletes. *Am J Sports Med.* 2007;35(9):1500–1506.
37. Almekinders LC, Gilbert JA. Healing of experimental muscle strains and the effects of nonsteroidal antiinflammatory medication. *Am J Sports Med.* 1986;14(4):303–308.
38. Reynolds JF, Noakes TD, Schwellnus MP, et al. Non-steroidal anti-inflammatory drugs fail to enhance healing of acute hamstring injuries treated with physiotherapy. *S Afr Med J.* 1995;85(6):517–522.
39. Rantanen J, Thorsson O, Wollmer P, et al. Effects of therapeutic ultrasound on the regeneration of skeletal myofibers after experimental muscle injury. *Am J Sports Med.* 1999;27(1):54–59.
40. Heiser TM, Weber J, Sullivan G, et al. Prophylaxis and management of hamstring muscle injuries in intercollegiate football players. *Am J Sports Med.* 1984;12(5):368–370.
41. Schneider-Kolsky ME, Hoving JL, Warren P, et al. A comparison between clinical assessment and magnetic resonance imaging of acute hamstring injuries. *Am J Sports Med.* 2006;34(6):1008–1015.
42. Verrall GM, Slavotinek JP, Barnes PG et al. Diagnostic and prognostic value of clinical findings in 83 athletes with posterior thigh injury: Comparison of clinical findings with magnetic resonance imaging documentation of hamstring muscle strain. *Am J Sports Med.* 2003;31(6):969–973.
43. Street CC, Burks RT. Chronic complete hamstring avulsion causing foot drop: A case report. *Am J Sports Med.* 2000;28(4):574–576.
44. Folsom GJ, Larson CM. Surgical treatment of acute versus chronic complete proximal hamstring ruptures: Results of a new allograft technique for chronic reconstructions. *Am J Sports Med.* 2008;36(1):104–109.
45. Blasier RB, Morawa LG. Complete rupture of the hamstring origin from a water skiing injury. *Am J Sports Med.* 1990;18(4):435–437.
46. Muscato M, Lim-Dunham J, Demos TC, et al. Avulsion fracture of the apophysis of the ischial tuberosity. *Orthopedics.* 2001;24(12):1127, 1198–1200.
47. Puranen J, Orava S. The hamstring syndrome. A new diagnosis of gluteal sciatic pain. *Am J Sports Med.* 1988;16(5):517–521.
48. Carmody C, Prietto C. Entrapment of the sciatic nerve as a late sequela of injury to the hamstring muscles: A case report. *J Bone Joint Surg Am.* 1995;77(7):1100–1102.
49. Chakravarthy J, Ramisetty N, Pimpalnerkar A, et al. Surgical repair of complete proximal hamstring tendon ruptures in water skiers and bull riders: A report of four cases and review of the literature. *Br J Sports Med.* 2005;39(8):569–572.
50. Thomsen NO, Jensen TT. Late repair of rupture of the hamstring tendons from the ischial tuberosity—A case report. *Acta Orthop Scand.* 1999;70(1):89–91.
51. Lempainen L, Sarimo J, Orava S. Recurrent and chronic complete ruptures of the proximal origin of the hamstring muscles repaired with fascia lata autograft augmentation. *Arthroscopy.* 2007;23(4):441·e1–441·e5.
52. Miller A, Stedman GH, Beisaw NE, et al. Sciatica caused by an avulsion fracture of the ischial tuberosity: A case report. *J Bone Joint Surg Am.* 1987;69(1):143–145.
53. Kujala UM, Orava S, Karpakka J, et al. Ischial tuberosity apophysitis and avulsion among athletes. *Int J Sports Med.* 1997;18(2):149–155.
54. Schlonsky J, Olix ML. Functional disability following avulsion fracture of the ischial epiphysis. Report of two cases. *J Bone Joint Surg Am.* 1972;54(3):641–644.
55. Barnes ST, Hinds RB. Pseudotumor of the ischium: A late manifestation of avulsion of the ischial epiphysis. *J Bone Joint Surg Am.* 1972;54(3):645–647.
56. Hamada G, Rida A. Ischial apophysiolysis (IAL). Report of a case and review of the literature. *Clin Orthop Relat Res.* 1963;31:117–130.
57. Servant CT, Jones CB. Displaced avulsion of the ischial apophysis: A hamstring injury requiring internal fixation. *Br J Sports Med.* 1998;32(3):255–257.
58. Gill DR, Clark WB. Avulsion of the ischial apophysis. *Aust NZ J Surg.* 1996;66(8): 564–565.

CHAPTER

19

Benton E. Heyworth
Benjamin A. MacArthur
Bryan T. Kelly

Anterior Hip Muscle Injuries

INTRODUCTION

Hip injuries in the athletic population, while less common than other injuries to the lower extremity,[1–3] are becoming recognized with increasing frequency. An important subset of these injuries includes conditions affecting the anterior muscles of the hip. Improved technology in diagnostic imaging, particularly magnetic resonance imaging (MRI), has led to the identification of a number of previously undiagnosed and underappreciated anterior muscle injuries primarily affecting competitive and recreational athletes. Despite these advances, because of the complex anatomy of the hip, these injuries continue to present diagnostic challenges for clinicians. A number of injuries to the hip region—such as sports hernia, osteitis pubis, acetabular labral tear, and femoral neck stress fracture—which are the subjects of other chapters of this text, can mask or confound the diagnosis of an anterior muscle injury and must be ruled out. For example, a competitive hurdler may have sustained an iliopsoas or sartorius muscle strain, but an underlying femoral neck stress fracture (which may have led to modifications in the athlete's hurdling form and represented an etiological factor in the muscle injury) could be associated with devastating sequelae if the diagnosis is delayed. Thus, familiarity with the range of hip conditions that occur in athletes, both acute and chronic, is essential for sports medicine specialists and general orthopedic surgeons alike.

This chapter will focus on three distinct forms of anterior hip muscle injury. First, apophyseal avulsion injuries, which specifically affect pediatric and adolescent patients, will be reviewed. The topics of the second section, which discusses rectus femoris and iliopsoas strains and ruptures, are essentially a continuation of the first subject as similar mechanisms of injury preceding apophyseal avulsion injury can lead, in adults, to injuries of the musculotendinous units originating from and inserting upon the stronger, ossified apophyses in the mature skeletal system. Finally, the topic of iliopsoas impingement (IPI), and the concomitant, associated injuries of the iliopsoas tendon and anterior acetabular labrum, will be explored. In each section, an analysis of epidemiological factors, clinical presentation, diagnostic approaches, and management strategies will guide the reader to a deeper and broader understanding of the topic of anterior hip muscle injuries.

APOPHYSEAL AVULSION INJURIES

Apophyseal avulsion injuries, while rare, are becoming increasingly recognized among young athletes. These injuries are unique to adolescents and are particularly prevalent among those involved in athletics such as football, soccer, gymnastics, dance, hockey, lacrosse, volleyball, and track and field.[4] In an analysis of 203 pelvic apophyseal avulsion injuries in 198 adolescent athletes, Rossi and Dragoni[5] found that soccer and gymnastics represented the most common sporting activities among their population. Injuries are typically seen in athletes between the ages of 10 and 25 years old, prior to the completion of skeletal maturation.[6]

The mechanism of apophyseal avulsion is most commonly a sudden, powerful contraction of the attached hip muscles, as is seen in a soccer kick, or a forceful stretch of these muscles, as with a gymnastics split. Because the apophyses of the femur and pelvis undergo ossification later than other areas of bone about the hip, these areas of attachment of hip and abdominal wall muscle groups are typically weaker than their tendinous attachments. As a result, the apophyses are vulnerable to repetitive, microtrauma-induced apophysitis or acute rupture. Thus, the same mechanism of injury that might result in a muscular strain in the adult patient is likely to cause avulsion or traction injuries to the inherently weaker, cartilaginous apophysis in a pediatric or adolescent patient. Similarly, the sort of repetitive overuse microtrauma that can cause tendonitis in an adult patient is likely to be associated with apophysitis in a younger athlete. Areas most commonly affected include the anterior superior iliac spine (ASIS) and the ischial tuberosity, where the sartorius muscle and the hamstring and adductor muscles originate, respectively.[7] Involvement of the anterior inferior iliac spine (AIIS), origin of the direct head of the rectus femoris, greater trochanter, into which the gluteus medius and minimus insert, or lesser trochanter, site of the iliopsoas insertion, may also be seen.

A thorough history of the associated injury, with specific attention to activity and leg position at the time of injury, provides crucial information about the area or areas likely to be affected. While sudden hip flexion during a dance routine might be associated with an avulsion of the ischial tuberosity, injury while punting a football with the hip in extension may lead the treating physician to consider the possibility of AIIS or ASIS avulsion. The hallmark presentation for acute apophyseal avulsion is an adolescent athlete who presents with acute onset of pain after an episode of strenuous activity. Patients may report feeling a "pop" followed by localized pain, swelling, and tenderness in the affected area. Patients will often hold the injured leg in a position that reduces tension on the involved muscle.[1]

On physical exam, careful palpation of the bony landmarks of the pelvis and proximal femur will reveal localized tenderness. Similarly, active or passive stretching of attached muscle groups will result in reproduction of pain at the site of attachment. As with any orthopaedic physical exam, it is helpful and appropriate to compare physical findings with the unaffected contralateral hip.

Evaluation of plain radiographs of the pelvis along with orthogonal views of the hip can give useful information with regards to the size and displacement of the avulsed fragment. However, radiographic evaluation may be more difficult in younger patients, and a high index of suspicion should be maintained even in the setting of negative radiographs if history and physical exam are suggestive of apophyseal injury, since secondary ossification centers may not yet be visible. MRI is a useful adjunctive imaging tool for younger patients, particularly when X-rays do not provide definitive diagnosis, for example with nondisplaced apophyseal avulsion injuries. Moreover, decisions related to the need for surgery, for which degree of displacement may be instructive, are assisted with the three-dimensional assessment capabilities of MRI over radiographs. However, as a general rule, plain films alone are sufficient to diagnose apophyseal avulsion in the majority of cases. Notably, frog-leg lateral radiographs should be ordered in all adolescents complaining of hip pain in order to rule out slipped capital femoral epiphysis.

The overwhelming majority of apophyseal injuries can be treated nonoperatively. Conservative management of nondisplaced and minimally displaced apophyseal fractures should typically include rest, ice, and protected weight bearing with crutches until the resolution of symptoms. In addition, physical therapy, which should be initiated after a short period of rest, is an important component of patient care. Therapy should begin with gentle stretching and passive range of motion exercises aimed at the prevention of stiffness. Strengthening exercises, which place significant load on the area of injury, should be avoided until pain is completely resolved.[8,9] Though minimally displaced fractures are initially considered nonsurgical problems, follow-up evaluation is needed to ensure appropriate healing and bony development at the site of injury as well as to monitor for recurrence of injury upon the patient's return to athletics.

On rare occasions, significant displacement of an avulsed fragment or persistent pain refractory to conservative measures dictate the need for surgical intervention.[10] There is some controversy in the existing literature as to precisely what degree of displacement warrants surgery.[8] While it is generally accepted that fractures that are either nondisplaced or minimally displaced should be treated nonoperatively, some authors have noted that fractures with any displacement are more likely to end in painful fibrous nonunion, which may limit function and eventually require delayed operative intervention.[11] In 1965, Howard and Piha[12] advocated fixation for displacement greater than 2 cm. Anderson et al.[1] echoed the use of this parameter in a 2001 review. The operative technique for fixation has been variably described. While some advocate open reduction internal fixation of the bony fragment, others suggest resection of the fragment and reattachment of the tendon origin.[11] Criteria for return to play should include radiographic evidence of bony healing and the absence of pain during activities similar to those performed in the sport. Time to recovery may vary with some patients being able to return to play in 6 weeks while others may require up to 6 months.

RECTUS FEMORIS AND ILIOPSOAS INJURIES

Injuries to the anterior muscles of the hip in adult athletes may often be seen as part of a simple epidemiological progression of the apophyseal avulsion injuries that affect children and adolescents. As the growing skeleton undergoes the normal process of ossification of apophyses, the strength of these bony protuberances exceed that of their originating and inserting musculotendinous units. As a result, similar mechanisms of injury preceding apophyseal injuries transmit abnormal forces to the relatively weaker tendons or muscles in the adult musculoskeletal system, leading to different sites of injury that affect younger patients.

Muscle strains are the most common injuries about the hip and groin resulting from athletic competition.[1] Anatomical structures that cross two joints, such as the rectus femoris, iliopsoas, and sartorius, are among the most frequently injured structures because of the tendency toward eccentric contractions, in which the muscle is contracting as it is lengthening.[1,13] The myotendinous junction is the most common site of injury, though the muscle belly injuries can occur as well.[1,13–16] One classification system for quadriceps strain injuries has been applied to strain injuries in other muscles.[16] In this system, a grade 1 injury represents a tear of limited number of muscle fibers. Grade 2 injury refers to the tearing of a moderate number of fibers without disruption of the muscle fascia. A grade 3 muscle strain involves tearing many fibers as well as part of the fascia. Grade 4 injury denotes a complete rupture of the musculotendinous unit with disruption of all fibers and fascia. Patients who present with more severe, higher grade injuries are more likely to suffer through a longer recovery and tend to have poorer long-term outcomes.

RECTUS FEMORIS INJURY

The rectus femoris is among the most well-studied anterior hip muscles in which strains occur, and because of its biarticular nature, it is the most commonly injured of the four individual quadriceps muscles.[17–19] In addition, the rectus femoris is involved in rapid, forceful contractions due to a high percentage of type II fast-twitch muscle fibers.[20] Sudden hip flexion, which may occur in running, sprinting, kicking a soccer ball, or certain maneuvers in gymnastics, may be the mechanism of action preceding the injury. However, more often, it is during an eccentric contraction phase, related to the regulation of hip extension or knee flexion, that the rectus femoris is injured.[21] It is also not uncommon for patients to be unaware of a traumatic event, and instead present primarily with a complaint of an anterior thigh mass,[22] in which case, soft-tissue sarcoma must be ruled out.

While the distal musculotendinous junction of the rectus femoris in the quadriceps complex is the most commonly described site of injury, proximal injuries of fibers running from both the direct head, which arises from the AIIS, and indirect or reflected head, which originates more broadly from the superior acetabular ridge, may occur as well. A recent study by Gamradt et al.[23] investigating proximal rectus femoris avulsion injuries in the National Football League (NFL) reported only ten cases from 1986 to 2006, which were described in the league registry underscoring the relative rarity of proximal avulsion injury relative to distal rectus femoris or quadriceps strains or tears.

However, in another series of seven cases among military personnel, three cases occurred at the distal myotendinous junction, three at the proximal myotendinous junction and one just distal to the proximal tendo-osseous junction at the AIIS.[22] A second report describes ten athletes with incomplete, intrasubstance tears at the junction of the tendon of the indirect head and its arising muscle fibers.[17] In this series, kicking and sprinting were the most common precipitating events, and two patients required surgical treatment, including excision of the entire rectus femoris muscle in one collegiate football player.[17]

Clinical presentation following rectus femoris strain can be somewhat variable. Pain may be acute or chronic, and it is generally moderately diffuse about the hip, groin, or thigh. Thigh pain may be either proximal or distal, depending on which myotendinous junction was injured. An anterior thigh mass is often grossly appreciable on physical inspection and ecchymosis is variably present. For proximal rectus femoris injuries, swelling and tenderness is palpable approximately 8 to 10 cm distal to the ASIS.[1] In cases of complete rupture, a palpable defect may be noted on physical exam.[16] Hip flexion and/or knee extension is associated with varying degrees of pain and weakness. MRI is the study of choice for assessing possible muscle strains, ruptures, or avulsion injuries, and should demonstrate acute edema (Fig. 19.1) and retracted muscle or tendon fibers (Fig. 19.2).

Treatment of acute rectus femoris injury, from simple strains to complete proximal avulsions, is generally nonoperative. Gamradt et al.[23] reported that all ten cases in the NFL were treated nonoperatively. The authors noted that the average time from injury to full return to play was 74 days, underscoring the considerable rehabilitation phase associated with recovery from these injuries. In some instances, operative management of severe or chronic cases has been described. A case report by Straw et al.[24] described a chronic rectus femoris muscle rupture in a 22-year-old soccer player that had been refractory to nonoperative management for 12 months. Prior to surgery, the patient was unable to sprint or kick. After a suture repair of the musculotendinous junction, the patient regained near normal strength and returned to play within 6 months. In another series of five athletes consisting of four professional soccer players and one hurdler, Irmola et al.[25] report surgical repair with two to four suture anchors followed by protective hip bracing at 45° of flexion for a week. At 8 weeks, patients began running and average recovery time for return to sport was 9 months. Notably, two of the five patients suffered from postoperative meralgia paresthetica. While not a controlled or comparative study, the authors concluded that the operative treatment of total proximal tendinous avulsions was a good treatment alternative to conservative care.

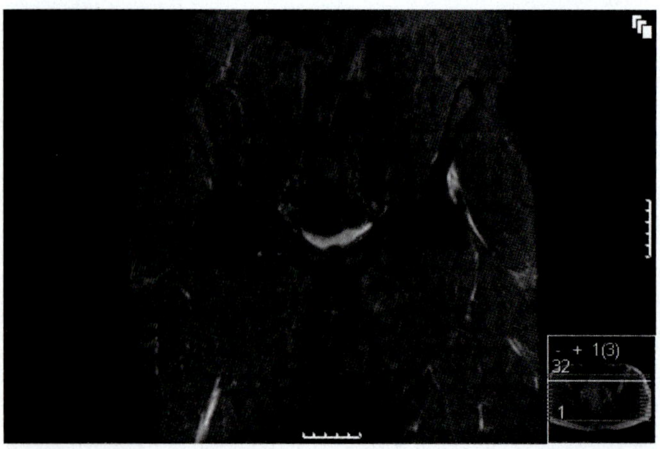

Figure 19.1. Coronal plane T2-weighted MRI image of the pelvis of a 24-year-old NFL linebacker who suffered an acute, proximal rectus femoris avulsion injury. The image demonstrates an acute edema pattern adjacent to the ASIS and superolateral acetabular brim, consistent with the described injury.

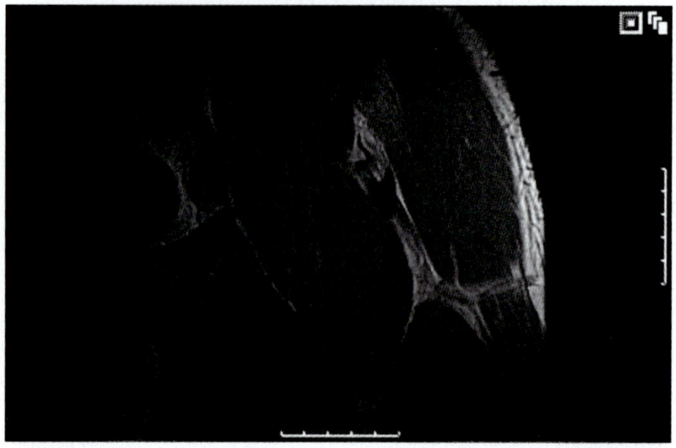

Figure 19.2. Coronal plane T1-weighted MRI image of the left hip of the same patient showing the avulsed, retracted direct head of the rectus femoris adjacent to the ASIS, with a thin shell of osseous fragment still attached to the muscle tendon.

One potential complication of rectus femoris injury is heterotopic ossification (HO), which can occur at the site of any significant muscle strain, contusion, or tendinous avulsion.[1,26] Reactive ossification of the soft tissues surrounding the site of injury may present as a mass, which can be difficult to distinguish from malignant neoplasm both clinically and radiographically. Standard radiographs (Fig. 19.3) and, in some cases, computed tomography (CT) imaging (Fig. 19.4) should be obtained to delineate the precise extent of an HO lesion, particularly if excision is considered. For variably calcified lesions or soft-tissue masses presenting any question or concern for neoplasm, Resnick et al.[26] advocated the use of a Tru-Cut needle biopsy of the lesion. In the case of a confirmed contusion or hematoma, nonsteroidal anti-inflammatory drugs may be useful for prevention of ossification. Treatment of HO is typically conservative; however, if the size or location of the mass causes it to interfere significantly with patient function, it can be excised. However, it is recommended that excision take place at least 6 months and preferably 12 months after the initial insult as this will decrease the likelihood of recurrence.[1]

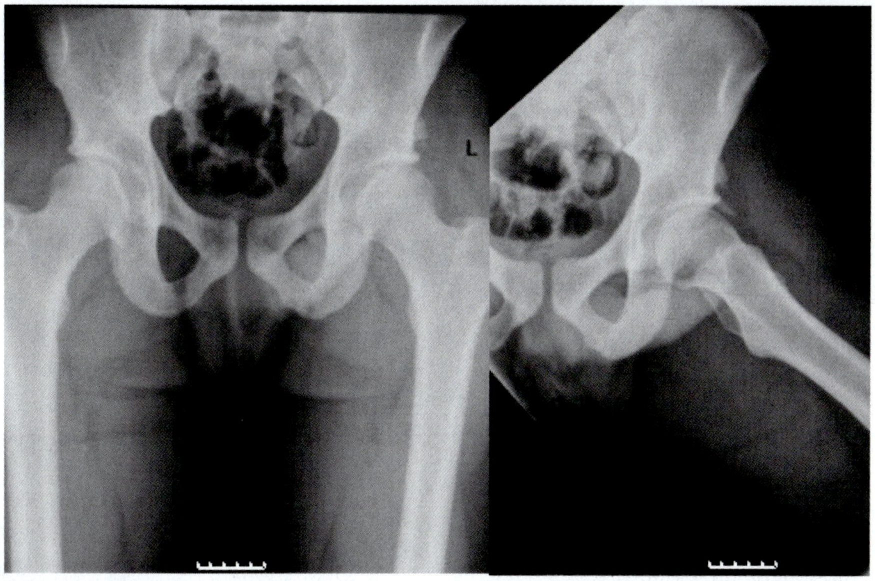

Figure 19.3. Six-month follow-up radiographs (**left**: anteroposterior pelvis; **right**: left hip frog-leg lateral) of the patient demonstrating focal regions of HO at the ASIS and superolateral brim of the acetabulum.

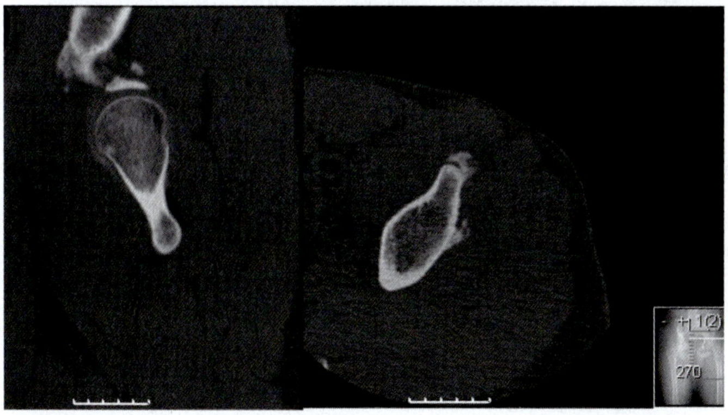

Figure 19.4. Six-month follow-up CT scan (**left**: left hip sagittal plane image; **right**: left hip axial plane image) shows similar findings to radiographs, with more detail of three-dimensional extent of bone formation.

ILIOPSOAS INJURY

A number of different conditions affecting athletes involve the iliopsoas musculotendinous unit, such as snapping hip (reviewed in another chapter in this text), IPI (described in a following section of this chapter), and iliopsoas strain, hematoma, or rupture. In a prospective study of 207 athletes with activity-induced groin pain lasting greater than 2 months, Holmich[27] found that one third of patients suffered from a primary iliopsoas injury, and among runners, iliopsoas injury represented the most common cause of groin pain. As the major flexor of the hip, the iliopsoas is particularly at risk for overuse injuries in runners.

The most common mechanism of injury for iliopsoas strain or rupture involves powerful hip flexion against resistance or passive hyperextension of the hip joint. When the lower limbs are aligned with the trunk, hip flexion is achieved through the contraction of the sartorius, rectus femoris, and several other muscles in addition to the iliopsoas. However, when the lower limbs are not in line with the trunk, hip flexion may depend on the action of the iliopsoas alone, resulting in a marked increase in muscle load.[28] As is the case with other muscle groups, eccentric loading is particularly likely to cause strain injuries to the iliopsoas. These types of injuries are especially prevalent among soccer players, runners, and gymnasts.[1,27] Soccer players who are forcefully blocked while kicking with the hip in extension are prone to this injury.

Clinical presentation of patients with iliopsoas injury is quite variable. Patients may complain of lower quadrant abdominal pain or groin pain that is made worse with hip flexion, especially flexion against resistance. Because of the typical pain distribution, iliopsoas injuries can mimic other important pathology including appendicitis, inguinal hernia, and gynecological conditions.[27] As such, a thorough history and physical examination are crucial in these patients.

The iliacus muscle may also undergo an isolated strain or tear. While iliacus rupture and hematoma have more commonly been described in association with anticoagulation medicines,[20,21,29,30] hemophilia,[31] or other bleeding disorders,[32] there are reports related to athletic activities as well.[32,33] One case report described the case of a healthy 24-year-old male who sustained a tear of iliacus fibers at the distal myotendinous junction following simple abdominal extension exercises.[33] Notably, a large hematoma surrounded the femoral neurovascular bundle and was associated with quadriceps weakness, diminished anterior thigh sensation in the distribution of the lateral femoral cutaneous and saphenous nerves, and an absent patellae tendon reflex. Conservative treatment resulted in full resolution of pain and neurologic signs and symptoms within 6 months. A second report described a gymnast who sustained proximal avulsion of the iliacus muscle from its pelvic origin on the iliac crest, which was also associated with paralysis of the femoral nerve.[32] Other reports, frequently citing gymnastics activities, have been published as well, and femoral nerve deficits are nearly universal.[34]

Physical examination for investigating possible iliopsoas or iliacus injury usually reveals tenderness to palpation in the groin or overlying the area of the tendon. Positioning the patients supine and asking them to attempt a straight leg raise while the examiner applies resistance and pressure over the iliacus fossa will intensify pain symptoms. In a report by Mozes et al.[28] on the diagnosis and treatment of various iliopsoas injuries seen in 40 soccer players, it was noted that all patients demonstrated this sign on physical examination. Additionally, when sitting with outstretched legs, patients with iliopsoas injury will experience pain and difficulty with any attempt to lift their heels off of the table. This is referred to as Ludlof sign. Injuries are often associated with significant soft-tissue swelling and femoral nerve palsy may be a concomitant finding in some cases.[1]

Radiographic evaluation of patients suspected to have iliopsoas injury may be necessary to rule out the possibility of intra-abdominal pathology. Plain radiographs may show signs of soft-tissue swelling and edema in the area of muscle strain but will frequently appear normal. MRI is the best imaging modality for clear depiction of the degree of soft-tissue damage. However, MRI is rarely necessary as the clinical history and physical findings are usually sufficient for diagnosis.

Management of iliopsoas strains or partial tears is generally nonoperative, consisting primarily of rest and directed physical therapy. Mozes et al.[28] reported successful treatment with corticosteroid and anesthetic injections into the iliopsoas tendon sheath in 40 soccer players with symptoms diagnosed by physical exam findings, with other entities being ruled out by radiographs and ultrasound. All players returned to play, though 25% required additional injections before significant symptomatic relief was obtained. Treatment of suspected proximal iliacus muscle or tendon avulsion has ranged from observation to use of retroperitoneal approaches for iliacus exploration, hematoma drainage, and/or femoral nerve exploration.[29–34] If the injury is associated with femoral nerve compromise, expeditious diagnostic workup, including either CT or MRI, followed by hematoma evacuation if present, is warranted.

ILIOPSOAS IMPINGEMENT

IPI has previously been described predominantly in patients who have undergone total hip arthroplasty (THA).[35–39] In these patients, anterior extrusion of cement or overhang of the acetabular cup has been associated with symptoms of iliopsoas irritation including groin pain with active hip flexion or flexion against resistance.[35,40] However, a recent study by Domb et al.[41] suggests that IPI may be seen in association with, and play a causative role in, a previously undescribed mechanism of anterior labral injury. In this study, 56 patients with anterior hip pain were found to have an anterior labral injury corresponding to the 3 o'clock position. Unlike labral injury associated with femoroacetabular impingement (FAI), which is typically anterosuperior in roughly the 1 o'clock or 2 o'clock position, these patients were found to have injury that was directly anterior, without any evidence of FAI, bony abnormality, trauma, or other known cause of labral pathology. MRI may demonstrate a focal adhesion of the psoas tendon to the labrum or an edema pattern deep to the psoas tendon and adjacent to the labrum, which may be torn, frayed, or partially delaminated (Fig. 19.5). Arthroscopic examination of the affected joint revealed a consistent, intimate relationship between the iliopsoas tendon and the site of pathology, with the inflamed tendon lying directly anterior to the injury in all cases (Figs. 19.6 & 19.7). The authors propose three theoretical explanations for the direct anterior labral tear described in the study.

First, the authors suggest that a tight, inflamed iliopsoas tendon causes impingement of the anterior labrum with the hip in extension.[41] This theory is based upon the anatomic and biomechanical function of the iliopsoas. In the native hip, the iliopsoas tendon runs around the iliopectineal eminence and femoral head at an obtuse angle that widens with hip extension. Because maximal pressure beneath the iliopsoas tendon occurs directly over the femoral head, the possibility exists that pressure and friction exerted on the femoral head and anterior labrum during hip motion could cause labral damage.[42] This mechanism would be particularly relevant in patients with a tight or inflamed iliopsoas since contact pressures would be significantly increased, further increasing the likelihood of labral impingement.

Second, the study described frictional contact, and the resulting adhesions between iliopsoas tendon and the anterior capsulolabral complex leads to a repetitive traction induced injury.[41] This mechanism would involve chronic inflammation of the tendon or bursa resulting in tissue injury and fibrotic scar

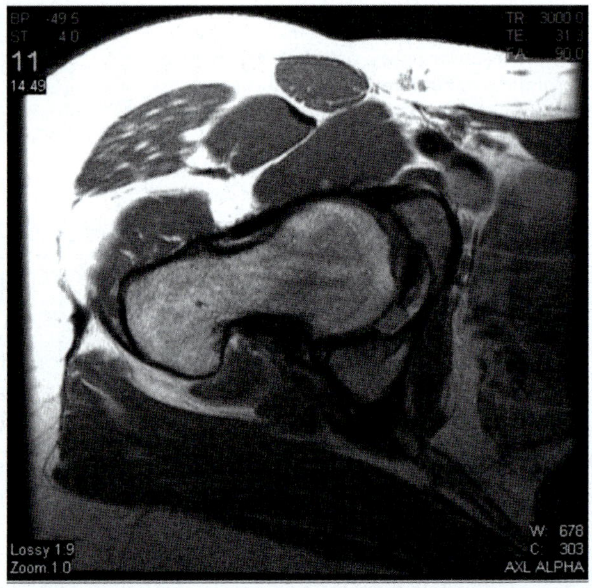

Figure 19.5. Preoperative axial plane MRI image of right hip of 20-year-old female gymnast with complaints of right anterior groin pain and weakness with right hip flexion. The image demonstrates a focal edema pattern between the anterior acetabulum and the psoas musculotendinous unit, with partial delamination of the labral attachment to the acetabulum.

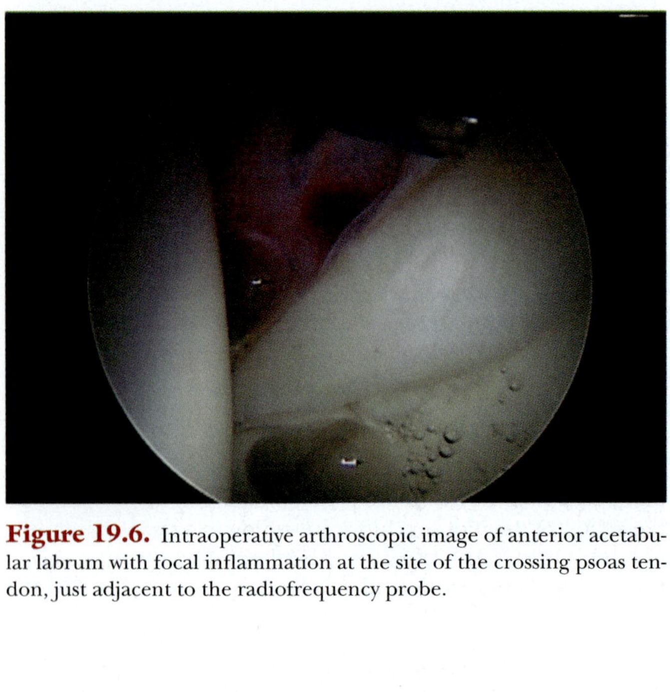

Figure 19.6. Intraoperative arthroscopic image of anterior acetabular labrum with focal inflammation at the site of the crossing psoas tendon, just adjacent to the radiofrequency probe.

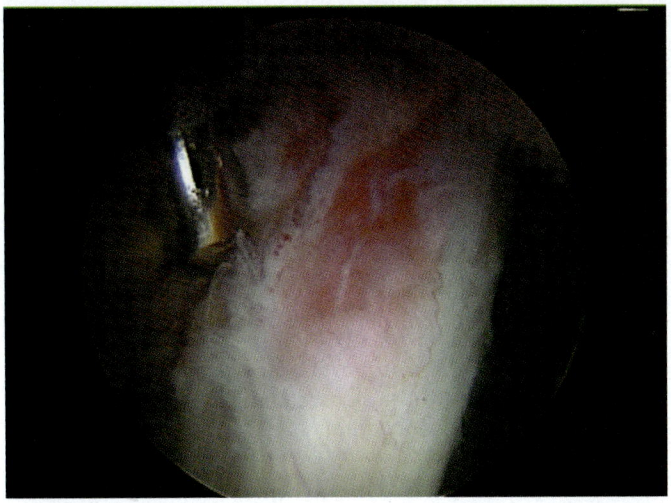

Figure 19.7. Intraoperative arthroscopic image of underside of psoas tendon after debridement of overlying capsule, demonstrating diffuse inflammation.

formation with adhesion of the tendon to the anterior capsule which lies just deep to it. Because the normal biomechanics of the iliopsoas involve lift off from the femoral head at 14° of flexion and from the iliopectineal eminence at 54°, this scarring and adhesion would result in repetitive traction on the capsulolabral complex with hip flexion, which would in turn cause injury to the anterior labrum in the characteristic 3 o'clock position.

Finally, Domb et al.[41] suggest that a hyperactive iliocapsularis muscle may create excessive traction on the anterior labrum resulting in injury. The iliocapsularis, a little known muscle, first described by Ganz et al.[43] was initially noted in patients with dysplasia and was consistently found in cadaveric specimens. The muscle originates on the anterior joint capsule and iliopectineal eminence and inserts just distal to the lesser trochanter. It is believed to act as an anterior stabilizer of the hip, which tightens the capsule upon contraction, and might thus be expected to demonstrate hypertrophy in patients with dysplastic or unstable hip joints. The authors thus propose that if the iliocapsularis was hyperactive or hypertrophied, its action to tighten the capsule might create excessive traction on the capsulolabral complex and induce a traction injury. Though the tendon overlying the labral injuries observed in the study is suspected to be the iliopsoas, the relative proximity of the iliocapsularis to the iliopsoas raises the possibility that the observed tendon may have belonged to the former in some cases.

A report by Yoshio et al.[42] described the tension of and pressure beneath the psoas muscle as the hip was moved from 0° to 90° of flexion in a cadaveric specimen. Of note, it was found that the femoral head, rather than the iliopectineal eminence, was the primary pulley over which the iliopsoas tendon rests. As a result, the pressure beneath the tendon was highest at the location of contact with the femoral head. Factors which the authors noted to be associated with higher pressures include a large femoral head, a tendon that is wide and thin at the point of contact with the femoral head, a small neck shaft angle, a high degree of femoral anteversion, and a relatively small angle at the level of the pulley. Domb et al.[41] cite these findings as evidence in support of IPI as an etiology for anterior labral injury and assert that the five factors described above may in fact be risk factors for the development of this particular pathology.

Domb et al.[41] also point to the well-described mechanism in arthroplasty patients, namely, impingement of the iliopsoas tendon on the anterior acetabular cup, as being analogous to the proposed mechanism of IPI on the anterior capsule–labral complex in their patient population. They point out that the anterior overhang of the acetabular cup may be similar to a large or deformed femoral head, which may cause the psoas tendon angle to be more acute than normal.[37]

As would be expected with IPI, all patients in the study by Domb et al.[41] presented with complaints of anterior hip pain and pain with active hip flexion. Hip snapping was reported by some patients as well. On physical examination, patients were noted to have focal tenderness to palpation over the iliopsoas. In addition, a positive impingement test was repeatedly demonstrated, with patients endorsing symptoms of pain with flexion, adduction, and internal rotation of the hip. Patients were also noted to have pain or apprehension with resisted straight leg raise.

Several series have described patients with IPI after THA undergoing injections about the iliopsoas tendon or iliopsoas tenotomy at the level of the acetabulum, with subsequent relief of symptoms.[34,35,41,42] For example, Dora et al.[40] noted relief of pain in 18 out of 22 cases treated with either tenotomy or revision of the acetabular component. Furthermore, the authors noted that the same functional results were achieved with tenotomy as were seen with acetabular component revision without subjecting the patient to the increased risk of a revision procedure. A report by Ala Eddine et al.[35] described nine cases of IPI treated first with infiltration of xylocaine and long acting steroid preparations, which was completely effective in four patients and partially effective in another. Patients who suffered a recurrence of pain were treated with tenotomy, with three patients experiencing complete relief and another patient experiencing partial relief. Thus, seven of the nine patients experienced complete relief of symptoms with either steroid injection or tenotomy. Based upon these reports, Domb et al.[41] assert that in patients with direct anterior labral injury believed to be associated with IPI, treatment with fractional lengthening—involving release of the tendinous portion of the musculotendinous unit (Fig. 19.8)—of the iliopsoas tendon at the level of the anterior acetabular brim may provide relief of symptoms.

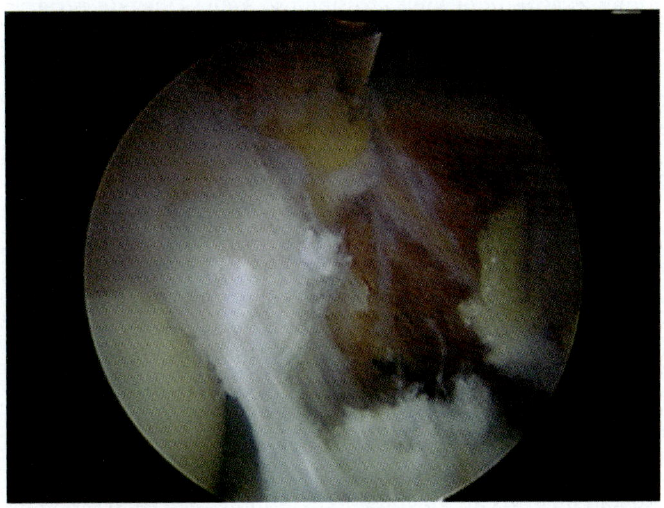

Figure 19.8. Intraoperative arthroscopic image of iliopsoas muscle, after release of inflamed tendinous portion of musculotendinous unit.

A review of the literature reveals several reports of release of the iliopsoas as a treatment for internal coxa saltans. Moderate success has been reported with open release.[39,44] In a report of 92 cases of coxa saltans treated with open iliopsoas fractional lengthening, Hoskins et al.[45] noted 89% patient satisfaction postoperatively. However, their series had a complication rate of 40% with the open technique. Arthroscopic release of the psoas tendon has also been described in the literature.[46–49] Techniques described vary from complete tenotomy at the site of insertion on the lesser trochanter to fractional lengthening through either the central or peripheral compartments. Domb et al.[41] report no complications at short-term follow-up. Long-term follow-up outcome measures with strength assessments of hip flexion and leg extension are being collected.

CONCLUSION

In summary, the anterior muscles of the hip may be involved in a wide variety of athletic injuries. In adolescents, prior to the onset of skeletal maturity, the cartilaginous apophyses about the hip are vulnerable to injury and avulsion with powerful contraction of the attached musculature. The ischial tuberosity, ASIS, AIIS, and greater and lesser trochanters are commonly affected. While clinical history and physical examination are crucial for proper diagnosis, radiographic evaluation or MRI is often useful for confirmation of clinical suspicion as well as characterization of the orientation and degree of separation of the avulsed fragment. While most cases are treated nonoperatively, some cases with significant displacement may be refractory to conservative management and consideration of operative fixation is appropriate. Minimally displaced fragments should be followed by an orthopaedist to ensure that adequate healing occurs.

Injuries similar in mechanism to those responsible for apophyseal avulsions in adolescents are likely to cause acute muscle strain or rupture in the skeletally mature adult. With the ossification of the apophyses, the musculotendinous junction becomes the weakest link in the musculoskeletal unit and is thus vulnerable to injury with forceful muscle contraction, especially eccentric contraction, where the muscle contracts during extension. The rectus femoris and iliopsoas represent the most commonly affected muscles and are at an increased risk for injury as a result of their crossing two joints. Imaging is rarely necessary for these patients since clinical history and physical exam are fairly specific and usually sufficient for diagnosis. In cases when imaging studies are desired for better delineation of the magnitude and character of soft-tissue injury, MRI is the most appropriate imaging modality. Rest, ice elevation, compression, and short-term use of NSAIDs are the cornerstone of muscle strain management, with gradual return to activity as pain subsides. In some cases of grade 4 complete muscle rupture, surgical reapproximation may be considered in patients with a prolonged treatment course and symptoms refractory to conservative measures.

IPI, which has been well described in THA patient populations, may represent a previously undescribed cause of anterior hip pain and labral injury in the native hip. Current evidence suggests a possible association between iliopsoas inflammation, hypertrophy, or scarring and anterior labral pathology. Research efforts are ongoing to determine the efficacy of combined arthroscopic labral debridement and fractional lengthening of the iliopsoas tendon. Further research is necessary to determine the overall prevalence of this condition and its relevance to the sports medicine community.

As a deep, anatomically complex junction between the axial and appendicular skeleton, the hip joint may be affected by a broad and varied range of pathology. As a result, hip conditions present frequent diagnostic challenges that demand a comprehensive understanding of their intra-articular and periarticular pathophysiology from sports medicine specialists and general orthopaedic surgeons alike. As this understanding continues to be propelled by new research and advancements in diagnostic technology, anterior muscle injuries of the hip are being recognized with increasing frequency in both competitive and recreational athletes. Early identification and proper treatment will lead to prevention of more significant injury and optimization of performance and return to play.

REFERENCES

1. Anderson K, Strickland SM, Warren R. Hip and groin injuries in athletes. *Am J Sports Med.* 2001;29(4):521–533.
2. DeLee JC, Farney WC. Incidence of injury in Texas high school football. *Am J Sports Med.* 1992;20(5):575–580.
3. Gomez E, DeLee JC, Farney WC. Incidence of injury in Texas girls' high school basketball. *Am J Sports Med.* 1996;24(5):684–687.
4. Frank JB, Jarit GJ, Bravman JT, et al. Lower extremity injuries in the skeletally immature athlete. *J Am Acad Orthop Surg.* 2007;15(6):356–366.
5. Rossi F, Dragoni S. Acute avulsion fractures of the pelvis in adolescent competitive athletes: Prevalence, location and sports distribution of 203 cases collected. *Skeletal Radiol.* 2001;30(3):127–131.
6. Waters PM, Millis MB. Hip and pelvic injuries in the young athlete. *Clin Sports Med.* 1988;7(3):513–526.
7. Fernbach SK, Wilkinson RH. Avulsion injuries of the pelvis and proximal femur. *AJR Am J Roentgenol.* 1981;137(3):581–584.
8. Metzmaker JN, Pappas AM. Avulsion fractures of the pelvis. *Am J Sports Med.* 1985;13(5):349–358.
9. Outerbridge AR, Micheli LJ. Overuse injuries in the young athlete. *Clin Sports Med.* 1995;14(3):503–516.
10. Kocher MS, Tucker R. Pediatric athlete hip disorders. *Clin Sports Med.* 2006;25(2):241–253, viii.
11. Wootton JR, Cross MJ, Holt KW. Avulsion of the ischial apophysis: The case for open reduction and internal fixation. *J Bone Joint Surg Br.* 1990;72(4):625–627.
12. Howard FM, Piha RJ. Fractures of the apophyses in adolescent athletes. *JAMA.* 1965;192:842–844.
13. Garrett WE Jr. Muscle strain injuries. *Am J Sports Med.* 1996;24(Suppl. 6):S2–S8.
14. Tidball JG, Salem G, Zernicke R. Site and mechanical conditions for failure of skeletal muscle in experimental strain injuries. *J Appl Physiol.* 1993;74(3):1280–1286.
15. Noonan TJ, Best TM, Seaber AV, et al. Identification of a threshold for skeletal muscle injury. *Am J Sports Med.* 1994;22(2):257–261.
16. Noonan TJ, Garrett WE Jr. Muscle strain injury: Diagnosis and treatment. *J Am Acad Orthop Surg.* 1999;7(4):262–269.
17. Hughes C IV, Hasselman CT, Best TM, et al. Incomplete, intrasubstance strain injuries of the rectus femoris muscle. *Am J Sports Med.* 1995;23(4):500–506.
18. Speer KP, Lohnes J, Garrett WE Jr. Radiographic imaging of muscle strain injury. *Am J Sports Med.* 1993;21(1):89, 95, discussion 96.
19. Zarins B, Ciullo JV. Acute muscle and tendon injuries in athletes. *Clin Sports Med.* 1983;2(1):167–182.
20. Garrett WE Jr, Califf JC, Bassett FH III. Histochemical correlates of hamstring injuries. *Am J Sports Med.* 1984;12(2):98–103.
21. Renstrom PA. Tendon and muscle injuries in the groin area. *Clin Sports Med.* 1992;11(4):815–831.
22. Temple HT, Kuklo TR, Sweet DE, et al. Rectus femoris muscle tear appearing as a pseudotumor. *Am J Sports Med.* 1998;26(4):544–548.
23. Gamradt SC, Brophy RH, Barnes R, et al. Nonoperative treatment for proximal avulsion of the rectus femoris in professional American football. *Am J Sports Med.* 2009;37(7):1370–1374.
24. Straw R, Colclough K, Geutjens G. Surgical repair of a chronic rupture of the rectus femoris muscle at the proximal musculotendinous junction in a soccer player. *Br J Sports Med.* 2003;37(2):182–184.
25. Irmola T, Heikkila JT, Orava S, et al. Total proximal tendon avulsion of the rectus femoris muscle. *Scand J Med Sci Sports.* 2007;17(4):378–382.
26. Resnick JM, Carrasco CH, Edeiken J, et al. Avulsion fracture of the anterior inferior iliac spine with abundant reactive ossification in the soft tissue. *Skeletal Radiol.* 1996;25(6):580–584.
27. Holmich P. Long-standing groin pain in sportspeople falls into three primary patterns, a "clinical entity" approach: A prospective study of 207 patients. *Br J Sports Med.* 2007;41(4):52, 247, 52, discussion 252.
28. Mozes M, Papa MZ, Zweig A, et al. Iliopsoas injury in soccer players. *Br J Sports Med.* 1985;19(3):168–170.
29. Sigler L, Raut PS, Vollman RW. Iliacus muscle hematoma: A complication of heparin administration. *Angiology.* 1970;21(2):114–115.

30. Fearn CB. Iliacus haematoma syndrome as a complication of anticoagulant therapy. *Br Med J.* 1968;4(5623):97–98.
31. Goodfellow J, Fearn CB, Matthews JM. Iliacus haematoma: A common complication of haemophilia. *J Bone Joint Surg Br.* 1967;49(4):748–756.
32. Green JP. Proximal avulsion of the iliacus with paralysis of the femoral nerve: Report of a case. *J Bone Joint Surg Br.* 1972;54(1):154–156.
33. Sanders SM, Schachter AK, Schweitzer M, et al. Iliacus muscle rupture with associated femoral nerve palsy after abdominal extension exercises: A case report. *Am J Sports Med.* 2006;34(5):837–839.
34. Tomishige M, Morita M. A case report: Tearing of the iliopsoas muscle caused by a fall from a handstand position. *Seikei Geka.* 1965;16(6):530–534.
35. Ala Eddine T, Remy F, Chantelot C, et al. Anterior iliopsoas impingement after total hip arthroplasty: Diagnosis and conservative treatment in 9 cases. *Rev Chir Orthop Reparatrice Appar Mot.* 2001;87(8):815–819.
36. Bricteux S, Beguin L, Fessy MH. Iliopsoas impingement in 12 patients with a total hip arthroplasty. *Rev Chir Orthop Reparatrice Appar Mot.* 2001;87(8):820–825.
37. Cyteval C, Sarrabere MP, Cottin A, et al. Iliopsoas impingement on the acetabular component: Radiologic and computed tomography findings of a rare hip prosthesis complication in eight cases. *J Comput Assist Tomogr.* 2003;27(2):183–188.
38. Meyer JD, Plotz W, Tillmann K, et al. Iliopsoas impingement after cementless total hip arthroplasty. Case reports. *Orthopade.* 2002;31(2):213–216.
39. Trousdale RT, Cabanela ME, Berry DJ. Anterior iliopsoas impingement after total hip arthroplasty. *J Arthroplasty.* 1995;10(4):546–549.
40. Dora C, Houweling M, Koch P, et al. Iliopsoas impingement after total hip replacement: The results of non-operative management, tenotomy or acetabular revision. *J Bone Joint Surg Br.* 2007;89(8):1031–1035.
41. Domb BG, Shindle MK, Asnis PD, et al. Iliopsoas impingement: A newly identified cause of labral pathology in the hip. In press.
42. Yoshio M, Murakami G, Sato T, et al. The function of the psoas major muscle: Passive kinetics and morphological studies using donated cadavers. *J Orthop Sci.* 2002;7(2):199–207.
43. Ward WT, Fleisch ID, Ganz R. Anatomy of the iliocapsularis muscle: Relevance to surgery of the hip. *Clin Orthop Relat Res.* 2000; 374:278–285.
44. Taylor GR, Clarke NM. Surgical release of the "snapping iliopsoas tendon." *J Bone Joint Surg Br.* 1995;77(6):881–883.
45. Hoskins JS, Burd TA, Allen WC. Surgical correction of internal coxa saltans: A 20-year consecutive study. *Am J Sports Med.* 2004;32(4):998–1001.
46. Wettstein M, Jung J, Dienst M. Arthroscopic psoas tenotomy. *Arthroscopy.* 2006;22(8):907.e1–907.e4.
47. Flanum ME, Keene JS, Blankenbaker DG, Desmet AA. Arthroscopic treatment of the painful "internal" snapping hip: results of a new endoscopic technique and imaging protocol. *Am J Sports Med.* 2007;35(5):770–779.
48. Byrd JW. Evaluation and management of the snapping iliopsoas tendon. *Instr Course Lect.* 2006;55:347–355.
49. Ilizaliturri VM Jr, Villalobos FE Jr, Chaidez PA, et al. Internal snapping hip syndrome: Treatment by endoscopic release of the iliopsoas tendon. *Arthroscopy.* 2005;21(11):1375–1380.

CHAPTER

20

Heidi Prather
Devyani Hunt

Sacroiliac Joint Problems

INTRODUCTION

When an athlete presents with complaints of posterior pelvic pain, the differential diagnosis is broad. At the center of this conundrum lies the sacroiliac joint (SIJ). Many researchers have studied the diagnostic criteria for SIJ dysfunction; however, none have been done in athletes specifically and not one test alone has been proven diagnostic. A constellation of history and physical exam findings can be suggestive. The gold standard for diagnosis has historically been an intra-articular block[1]; however, this is problematic due to the fact that SIJ dysfunction is also caused by extra-articular sources, such as ligaments and muscles.

In an athlete, significant repetitive forces are transferred across the SIJ during sports participation. In order to perform at this high level, the structures that surround and control the SIJ must work in perfect concert and in the most efficient manner. When this system is challenged beyond its capability, pain and dysfunction can occur.

Other areas of consideration that contribute to posterior pelvic pain are the structures that influence the SIJ. Since the pelvis is a ring and articulates with the spine above and the hip joint below, the function of these joints and structures must be considered and any abnormal forces they transfer through the pelvis must be taken into account. Researchers are attempting to qualify the spine–pelvis–hip connection; however, given the complexity of this relationship it remains minimally investigated.

A subset of athletes is at higher risk for SIJ injury. Gymnasts, skaters, golfers, and rowers are examples of athletes who perform asymmetric loading through the SIJ. The combination of repetitive stress and shear forces across the joint puts these athletes at risk for injury. Trauma has also been implicated in a large majority of patients with SIJ pain.[2]

ANATOMY AND BIOMECHANICS

The SIJ is "L" or "C" shaped with two lever arms that interlock at the second sacral level. The SIJ has several joint classifications including a synovial joint, synarthrosis, and amphiarthrosis. The sacral side of the SIJ is lined by thick hyaline cartilage, while the ilial side is lined with fibrocartilage. Both intra and inter individual differences in shape of the joint exist. The anterior fibrous capsule is consistent in most joints, but the posterior capsule is thinner and may have multiple plications. Up to 35% of the population has accessory articulations at the SIJ that develop as a result of degenerative changes over time.[3] Joint stability is aided by ligaments located intra-articularly and periarticularly. The iliolumbar ligament also affects the joint by preventing anterior translation and rotation of L5.

The posterior SIJ is innervated by L3–S3 sacral roots, while the anterior joint receives innervation from L2–S2 roots. Fortin et al.[4] described the dorsal rami of S1 to be the primary innervator of the posterior SIJ ligament. SIJ pain may present in variable regions of the pelvis and lower extremity. This may be due, in part, to its innervation from multiple root levels. Fortin's description of SIJ distribution of pain localized to the buttocks near the posterior superior iliac spine (PSIS) with or without radiation into the groin or lower extremity remains to be the best characterization of SIJ pain.

Vleeming et al.[5,6] best describe the subtle motion changes that occur at the SIJ as a "self-locking mechanism." Stability of the interlocking mechanism is made up of four components. The first two components are form and force closure. Form closure refers to joint surfaces that congruently fit together and require no extra forces to maintain stability. Force closure refers to the forces provided by muscles and ligaments around a joint that assist in providing joint stability. Congruency in form and force closure is necessary to maximize joint stability. Breakdown in either component can lead to less joint stability. The SIJ can vary from side to side in individuals. As a result, form and force closure providing stability may differ as well. An individual's functional demands such as loading with asymmetrical force can lead to breakdown or secondary adaptive patterns that facilitate dysfunction or injury. In general, women tend to have less congruent or form closure as compared to men and require a greater degree of balanced force closure to provide stability. Motor control is the third component[7] and refers to the timing and sequencing of muscle activation and release to facilitate load transfer. The fourth component is emotions and awareness. This refers to the concept that emotions can play favorably or unfavorably on motor control. Each component contributes to joint stability and efficiency.

Proper functioning of the joints surrounding the pelvis is key for cohesive mechanics at the pelvis. Specific direct interrelationships include the ilium that articulates with the sacrum at the SIJ, the lumbar spine that articulates with the sacrum anteriorly via the lumbar disc and posteriorly via the L5–S1 facets. Other joints of the pelvis that indirectly affect the SIJ include the pubic symphysis and the hip. The pelvis serves as the central base through which forces are transmitted both directly and indirectly. Asymmetrical shear and torsional force transmission across the pelvis can lead to SIJ dysfunction. The muscles of the hip, pelvis, and lumbar spine provide indirect motion and load transfer at the SIJ. Abdominal muscles affect motion at the ilium, pubis, and lumbar spine. The psoas connects the thoracolumbar fascia with the lower extremity and may restrict lumbopelvic rhythm. The hamstring and gluteals directly affect the position of the ilium via their attachments at the sacrum and ilium. Muscles functioning in a lengthened or shortened position are not able to provide maximal force absorption. Abdominals firing in a lengthened position do not efficiently absorb forces that affect stability at the lumbar spine and pubic symphysis. Balancing muscle length and strength with coordination of muscle activation is key in maintaining stability.

The thoracolumbar fascia is an important structure that assists in providing SI joint stability during load transmission from the lower extremity through the pelvis, lumbar spine, and abdominals. The superficial lamina of the thoracolumbar fascia facilitates transmission of forces from the lower extremity to the contralateral latissimus dorsi. These forces cross at the level of the sacrum. This transitional region may be a potential area of breakdown.[8]

Studies have shown various ranges of motion but most agree that approximately 4° of rotation and 1.6 mm of translation occurs.[9] The amount of joint motion decreases with age. Women develop degenerative changes that restrict motion at age 50, while men develop them around age 40. With aging, degenerative changes direct the joint into a relative hypomobile state. Often, motion lost at the SIJ is attempted to be regained at another joint such as the hip, lumbosacral segments, and pubic symphysis. Though changes in motion at the SIJ may not cause direct injury to the joint, they place peripheral joints at risk for altered adaptive patterns. Changes in adaptive patterns and mechanics may make these joints more susceptible to injury.

Though the natural degenerative changes that take place must be recognized in both genders, special consideration must be given to women. Women face a constitution of physiological changes across the life span and place them at increased risk of injury. For example, the leading cause of low back and posterior pelvic pain during pregnancy is SIJ dysfunction.[10] This is related to the hormonal changes that promote joint laxity and the change in force distribution related to a growing fetus. Structural differences between men and women also need consideration. The bony pelvis of the female is broader than that of the male. The lower extremity extends from the pelvis including the femur articulating with the acetabulum at the hip joint. Both greater femoral neck anteversion and shorter lower extremity limb length lead to a lower center of gravity for women as compared to men.[11] This alignment suggests different adaptive or firing patterns in women versus men, but not necessarily increased risk for injury.[12] Though the pelvis is inherently a stable ring for both genders, in general, women require more extrinsic forces to assist with stability (muscle activation and ligament stiffness) than men.

Altered lower extremity and pelvic mechanics can then alter pelvic floor function, and in women lead to secondary pelvic pain. An example of an adaptive pattern is overload of the obturator internus. This muscle functions as a primary hip external rotator and abductor. If the gluteus medius is inhibited, the obturator internus is recruited as a hip abductor and may not be strong enough to respond to the load demand or repetition. As a result, an overuse syndrome may develop with pain in the groin and pelvic floor as the primary symptom. Other pelvic floor muscles such as the levator ani group must transfer load forces directly and indirectly across the SIJ and pubic symphysis.

Understanding the anatomy and the complexity of the biomechanics of the hip, pelvis, and lumbar spine, and their relationships to each other is essential in devising a comprehensive treatment program. In isolation, biomechanical changes that lead to overuse injuries in each of these regions are fairly well understood. How they overlap with one another has not fully been vetted in the literature. Also, patients with coexisting disorders presenting with overlapping symptoms can go unrecognized due to the known natural course and degenerative conditions expected with age and trauma especially in patients with posterior pelvic pain. For example, a 30-year-old long-distance runner with posterior pelvic pain may have symptoms from both a herniated disc at L5–S1 and cam type hip impingement associated with an acetabular labral tear. Determining which condition is the "driver" or instigator of the primary complaint becomes the dilemma for the health care provider. The specific biomechanical requirements and adaptive changes that occur in patients with posterior pelvic pain have not been studied in athletes. This discussion is limited to the SIJ, however, the biomechanical changes that can occur at the lumbar spine and hip as a result of a primary injury, degenerative condition, as well as adaptive pattern of movement should always be considered.

HISTORY AND PRESENTATION

Athletes experiencing posterior pelvic pain may present with a wide variety of complaints. Gluteal pain near or surrounding the PSIS is the most common region as described by Fortin et al.[13,14] Other symptoms include groin pain, pain radiating into the lower extremity, numbness, and clicking or popping in the posterior pelvis. Pain may be reported with popping and/or clicking with transitional activities such as getting up from a chair or with sport-specific activities that require unilateral loading or torsion through the pelvis and lower extremity. In particular hurdlers, skaters, and bowlers are at risk because of the repetitive asymmetric load and torsion required. Two studies have been published regarding the risk of SIJ dysfunction in rowers related to the mechanics of rowing.[15,16] In addition to sport-specific activities, some exercise routines including step aerobics, stair stepper, and elliptical trainer can lend themselves to repetitive overload if the exerciser's technique or adaptive pattern allows for asymmetrical shear and torsional forces through the pelvis and lower extremities. Trauma including a direct fall onto or blow to the pelvis is an important historical point to note when evaluating an athlete with posterior pelvic pain. Bernard and Kirkaldy-Willis[2] reported that 58% of those with SIJ pain by history and physical examination presented with a history of trauma. Similarly, Chou et al.[17] found that 44% of patients who experienced pain relief with a fluoroscopically guided SIJ steroid injection had a history of trauma.

There are several similarities in pain distribution and sensation of clicking and/or popping for patients presenting with SIJ pain and early intra-articular hip disorders such as acetabular labral tears with and without hip deformity (femoroacetabular impingement and developmental hip dysplasia).[18]

The examiner must clarify with the patient the location of the pop or click and precise distribution of pain. Though it has not been investigated in the literature, there is the potential for SIJ pain and symptomatic early intra-articular hip disorders to coexist. There is significant overlap in presentation of both conditions.[18,19] Burnett et al.[18] found that 38% of patients treated for hip labral tears had posterior pelvic pain. Five of the sixty-six patients had treatment for a lumbar spine condition prior to labral tear diagnosis. Patients with primary degenerative hip disorders can present with groin and posterior pelvic pain. Nunley et al.[20] reported that 16.1% of patients treated for hip dysplasia complained of posterior pelvic pain associated with lateral hip or groin pain. Fifty percent of acetabular labral tears presenting with buttock pain associated with lateral groin pain were found to have resolution of their symptoms 15 months postarthroscopy.[21] Further, Clohisy et al.[22] reported that 87% of patients presenting with femoral acetabular impingement requiring surgical intervention complained of posterior pelvic pain associated with lateral hip or groin pain. Patients with primary degenerative hip disorders can also complain of buttock pain. Lesher et al.[23] reported that patients responding to intra-articular hip injection reported pain in the groin, lateral hip, and buttock region.

In addition to hip pain, low back pain (LBP) related to degenerative conditions can present in similar distributions. In caring for the athlete with posterior pelvic pain, the history and pain distribution provides important information to guide the diagnostic evaluation and treatment. Because of the overlap in symptoms, the specialists must often rely on their individual experiences to direct care.

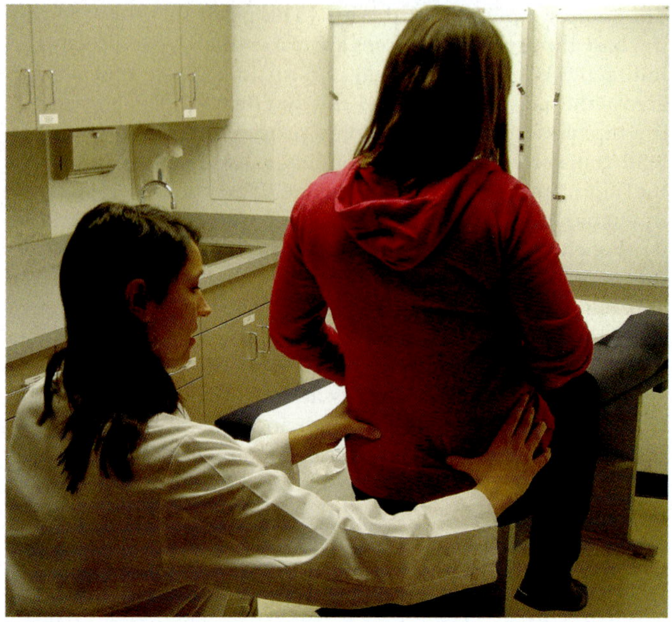

Figure 20.1. Gillet examination.

PHYSICAL EXAMINATION

Just as the presentation of SIJ pain is varied, so can the physical examination findings.

Because of this variability and possibility of coexisting conditions the physical examination should include evaluation of the joints, muscle, fascia, and neurological structures of the spine, hip, and pelvis. Unfortunately, some of the physical findings may be subtle. Examples include recognizing imbalance between muscle length and strength and asymmetry in muscle recruitment patterns that affect quality of motion. The physical exam should also include the usual gait analysis, neurological, postural, joint range of motion, and manual muscle strength evaluation. Recognizing postural changes that may be asymptomatic in the lower extremity may give better clues to what is causing the proximal posterior pelvic pain. For example, excessive foot pronation on one side may facilitate genu valgus at the knee, internal rotation at the hip, and an iliac crest that appears lower than the contralateral side. Load transmission through the pelvis and lower extremity is assumed to be compromised in this setting, which may facilitate SIJ pain. The Gillet test assesses side-to-side ilial-sacral motion (Fig. 20.1). The examiner assesses for posterior iliac rotation associated with hip flexion and single leg stance on the contralateral lower extremity. Lack of posterior rotation is a positive test but does not necessarily indicate the side of pain or dysfunction. Hip range of motion should be assessed in both supine and prone and noted for range of motion limits and asymmetries from side to side. This can help differentiate bony deformity or arthritic conditions from soft tissue restrictions. Range of motion of the lumbar spine should be assessed for the quantity of motion as well as positions of discomfort. Straight leg raise in both the seated and supine position will assist in detecting pain that is neurological in origin. Observation and palpation of bony landmarks in weight-bearing and non-weight-bearing positions are helpful. Asymmetric lumbopelvic rhythm in standing and/or sitting may identify problem areas to address. Researchers have found that the multifidus and gluteus maximus firing is delayed on the symptomatic side of patients with SIJ pain, suggesting an alteration of load transfer through the pelvis.[24] The active straight leg test has been shown to be reliable in examining patients with posterior pelvic pain (Fig. 20.2). Though this maneuver is not specific and assesses the patient in a non-weight-bearing position, the authors utilize this test to assess lumbopelvic stability. It is also important to determine if a functional or anatomic leg length discrepancy exists in order to prescribe or avoid heel lifts. Patients often have pain on palpation along the PSIS and sacral sulci.[25,26] Other tender areas may exist along the posterior pelvis, iliotibial band region, greater trochanter of the femur, and iliopsoas. Several provocative SIJ techniques can be very helpful when positive. However, a negative test does not exclude the diagnosis. Examples of tests utilized to provoke

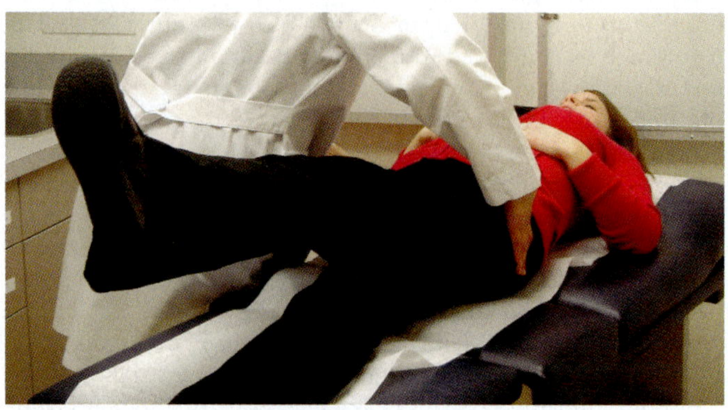

Figure 20.2. Active straight leg raise (ASLR).

TABLE 20.1 Provocative Physical Examination Tests

Provocative Tests for SIJ Pain	*Provocative Tests for Intra-articular Hip Disorders*
FABER/Patrick test	FABER/Patrick test
Pelvic compression	Log roll
Sacral thrust	Hip distraction
Gaenslen test	Hip impingement
Thigh thrust	Resisted active straight leg raise
Ilial distraction	

posterior pelvic pain are listed in the first column of Table 20.1. The authors recommend combining these with tests listed in the second column of Table 20.1 that are utilized to provoke pain related to intra-articular hip disorders. Inclusion of these may help detect coexisting conditions.

No one specific physical examination finding or test has been found to be sensitive or specific for diagnosing SIJ pain and validated by SIJ injection.[1,25,28] Dreyfuss et al.[25] studied 12 SIJ "tests" to determine their sensitivity/specificity for SIJ pain by the patient's response to fluoroscopically guided SIJ injection. No one specific examination technique or grouping of techniques was particularly sensitive or specific for SIJ pain. Several studies[29–31] have found good interrater reliability in some pain provocative tests for SIJ pain, but no consensus that one test is most sensitive or specific for SIJ pain. Some correlation was found if a number of a series of tests were found to be positive.[29,31] However, the physical examination maneuvers tested varied between studies. Laslett et al.[32] correlated individual provocative examination tests with fluoroscopically guided SIJ injections. Individual test sensitivity was 0.6 to 0.88, while individual test specificity was 0.69 to 0.81. The prevalence of one positive test was 29% to 50%. If more than three tests were found to provoke pain, then the sensitivity increased to 93% and the specificity improved to 78%.

In summary, the physical examination of patients with SIJ pain must include the spine, pelvis, hip, and lower extremity. No one physical examination maneuver is sensitive or specific for SIJ pain. The authors recommend combining gait analysis, lumbar spine and hip range of motion, quality of motion observation, neurological examination, and provocative tests to determine the next steps to be taken in the evaluation and treatment of the patient with posterior pelvic pain.

DIFFERENTIAL DIAGNOSIS

The differential diagnosis for posterior pelvic pain is variable. Inflammation of the SIJ may occur as a result of metabolic changes, arthritis, trauma, or infection. Primary tumors of the SIJ can occur but are rare. Bone graft harvesting near the joint can result in iatrogenic instability. An increased density on the ilial side of the inferior SIJ known as osteitis condensans occurs in 2.2% of the multiparous female population and is usually self-limiting. Sacroiliitis may develop as a part of pelvic inflammatory disease and should be considered when pain remains a persistent problem. Instability related to hormonal changes and evolving load changes during pregnancy is another cause for pain.

Most commonly, SIJ pain is considered to be idiopathic. For athletes, this is the most common scenario. The authors recommend that the athlete should be fully assessed for lumbar spine and hip disorders that may contribute to posterior pelvic pain. Addressing these adjacent region disorders assists in both diagnosis and specific treatment planning.

DIAGNOSTICS

IMAGING

Idiopathic posterior pelvic pain can often be determined by exclusion. Imaging is important to determine if fracture, infection, tumor, or significant inflammation or degenerative changes have occurred, but are not always conclusive for the source of pain. The preferred X-ray evaluation of the SIJ is taken at 25° to 30° angle to the anterior/posterior plane. The majority of X-rays in patients with posterior pelvic pain related to the SIJ will be normal. The usual patterns of aging may be noted with sclerotic changes initially presenting on the ilial side of the joint. Sclerotic changes exclusively noted on the sacral side of the joint should serve as an indicator to evaluate the patient further for metabolic or inflammatory etiologies of pain and X-ray findings. Computed tomography (CT) can define early joint narrowing and bony abnormalities such as fracture that is not easily visible on X-ray. Bone scan and/or single photon emission CT are useful in identifying fractures, tumor, or infection. MRI is the most sensitive in detecting inflammatory changes in the SIJ. Newer technology geared toward assessing joint stresses utilizes color Doppler imaging (CDI). Buyruk et al.[33] have measured SIJ stiffness with CDI. Patients with posterior pelvic following childbirth were found to have greater asymmetry of stiffness across the SIJ as compared to controls. Further studies showed this technique to be a reliable[34] and valid method[35] to measure SIJ stiffness.

CDI appears to be a useful instrument to gain objective evidence regarding the SIJ but is currently not widely used for this purpose. Imaging will rarely clearly define idiopathic SIJ dysfunction and pain. Despite this, it is important to obtain imaging to rule out other sources of pain.

UTILIZATION OF INJECTIONS IN THE DIAGNOSTIC WORKUP

If diagnostic imaging is often normal and no gold standard for physical examination exists, how does the health care provider make the diagnosis of SIJ pain? The answer is not simple. A consensus of several authors is to recommend the following: SIJ pain is indicated when there is no neurological deficit, no dural tension signs, no objective testing indicating medical etiologies for pain, no evidence of lumbar pain, and 75% relief with fluoroscopically guided contrast enhanced intra-articular SIJ injection.[1,25,26,36]

There is some evidence that not all SIJ pain is exclusively intra-articular in origin. Ligaments extrinsic to the SIJ itself but key in providing pelvic stability are thought to contribute to SIJ pain. In particular, the long dorsal sacroiliac ligament and sacrotuberous ligament play a dynamic role in providing stability but may also contribute to pain.[37–39] Currently, there is not a standard method to consistently administer a periarticular injection and therefore not helpful from a diagnostic standpoint.

TREATMENT

Treatment for the athlete with posterior pelvic pain due to SIJ dysfunction should be individualized based on the athlete's mechanism of injury, biomechanical deficits, and directional preference of pain-free motion with the ultimate goal of return to sport or exercise.

ACUTE PHASE (1 TO 3 DAYS)

Acute injury is often associated with a direct trauma or marked increase in intensity, frequency, or duration of a specific activity. Often, SIJ pain presents as a progressive problem with fluctuations in symptoms that the athlete may only experience symptoms during certain activities including sports or exercise. As with other musculoskeletal injuries, the usual principles of ice, relative rest, and analgesics should be implemented. Activities that provoke pain should be avoided during this phase. These may include activities that require single leg stance like bowling, skating, running, and stair stepper. Correcting asymmetries in muscle length or stiffness should start as soon as possible and progress within pain-free limits. Manual medicine techniques can assist in gaining motion even in the acute phase of recovery. A variety of treatments administered by a number of manually trained practitioners can be included within the mobilization category including high velocity low amplitude, low velocity high amplitude, physical therapy joint mobilization, muscle energy, and active release therapy. If an SIJ appears to require recurrent joint mobilization, a significant muscle imbalance may still exist. Muscle energy techniques are particularly helpful as they require patient activation of muscle groups and therefore, pain tolerance is easily monitored. Treatment for patients with significant muscle weakness and/or poor endurance may need to focus on stabilization through strengthening rather than recurrent mobilization. Special care should be taken with early treatment of the pregnant athlete, as aggressive stretching or mobilization can further aggravate symptoms secondary to pregnancy related hypermobility. Though there is considerable focus on gaining range of motion during this phase and continuing into the recovery phase, it is important to differentiate hip range of motion limits that are related to pain or soft tissue restrictions versus limitations related to bony deformity (Femoral acetabular impingement (FAI) and Developmental dysplasia of the hip (DDH)).

RECOVERY PHASE (3 DAYS TO 8 WEEKS)

Once pain has been controlled and the injured area has been rested, correction of the functional biomechanical deficit and tissue overload complex[40] becomes the focus of rehabilitation. Balancing lower extremity muscle length and strength is important because of direct and indirect force transmission across the ilium and sacrum. Muscle length must first be restored. For example, if the iliopsoas is in a shortened position it leads to an anteriorly rotated ilium. Hamstring strengthening cannot be accomplished until the iliopsoas is restored to activating at a biomechanically efficient length as an anterior pelvic tilt forces the hamstring to work in a lengthened position. The converse can occur as well. If the hamstring is working in a shortened position, it cannot work at maximum efficiency. The hamstring is a key muscle to provide stability to the SIJ because of its direct attachment and/or fascial connections to the sacrotuberous ligament and therefore, restoration of appropriate strength is a key to successful outcome. Other muscles commonly found to be working in a shortened position include the rectus femoris, tensor fascia lata, adductors, quadratus lumborum, latissimus dorsi,[41] and obturator internus. As muscle length is restored, muscle strengthening can progress. Neuromuscular re-education and facilitation techniques are helpful with this process. Closed kinetic chain strengthening should be attempted first and incorporated into the lumbopelvic stabilization program. As trunk strengthening improves, adding multiplanar strengthening exercises will facilitate return to functional activities (Fig. 20.3). Muscles commonly found to be weak include the gluteus medius, gluteus maximus, lower abdominals, and hamstrings.

Though maintaining individual muscle flexibility and strength is important, retraining of multiple muscle groups to fire in coordination is the key to a successful recovery. This can be facilitated with lumbopelvic stabilization, advanced proprioceptive re-education, plyometrics and exercise or sport-specific activities. Simulating sport-specific activities in the therapeutic exercise program is also a key. Further, education regarding proper ergonomics in activities of daily living and work environment should be included. Careful attention to training techniques must also be incorporated into the program for those active in sports and exercise. Return to sporting activities is indicated when a pain-free state without medications is achieved. Proper muscle balance in flexibility and strength should remain a part of the maintenance program. Careful monitoring during initial return can prevent reinjury.

SACROILIAC JOINT BELTS

SIJ belts can be used to provide compression across the SIJ. In turn, this will provide proprioceptive feedback to the gluteal muscles. Vleeming et al.[42] reported that SIJ belts applied

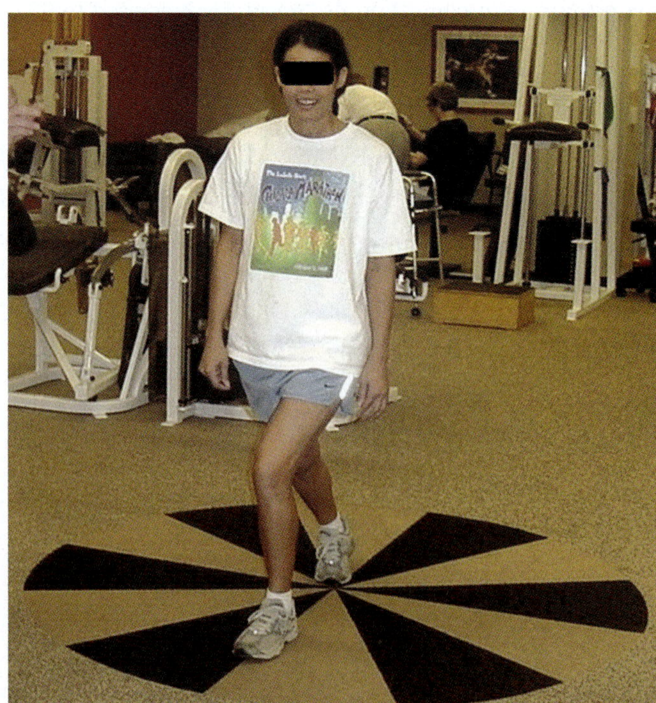

Figure 20.3. Matrix testing.

to cadaver models reduced SIJ rotation by 30%. SIJ belts can be especially helpful in patients with SIJ hypermobility or significant muscle weakness. Care must be taken to ensure that the patient is able to apply the belt appropriately. The SIJ belt should be secured posteriorly across the sacral base and anteriorly inferior to the anterior superior iliac spines (Fig. 20.4). Patients are often recommended to wear the belt during walking and standing activities. However, patients with significant pain and weakness often find the belt helpful in reducing symptoms when worn during sedentary activities as well.

ORTHOTICS

Other treatment considerations include orthotics and shoe modifications. A shoe lift to correct a functional leg length discrepancy can be helpful in the acute setting to manage pain with weight bearing or ambulation. Shoe lifts should be approached with caution, as functional leg length discrepancy should be corrected with muscle rebalancing and not an orthotic. An inappropriate shoe lift can promote adaptive muscle imbalances, which may initially be asymptomatic but cause problems because of a shift in force transmission which ultimately can change wear and tear pattern in the future. By contrast, anatomical leg length discrepancies should be determined as early in treatment as possible so that the appropriate modifications can be completed.

THERAPEUTIC INJECTIONS

SIJ injections can be used as an adjunct treatment when progress with recovery plateaus or the physical therapy program cannot be advanced because of pain provocation. The utilization of image (fluoroscopic of CT) guidance is important to ensure the accuracy of the placement of the medication as well as avoid complications (Fig. 20.5). Rosenberg et al.[43] reviewed the accuracy of blind placement of the needle presumably into the SIJ. Of 37 blind injections, 22% were placed within the SIJ confirmed on CT, while 24% showed epidural flow of contrast and 44% demonstrated dorsal sacral foraminal flow. Early reports of US guidance show promise.[44] Potential benefits include reduced radiation exposure and reduced cost. No prospective studies are available at this time regarding the therapeutic benefit of SIJ injections in the active athletic population. In a retrospective review of 31 patients with 94-week follow-up, SIJ injections improved pain function and work status.[45] If needed, injections can be an important adjunct treatment utilized to help speed the recovery and return to sport or exercise for the athlete.

Advancement to the maintenance phase of treatment begins with an absence of pain, inflammation, functional joint and myofascial dysfunction, and return of approximately 75% of strength and flexibility as judged per the patient's preinjury baseline. Normal activities of daily living, especially walking, should not provoke symptoms.[46]

MAINTENANCE PHASE

During this phase, the rehabilitation program focuses on advancing the strengthening program while maintaining appropriate muscle length. The exercise program should be concise, specific to the individual's functional requirements, and simulate the individual's activities. For example, side lying hip abduction as a form of gluteus medius strengthening may not be aggressive enough for a rock climber. The rock climber will need a gluteus medius strengthening exercise that incorporates multiple planes in a weight-bearing position. This is also the time to review specific exercises or activities that should be avoided. Athletes with reduced hip flexion due to hip deformity should not aggressively stretch the hip musculature in attempts to improve hip flexion. Even if the hip is asymptomatic, aggressive stretching across a joint with inherent bony limitation will increase stress across the SIJ as well as potentially initiate intra-articular hip pain. At this

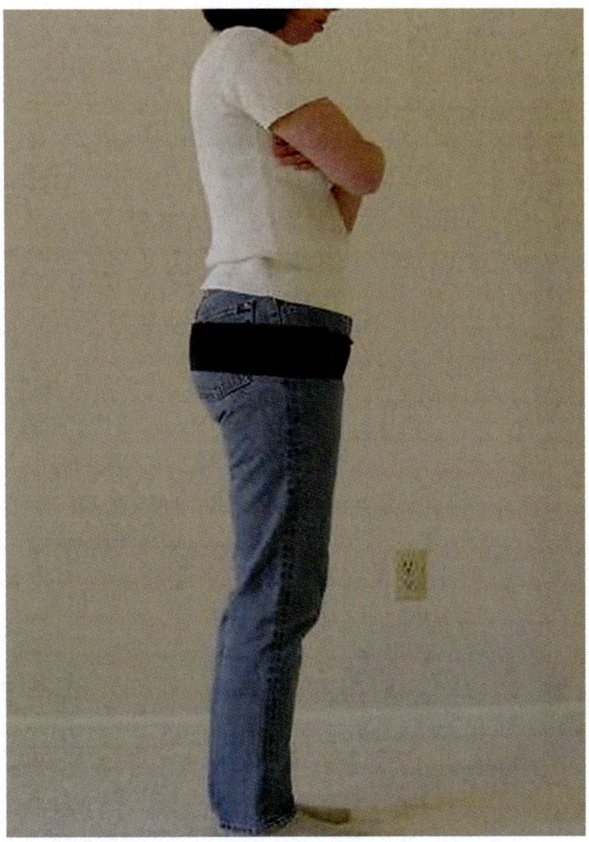

Figure 20.4. SIJ belt.

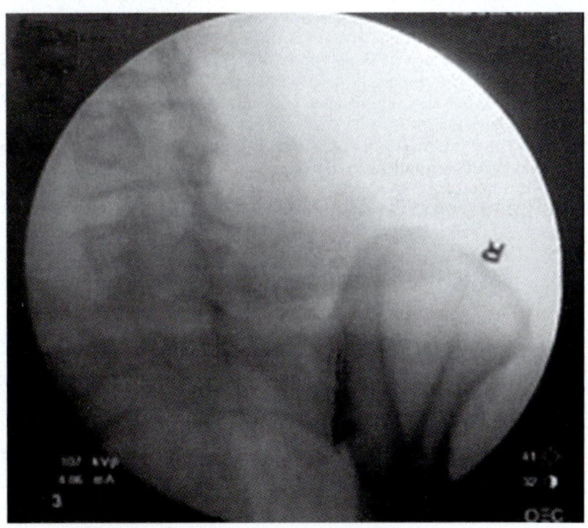

Figure 20.5. SIJ injection under fluoroscopy.

time, aerobic conditioning should be advanced while monitoring return to usual sport/exercise activities. The exercise prescription should fit the individual.

CONCLUSION

For athletes with low back pain, posterior pelvic or gluteal pain, and groin pain, SIJ pain should be considered as part of the differential diagnosis. SIJ stability plays an important role in providing a base that facilitates appropriate motor control to successfully compete and participate in sports and exercise. Because there are no good gold standards for diagnosis or treatment of this condition, the diagnosis is often achieved by process of elimination. Further, treatment is often directed by the health care provider's understanding of the integrated biomechanics of the spine, hips, and pelvis. Disorders that influence SIJ mechanics including lumbar radiculopathy or intra-articular hip pathology need to be properly evaluated and treated. Research describing the biomechanics of the SIJ continues to add to our understanding of its function. Further studies are needed to follow long-term outcomes in athletes with SIJ pain to better provide prevention and treatment options.

REFERENCES

1. Maigne JY, Aivaliklis A, Pfefer F. Results of sacroiliac joint double block and value of sacroiliac pain provocation tests in 54 patients with low back pain. *Spine.* 1996;21(16): 1889–1892.
2. Bernard TN, Jr, Kirkaldy-Willis WH. Recognizing specific characteristics of nonspecific low back pain. *Clin Orthop Relat Res.* 1987(217):266–280.
3. Bernard TN Jr, Cassidy JD. The sacroiliac joint syndrome: Pathophysiology, diagnosis, and management. In: Frymoyer JW, ed. *The Adult Spine: Principles and Practice.* New York: Raven Press; 1991.
4. Fortin JD, Kissling RO, O'Connor BL, et al. Sacroiliac joint innervation and pain. *Am J Orthop.* 1999;28(12):687–690.
5. Vleeming A, Stoeckart R, Volkers AC, et al. Relation between form and function in the sacroiliac joint. Part I. Clinical anatomical aspects. *Spine.* 1990;15(2):130–132.
6. Vleeming A, Volkers AC, Snijders CJ, et al. Relation between form and function in the sacroiliac joint. Part II. Biomechanical aspects. *Spine.* 1990;15(2):133–136.
7. Lee DG. An integrated model of "joint" function and its clinical application. In: *4th Interdisciplinary World Congress on Low Back and Pelvic Pain.* Montreal, QC, Canada; 2001.
8. Vleeming A, Pool-Goudzwaard AL, Stoeckart R, et al. The posterior layer of the thoracolumbar fascia: Its function in load transfer from spine to legs. *Spine.* 1995;20(7):753–758.
9. Vleeming A, Van Wingerden JP, Dijkstra P. Mobility of the sacroiliac joint in the elderly: A kinetic and radiology study. *Clin Biomech.* 1991;6:161–168.
10. Ostgaard HC, Roos-Hansson E, Zetherstrom G. Regression of back and posterior pelvic pain after pregnancy. *Spine.* 1996;21(23):2777–2780.
11. Sady S, Freedson P. Body composition and structural compositions of female and male athletes. *Clin Sports Med.* 1984;3:755–777.
12. Ciullo J. Lower extremity injuries. In: Pearl A, ed. *The Athletic Female.* Champaign, IL: Human Kinetics Publishers; 1993, pp. 267–288.
13. Fortin JD, Aprill CN, Ponthieux B, et al. Sacroiliac joint: Pain referral maps upon applying a new injection/arthrography technique. Part II: Clinical evaluation. *Spine.* 1994;19(13):1483–1489.
14. Fortin JD, Dwyer AP, West S, et al. Sacroiliac joint: Pain referral maps upon applying a new injection/arthrography technique. Part I: Asymptomatic volunteers. *Spine.* 1994;19(13):1475–1482.
15. Rumball JS, Lebrun CM, Di Ciacca SR, et al. Rowing injuries. *Sports Med.* 2005;35(6):537–555.
16. Timm KE. Sacroiliac joint dysfunction in elite rowers. *J Orthop Sports Phys Ther.* 1999;29(5):288–293.
17. Chou LH, Slipman CW, Bhagia SM, et al. Inciting events initiating injection-proven sacroiliac joint syndrome. *Pain Med.* 2004;5(1):26–32.
18. Burnett RS, Della Rocca GJ, Prather H, et al. Clinical presentation of patients with tears of the acetabular labrum. *J Bone Joint Surg Am.* 2006;88(7):1448–1457.
19. Hunt D, Clohisy J, Prather H. Acetabular labral tears of the hip in women. *Phys Med Rehabil Clin N Am.* 2007;18(3):497–520, ix–x.
20. Nunley R, Schoenecker P, Hunt D, et al. Clinical presentation of developmental Dysplasia of the hip in the skeletally mature patient. *J Bone Joint Surg Am.* 2009; In press.
21. Prather H, Spitznagle TM, Dugan SA. Recognizing and treating pelvic pain and pelvic floor dysfunction. *Phys Med Rehabil Clin N Am.* 2007;18(3):477–96, ix.
22. Clohisy JC, Knaus ER, Hunt DM, et al. Clinical presentation of patients with symptomatic anterior hip impingement. *Clin Orthop Relat Res.* 2009;467(3):638–644.
23. Lesher JM, Dreyfuss P, Hager N, et al. Hip joint pain referral patterns: A descriptive study. *Pain Med.* 2008;9(1):22–25.
24. Hungerford B, Gilleard W, Hodges P. Evidence of altered lumbopelvic muscle recruitment in the presence of sacroiliac joint pain. *Spine.* 2003;28(14):1593–1600.
25. Dreyfuss P, Michaelsen M, Pauza K, et al. The value of medical history and physical examination in diagnosing sacroiliac joint pain. *Spine.* 1996;21(22): 2594–2602.
26. Slipman CW, Sterenfeld EB, Chou LH, et al. The predictive value of provocative sacroiliac joint stress maneuvers in the diagnosis of sacroiliac joint syndrome. *Arch Phys Med Rehabil.* 1998;79(3):288–292.
27. Schwarzer AC, Aprill CN, Bogduk N. The sacroiliac joint in chronic low back pain. *Spine.* 1995;20(1):31–37.
28. Slipman CW, Jackson HB, Lipetz JS, et al. Sacroiliac joint pain referral zones. *Arch Phys Med Rehabil.* 2000;81(3):334–338.
29. Arab AM, Abdollahi I, Joghataei MT, et al. Inter- and intra-examiner reliability of single and composites of selected motion palpation and pain provocation tests for sacroiliac joint. *Man Ther.* 2009;14(2):213–221.
30. Kokmeyer DJ, Van der Wurff P, Aufdemkampe G, et al. The reliability of multitest regimens with sacroiliac pain provocation tests. *J Manipulative Physiol Ther.* 2002;25(1):42–48.
31. Robinson HS, Brox JI, Robinson R, et al. The reliability of selected motion- and pain provocation tests for the sacroiliac joint. *Man Ther.* 2007;12(1):72–79.
32. Laslett M, Aprill CN, McDonald B, et al. Diagnosis of sacroiliac joint pain: Validity of individual provocation tests and composites of tests. *Man Ther.* 2005;10(3): 207–218.
33. Buyruk HM, Stam HJ, Snijders CJ, et al. Measurement of sacroiliac joint stiffness with color Doppler imaging and the importance or asymmetric stiffness in sacroiliac pathology. In: Vleeming A, Mooney V, Dorman TA, et al., eds. *Movement, Stability, and Low Back Pain: The Essential Role of the Pelvis.* New York: Churchill Livingston; 1999.
34. Damen L, Stijnen T, Roebroeck ME, et al. Reliability of sacroiliac joint laxity measurement with Doppler imaging of vibrations. *Ultrasound Med Biol.* 2002;28(4):407–414.
35. Vlaanderen E, Conza NE, Snijders CJ, et al.. Low back pain, the stiffness of the sacroiliac joint: A new method using ultrasound. *Ultrasound Med Biol.* 2005;31(1):39–44.
36. Dreyfuss P, Cole A, Pauza K. Sacroiliac joint injection techniques. *Phys Med Rehabil Clin N Am.* 1995;6:785–813.
37. Vleeming A, Pool-Goudzwaard AL, Hammudoghlu D, et al. The function of the long dorsal sacroiliac ligament: Its implication for understanding low back pain. *Spine.* 1996;21(5): 556–562.
38. Vleeming A, Stoeckart R, Snijders C. The sacrotuberous ligament: A conceptual approach to its dynamic role in stabilizing the sacro-iliac joint. *Clin Biomech.* 1989;4:201–203.
39. van Wingerden JP, Vleeming A, Snijders C, et al. A functional-anatomical approach to the spine-pelvis mechanism: Interaction between the biceps femoris muscle and the sacrotuberous ligament. *Eur Spine J.* 1993;2:140–144.
40. Herring SA. Rehabilitation of muscle injuries. *Med Sci Sports Exerc.* 1990;22(4):453–456.
41. Geraci M. Rehabilitation of the hip and pelvis. In: Kibler W, Herring S, Press J, eds. *Functional Rehabilitation of Sports and Musculoskeletal Medicine.* Maryland, MD: Aspen Publishers; 1998, pp. 216–243.
42. Vleeming A, Buyruk HM, Stoeckart R, et al. An integrated therapy for peripartum pelvic instability: A study of the biomechanical effects of pelvic belts. *Am J Obstet Gynecol.* 1992;166(4):1243–1247.
43. Rosenberg JM, Quint TJ, de Rosayro AM. Computerized tomographic localization of clinically-guided sacroiliac joint injections. *Clin J Pain.* 2000;16(1):18–21.
44. Pekkafal M, Kralp M, Baekim C, et al. Sacroiliac joint injections performed with sonographic guidance. *J Ultrasound Med.* 2003;22:553–559.
45. Slipman CW, Lipetz JS, Plastaras CT, et al. Fluoroscopically guided therapeutic sacroiliac joint injections for sacroiliac joint syndrome. *Am J Phys Med Rehabil.* 2001;80(6):425–432.
46. Prather H. Sacroiliac joint pain: Practical management. *Clin J Sport Med.* 2003;13(4): 252–255.

CHAPTER

21

Christopher M. Larson
Gary B. Fetzer
Brett Wolters
Hollis M. Fritts

Stress Fractures of the Pelvic Ring and Hip

INTRODUCTION

Stress fractures of the pelvic ring and hip are not common. However, with increasing repots in the literature, there has been increased awareness of these injuries as an etiology of low back and buttock pain, and groin pain in patients. In general, there are two types of stress fractures: insufficiency-type stress fractures and fatigue-type stress fractures. Insufficiency fractures result from physiologic (normal) stresses within abnormal bone (e.g., osteoporotic bone). Insufficiency fractures are typically seen in older populations, and have been reported to be associated with postmenopausal osteoporosis, patients with history of radiation to the pelvis, corticosteroid-induced osteopenia, secondary osteoporosis (hyperparathyroidism, renal osteodystrophy, lumbosacral fusion, and Paget disease), rheumatoid arthritis, osteomalacia, transient osteoporosis associated with pregnancy and lactation, and osteopenia secondary to the female athletic triad. Fatigue-type stress fractures are the result of mechanical overload (repetitive loading) within a normal bone. In athletes, there may be a combination of insufficiency- and fatigue-type mechanisms. These generally occur in a younger, more active population such as distance runners and military recruits. The incidence of stress fractures ranges from 0.3% to 8% in the military population.[1] While in a sports medicine clinic, approximately 10% of all injuries seen are stress fractures. Specifically, runners presenting to a sports medicine clinic with stress fractures can make up 15% of all the injuries seen.[2] This chapter will discuss stress fractures of the femoral neck and pelvic ring.

FEMORAL NECK STRESS FRACTURES

EPIDEMIOLOGY AND CLASSIFICATION

Femoral neck stress fractures account for approximately 5% of all stress fractures.[3] Most of these fractures are seen in skeletally mature individuals, however, more recently children and adolescents have been reported to develop femoral neck stress fractures.[4–7] In a large Finnish study of male military recruits, body mass index, neck shaft angle, and leg dominance were not shown to correlate with the development of femoral neck stress fractures.[8] The development of femoral neck stress fractures has been reported to be due to a decrease in the absorption effect of the abductor musculature and secondary muscle fatigue with a compensatory alteration in gait pattern.[9–11]

Based upon the radiographic presentation of 54 femoral neck stress fractures, one study felt that previous classifications were inadequate.[1] They found a combination of a biomechanical model and the degrees of displacement to be more clinically useful. They divided their classification into stages of tension- and compression-sided fractures. Initially, tension-sided fractures have normal radiographs with positive bone scans on the tension side of the neck. Later, the fracture exhibits either endosteal or periosteal callus or a tension-sided fracture line without displacement. In the final stages, complete displacement of the femoral neck fracture is seen. Compression-sided stress fractures initially exhibit sclerosis on the medial side of the neck. In this stage, a negative plain radiograph with a positive bone scan on the compression side is commonly seen. Later, sclerosis is seen on plain radiographs, followed by a compression-sided cortical break. Finally, compression-sided widening of the fracture line is seen. In this series no fracture, either compression- or tension-sided, went on to displacement.

Compression-sided fractures are commonly seen in athletes, while tension-sided stress fractures have historically been reported in the elderly population. Recently, Provencher et al.[12] reported on tension-sided femoral neck stress fractures seen in the adult military population. As with the adult population, most femoral neck stress fractures in children are compression-sided, however, a recent report demonstrated a tensile-sided femoral neck stress fracture in a child.[5–7]

CLINICAL PRESENTATION AND DIAGNOSIS

Femoral neck stress fractures usually present with an insidious onset of vague anterior thigh and groin pain with weight bearing. Pain noted about the posterior aspect of the hip joint and greater trochanter is a less frequent presentation.[8,12] Patients usually report a recent change in their activity, equipment, or training intensity level. Pain may be exacerbated by hopping on the affected leg or running long distances. In more advanced stages, the pain occurs earlier during these activities and often requires longer recovery periods. Patients may report a history of previous stress fractures and acute severe pain should alert the clinician that a displaced fracture may be present.

On physical examination, patients will typically demonstrate a full range of motions of the affected hip with a mildly antalgic gait. Groin or deep lateral hip pain may be elicited at the end ranges of hip internal and external rotations. Hip flexion and axial compression, and a single leg hop test may recreate the patient's groin pain. Patients less commonly have palpable pain or swelling in the inguinal region.[1,12]

IMAGING

The vague symptoms associated with femoral neck stress fractures often lead to a delay in the diagnosis.[13] Radiographs, initially, are normal and it has been reported that 75% of femoral neck stress fractures are missed because they do not appear on plain radiographs.[13] The delay in diagnosis and the resulting inadequate treatment may lead to a progression of the fracture and ultimately fracture displacement.

Radiographs, including anteroposterior (AP) and Frog leg or cross-table lateral views of the affected hip, are taken as a screening tool. Femoral neck stress fractures typically demonstrate a gradual alteration in the trabeculae of the femoral neck on plain radiographs.[9] Historically, bone scans were

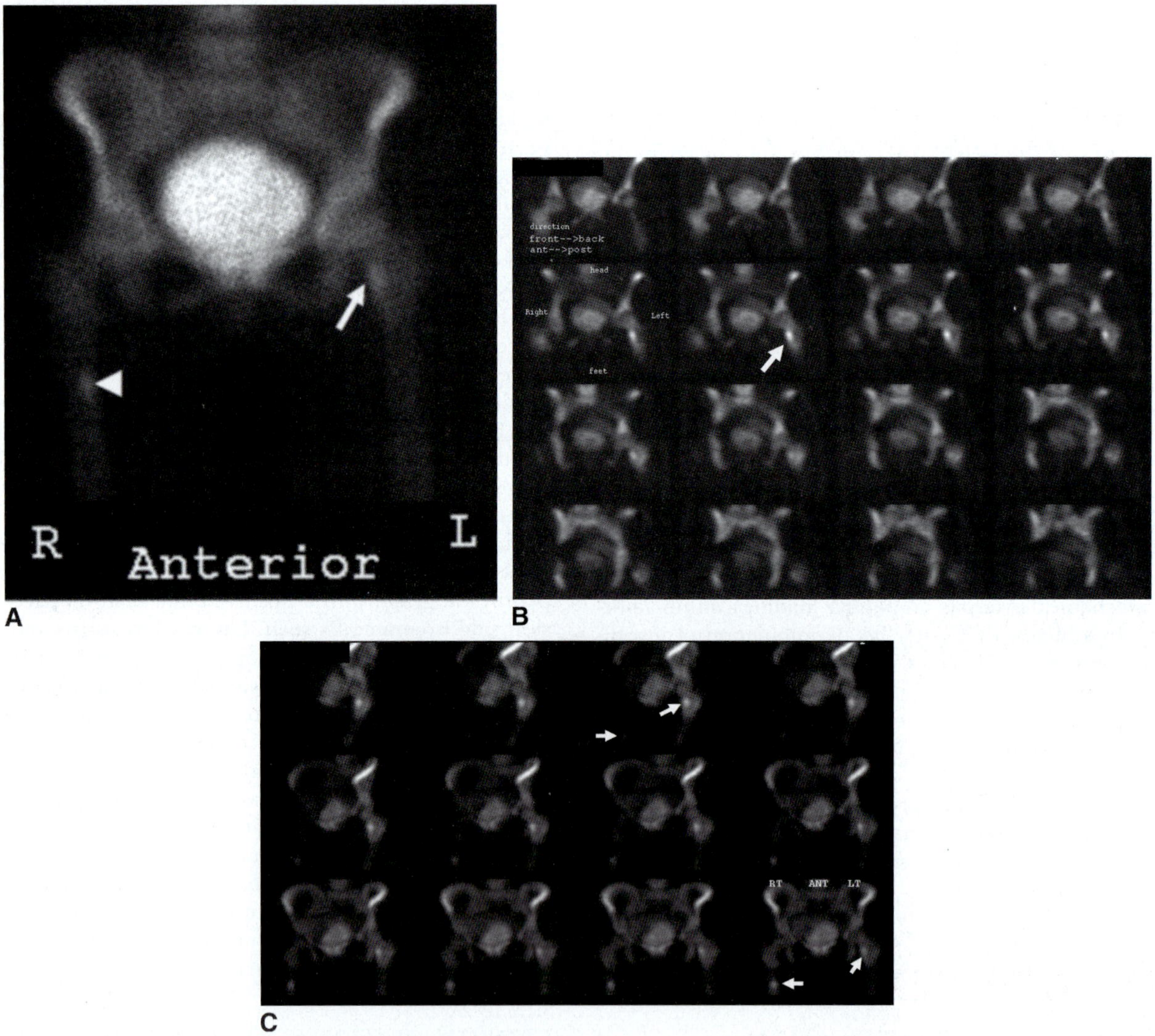

Figure 21.1. Thirty-one-year-old female runner training for marathon with 2 weeks of bilateral hip and proximal right thigh pain. Anterior and posterior scintigrams **(A)** show focal uptake at the medial left femoral neck, consistent with incomplete stress fracture (*arrow*), and another focal stress reaction/fracture of the contralateral right medial subtrochanteric region (*arrowhead*). Sequential slices of coronal SPECT images **(B)** further define the location of the stress fracture to the anteromedial left femoral neck (*arrow*). SPECT imaging allows postprocessing reconstruction to 3D volume images that can be rotated **(C)** which even more visually shows uptake consistent with stress fractures at the anteromedial left femoral neck and right femoral anteromedial subtrochanteric region (*arrows*).

recommended (Fig. 21.1) to make the correct diagnosis, as this imaging modality may be positive several days after the onset of symptoms.[14] More recently, magnetic resonance imaging (MRI) is emerging as the gold standard secondary to a higher degree of specificity (Fig. 21.2).

TREATMENT AND OUTCOMES

Treatment strategies are primarily based on the classification of the fracture. Harmon[15] has developed a protocol for the treatment of femoral neck stress fractures. Compression-sided lesions only seen on the MRI as bone edema are treated with protected weight-bearing activity until the patient is asymptomatic, followed by a gradual increase in the activity over the course of 4 to 6 weeks. After this time period, the patient may resume full activity if pain free. If during the increase in activity a relapse of symptoms occurs, the patient is instructed to return to pain-free activity. When a fracture line less than 50% of the width of the femoral neck is present, patients should remain nonweight bearing on crutches until they are asymptomatic (typically 4 to 6 weeks). If the patient is not improving then additional radiographic studies should be obtained to evaluate

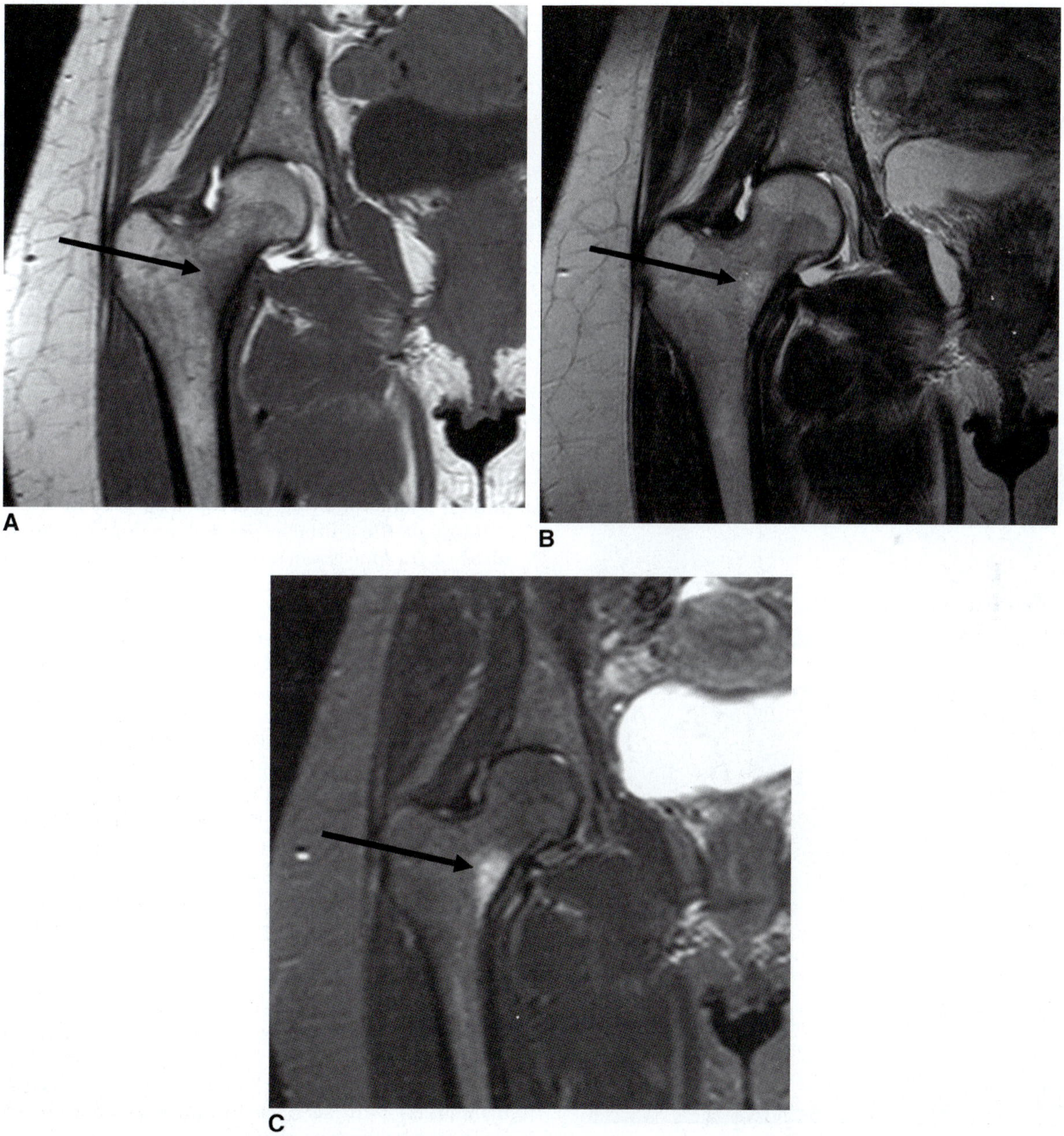

Figure 21.2. Forty-five-year-old female with right hip pain 2 weeks prior to running a 5 km race. MR arthrogram was performed. A coronal T1 image **(A)** shows decreased signal intensity of the marrow of the medial aspect of the right femoral neck (*arrow*). A coronal STIR image **(B)** shows increase in signal intensity. This signal intensity pattern is consistent with early stage stress reaction/fracture. A coronal STIR image **(C)** of 6 month follow-up MRI shows resolution of bone marrow edema.

fracture healing or progression. When a fracture line extends over 50% of the femoral neck width, then orthopaedic consultation should be obtained, as the incidence of displacement increases dramatically. Percutaneous pinning may be considered in this situation.

Surgical treatment is considered for tension-sided fractures or failed nonoperative treatment of compression-sided fractures with percutaneous pinning of the affected hip (Fig. 21.3).[1] Displaced femoral neck stress fractures require emergent closed or open reduction and percutaneous pinning to minimize the risk of avascular necrosis and nonunion. Displaced nonunions may benefit from vascularized bone grafting.[16] A high index of suspicion and appropriate treatment has been shown to minimize complications as a result of femoral neck stress fractures. In 2006, Pihlajamaki et al.[8] reported the long-term outcomes of nondisplaced femoral neck fatigue fractures in a young, adult male military population. With proper conservative management, no patient developed a displaced fracture or avascular necrosis, nor did they find an increased incidence of hip osteoarthritis at mean 18.3 years follow-up. In 2006, Pihlajamaki et al. reported on 19 patients over a 20-year period with displaced femoral neck stress fractures. Among the patients with displaced femoral neck stress fractures, a very high incidence of delayed or nonunion, avascular necrosis, and osteoarthritis was seen.[17] They reported that almost every patient had prodromal symptoms. The Finnish army subsequently implemented a policy regarding hip pain: "Conscripts complaining of pains in the hip, the proximal part of the femur or groin associated with or following physical activity were to be promptly referred for bone scans or MRI at the main military hospital." As a result, the army increased detection of femoral neck stress fractures from 13.2/100,000 service years to 53.2/100,000 service years. In addition, the rate of Garden IV displaced femoral neck stress fractures decreased from 3.8/100,000 service years to 0/100,000 service years. They concluded that by increasing awareness of this injury, early diagnosis and treatment can prevent displacement of these fractures. Few complications have been reported in skeletally immature individuals with femoral neck stress fractures.[10]

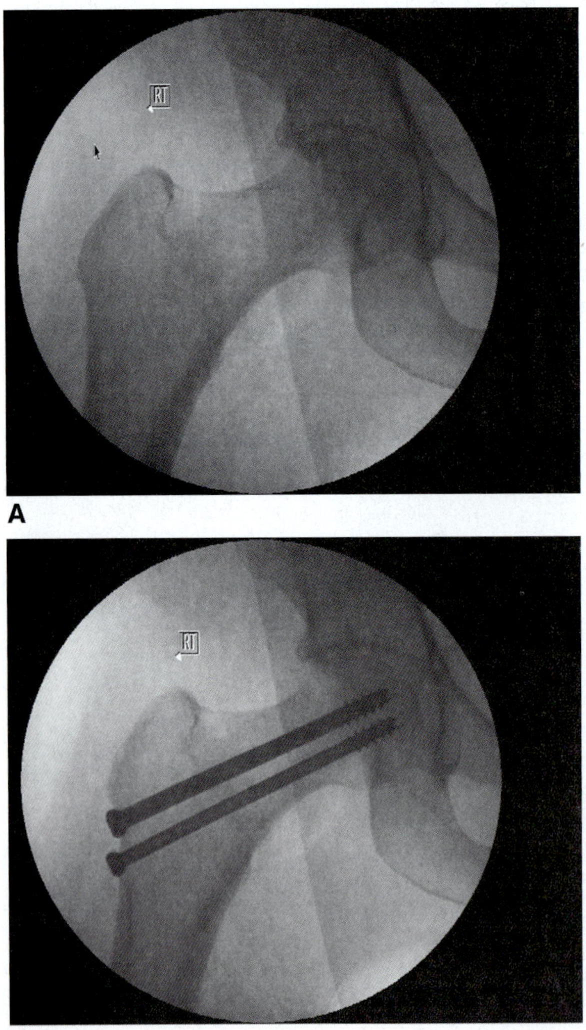

Figure 21.3. **A:** Forty-five-year-old female who continued to have pain after being treated for a compression-sided femoral neck stress fracture. Repeat radiographs revealed extension to the tension side. **B:** Intraoperative radiographs of the hip after percutaneous screw fixation with three cannulated screws.

PELVIC STRESS INJURIES

EPIDEMIOLOGY AND CLASSIFICATION

Pelvic stress fractures are uncommon injuries. Running athletes[18–22] and military recruits[23–28] are typical populations that are at increased risk for this injury. Pelvic ring stress fractures have also been reported during pregnancy or the postpartum period[29–36] and following total hip arthroplasty.[37–43]

Most of the initial reports describing fatigue-type fractures of the pelvis were in military recruits.[23–28] Meurman[28] reported one of the largest series of pubic stress fractures among 630 stress fractures in Finnish soldiers. In this population, stress fractures are believed to result from the onset of repetitive training activity commonly seen in basic training of military recruits. Selakaovich and Love[23] hypothesized that the precipitating factor is the repeated pull of the adductor muscle and hamstring complexes in unconditioned individuals.

Athletes, in particular, long-distance runners, are a significantly at risk population.[18–22] The precise incidence of pelvic stress fractures in running athletes is unknown. In a recent review of the literature, pelvic stress fractures represented about 1.25% of all stress fractures in running athletes.[19] In a report of 11 patients with 12 pubic rami fractures, all athletes were runners, with 9 of the 11 being distance or marathon runners.[20]

Pelvic ring fractures are also reported to occur during pregnancy.[29–36] Risk factors reported in the literature include vaginal delivery, increased birth weight, increased lumbar lordosis, excessive maternal weight gain, and selected obstetric maneuvers.[30,32] It has been hypothesized that breech position and constant pressure against the superior rami, and transient osteoporosis of the hip could account for this fracture.[29,31] Pubic insufficiency fractures have also been reported following total hip arthroplasty.[37–43]

Pelvis stress fractures occur in both males and females, with an increased prevalence among women. Differences in pelvis geometry and gait have been reported to account for this gender disparity.[20,44] It has been suggested that increased content of cancellous bone within the pelvis and the greater sensitivity of cancellous bone to estrogen deficiencies play a role.[44] It has also been hypothesized that tensile forces on the medial portion of the pubic rami are produced by strong musculature moments on the lateral part of the pubic rami and ischium with hip extension. Inferior pubic rami fractures are reported to be more common than superior rami fractures.[19,20,23] Pubic symphysis stress injury ("Osteitis Pubis") is another overuse injury of the pelvic ring.[44] This diagnosis must also be considered in the differential diagnosis of pelvic stress fractures, and can be associated with "athletic pubalgia."

CLINICAL PRESENTATION AND DIAGNOSIS

The clinical history is extremely important in making the diagnosis, and a high index of suspicion is necessary. Pain is the most common complaint, and is typically localized to the inguinal region.[18,19,44] Initially, pain is activity-related and resolves with rest, but with continued insult, symptoms can occur at rest. In the training athlete, the onset of symptoms is typically several weeks to months after starting a new training program or after a significant change in an existing training program. Eliciting the details of their training program is important, including changes in training schedule or technique, increases in mileage, and changes in footwear or running surfaces.[19]

Physical examination may reveal an antalgic gait. Pain or inability to stand unsupported on the leg of the affected side is a positive "standing test."[18] Noakes et al.[18,45] noted that diagnosis of a pelvic stress fracture can be confidently made, even when the radiograph is normal, when there is: groin pain of sufficient severity to prevent running, a positive "standing test" or "Hop test," and exquisite tenderness localized to the affected pubic rami.

IMAGING

Plain radiographs are initially obtained. An AP view of the pelvis should be obtained and additional views, such as inlet/outlet views or Judet views, may also be beneficial. Findings of a stress fracture include increased sclerosis with or without radiographic lucency. It is important to remember that normal radiographs do not exclude a stress fracture, especially if the clinical suspicion is high. Noakes et al.[18] reported that only five of 13 clinically diagnosed pelvic stress fractures in their series had abnormal initial radiographs.

If the clinical suspicion is high, treatment should proceed, with follow-up radiographs in approximately 2 weeks. For the in-season athlete, it is reasonable to consider further imaging modalities to confirm the diagnosis. MRI and bone scintigraphy are useful modalities.[14,46] A bone scan will show increased uptake in the area of the stress fracture (Fig. 21.4). Bone scans, however, are very nonspecific, and MRI is emerging as the imaging modality of choice (Fig. 21.5). Bony edema is observed as a low intensity signal on T1-weighted sequences and high signal on T2-weighted sequences. Fracture lines are observed as linear low-intensity signals on both T1- and T2-weighed sequences.

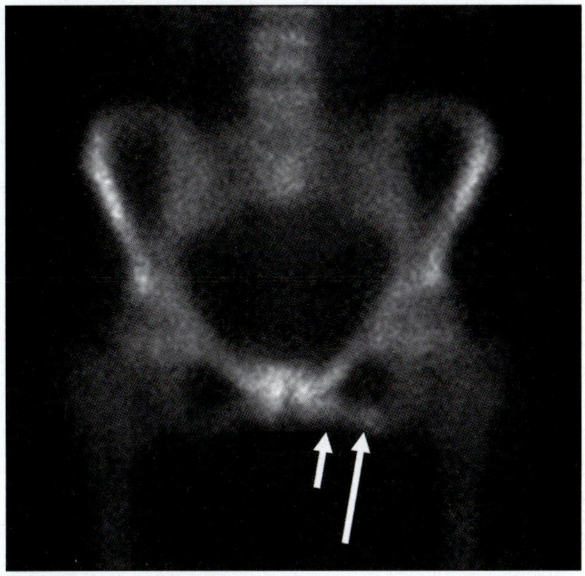
A

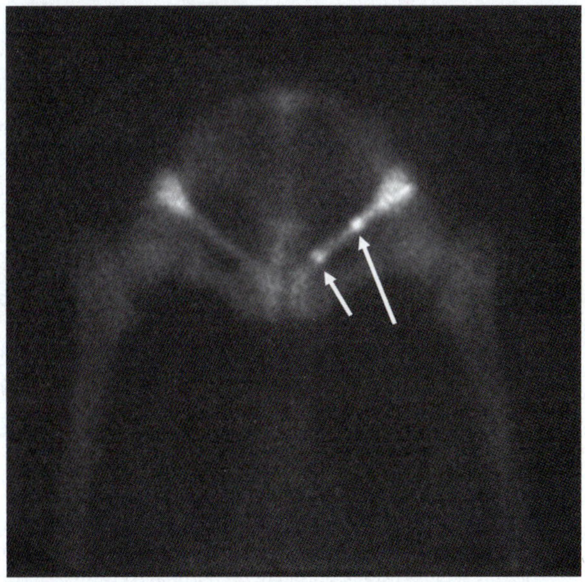
B

Figure 21.4. Twenty-three-year-old female training for marathon with left groin pain 1 week before the race. Anterior scintigram of bone scan **(A)** shows focal uptake at the left inferior pubic ramus (*long arrow*), and more subtly, increased uptake of the inferior pubic ramus nearer the symphysis pubis (*short arrow*). A TOD (tail-on-detector) scintigram **(B)** better delineates the two foci of uptake (*arrows*) in the left inferior pubic ramus consistent with two stress fractures.

TREATMENT AND OUTCOMES

Pubic rami stress fractures are typically treated with relative rest and activity modification.[18–20,23,31,37,44] Although, there is a low risk of complications, delayed union or nonunion can occur without adequate cessation of inciting activity. For most patients, symptoms resolve over a period 3 to 8 weeks.[30,44] Most importantly, errors in training, improper equipment, as well as nutritional or hormonal deficiencies must be corrected.

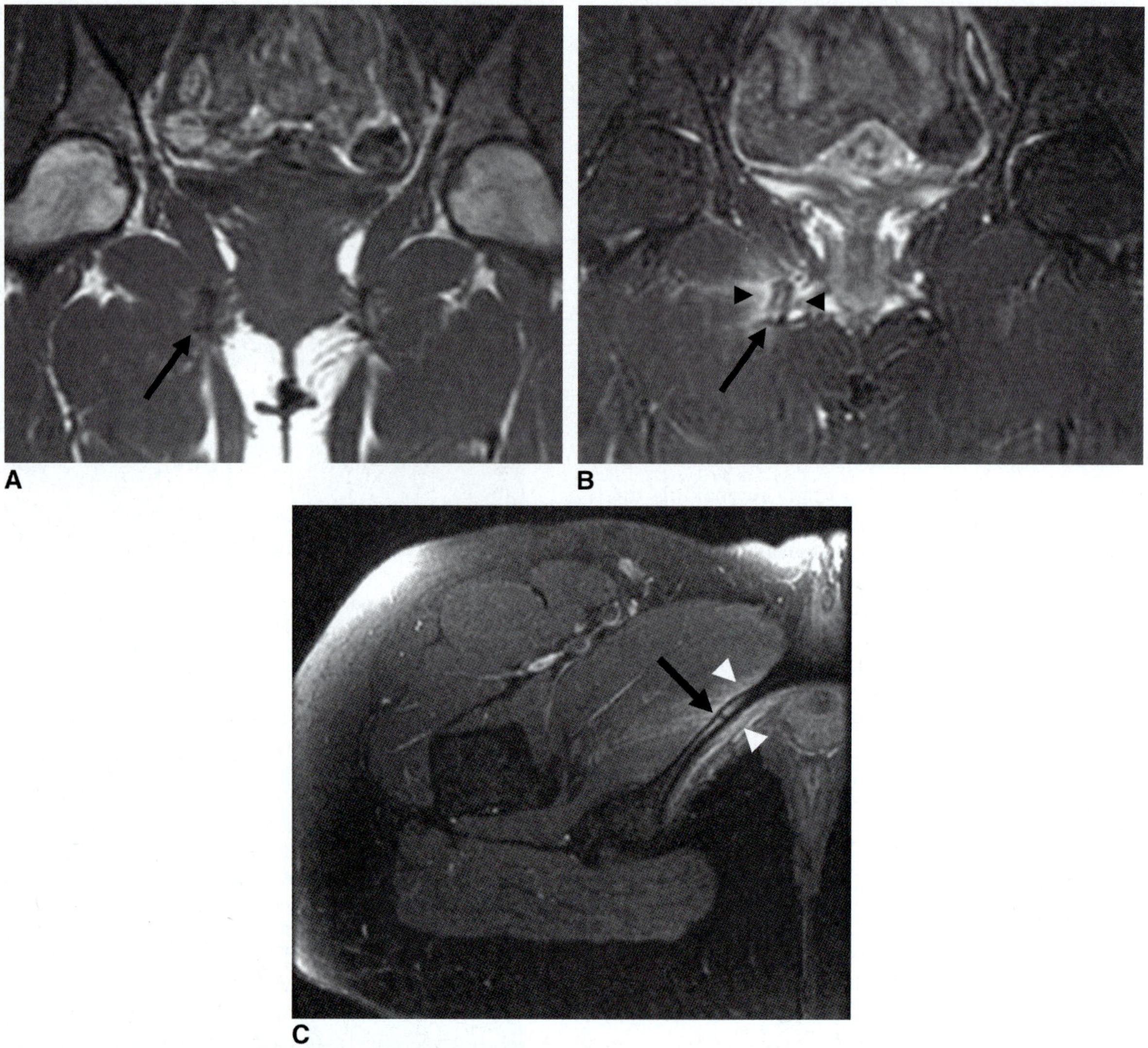

Figure 21.5. Twenty-six-year-old female runner with right hip pain for 5 days. Decreased signal intensity on coronal T1 image **(A)** and increased signal intensity on coronal STIR image **(B)** of marrow of the right inferior pubic ramus (*arrow*) reflects abnormal bone marrow edema, associated with surrounding soft tissue edema seen as increased signal on coronal STIR image (*arrowheads*). Axial T2 fat-suppressed image **(C)** shows a nondisplaced stress fracture (*arrow*), adjacent bone marrow edema, and soft tissue edema (*arrowheads*).

STRESS INJURIES OF THE SACRUM

EPIDEMIOLOGY AND CLASSIFICATION

Similar to other stress fractures, there are fatigue- and insufficiency-types. The true incidence of sacral stress fractures is unknown, as most of the data in the literature is based on case reports and small series.[47–61] Sacral insufficiency fractures are a well described in the elderly population.[50,56,57] Weber et al.[50] performed a review of the literature and reported that 93% of the sacral insufficiency-type fractures were in females. Nearly 2% of women aged 55 years, who presented to the hospital with low back pain, were found to have sacral insufficiency fractures.[50] Risk factors for sacral insufficiency-type fractures include osteoporosis, steroid-induced osteopenia, history of radiation therapy to the pelvis, and secondary osteoporosis.[50,53,56,57]

Fatigue-type fractures are less common. Athletic populations (distance runners) and military personnel are at increased risk due to the strenuous and repetitive activity demands.[47,48,51,54,55,58,60,61] Fatigue-type stress fractures of the sacrum represented <2% of injuries in a series of 320 athletes with stress fractures.[2] One review noted that 90% of sacral fatigue-type fractures were in runners with a mean age of 26 years.[47] Volpin et al.[48] reported only three sacral stress fractures in 194 military recruits during basic training. Significant risk factors for this injury include a rapid increase in a training regimen, nutritional and metabolic abnormalties, and leg length discrepancy.[49,60–62] Many athletes with fatigue-type sacral fractures have been found to have low bone density on DEXA scan, which indicates a component of insufficiency-type stress injury.[61]

Currently, there is no specific classification system to describe sacral stress fractures. The classification system described by Denis et al.[63] used to describe traumatic sacral fractures, however, may be applied. Zone 1 is the area lateral to the sacral foramina, known as the sacral ala, and are usually not associated with any neurologic symptoms. Zone 2 includes the sacral formina and has a higher prevalence of associated neurologic symptoms. Zone 3 is the sacral body and includes the central canal and also has a higher incidence of neurologic symptoms compared to sacral ala fractures. Typically, sacral stress fractures are most commonly found in the sacral ala (Zone 1).[50] Insufficiency-type fractures are typically vertical (parallel to the sacroiliac [SI] joints), with a horizontal component occasionally seen.[50,64]

DIAGNOSIS/CLINICAL PRESENTATION

Diagnosis of sacral stress fractures requires a high index of suspicion, and low back pain or buttock pain is a common complaint.[47,49,52,55,58] Symptoms are exacerbated by weight-bearing activities and relieved by rest. Unilateral symptoms are more common with fatigue-type injuries. Radicular symptoms are uncommon but may be present if fractures involve the sacral foramina, central canal, or if callus formation abuts lumbosacral nerve roots.[64] Groin pain and anterior thigh pain are less commonly noted.[47]

Physical examination may reveal an antalgic gait and pain with deep palpation along the posterior aspect of the sacrum or with lateral pelvis compression. A thorough neurovascular examination is important to identify subtle changes in neurologic function. FABER test (Patrick test) is performed with the patient supine. The foot of the affected side is placed on the contralateral knee. Pain in the groin suggested hip joint pathology rather than lumbar spine pathology. Posterior pain with application of pressure to the flexed knee and the contralateral anterior superior iliac spine (ASIS) suggests sacral or SI pathology. Gaenslen test is performed with the patient supine, with maximal hip flexion on one side and the opposite hip extended. This maneuver stresses both SI joints simultaneously.

IMAGING

AP and lateral views of the lumbosacral spine, AP pelvis, as well as inlet and outlet views of the pelvis, are useful views to obtain for radiographic assessment. Although initial plain radiographs are usually normal, they are useful to rule out other disorders.[47,49,50,52,55,65] The complex geometry and overlying bowel gas shadows complicate accurate interpretation.[51,55] Delayed radiographs may demonstrate radiographic changes, such as fracture lucency or callus, but there still must be a 30% to 50% change in trabecular bone density to be appreciated.[49] Kiuru et al.[65] have reported that plain radiography has a sensitivity and specificity of 37% and 79%, respectively, for diagnosing a sacral stress fracture. Several reports have noted the majority of patients ultimately diagnosed with sacral stress fractures had normal initial plain radiographs.[47,49,50]

Technetium-99 m bone scans are reported to have a sensitivity approaching 100% for the diagnosis of sacral stress fractures, with poor specificity (Fig. 21.6).[47,49,50,52,54,62,64,65] Bone scans usually show increased uptake at the fracture site location, and can be positive as early as 72 h after the onset of symptoms.[14,49,52] Appearance on the bone scan ranges from ill-defined area of radiotracer uptake in the sacral ala to focal linear uptake. The classic "Honda sign" is a H-shaped area of increased tracer uptake in the sacrum and is pathognomonic of bilateral insufficiency fractures.[50,51,53,56,62,64]

MRI is reported by some to be the gold standard in the radiographic diagnosis of sacral stress fractures (Figs. 21.7 & 21.8).[51,52,54,55,58,60] The advantages of MR examination of these patients are the greater soft tissue detail and no radiation exposure. The earliest MRI finding is typically an area of low signal on T1-weighted images and high intensity signal on T2-weighted fat-suppressed sequences.[51,52] A linear low intensity (void line), which represents the actual fracture line, may be seen on both the T1- and T2-weighted sequences.[51]

Interestingly, sacral fatigue-type stress fractures and insufficiency-type fractures are reported to show different patterns. Insufficiency-type fractures of the sacrum show edema and fracture parallel to the SI joint[51,56,64] whereas, fatigue-type fractures typically seen in the upper-most part of the sacral ala, occasionally extending to the first and second sacral foramina.[51,55,56,64] Recently, there has been some concern about the time frame, and bony changes will become evident on MR examination. Fredericson et al.[54] recently reported two cases of sacral fatigue-type fractures, where the initial MRI was negative for stress fracture. If clinical suspicion is high, a bone scan can be obtained and treatment for suspected sacral stress fracture should proceed, with repeat imaging to confirm or deny the diagnosis.

Computed topography (CT) examination is also a potential imaging modality.[47,49,50,54,55,58] Weber et al. utilized CT examination for diagnosis of all 20 of their insufficiency-type sacral fractures. However, Johnson et al.[49] reported that in only three sixth of the patients did the primary CT reading successfully identify the site of the lesions in their athletic population. The radiation exposure of CT scans is much higher than that of conventional radiographs, however, CT scans are less expensive than MRI.

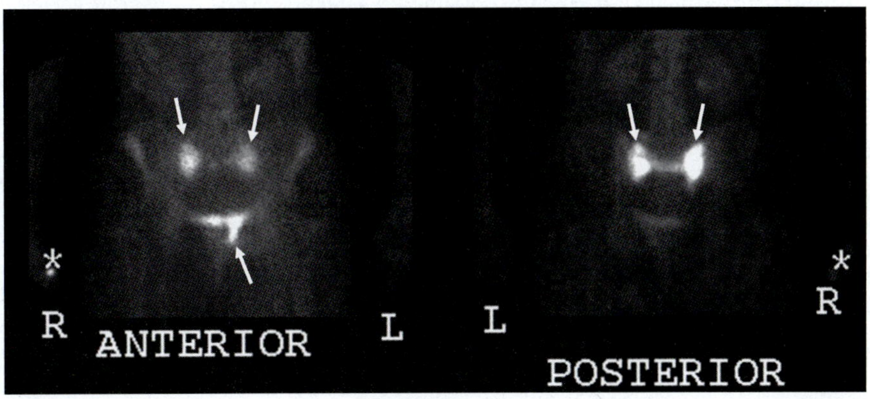

Figure 21.6. Seventy-six-year-old female with posterior pelvic and left anterior groin pain. Anterior and posterior bone scan scintigrams document marked increased uptake of bilateral sacral alae and the left pubis (*arrows*). The location of these findings in this age group is consistent with insufficiency fractures.

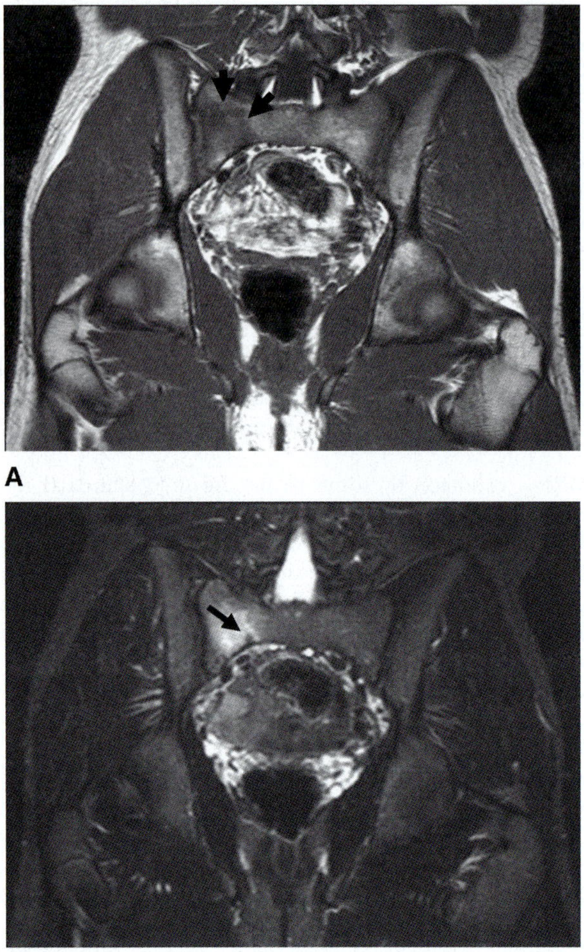

Figure 21.7. Fourteen-year-old male with right upper buttock pain for 2 weeks since running in the track. Coronal T1 image **(A)** shows decreased signal intensity in marrow of the right sacral alae (*arrows*). Corresponding coronal STIR image **(B)** shows a small low signal intensity stress fracture (*arrow*) associated with surrounding increased signal of adjacent bone marrow edema.

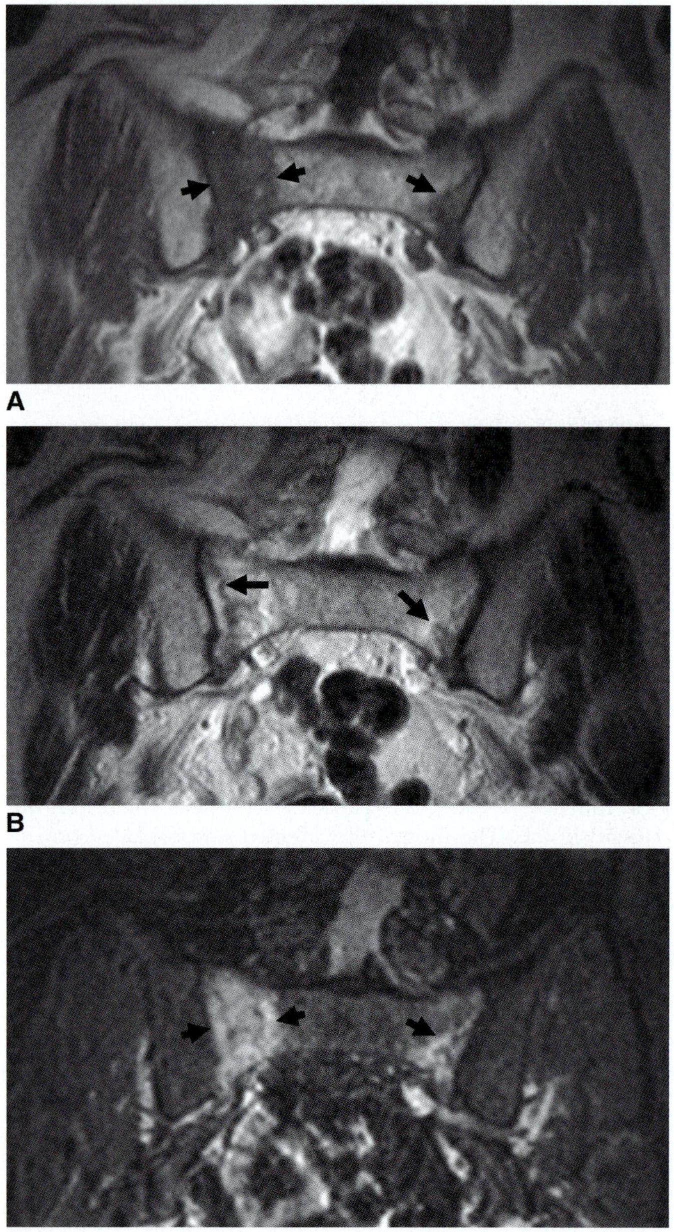

Figure 21.8. Eighty-five-year-old female with 6 weeks of severe pelvic/buttock pain since injury bending down. Coronal T1 image **(A)** through the sacrum and sacroiliac joints shows decreased signal intensity of marrow of bilateral sacral alae, right greater than left (*arrows*). Coronal STIR image **(B, C)** show increased signal intensity of the bone marrow edema with contained foci of serpiginous decreased signal intensity which represent bilateral sacral insufficiency fractures, right greater than left (*arrows*).

TREATMENT AND OUTCOMES

Treatment of sacral insufficiency or fatigue fractures is typically nonoperative.[47–50,55,56,61,62,64,66] Frequently, some time passes before the diagnosis is confirmed either via MRI or bone scan. Initial treatment involves "relative rest" with protected weight bearing with crutches as needed. Low-impact activities are a good transition back to activity/sport (e.g., pool running, stationary bike). Gradual return to sport is based on a pain-free activity level.

Patients typically return to normal activity levels in 4 to 6 weeks with up to 7 months recovery time for fatigue-type fractures.[47–49,55,67] Treatment must also address estrogen deficiency states, deficient dietary intake of calcium, eating disorders, and any underlying metabolic bone disease.[52,62,64] It is also recommended by some that any female with a stress fracture must be evaluated for the female athlete triad, which consists of amenorrhea, an eating disorder, and osteoporosis.[52] Upon return to sports, training issues such as footwear, training surface, cross training, core strengthening, and modification/evaluation of exercise technique and training method should be addressed.

Insufficiency fractures are treated similarly. As most insufficiency fractures are in the elderly, physical debilitation may complicate mobilization. A short period of bed rest may be necessary with oral analgesics. Early mobilization is emphasized with ambulatory aids as necessary. Weber et al.[50] reported pain resolution in about 4 to 6 weeks, with complete resolutions of symptoms in all patients by 9 months. Bone density testing may be appropriate in some individuals if insufficiency fracture is suspected. Estrogen deficiencies, deficient dietary intake of calcium, eating disorders, or other metabolic bone diseases must also be addressed.[64]

ACETABULAR AND ILIAC STRESS FRACTURES

Acetabular and iliac stress fractures are much less common than the above noted stress fractures, but deserve mention and should be included in the differential diagnosis of hip pain. Acetabular and iliac stress fractures are usually insufficiency-type stress fractures in elderly women.[68–71] These are often associated with other insufficiency stress fractures such as sacral and rami stress fractures, and may be confused with metastatic disease.[71] One report, however, noted 12 acetabular stress fractures in 178 military endurance trainees presenting with hip pain.[72] Another report described an iliac stress fracture in a young female runner.[73] Plain radiographs are typically normal or reveal ill- defined medullary sclerosis.[70] Both MRI and bone scan can be diagnostic for acetabular and iliac stress fractures.[68,69,71,72] Treatment for acetabular and iliac stress fractures focus on relative rest and gradual return to activity after workup for training errors and possible underlying osteoporosis and metabolic abnormalities. Displacement is rare, however, intra-articular acetabular stress fractures may warrant more stringent weight-bearing restrictions as protrusio acetabuli has been reported.[68]

CONCLUSIONS

Stress fractures about the hip and pelvis occur in both young athletic and elderly populations. Although pelvic ring stress fractures are typically self-limited, femoral neck stress fractures can have grave consequences if not treated in a timely manner. A high index of suspicion and appropriate imaging studies and treatment can help to minimize disability and morbidity as a result of these injuries.

REFERENCES

1. Fullerton LR Jr, Snowdy HA. Femoral neck stress fractures. *Am J Sports Med.* 1988;16:365–377.
2. Matheson GO, Clement DB, McKenzie DC, et al. Stress fractures in athletes: A study of 320 cases. *Am J Sports Med.* 1987;15:46–58.
3. Clement DB, Ammann W, Taunton JER, et al. Exercise-induced stress injuries to the femur. *Int J Sports Med.* 1993;14:347–352.
4. Bailie DS, Lamprecht DE. Bilateral femoral neck stress fractures in an adolescent male runner: A case report. *Am J Sports Med.* 2001;29:811–813.
5. Coldwell D, Gross GW, Boal DK. Stress fracture of the femoral neck in a child (stress fracture). *Pediatr Radiol.* 1984;14:174–176.
6. Meaney JE, Carty H. Femoral stress fractures in children. *Skeletal Radiol.* 1992;21:173–176.
7. Lehman RA, Shah SA. Tension-sided femoral neck stress fracture in a skeletally immature patient: A case report. *J Bone Joint Surg Am.* 2004;86:1292–1295.
8. Pihlajamaki HK, Ruohola JP, Weckstrom M, et al. Long-term outcome of undisplaced fatigue fractures of the femoral neck in young male adults. *J Bone Joint Surg Br.* 2006;88:1574–1579.
9. Blickenstaff LD, Morris JM. Fatigue fracture of the femoral neck. *J Bone Joint Surg Am.* 1966;48:1031–1047.
10. St Pierre P, Staheili LT, Smith JB, et al. Femoral neck stress fractures in children and adolescents. *J Pediatr Orthop.* 1995;15:470–473.
11. Daffner RH, Pavlov H. Stress fractures: Current concepts. *Am J Roentgenol.* 1992;159:245–252.
12. Provencher MT, Baldwin AJ, Gorman JD, et al. Atypical tensile-sided femoral neck stress fractures: The value of magnetic resonance imaging. *Am J Sports Med.* 2004;32(6):1528–1534.
13. Johansson C, Ekenman I, Tornkvist H, et al. Stress fractures of the femoral neck in athletes: The consequence of a delay in diagnosis. *Am J Sports Med.* 1990;18:524–528.
14. Prather JL, Nusynowitz ML, Snowdy HA, et al. Scintigraphic finding in stress fractures. *J Bone Joint Surg Am.* 1977;59:869–874.
15. Harmon KG. Lower extremity stress fractures. *Clin J Sport Med.* 2003;13:358–364.
16. Mendez AA, Eyster RL. Displaced nonunion stress fracture of the femoral neck treated with internal fixation and bone graft: A case report and review of the literature. *Am J Sports Med.* 1992;20(2):230–233.
17. Pihlajamaki HK, Ruohola JP, Kiuru MJ, et al. Displaced femoral neck fatigue fractures in military recruits. *J Bone Joint Surg Am.* 2006;88(9):1989–1997.
18. Noakes TD, Smith JA, Lindenberg G, et al. Pelvic stress fractures in long distance runners. *Am J Sports Med.* 1985;13(2):120–123.
19. Latshaw RF, Kantner TR, Kalenak A, et al. A pelvic stress fracture in a female jogger: A case report. *Am J Sports Med.* 1981;9(1):54–56.
20. Pavlov H, Nelson TL, Warren RF, et al. Stress fractures of the pubic ramus: A report of twelve cases. *J Bone Joint Surg Am.* 1982;64(7):1020–1025.
21. Tehranzadeh J, Kurth A, Elyaderani M, et al. Combined pelvic stress fracture and avulsion of adductor longus in a middle distance runner. *Am J Sports Med.* 1981;9:54–56.
22. Orava S, Puranen J, Ala-Ketola L. Stress fractures caused by physical exercise. *Acta Orthop Scand.* 1978;49:19–27.
23. Selakaovich W, Love L. Stress fractures of the pubic ramus. *J Bone Joint Surg Am.* 1954;36(3):573–576.
24. Jones DB. March fracture of the inferior pubic ramus. *Radiology.* 1943;41:586–588.
25. Nickerson SH. March fracture or insufficiency fracture. *Am J Surg.* 1943;62:154–164.
26. Wachsmuth W. Zur Atiologie der schleichenden fraketuren. *Chirurg.* 1937;9:16–24.
27. Leveton AL. March (fatigue) fractures of the long bones of the lower extremity and pelvis. *Am J Surg.* 1946;71:222–232.
28. Meurman KO. Stress fracture of the pubic arch in military recruits. *Br J Radiol.* 1980;53:521–524.
29. Howard FM, Meany RP. Stress fracture of the pelvis during pregnancy. *J Bone Joint Surg Am.* 1961;43(4):538–540.
30. Alonso-Burgos A, Royo P, Diaz L, et al. Labor-related sacral and pubic fractures: A case report. *J Bone Joint Surg.* 2007;89:396–398.
31. Brodell JS, Burns JE, Heiple KG. Transient osteoporosis of the hip of pregnancy: Two cases complicated by pathologic fracture. *J Bone Joint Surg Am.* 1989;71(8):1252–1257.
32. Leroux JL, Denat B, Thomas E, et al. Sacral insufficiency fractures presenting as acute low-back pain: Biomechanical aspects. *Spine.* 1993;18:2502–2506.
33. Schmid L, Pfirrmann C, Hess T, et al. Bilateral fracture of the sacrum associated with pregnancy: A case report. *Osteoporos Int.* 1999;10:91–93.
34. Sibilia J, Javier RM, Werle C, et al. Fracture of the sacrum in the absence of osteoporosis of pregnancy: A rare skeletal complication of the postpartum. *Br J Obstet Gynecol.* 1999;106:1096–1097.
35. Hoang TA, Nguyen TH, Daffner RH, et al. Case report 491: Stress fracture of the right sacrum. *Skeletal Radiol.* 1988;17:364–367.
36. Thienpont E, Simon JP, Fabry G. Sacral stress fracture during pregnancy—A case report. *Acta Orthop Scand.* 1999;70:525–526.
37. Christiansen CG, Kassim RA, Callaghan JJ, et al. Pubic ramus insufficiency fractures following total hip arthroplasty: A report of six cases. *J Bone Joint Surg Am.* 2003;85(9):1819–1822.
38. Launder WJ, Hungerford DS. Stress fractures of the pubis after total hip arthroplasty. *Clin Orthop.* 1981;159:183–185.
39. Hallel T, Malkin C. Fatigue fracture of the pubic ramus following total hip arthroplasty with unusual delayed healing. *Clin Orthop.* 1982;166:162–164.
40. Marmor L. Stress fracture of the pubic ramus stimulating a loose total hip replacement. *Clin Orthop.* 1976;121:103–104.
41. Oh I, Hardacre JA. Fatigue fracture of the inferior pubic ramus following total hip replacement for congenital hip dislocation. *Clin Orthop.* 1980;147:154–156.
42. McElfrash EC, Coventry MB. Femoral and pelvic fractures after total hip arthroplasty. *J Bone Joint Surg Am.* 1974;56:483–492.
43. Cracchiolo A. Stress fractures of the pelvis as a cause of hip pain following total hip and knee arthroplasty. *Arthritis Rheum.* 1981;24:740–742.
44. Miller C, Major N, Toth A. Pelvic stress injuries in the athlete: Management and prevention. *Sports Med.* 2003;33(13):1003–1012.
45. Callahan LR. Stress fractures in women. *Clin Sports Med.* 2000;19(2):303–314.
46. Rizzo PF, Gould ES, Lyden JP, et al. Diagnosis of occult fractures about the hip: Magnetic resonance imaging compared with bone-scanning. *J Bone Joint Surg Am.* 1993;75:395–401.
47. Shah MK, Stewart GW. Sacral stress fractures. *Spine.* 2002;27(4):104–108.
48. Volpin G, Milgrom C, Goldsher D, et al. Stress fractures of the sacrum following strenuous activity. *Clin Orthop.* 1989;243:184–188.
49. Johnson AW, Weiss CB Jr, Stento K, et al. Stress fractures of the sacrum: An atypical course of low back pain in the female athlete. *Am J Sports Med.* 2001;29(4):498–508.
50. Weber M, Hasler P, Gerber H. Insufficiency fractures of the sacrum: Twenty cases and review of the literature. *Spine.* 1993;18(16):2507–2512.
51. Ahovuo JA, Kiuru MJ, Visuri T. Fatigue stress fractures of the sacrum: Diagnosis with MR imaging. *Eur Radiol.* 2004;14:500–505.
52. Featherstone T. Magnetic resonance imaging in the diagnosis of sacral stress fracture. *Br J Sports Med.* 1999;33:276–277.
53. Fanciullo JJ, Bell CL. Stress fractures of the sacrum and lower extremity. *Curr Opin Rheumatol.* 1996;8:158–162.
54. Fredericson M, Moore W, Biswal S. Sacral stress fractures: Magnetic resonance imaging not always definitive for early stage injuries. A report of 2 cases. *Am J Sports Med.* 2007;35(5):835–839.
55. Major NM, Helms CA. Sacral stress fractures in long-distance runners. *Am J Roentgenol.* 2000;174:727–729.
56. Tsiridis E, Upadhyay N, Giannoudis PV. Sacral insufficiency fractures: Current concepts of management. *Osteoporos Int.* 2006;17:1716–1725.
57. Newhouse KE, El-Khoury GY, Buckwalter JA. Occult sacral fractures in osteopenic patients. *J Bone Joint Surg Am.* 1992;74(10):1472–1477.

58. Eller DJ, Katz DS, Bergman AG, et al. Sacral stress fractures in long-distance runners. *Clin J Sport Med.* 1997;7(3):222–225.
59. Czamecki DJ, Till EW, Minikel JL. Unique sacral stress fracture in a runner. *Am J Roentgenol.* 1988;151:1255.
60. Fredericson M, Salamancha L, Beaulieu C. Sacral stress fractures: Tracking down nonspecific pain in distance runners. *Physician Sports Med.* 2003;31:31–42.
61. Crockett HC, Wright JM, Madsen MW, et al. Sacral stress fracture in an elite college basketball player after the use of a jumping machine. *Am J Sports Med.* 1999;27(4):526–528.
62. Haun DW, Kettner NW, Yochum TR, et al. Sacral fatigue fracture in a female runner: A case report. *J Manipulative Physiol Ther.* 2007;30(3):228–233.
63. Denis F, Davis S, Comfort T. Sacral Fractures: An important problem. Retrospective analysis of 236 cases. *Clin Orthop.* 1988;227:67–81.
64. Lin J, Lane JM. Sacral stress fractures. *J Womens Health.* 2003;12:879–888.
65. Kiuru MJ, Pihlajamaki HK, Hietanen HJ, et al. MR imaging, bone scintigraphy, and radiography in bone stress injuries of the pelvis and the lower extremity. *Acta Radiol.* 2002;43:207–212.
66. Atwell EA, Jackson DW. Stress fractures of the sacrum in runners: Two case reports. *Am J Sports Med.* 1991;19(5):531–533.
67. McFarland EG, Giangarra C. Sacral stress fractures in athletes. *Clin Orthop.* 1996;329:240–243.
68. Yamamoto T, Schneider R, Iwamoto Y, et al. Rapid acetabular osteolysis secondary to subchondral insufficiency fracture. *J Rheumatol.* 2007;34(3):592–595.
69. Otte MT, Helms CA, Fritz RC. MR imaging of supra-acetabular insufficiency fractures. *Skeletal Radiol.* 1997;26(5):279–283.
70. Davies AM, Bradley SA. Iliac insufficiency fractures. *Br J Radiol.* 1991;64 (760):305–309.
71. Hauge MD, Copper KL, Litin SC. Insufficiency fractures of the pelvis that simulate metastatic disease. *Mayo Clin Proc.* 1988;63(8):807–812.
72. Williams TR, Puckett ML, Denison G, et al. Acetabular stress fractures in military endurance athletes and recruits: Incidence and MRI and scintigraphic findings. *Skeletal Radiol.* 2002;31(5):277–281. Epub 2002 April 4.
73. Atlihan D, Quick DC, Guanche CA. Stress fracture of the iliac bone in a young female runner. *Orthopedics.* 2003;26(7):729–730.

CHAPTER

22

Greg Lovell

Osteitis Pubis: Pubic Symphysis Joint Injury in Athletes

INTRODUCTION

Since its early descriptions nearly 100 years ago, osteitis pubis has provided clinicians with many dilemmas. While recent anatomical and radiological studies are beginning to clarify a poorly understood and confusing region, the pathophysiology of painful groin conditions remains difficult to interpret. The mixture of terminology used in groin conditions has been problematic in both research and treatment. In addition, multiple pathologies have been found to coexist, creating significant management difficulties. Despite research intensifying in recent years, there are few basic science studies and the clinician is provided with only limited evidence to guide the assessment, investigation, and management.[1,2] This chapter will review some of the current concepts on athletes who present with pain directly related to the pubic symphysis and provide some guidance for the clinician until further research and evidence improves our present level of knowledge.

HISTORY

Following Beer's 1924 description of "periostitis of the symphysis,"[3] by the 1940s, the term *osteitis pubis* was being used for a postsurgical painful disorder of the pubic symphysis associated with joint erosion on X-ray. While papers reported and discussed the possible etiology, causes, and treatment of osteitis pubis, several papers were published describing the same clinical and radiological features occurring after pelvic trauma.[4,5] In 1953, Adams and Chandler[6] coined the term "traumatic osteitis pubis" after describing the onset in a runner and after noting the above reports following trauma. In 1961, Schnute[7] described a case of a male acrobatic dancer with episodic pubic and adductor pain related to activity and with radiological changes at the pubic symphysis. Howse[8] presented a case of osteitis pubis of traumatic origin in an Olympic road walker; however, some unusual features were present suggesting there was an infective etiology. The first report of "osteitis pubis in athletes" was given by Cochrane[9] in 1971 in three soccer players who began to feel discomfort in the groin which became worse as they continued to train and play—more typical of recent descriptions in athletes. Radiological changes of osteitis pubis were noted and other extensive investigations were normal. Cochrane suggested that osteitis pubis may be an example of an overuse injury. Further reports in athletes then began to appear in the literature. Harris and Murray[10] noted in 1974 that not only were there plain X-ray changes at the pubic symphysis in athletes with groin pain but also in physically active individuals.

Koch and Jackson[11] described two runners with groin pain who had normal plain X-rays. Bone scans showed increased uptake at the pubic symphysis leading them to describe this condition as "pubic symphysitis," which may be "a precursor to osteitis pubis or a subtle variant." In 1991, two significant patient series were published—Fricker et al.[12] on 59 patients and Shaker et al.[13] on 78 soccer players. Fricker described the condition as "osteitis pubis in athletes" while Shaker preferred the term "aseptic traumatic osteitis pubis." In a radiology paper, Tuite and DeSmet[14] noted that osteitis pubis was a description of a group of conditions with a similar clinical picture of localized pain and tenderness at the pubic symphysis with plain radiology showing joint irregularity, erosions, and sclerosis. Similarly, Hölmich[15] recognized that this condition was not related to surgery and did not involve infection, and he reported in 1997 that "the diagnosis of osteitis pubis is often used to describe athletes with groin pain and X-ray changes similar to osteitis pubis secondary to surgery." Hölmich noted that the symptoms and signs were adductor related and suggested the descriptive term "adductor-related groin pain in athletes." Further, in 2007, he recommended that osteitis pubis should only be used as a term to describe a "radiologic sign" (of the typical changes seen in osteitis pubis).[16] With the development of magnetic resonance imaging (MRI) of the groin, a large series of Australian footballers was screened and imaged by Verrall et al. in 2001.[17] In this report, a significant association was found between increased signal on T2 fat suppressed MRI (bone marrow edema [BME]) at the pubic symphysis and athletes with groin pain. Following on from Ekberg et al.,[18] who also noted similar findings and suggested that microfracture may be the underlying cause, Verrall et al.[17] proposed the term "pubic bone stress injury" to describe the condition.

Another condition causing groin pain in athletes is that which is associated with injury to the inguinal canal/rectus abdominis region. Nomenclature used for this condition has included *pubalgia, Gilmore's groin, sportsman's hernia, sports hernia, incipient inguinal hernia,* and *primary abdominal musculofascial abnormality.* Unfortunately, this terminology has been confused and entwined with that of osteitis pubis.

In summary, in the absence of findings consistent with infection, underlying disease (e.g., rheumatological), or a relationship to surgery, the condition in athletes that we have been describing as osteitis pubis is perhaps more suggestive of pubic bone stress with a pubic symphysis joint injury secondary to athletic activity. Given this description, "pubic symphysis joint injury" will be predominantly used in this text; however, "osteitis pubis" will still be used in its historical context (Table 22.1).

ANATOMY

DEFINITION

The pubic symphysis joint consists of two pubic bones (each consisting of a pubic body and superior and inferior rami) and an intervening fibrocartilaginous disc. Functionally, the pubic symphysis is described as a secondary cartilaginous (fibrocartilage) joint and, biomechanically, while beginning as a synchondrosis, it develops into a nonsynovial amphiarthrodial joint.[19]

DEVELOPMENT

The centers of chondrification arise in the primitive sclero-blastema and grow together in the midline, thus forming the precursor of the pubic symphysis—from the Greek sumphuein, causing to grow together. A complete cartilaginous pelvis is present by the second month of development. The symphysis then appears at a point where the dense mesenchyme cavitates and differentiates into hyaline cartilage and the fibrocartilaginous disc. Secondary centers of ossification occur at puberty on the superior and inferior aspects of the ventral surface of each pubic bone near the symphyseal face. Although erratic in their development, they tend to meet and fuse along the ventral border of each pubic bone in the early 20s.[20]

TABLE 22.1 History of Osteitis Pubis Terminology

Year	*Author*	*Terminology*
1924	Beer	Periostitis of the symphysis
1934	Burman et al.	Adolescent osteochondritis of the symphysis pubis
1953	Adams and Chandler	Traumatic osteitis pubis
1971	Cochrane	Osteitis pubis in athletes
1981	Koch and Jackson	Pubic symphysitis
1991	Shaker et al.	Traumatic aseptic osteitis pubis
1997	Hölmich	Adductor-related groin pain
2001	Verrall et al.	Pubic bone stress injury

The joint is wedge shaped, wider anteriorly than posteriorly, and the articular surfaces are oval. The pubic bodies are covered with hyaline cartilage. This cartilage is initially quite thick and begins to become thinner in the teenage years until finally only a small segment is left in the adult (1 to 2 mm). The osteocartilaginous border is initially smooth, then develops irregularities (interdigitations) that slowly even out after 23 to 25 years of age.[21] A median cleft develops in the postero-superior portion of the symphysial cleft in the second year of life. Putschar termed these as "primary clefts." He also noted "secondary clefts" that followed an eccentric course between the hyaline cartilage covering the pubic bone and the fibrous cartilage forming the symphysial disc and thought that these were traumatically modified clefts. When present, he noted that, unlike primary clefts, these secondary clefts acquired a synovial lining.

The symphysis has been described as being richly innervated with branches from the pudendal and genitofemoral nerves. Its blood supply is derived from branches of all major vessels in the area including the obturator, the internal pudendal, inferior epigastric, and medial circumflex arteries.[19]

Goncalves da Rocha and Chopard[22] noted that while classically the symphysis pubis has been described as avascular, other articular discs such as knee menisci and intervertebral discs have been found to have peripheral blood vessels. They therefore studied the pubic disc in Wistar rats and found that the disc was well vascularized in the rim and ligaments by branches from the obturator and inferior epigastric arteries which formed a vascular plexus. From this arterial circle, branches supplied the pubic bone, muscle attachments, and articular tissues to supply the pubic ligaments and the fibrous rim of the interpubic disc. There were marrow contacts between the interpubic disc and subchondral bone. The authors also noted that the disc had an inner portion of fibrocartilage and an outer rim of fibrous tissue (dense connective tissue). This would suggest that it would have both a compression and tension function as pure tension would result in only connective tissue forming. Human studies are needed to confirm the value of these interesting findings.

LIGAMENTS

The joint is held together by four ligaments (superior, inferior, anterior, and posterior) which form a continuous circumferential envelope. The anterior ligament is the thickest and its decussating fibers intrude into the pubic disc and blend with the rectus abdominis and adductor aponeurosis.[19,20] The inferior (arcuate) ligament is thought to contribute the most to the stability of the joint.[19] Sutro[20] has also noted clefts and cysts within the ligaments. When examining for movement at the symphysis, he found that slight movement occurred in an anterior direction but separation was particularly difficult.

MUSCLE INSERTIONS

Recently, a cadaveric and MRI study has confirmed continuation of the rectus abdominis tendon and aponeurosis around the anterior pubic symphysis, merging with the capsular tissues and fibrocartilage disc and continuous with the origin of the adductor longus.[23] In 53% of the specimens, the tendinous and the muscular parts of adductor longus attached to the pubic symphysis capsular tissues and, in the remaining 47%, only muscular parts had symphyseal attachments (although in males, the results were 38% and 62%, respectively). The adductor brevis origin was involved in the capsular tissues in 41% of cases. In only one specimen, the gracilis was found to be attached to the pubic symphysis capsular tissues. In all other cases, the adductor magnus and gracilis were attached to the pubis but not the capsule. Another report found the same finding of continuation of the rectus abdominis and adductor longus leading the authors to use the term "rectus abdominis/adductor aponeurotic plate."[24] Earlier, a letter by Gibbon[25] had reported that an early French anatomical text based on nonembalmed cadavers showed a vertical ligamentous continuation of the rectus sheath inserting onto the pubic margin and being inseparable from the fused adductor longus and brevis origins. Gibbon felt that MRI evidence supported this notion of a common adductor-rectus abdominis anatomical and functional unit and, in athletes, he found features suggestive of a shear injury to this complex. Illustrations of this area are depicted in Figures 22.1 and 22.2.

To complicate the above mentioned anatomical findings, in a paper on cadaver dissections of the proximal adductor longus, 25% were found to have anatomical anomalies such as fusion of the adductor longus and gracilis tendons, projections of the tendinous fibers distally, and tendon fibers present on the posterior surface of the muscle.[26] The authors suggested that this may partially explain the difficulty in localizing the site of injury.

ETIOLOGY—RISK FACTORS, BIOMECHANICS, MRI FINDINGS, AND HISTOPATHOLOGY

RISK FACTORS

A recent systematic review of the risk factors for groin strain (all causes) highlighted many limitations of the studies including issues of methodology, definitions, validity, and lack of control of many confounding variables.[27] Overall, there was support for an association with previous injury, sport-specific training and preseason load, decreased adductor/abductor strength ratio, and individual risk factors such as femoral diameter, body mass index, increasing age, and more sports experience. The authors found that there was no strong evidence to support a causal association for any of these risk factors.

Hip range of motion is often quoted as an important factor in osteitis pubis. Hölmich et al.[28] noted a reduced range of hip abduction in athletes with groin pain; however, both of the study treatment groups improved over the course of the study (one had stretching as part of the program and the other group had no stretching in their rehabilitation). Verrall et al.[29] found hip range of motion (combined internal and external rotation in hip flexion) to be reduced in athletes with pubic bone stress injury and no difference was found between asymptomatic individuals and those with previous groin pain. When some of the asymptomatic athletes were subsequently followed, those that developed a groin injury had a smaller initial total hip range of motion.[30] Further work is needed to clarify the relationship between hip range of motion and pubic symphysis joint injury.

BIOMECHANICS

The literature on biomechanical factors in pubic symphysis injury is sparse. Dalstra and Huiskes[31] reported that there was a compressive load of 115% of body weight at the pubic symphysis occurring at the beginning of the swing phase during walking. This accords with the anatomical finding of a fibrocartilage disk primarily designed for resisting compressive forces. The finding of a fibrous rim in rats (noted above) would indicate that some tension forces also occur at this joint. Wang and Dumas[32] found that the compression stiffness was higher than the tensile stiffness and that the shear stiffness was higher in the superior–inferior direction than the anterior–posterior direction. During a study on the soccer in-step kick, the hip adductors were found to be activated at 81% of their maximum voluntary isometric contraction.[33] An EMG study on hip adductor strength found a breakpoint (point between the outputs

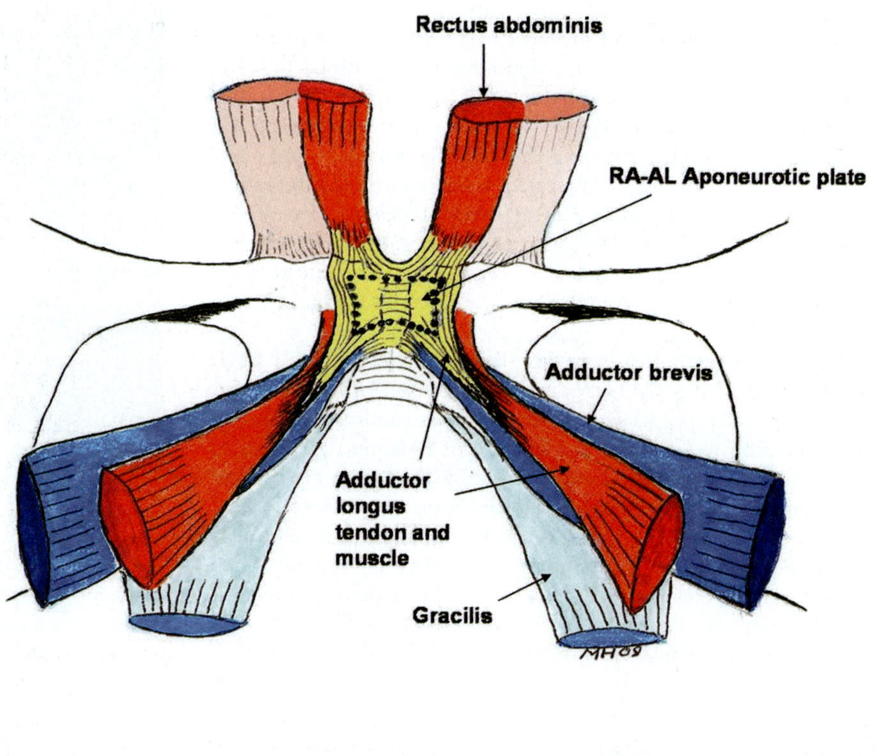

Figure 22.1. Illustration of muscle origins and aponeurotic plate at the pubic symphysis, frontal view. Central dotted area is shown as a cross section in Figure 22.2. (Courtesy of Dr. Michael Hammerton.)

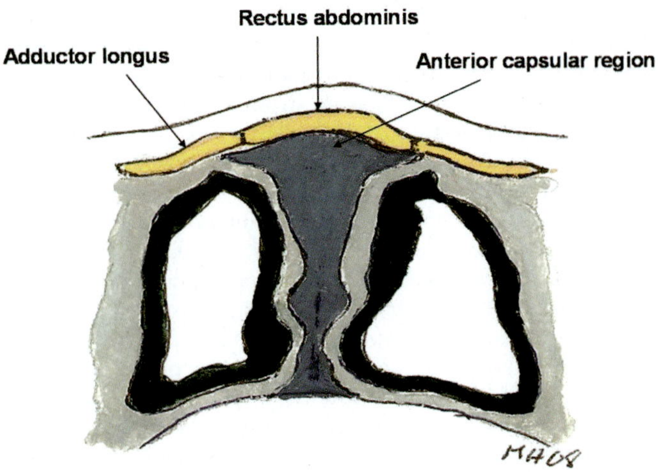

Figure 22.2. Illustration of a cross section of the pubic symphysis below the pubic tubercles demonstrating the proximity of the rectus abdominis, adductor longus, and the anterior capsular region of the joint. (Courtesy of Dr. Michael Hammerton.)

decreasing steeply during the initial contractions followed by a stable level) after around 30 maximal contractions.[34] This information may be useful when developing training programs. Using an MRI technique to examine the lower limb muscles before and after 100 kicks in a small group of Australian rules footballers, significant increases in signal intensity were found in the adductor longus and gracilis muscles in the kicking leg (30% and 49%, respectively). Minimal increases were found in the stance leg.[35] Overall, these studies suggest that compression and tension at the pubic symphysis in association with adductor muscle strength and fatigue and the kicking action may be important factors in groin injuries.

MAGNETIC RESONANCE IMAGING

MRI enables us to gain further insights into the anatomy and pathology of an injury. One of the early reports on MRI on 11 athletes with chronic groin pain compared bone scanning with MRI.[18] In this report, all athletes had abnormal plain radiographs showing erosions and irregular margins with bone scans showing increased uptake at the pubic symphysis. MRI examination was abnormal in all cases. The symphysis was found to be broad and irregular corresponding to the abnormal bone scan. The superior capsule was hypertrophied. The most interesting finding was high signal in T2-weighted images in eight of the patients in the region of the superior pubic ramus. Correlating these findings with the clinical picture led the authors to speculate that a microfracture was the primary lesion in these athletes.

In a cross-sectional study describing the incidence of BME in Australian rules (AFL) footballers, 72% were found to have BME near the pubic symphysis.[17] An association was found between finding a significant amount of BME and groin pain. The hypothesis proposed was that the BME was likely to be due to a tension bone stress injury. However, in one study following elite soccer players over a 4-month period, substantial amounts of BME were found in asymptomatic athletes.[36] Further, in a report on athletes with surgically treated pubalgia, changes of pubic BME were found in 70% of the athletes.[37] Similarly, in a study of army recruits using MR to image lower limbs, only 40% of 75 bone stress reactions became symptomatic.[38] These studies suggest that while pubic BME probably reflects bony stress changes, these changes may not be the source of an athlete's groin pain.

Recent MR studies have looked more closely at the pubic symphysis in an attempt to determine the underlying pathological abnormality. When the pubic symphysis was injected with local anesthetic, corticosteroid, and contrast in a group of 16 athletes with clinical osteitis pubis, all reported immediate pain relief.[39] Contrast was found to extrude from the disc in 12 of the patients indicating a loss of disc morphology (secondary cleft sign). Researchers at the same center found that the secondary cleft sign (best demonstrated on coronal STIR MRI) was a marker of the symptomatic side in athletes with groin pain (Fig. 22.3).[40] In this study, four of the six athletes with osteitis pubis had evidence of a secondary cleft. A secondary cleft sign was not found in their reference group of 70 athletes. The secondary cleft was thought to be an extension of the disc between fascial planes leading the authors to suggest that injury at the inferior pubis may continue to a tendon tear and progress to florid osteitis pubis (Fig. 22.4). The lack of finding of a secondary cleft in some athletes with osteitis pubis was thought to be consistent with the multifactorial causes for this condition. In a study on 100 soccer players with groin pain and 100 controls using a definition of abnormal BME remote from the adductor attachment for osteitis pubis and the secondary cleft sign as an indicator of adductor microtear, adductor dysfunction was found to be more common than osteitis pubis.[41] Most cases of osteitis pubis also had an adductor microtear. None of the controls had a secondary cleft sign or BME. This latter finding is intriguing and is in contrast with other studies that have found abnormal BME in asymptomatic athletes.[17,36,42]

Correlational analysis of MRI and clinical findings in 22 athletes with osteitis pubis by Kunduracioglu et al.[43] showed that

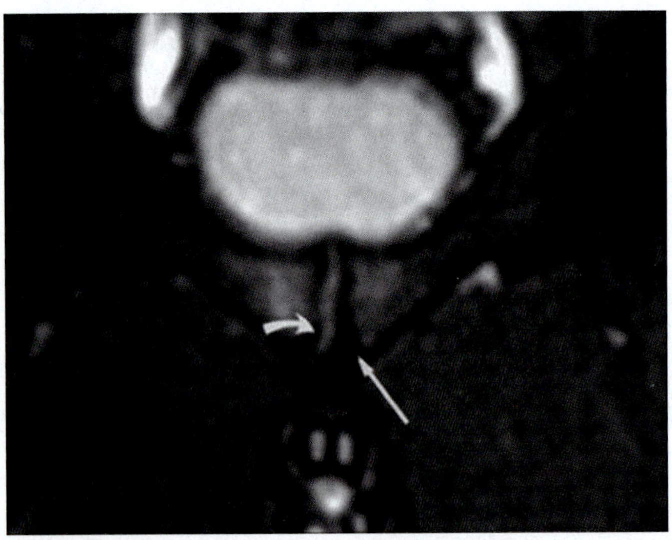

Figure 22.3. Coronal STIR (2000/20/160) image demonstrates a secondary cleft (*curved arrow*) on the right side. Extent of the cleft is slightly less at MRI than at symphyseal cleft injection. Parasymphyseal bone edema and articular surface irregularity indicate osteitis pubis. Thickening of the adductor aponeurosis (*straight arrow*) is noted on the left side. (From Brennan D, O'Connell MJ, Ryan M, et al. Secondary cleft sign as a marker of injury in athletes with groin pain: MR image appearance and interpretation. *Radiology.* 2005;235(1):162–167.)

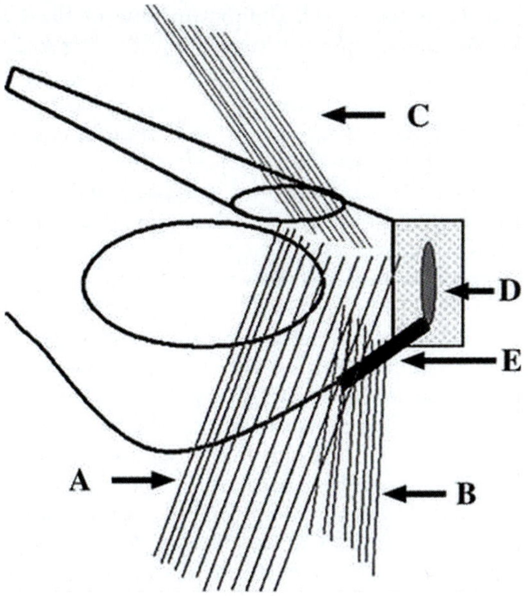

Figure 22.4. Frontal diagram shows anatomy of the symphysis pubis and the appearance of the secondary cleft. (*A*) Hip adductor aponeurosis; (*B*) gracilis aponeurosis; (*C*) conjoined tendon aponeurosis; (*D*) central physiologic cleft of the fibrocartilaginous disk; (*E*) secondary cleft. (From Brennan D, O'Connell MJ, Ryan M, et al. Secondary cleft sign as a marker of injury in athletes with groin pain: MR image appearance and interpretation. *Radiology.* 2005;235(1):162–167.)

subchondral BME, fluid in the symphysis joint, and periarticular edema were the most reliable MRI findings if the history of pain was less than 6 months while subchondral sclerosis, subchondral resorption and bony margin irregularities, and pubic beaking were the most reliable findings if pain had been present for more than 6 months. Similar changes are reported in the spine where marrow changes have been shown to correspond to endplate disruption. Pubic joint injury may thus involve a similar mechanism of avulsion fracturing at the osteochondral junction and degenerative chondral fissuring due to shear stresses.[44]

As MRI of the pubic region becomes more clearly defined, the different pathological conditions found may lead to more appropriate clinical decision making.

HISTOPATHOLOGY

Histopathological findings are limited in osteitis pubis with most reports coming from surgical procedures. Coventry and Mitchell[45] initially described finding marrow fibrosis and inflammatory exudate. In acute cases, they noted mild periostitis and extensive necrosis of cartilage and bone. In athletic osteitis pubis, there are two reports from wedge resection procedures in which histological findings are described.[46,47] Both found chronic nonspecific inflammatory tissue and areas of fibrosis. There were no signs of infection. In a recent series of 23 cases of curettage of the pubic symphysis, 15 had histology reported.[48] Degenerative cartilage was noted with no sign of inflammatory infiltrate. An early study (1955) on the theory of impaired circulation at the pubic symphysis involved injecting contrast material into the venous sinuses followed by X-ray.[49] Dilated tortuous vessels and slow rates of transit were found in patients with osteitis pubis. This led to anticoagulants being used as a treatment; however, this line of enquiry has not been further pursued. A report on biopsies of the bony pubis area showing increased bone signal on T2 MRI scans described woven bone with no signs of inflammation.[50]

More recently, Benjamin and McGonagle[51] described finding significant degenerative changes at large entheses such as the adductor longus (which was not found to be a synovio–entheseal complex). Changes were thought to be typical of a degenerative arthritis. He described fissuring at the origin of adductor longus that would reflect mechanical damage to collagen, which is followed by local loss of proteoglycans.

These findings indicate that pubic symphysis joint injury results in degenerative changes in cartilage and the disc. Whether these are due to chronic compressive/tension changes or whether they are the result of instability at the joint remains to be determined. The bone biopsy samples confirm MRI evidence of pubic bone stress which appears to be a prerequisite for the development of joint injury.

SUMMARY

Pubic BME is present in asymptomatic athletes, in athletes with osteitis pubis, and when there are other causes for athletic groin pain. This likely reflects a degree of bone stress reaction occurring in the pelvis in athletes. In symptomatic athletes with osteitis pubis, there are associated injuries at the pubic symphysis joint. Curettings have shown joint cartilage damage which is confirmed by plain X-ray and MRI evidence of joint erosions. Injection of anesthetic into the pubic symphysis clearly relieves the pain of this pubic joint injury and is a useful diagnostic measure.[39] Evidence of disc extravasation after contrast injection (secondary cleft sign) confirms earlier anatomical reports of joint injury causing traumatically modified clefts. Recent work suggests that these clefts may interfere with the aponeurotic plate formed by the rectus abdominis and adductor tendons; however, it is still unclear whether the clefts are caused by an initial disc injury or occur secondarily from an aponeurotic injury. The above information suggests that osteitis pubis in athletes would now be better described as a pubic symphysis joint injury with the pubic bone stress noted on MRI reflecting chronic biomechanical stress around the joint and that this injury may be associated with tears to the rectus abdominis/adductor aponeurotic plate. The constellation of pubic bone stress and joint injury would lend support to many authors' speculation on patterns of muscle fatigue, overuse, and overload as the cause of injury around the pubic symphysis.

CLINICAL ASSESSMENT

GROIN PAIN IN ATHLETES

Groin injury is reported in many sports but appears to be particularly of concern in football codes (soccer, Australian rules football), ice hockey, and callisthenics.[27] When reported, the definition of groin injuries can include adductor muscle or tendon injury, lower abdominal muscle injury, osteitis pubis, hernia, and many other causes of groin pain. This diversity will likely account for the large variation in injury rates from 0.2 to 5.17 injuries/1,000 participation hours.[27]

If an athlete presents with groin pain, the clinician must consider a wide differential diagnosis ranging from simple muscle strains to significant rheumatological conditions.[52,53] While being mindful of a large differential, some conditions are clearly more common and include adductor musculo-tendon injuries, hip joint lesions, sports hernia and rectus abdominis tendon insertion pathology, stress fractures of the pelvis (particularly in military recruits and long distance runners), and iliopsoas injury. Less common conditions to consider are pain referred from the spine or systemic disorders such as ankylosing spondylitis. Several authors have also reported finding multiple coexisting pathologies in athletes with chronic groin pain.[54–56]

CLINICAL FEATURES OF OSTEITIS PUBIS

In three large case series of athletes presenting with chronic groin pain, osteitis pubis (or adductor-related groin pain) features prominently as a clinical problem (Table 22.2).[16,55,56] From the many case reports and series over the years, the typical history given for osteitis pubis in athletes is of a gradual onset of pubic pain initially after sports activity. Gradually, pain interferes with sport and can finally become debilitating during daily activities. Often, pain is exacerbated by sit-ups, coughing, or sneezing. The football codes are the most commonly reported associated sports. Here, pain is noticed with sprinting and kicking. Clinical examination reveals pubic symphysis tenderness and pain with resisted hip adduction.

The results of four large case series that have described clinical findings in patients with osteitis pubis (using similar definitions but different terms for pubic symphysis joint injury) are presented in Table 22.3.[12,13,17,28] Surprisingly, unilateral adductor pain is reported as being the most common presenting symptom, and acute onset of pain is reported in up to 35% of cases. Usually, pubic tenderness is thought to be required for a diagnosis; however, in these series, up to 30% of cases did not have this finding. These findings, no doubt, reflect the difficulty in diagnosis between pubic lesions and adductor lesions and our evolving understanding of osteitis pubis.

BACKGROUND TO CLINICAL ASSESSMENT

Different grading scales have been used to assess an athlete's disability making consistency in analyzing reports difficult. One study used a grading classification based around unilateral and bilateral symptomatology which was found to be useful for predicting return to sport.[57] Others have used a modification of the Nirschl overuse pain scale using gradings such as no pain, pain before or after activity, pain during and impairing activity, and inability to play or train due to pain. This latter grading appears to be more useful. Combining one of these systems with a visual analog scale is valuable when trying to assess an athlete's progress.

Hölmich et al.[58] have evaluated the standard clinical examination tests for athletes with groin pain, finding good reliability for reproducing pain on palpation at the pubic symphysis, adductor longus, rectus abdominis, and psoas and for pain with resisted testing of adduction, functional testing of the abdominal muscles, and passive stretching of the adductors and psoas. The only test that was not reliable was that for assessing psoas strength—resisted hip flexion at 90° with the patient supine. Another test that has been described but not validated for psoas strength and pain is performed by resisting hip flexion with the knee in extension when the patient is sitting on the bed (Ludloff sign/test).[59] At the Australian Institute of Sport, we have found this test useful when assessing and following gymnasts with psoas injuries. Looking particularly at pubic pain provocation tests, another group found only moderate sensitivity but good predictive values (67% to 93%) for the single adductor, squeeze, and bilateral adductor tests (single leg resisted femoral adduction, "squeeze" test of femoral adduction in hip and knee flexion, and bilateral resisted femoral adduction in knee extension and slight hip flexion, respectively).[60] If all three tests were positive, there was a high likelihood that the athlete would have parasymphyseal pubic BME on MRI. A study using a hand dynamometer found that the most reliable position for measurement of hip adduction strength was in the supine position with hip flexion and knee flexion (approximately 45° and 90°) with the feet flat on the couch.[61] Interestingly, one study found that adductor-related groin pain may be relieved when using a pelvic belt while testing for adduction pain. The authors suggested that adductor tendonitis may not always be the cause of isometric hip adduction pain.[62] If hip adduction pain is relieved with pelvic stabilization, then it is likely that pain is arising from another site such as the pubic symphysis joint. These studies give the practitioner some confidence in clinical examination.

CLINICAL APPROACH

The evidence base is limited; however, the author's current practices include

- Consider a wide differential diagnosis. Look specifically for symptoms such as night pain, increasing pain despite reduction of activity, and symptoms from systemic, joint, urological, gynecological, spinal, gastrointestinal, and dermatological disorders.
- Obtain a clear history of the pain, including site and provoking and relieving factors.

TABLE 22.2 Top Five Diagnoses in Athletes with Chronic Groin Pain from Three Case Series

	Lovell (1995) N = 189	*Hölmich (2007) N = 207*	*Bradshaw (2007) N = 218*
1	Incipient hernia	Adductor-related groin pain	Hip joint pathology
2	Adductor tendonopathy	Iliopsoas-related pain	Osteitis pubis
3	Osteitis pubis	Sports hernia	Psoas pathology
4	Pubic instability	Pelvic floor-related pain	Stress fracture (neck of femur)
5	Iliopsoas tendonopathy	Rectus abdominis-related pain	Referred pain

TABLE 22.3 Case Series that Describe Clinical Symptoms and Signs of "Osteitis Pubis"

	Fricker et al. (1991)	*Shaker et al. (1991)*	*Verrall et al. (2001)*	*Hölmich et al. (1999)*
Diagnosis	Osteitis pubis	Aseptic traumatic osteitis pubis	Pubic bone stress injury	Adductor-related groin pain
N	50 (males) runners, footballers, others	78 (males) Soccer players	52 (males) AFL players + referees	68 (males) soccer players
Age (years, mean)	30	22	22	30
Site of pain, %				
Unilateral	59[a]	57	75	71
Bilateral	24[a]	18	25	29
Pubic	40[a]		19	
Adductor	80[a]		81	
Lower abdomen or pubic symphysis	40[a]	25		
Gradual onset, %	74%	65%	not stated	57%
Duration of symptoms (months, mean)	10 months	3 months	not stated	10 months (median)
Tenderness—site, %				
Pubic symphysis	70	92	85	
Superior pubic ramus	36		73	
Adductor	42	8	29	100
Adduction pain, %	12	70	not stated	100

[a]More than one site.

- Use a pain activity grading scale and a visual analogue pain scale to rate symptoms.
- Full clinical examination will include abdominal palpation, palpation of the pubic symphysis, hernial orifices, and scrotum, musculoskeletal assessment of muscle origins (adductors, rectus abdominis) and insertions (ilio-psoas), hip joint examination, spinal assessment, and neurological assessment. Any other area should be examined as directed by the clinical history. Careful clinical examination is required to differentiate the two main differential diagnoses for pubic symphysis joint injury of inguinal/rectus abdominis-related pain and adductor tendon injury.
- For a clinical diagnosis of pubic symphysis joint injury, search for tenderness directly over the pubic symphysis. Examine the adductor origins and musculotendinous junction of adductor longus. Adductor longus is usually prominent when the patient has the hip in flexion, abduction, and external rotation (Fig. 22.5). In this position, the examiner can more easily localize the patient's pain by careful palpation of the adductor longus origin and musculotendinous junction region, the pectineus origin along the superior pubic ramus and the gracilis at the inferior pubic ramus, and for bony tenderness at these sites. Passive hip adduction is usually painful only in severe cases. All patients should initially have pain with resisted hip adduction using one of the pain provocation tests (Fig. 22.6 shows the "squeeze" test). Adduction strength can also be assessed in one of these positions and also by resisted adduction when the patients are lying on their side (gluteal strength can also be assessed in this

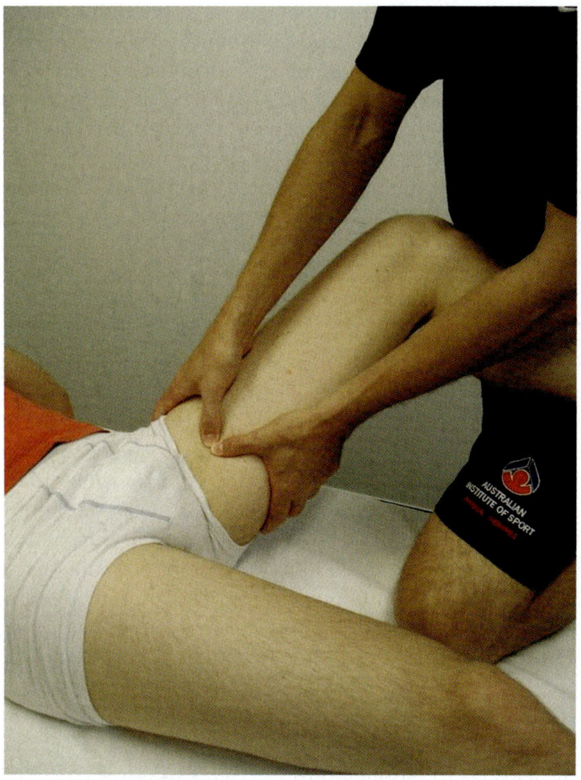

Figure 22.5. Palpation of the adductor longus. (Courtesy of AIS Dept of Sports Medicine.)

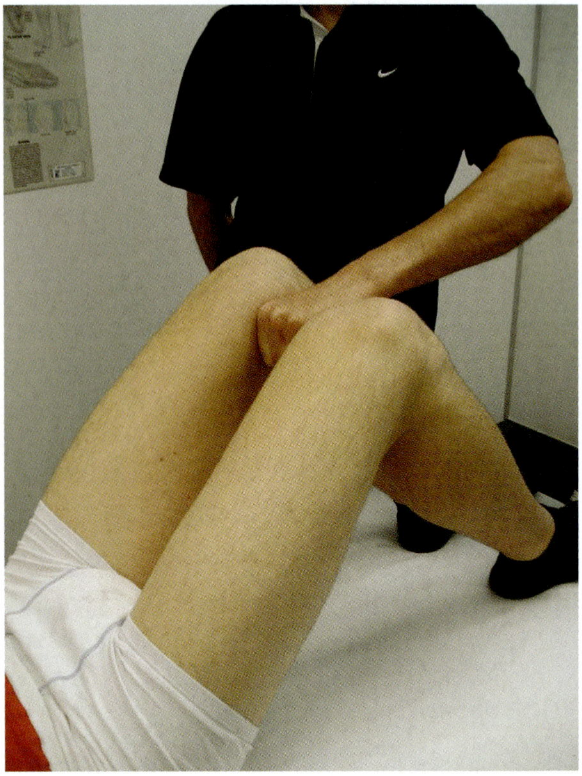

Figure 22.6. "Squeeze" test at 45° hip flexion (Courtesy of AIS Dept of Sports Medicine.)

position).[63] Local anesthetic injection into the pubic symphysis can be used to confirm a diagnosis in difficult cases.

- Coexisting pathologies and anatomical anomalies can be found in athletes with chronic groin pain and, therefore, during examination, the clinician should try to carefully reproduce the patient's pain by palpation or by using provocative maneuvers. Using current diagnostic criteria, the clinician can then determine the diagnosis(es) which will more readily guide the investigation and management process (Fig. 22.7).

INVESTIGATIONS

History and examination may suggest a narrow differential diagnosis and investigations will then need to be considered. When clinical examination suggests that an athlete may have a pubic symphysis joint injury, the clinician also needs to consider the multiple causes of this condition apart from sports injury—infectious, noninfectious (secondary to surgery), or rheumatological. A complete blood picture, erythrocyte sedimentation rate, C-reactive protein, rheumatoid factor, antinuclear antibody, and HLA B-27 will need to be considered if a rheumatological cause is suspected.[64]

Septic arthritis of the pubic symphysis is rare; however, in a review of 100 cases of septic arthritis of the pubic symphysis, athletes comprised the second most common risk group.[65] Typical features described were fever (74% of cases), pubic tenderness (88%), and a painful gait (59%). Only 35% had an elevated white cell count; however, the ESR was usually elevated and when blood cultures were performed, they were positive in 73% of cases. Needle aspiration yielded positive findings in 86% with the majority being *Staphylococcus aureus* and *Pseudomonas*.[65] Diagnosis can often be delayed indicating that if there is a clinical suspicion of infection, labeled white cell scan and CT guided aspiration would be appropriate.[64]

In most athletes, serological investigation is not necessary but should be considered if the rehabilitation progress is not proceeding as expected. In difficult cases, injection of local anesthetic, preferably under radiological control, has been found to reproduce and alleviate pain from the pubic symphysis.[39]

RADIOLOGY

The radiological approach to the athlete with chronic groin pain is relatively straightforward; however, the clinical interpretation of the complex information obtained may prove difficult due to the current changing state of the anatomical and pathological understanding of the tissues involved. After identifying the likely differential diagnoses, the clinician must then decide, in conjunction with the athlete, on the need for and appropriateness of radiological investigation. At an elite level, an athlete may require earlier and more extensive investigation due to factors such as the risk of continuing to compete and pressure of important competitions. Other athletes may be satisfied to proceed with an initial clinical diagnosis and only undergo imaging if there has been a poor response to treatment. Some differential diagnoses such as femoral neck stress fracture may warrant an early and aggressive approach to imaging. Different diagnoses will require different approaches to radiological investigation and not all practitioners may have access to tools such as MRI. Some consideration should be given to the radiation dose when using plain X-ray (pelvis, flamingo views, and hips), bone scans, and CT as many athletes have numerous investigations throughout their career.[66] All these factors require the physician to carefully determine the most appropriate investigative path. The main differential diagnoses have been noted earlier (Fig. 22.7), and this figure also suggests the most appropriate investigations for those conditions. In the area of osteitis pubis, the most useful investigations are plain X-ray, bone scan, and MRI. While ultrasound is useful for detecting tendonopathic changes and for hernia, it has a limited role in osteitis pubis.[44]

PLAIN X-RAY

Plain X-ray of the pelvis (giving the clinician a view of the pubic symphysis, rami, hip joints, sacro-iliac joints, and lower lumbar spine) should be the initial investigation of the athlete with groin pain. As noted earlier, plain X-ray was initially the primary investigation used to confirm a diagnosis of osteitis pubis. Coventry and Mitchell[45] succinctly described the findings as follows: "While early X-rays may be normal, after 2 to 3 weeks a blurriness of the borders of the pubic symphysis occurs. Erosions or progressive decalcification follows until a destructive or lytic phase is apparent. Woolly or a moth-eaten rarefaction may continue with a u-shaped area of loss of bone and cartilage formed. This phase lasts 4 to 6 weeks although it may be 8 to 12 months before regenerative changes are seen. Occasionally it may extend to the rami and tuberosities of the ischium. Eventually the bone contours return to normal."

In a group of soccer players and other athletes with groin pain, Harris and Murray[10] described the radiological changes

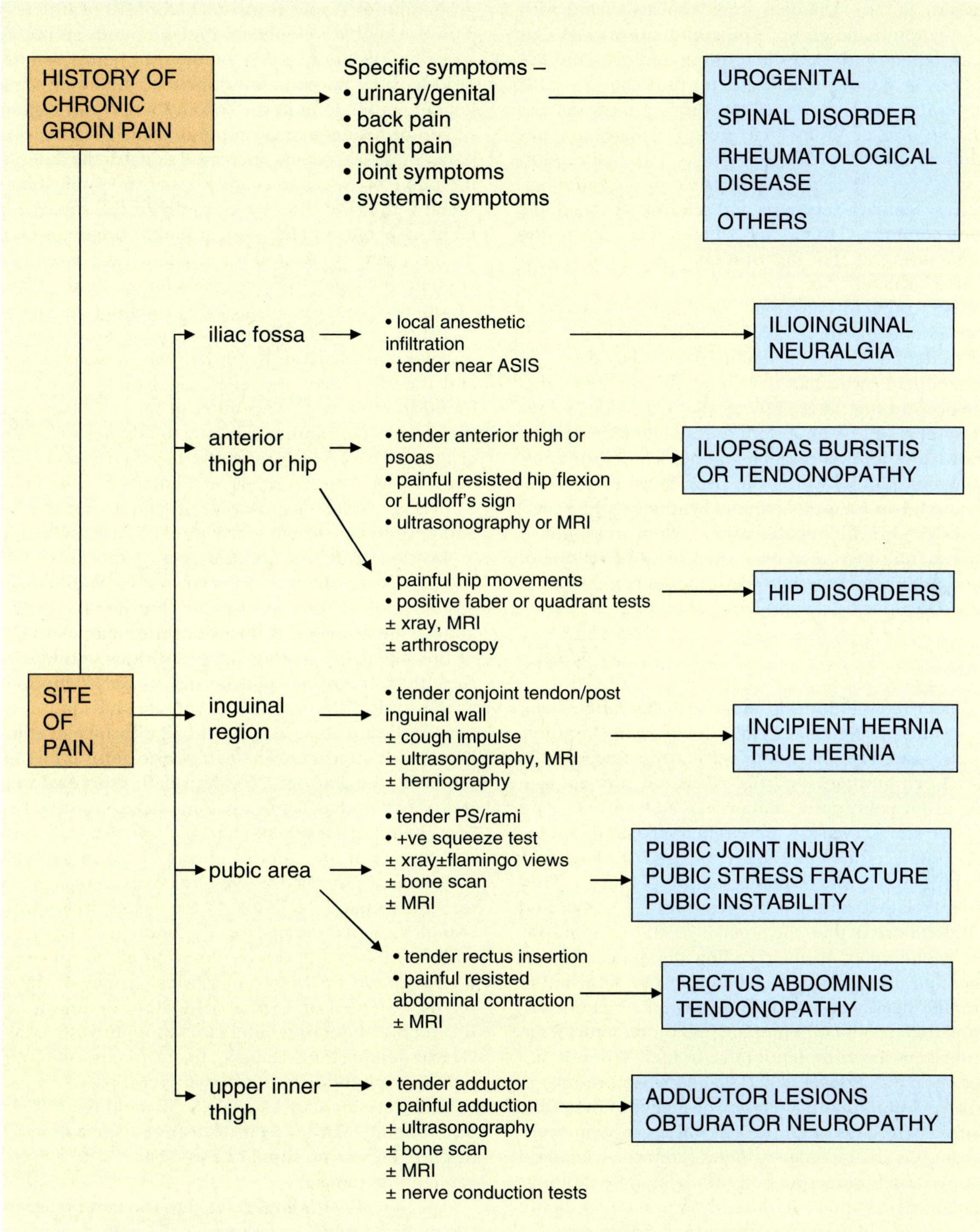

Figure 22.7. Differential diagnosis of chronic groin pain. (Adapted from Lovell G. The diagnosis of chronic groin pain in athletes: A review of 189 cases. *Aust J Sci Med Sport.* 1995;27:76–79.) ASIS, anterior superior iliac spine; Ludloff test/sign—see text, Faber, hip flexion, abduction, and external rotation; PS, pubic symphysis.

as similar to osteitis pubis with marginal irregularity, widening and instability at the pubic symphysis. In their control series of patients undergoing plain pelvic X-rays, 53% of those that played a high level of sport had abnormalities at the pubic symphysis whereas in only 9% of those that had a low level of activity, changes were found. Their injury group had a high incidence of pubic instability on flamingo view X-rays and there were also a high number with changes at the sacroiliac joint. Similarly, Besjakov et al.[67] reviewed plain pelvic X-rays of athletes and two control groups and concluded that athletes showed abnormal pubic symphysis changes more frequently and these changes were more severe. However, the activity of the age matched controls was not known. Changes were also associated with aging in the asymptomatic group. The authors proposed that a grading scale based on the sizes of erosions and cysts and the presence of bony beaking may be useful for physicians.

When reviewing plain X-rays of the pubic symphysis, the physician should also be aware that growth changes are not complete until around 23 to 25 years of age. This may lead to some confusion over the clinical significance of the radiological appearances. Similarly, erosions and sclerosis at the pubic symphysis are commonly found in patients with ankylosing spondylitis reminding us that this possibility should always be considered in an athlete.

Plain X-rays of pubic displacement on flamingo views have been used to define instability at the pubic symphysis, with >2 mm used to define vertical instability. This is based on the work of Chamberlain[68] who had developed this method originally for demonstrating instability of the sacro-iliac joints. Clinically, instability will be important as rehabilitation may be more difficult if the joint is unstable. Some centers routinely take these views in athletes with groin pain, however anecdotally they seem to be only a useful adjunct in athletes with recurring symptoms or difficult rehabilitation. When instability is present, however, it is often seen only when standing on one of the limbs (and not the other), thus providing some useful clinical information for specific rehabilitation exercises.

BONE SCAN

The triple phase Technetium-99c bone scan has often been used as the second line of investigation for pain in the pubic region. It is also useful for excluding pelvic stress fractures. As noted earlier, Koch and Jackson[11] described two runners with longstanding groin pain, pubic tenderness, and normal plain X-rays with bone scans revealing increased uptake at the pubic symphysis. Le Jeune et al.[69] in 1984, compared "radiography and scintigraphy" in 32 cases of pubic pain in sportsmen. They found good correlation between the scans, plain X-rays, and symptoms and reported that the uptake in the scintigraphy followed the evolution of pain preceding the appearance of X-ray changes and disappearing well before X-rays returned to normal. They felt that it was useful to confirm the diagnosis of pubic pain and that it could differentiate pubic joint injury from adductor and rectus insertion tendonitis. In their series of athletes with osteitis pubis, Fricker et al.[12] had bone scan results on 36 patients. They found that bilateral involvement of the pubic symphysis on the scans was often present when symptoms were unilateral; however, in the male athletes, abnormal bilateral uptake on scans closely corresponded with bilateral symptoms. They felt that increased uptake in the early flow and blood pool phase was associated with a shorter duration of symptoms.

Clinically, a bone scan is useful when symptoms are unclear and localization of pain is difficult, when there may be suspicion of a rheumatological disease such as ankylosing spondylitis, or when there may be suspicion of a bony disorder such as a stress fracture.

MRI

MRI has expanded the ability to investigate groin pain by allowing identification of numerous disorders and injuries in one investigative procedure without radiation exposure. It is now widely recommended as the diagnostic modality of choice in groin injuries. A specific protocol for MRI of athletes with groin pain has been developed and recommends an initial sequence surveying the entire pelvis, followed by both fat-suppressed and fluid-sensitive and non-fat-suppressed anatomic sequences and imaging of the joint in the coronal, axial, and sagittal planes.[70]

Abnormalities that are commonly seen in athletes on MRI are parasymphyseal edema, increased signal at the anterior cortex of the pubic body, erosions and cysts at the pubic joint, increased signal within the disc, hypertrophy of the superior pubic ligament, a secondary cleft sign, adductor origin and musculo-tendinous changes, disruption of the rectus abdominis/adductor aponeurotic plate, muscle signal changes in the rectus abdominis or adductors, inguinal hernia, and hip joint changes.

Parasymphyseal BME indicates pubic bone stress. This can be unilateral or bilateral. It can be seen in asymptomatic athletes and therefore may not reflect significant pathology. It is also found in association with other groin pathology and has been shown to occur more commonly in athletes when symptoms of groin pain have been present for less than 6 months. Focal bone marrow signal with a linear hypointensity (that may extend to a cortical surface) is indicative of a pubic ramus stress fracture and periosteal new bone formation will usually be apparent.

Erosions and subchondral cysts at the pubic joint, similar to plain X-ray changes, indicate pubic symphysis joint injury (osteitis pubis). Increased pubic disc signal clearly represents abnormal pathology as this is not normally seen. Hypertrophy of the superior pubic ligament indicates significant stresses at the joint and possibly reflects some increased motion occurring at the joint. The secondary cleft sign has only recently been described and its exact clinical significance is still unknown; however, it appears to indicate a disc/joint injury and may be similar to the synovial secondary clefts described in pubic joint injury by Putschar. Clinically, it has been shown to be consistent with the reported side of pain.

Changes at the anterior cortex of the pubic body near the adductor origin suggest stress reaction associated with adductor enthesopathy or injury to the rectus abdominis/adductor complex. Signal changes at the adductor origin will confirm adductor injury and can be seen without bony changes.

Disruption of the tenoperiosteal tissues of the pubic symphysis, best seen on sagittal MRI views, demonstrates injury to the rectus abdominis/adductor aponeurosis. Axial views can clearly demonstrate changes to the rectus abdominis muscle bulk (atrophy) due to injury to this complex.

Extensive increased signal on T2-weighted MRI with tendon discontinuity can be seen in pectineus or adductor complete or partial tears and should be associated with a more clear and acute injury pattern.

Specific MRI findings related to the main diagnoses around the pubic symphysis are shown in Table 22.4.

CLINICAL APPROACH TO INVESTIGATION

- In an athlete with specific clinical findings suggestive of a pubic symphysis joint injury and no other likely diagnoses, investigation is not always necessary initially.
- If the athlete's pain does not improve (or in an athlete with a need for early diagnostic confirmation), radiological investigation should begin with a plain X-ray film of the pelvis (including flamingo views when there has been a lengthy or changing symptomatology) followed by an MRI of the pubic symphysis and pelvis. Apart from excluding other diagnoses,

TABLE 22.4	MRI Abnormalities Seen at the Pubic Symphysis
Pubic symphysis joint injury (osteitis pubis)	• Increased signal in pubic bone marrow • Erosions, cysts • Increased signal within joint • Secondary cleft sign
Rectus abdominis/adductor common tendon injury	• Increased signal at anterior cortex at adductor origin • Disruption to adductor origin or rectus abdominis origin • Tenoperiosteal disruption on sagittal views • Secondary cleft sign
Adductor enthesopathy	• Increased signal at anterior cortex at adductor origin • High signal tendon origin

Source: Adapted from Omar IM, Kavanagh EC, Koulouris G, et al. Athletic pubalgia and the "sports hernia": Optimal MR imaging of the pubic symphysis region and pictorial review of MR technique and findings. Available at: http://www.bone.tju.edu/download/pubalgia.pdf (Accessed August 4, 2009).

MRI will give pertinent information regarding injury to the pubic joint, rectus abdominis/adductor aponeurotic plate, and adductor origins.

- When pain is persisting, the clinician should again consider other diagnoses and further laboratory investigations (e.g., for rheumatological disorders or septic arthritis). An ultrasound of the groin may be useful when considering inguinal hernia as a possible diagnosis or a bone scan may be necessary to seek other bony pathologies.
- If rehabilitation continues to be slow, injection of the pubic symphysis with local anesthetic (possibly with corticosteroid) under radiological guidance is worthwhile to confirm it as the source of pain and possibly improve rehabilitation.

MANAGEMENT

Using a pubic bone stress and joint injury model, the two principles to guide rehabilitation will then be first to manage the load placed on the pelvis by reducing activity and secondly to manage pain from the pubic symphysis and/or the aponeurotic plate. Load reduction will depend on the severity of pain and the disability associated with sport and will therefore range from total rest from activity to reductions in training load. Management of pain will range from rest, analgesics, or nonsteroidal anti-inflammatory drugs (NSAIDs) to corticosteroid injection before considering commencing an appropriate rehabilitation plan to support and strengthen musculature around the joint. In elite athletes, early investigation with MRI may be useful. The close relationship of the rectus abdominis, the pubic symphysis, the inguinal canal, and the adductor origins combined with some anatomical variants may make clear differentiation of pathology difficult. Management may therefore need to be more globally directed at first.

All practitioners should recommend a conservative program initially. While the prognosis of osteitis pubis is usually reported to be excellent, a close look at the reported case series is quite illuminating and paints a slightly different picture (Table 22.5).[12,13,28,71]

Across these studies, the return to sport rate varies from 14% to 100% (with 19% of this 100% still symptomatic). The only program supported by a randomized controlled study (for athletes with adductor-related groin pain) is a specifically structured exercise program by Hölmich et al.[28] This study described an "active training" (AT) program consisting of two phases, the first requiring two static and two dynamic adductor exercises to be done three times a week for 2 weeks and the second of eight exercises involving the hip adductors, abductors, flexors, and extensors, the lower back and side skating all performed three times a week for a further 4 weeks (with the first phase exercises being continued on the alternate days during the second phase). Adductor stretching was not allowed in this group. This was compared to a "physiotherapy treatment without active therapy program" (PT) of stretching, friction massage, laser therapy, and transcutaneous electrical nerve stimulation treatment. Both groups were allowed to return to pain-free activity at 6 weeks followed by the same return to sport protocol. The results (Table 22.5) indicate that 79% of the AT group returned to sport compared to 14% of the PT group (odds ratio 12.7 for the AT group [95% CI 3.4 to 47.2]). A follow-up report recommended exercising only to the point where pain begins, reducing the exercise intensity if the athlete experienced more pain, and emphasized that stretching of the adductors was to be avoided.[72] This program forms the basis of our current rehabilitation of athletes with adductor-related groin pain and osteitis pubis.

TABLE 22.5 Results of Conservative Treatment Programs

	Fricker et al. (1991)	*Shaker et al. (1991)*	*Verrall et al. (2007)*	*Hölmich et al. (1999)*
N	50 (mixed sports, males)	78 (soccer, males)	27 (AFL, males)	68 (soccer, males)
Follow-up (months)	17.5 (for 39 patients)	>18	24	7
Return to sport (%)	51% (20/39)	75%	100% (74% same level, 81% asymptomatic)	79% in AT group vs. 14% in PT group (see text)
Time to return to sport (months)	9.6	Not stated	5–24	4.5 (median)
Recurrence	25% (5/22)	25%		

Hogan[73,74] developed a similar program around an initial period of rest from pain, structured abdominal and adductor exercises and a graduated return to sport with progression depending on meeting the specific clinical criteria of avoiding pain during and after exercise, addressing adductor muscle guarding, and by using pubic symphysis stress tests and isometric adductor and rectus abdominis contractions to monitor exercise progression. Wollin and Lovell[75] have further modified this program and developed return-to-sport milestones based on physiologic data that were found to be useful for players in an elite junior soccer squad (Table 22.6). This resulted in a return to competitive sport between 10 and 16 weeks. Another protocol based around the premise of pubic bone stress has been reported and begins with an extended period of rest (3 months).[71] This does not seem to offer any advantages over the above mentioned programs.

In addition, an EMG study found that transversus abdominis activation was delayed in athletes with chronic groin pain supporting lower abdominal exercise retraining as a useful component in rehabilitation.[76] This is similar to an earlier finding in surgically treated athletes with inguinal pain.[77] As an adjunct to therapy, compression shorts have been found to be a useful addition during rehabilitation of groin pain.[78]

If compliant with the above programs, most athletes will be able to fully return to sport in 10 to 16 weeks from the commencement of a specific exercise rehabilitation regime.

Because of the management ramifications, it is important to differentiate between pubic joint injury and the inguinal-related groin pain (incipient hernia and rectus abdominis insertion injury) of athletes. A randomized clinical trial of treatment for 66 male soccer players with inguinal groin pain (which was verified as incipient hernia by herniography or by pain relief from an ilio-inguinal nerve block) found that surgical treatment clearly surpassed two different conservative rehabilitation programs and a control group.[79] Numerous other case reports and series support surgical intervention in this group of athletes. Therefore, if rehabilitation is not progressing satisfactorily, the clinician should carefully reexamine the athlete and reconsider the possibility of inguinal pathology either clinically or by further investigation. Similarly, investigation with MRI can be useful to determine if there is adductor tendon pathology that would be amenable to other therapeutic modalities such as corticosteroid injection or tenotomy (also see below). If the diagnosis is in doubt injection of the pubic symphysis with local anesthetic under radiological control appears to be a useful diagnostic intervention.

NSAIDs are commonly used initially to resolve pain; however, their role in this condition has not been specifically investigated. Since some surgical reports have shown chronic inflammation, NSAIDs may have a role initially; however, they are unlikely to be of value for ongoing management if there is significant bone stress. Conversely, if MRI reveals more chronic pathology without bone edema, NSAIDs or paracetamol (acetaminophen) may be of use in a similar manner to their use in osteoarthritis, enabling athletes to continue playing or be able to make better progress in their rehabilitation. During the rehabilitation process, pain is one of the usual assessment criteria and if this is masked by NSAIDs, assessment of progress may be compromised.

Soon after corticosteroids were introduced into medical practice, they were trialed in patients with osteitis pubis following urological surgery, with some very promising results.[80]

TABLE 22.6 Outline of a Specific Rehabilitation Program

Module I	*Pain reduction phase* • IU pelvic muscle training in RTUS as applicable • Static IU exercises • Low level dynamic IU exercises • Isometric hip adduction *Progress to module II:* • 20% increase in squeeze test strength pain-free
Module II	*Early dynamic phase* • Moderate dynamic IU exercises • Isolated gluteal exercises • Early integrated OU and IU exercise • Elastic band exercises, hip FLEX/EXT/ABD/ADD • Stationary cycling *Progress to module III:* • Adequate single leg hip/pelvic control and full abduction on lateral lunges
Module III	*Dynamic phase* • Skating on slide board • Large ROM adductor exercise • Moderate level integrated OU/IU exercise • Stationary cycling • Basic running program • Frequency—alternate days *Progress to module IV "advanced" phase* • 3 × 12 reps 3 kg hip adduction between tables • Completed basic running program (5 km)
Module IV	*Advanced phase* • Stationary cycling • Advanced running program • Skating on slide board • "Sprint" skating on slide board • Large ROM adductor exercise • Frequency—alternate days *Return to football* • 3 × 12 reps 6 kg hip adduction between tables • Slide-board skating 5 × 1 min full length board • Completed advanced running program

IU, inner unit pelvic muscles (transversus abd, pelvic floor, and multifidus), exercises done daily; OU, outer unit pelvic muscles (gluteals, adductors, obliques, and rectus abdominis), exercises done alternate days; RTUS, real-time ultrasound; FLEX, flexion; EXT, extension; ABD, abduction; ADD, adduction; ROM, range of motion. *Source*: Updated from Wollin M, Lovell G. Osteitis pubis in four young football players: A case series demonstrating successful rehabilitation. *Phys Ther Sport.* 2006;7(3):153–160.

Using high doses, the metabolic side-effects were soon noticed and their use was cautioned. In a group of athletes with osteitis pubis on clinical and radiologic grounds, Holt et al.[81] reported on their use in 1995. In this case report on nine athletes, eight required two injections and one needed three injections, leading the authors to suggest that corticosteroids may be useful if symptoms do not improve over 7 to 10 days. While three of the nine athletes returned to sport within a month from onset of treatment, the remainder returned in 3 to 6 months. This is not clearly better than an active conservative program. Corticosteroid injection (with anesthetic) into the symphyseal cleft has been reported in a group of 16 athletes with osteitis pubis.[39] During follow-up, ten had pain relief at 2 weeks but only five at 2 months. In a similar study, 24 athletes were injected and MRI findings of enthesopathy were used to divide the athletes into two groups.[82] Follow-up at 6 weeks and 1 year showed that if the MRI showed no abnormality, there was a good response. If an abnormality was found, there was a poor response to treatment. There have been no controlled studies on the use of corticosteroids in athletes; however, it is likely that results will be similar to other reports in musculoskeletal medicine where they provide only short-term symptom relief.

There has been one report on the use of prolotherapy in elite rugby and soccer players who had failed a conservative program (details of the program were not specified).[83] Using a solution of 12.5% dextrose, eight injection points, and injections every month until pain was resolved, 22 out of 24 athletes were playing fully at 3 months. VAS scores changed from 6.3 initially to 1.0 at 1 month after initial treatment. Treatments were repeated at monthly intervals if pain was still present with the number of treatments ranging from 1 to 6. These results are promising; however, there was no placebo arm to the trial and patients were instructed to do abdominal and adductor strengthening and stretching as tolerated. While the authors note the lack of understanding of placebo use in prolotherapy, they acknowledge that needling alone produced equivalent results to prolotherapy in a trial on low back pain. Considering these results, when the number of treatments that were required to reach a pain-free or steady state is summated, the mean time to return to pain-free sport was 12 weeks. While this is slightly faster than the structured exercise program outlined earlier, further investigation is needed.

The description of the successful use of bisphosphonates in three cases of osteitis pubis (one related to a spondyloarthropathy) has prompted an interest in this therapy for athletes with osteitis pubis.[84] The rationale for the use of these agents lies in their ability to localize to sites of active bone turnover and their potential anti-inflammatory properties. In a review article, joint erosion was described as being dependant on proinflammatory cytokines and osteoclast activity and, further to that, several animal studies showed that bisphosphonates were a useful adjuvant treatment in arthritis and may also be chondroprotective.[85] Another report has found their use of value in female basketballers with tibial stress reactions.[86] Anecdotally, bisphosphonates, both oral and intravenously, have been tried on athletes with recalcitrant osteitis pubis in the football codes with success; however, there are no published reports to date. Although these drugs have been used safely for a number of years in osteoporosis therapy and in other disorders, recent reports of mandibular osteonecrosis associated with their use should direct the clinician to ensure that an athlete is well informed, perhaps even recommending dental review prior to use.

After venous congestion was proposed and noted in patients with postsurgical osteitis pubis,[49] anticoagulant therapy was reported and found to be successful.[87] There have been no reports of their use in athletes with groin pain but this may be due to the uncertainty of the pathology described and also because most cases occur in contact sports, making their use inappropriate.

PUBIC INSTABILITY

Excess motion at the pubic symphysis is termed pubic instability and the diagnosis is made on imaging findings (see above). Not all athletes with joint injury develop pubic instability; however, as noted earlier, it should be suspected if an athlete has recurring symptoms or changing symptoms around the groin. Instability can also be acute after trauma or related to pregnancy and childbirth. Treatment should initially be the same with a specific exercise program and should also focus on stability exercises involving the leg demonstrating the instability on flamingo view X-rays. In recalcitrant cases, surgical fixation can be considered (see below). While a pelvic support belt is often used, a prospective randomized study on pregnant females with symphysis pubis dysfunction found that neither a rigid nor a nonrigid pelvic support belt was better than exercise and advice.[88]

SURGERY

If conservative measures fail, an athlete will either need to withdraw from sport or consider one of the surgical options. Mandelbaum and Mora[64] have noted that their clinic patients are considered for surgery only if they have undergone 9 months of observation, physiotherapy, NSAID treatment, and three corticosteroid injections into the pubic symphysis and have also been reviewed for a sports hernia. It would also be worthwhile to ensure that the conservative exercise program tried has been the specific "Hölmich" style program outlined above and that a complete differential diagnosis with appropriate investigation has also been considered. In our clinic, most apparent treatment failures have been due to poorly designed rehabilitation programs or poor patient compliance with the program.

The different surgical procedures proposed for recalcitrant osteitis pubis in athletes have included adductor tenotomy, possibly with rectus abdominis repair,[89,90] wedge resection of the symphysis pubis,[46] wedge resection and arthrodesis,[47] symphyseal curettage,[48,91] and extraperitoneal endoscopic mesh repair.[92] All papers based on these procedures are case reports or series and therefore provide only Level IV evidence. Surgical treatment should be only approached after careful case assessment using similar criteria to that noted above. In a case report on two patients, Moore et al.[93] described disabling symptoms of posterior instability after resection of the pubic symphysis and commented that arthrodesis may be a better option than resection. In the paper on arthrodesis by Williams et al., all athletes had evidence of pubic instability on flamingo view X-rays suggesting that this may be the more appropriate procedure for this group of athletes. Symphyseal curettage and endoscopic mesh repair are less invasive procedures and, at this stage, seem the most appropriate first line procedures for athletes without instability.

Adductor tenotomy is a commonly used procedure in adductor-related groin pain and it is surprising that, other than several case reports/series, no authors have studied this in a more controlled manner. The role of this procedure therefore remains ill defined, but it may be most useful in athletes with MRI confirmed adductor tendonopathy.

Treatment results of and recommendations for rectus abdominis/adductor aponeurosis plate injuries identified on MRI are still not clear. Pelvic floor/inguinal repairs consistently report good results despite many techniques not addressing injuries to the rectus or adductors. This pathology should be carefully considered on finding superior pubic or inguinal symptomatology, a failed response to a specific exercise program, or abnormal findings on ultrasound or MRI.

KEY POINTS ON MANAGEMENT

- There should be an initial period of rest (1 to 3 weeks) from all activity to reduce pain.
- Prescribe a specific strengthening exercise program and monitor progress using activity-related pain and a pain provocation test such as the "squeeze test." Advise the athlete that the program will take 12 to 16 weeks before he or she can fully return to sport. Use of compression shorts is useful during rehabilitation. Following return to sport, some groin rehabilitation exercises should be continued.
- During a competitive sporting season, consider modifying the training load while continuing to play with analgesia (particularly if symptoms are chronic and there is minimal BME on MRI of the pubic symphysis).
- If pain is not improving after 2 to 3 weeks, review the diagnosis(es), consider further investigation, or confirm the diagnosis with injection of anesthetic (possibly with corticosteroid) into the pubic symphysis joint.
- If progress remains poor at 4 to 6 weeks, consider compliance issues or intervention using bisphosphonate therapy or prolotherapy.
- With multiple pathology coexisting such as
- A summary of the evidence (based on NHMRC guidelines[94]) for management is shown in Table 22.7.

  – An incipient inguinal hernia—surgery should be considered prior to an exercise program
  – Adductor tendonopathy—consider local corticosteroid injection and an appropriate tendonopathy strengthening program
  – Pubic instability—use a tailored exercise program

- If pain is recalcitrant, consider a longer period of withdrawal from sport or a surgical option.

TABLE 22.7 **Levels of Evidence (using NH&MRC Guidelines) for the Treatment of Osteitis Pubis in Athletes**

Treatment	*Levels of Evidence*			
	1	*2*	*3*	*4*
Specific exercise program		*		
Compression shorts		*		
NSAIDs				*
Corticosteroids				*
Prolotherapy				*
Bisphosphonates				*
Warfarin				*
Surgery—pubic symphysis curettage, mesh repair, adductor tenotomy, symphyseal resection, symphyseal stabilization				*
Surgery—inguinal (not for osteitis pubis)		*		

SUMMARY/CONCLUSION

The term osteitis pubis in athletes was based on finding a similar radiological pattern in athletes with groin pain to that of an unusual condition at the pubic symphysis following urological surgery. In athletes with groin pain, recent anatomical and MRI studies have shown pubic bone stress, pubic symphysis joint injury, tears at the rectus abdominis–adductor common aponeurosis, and injury to the surrounding structures. In athletes, the term osteitis pubis should now be described as a pubic symphysis joint injury that can be associated with injury to the rectus abdominis–adductor common aponeurosis. Diagnosis can be determined by careful clinical examination, joint injection, and typical radiological features and management should initially be undertaken using a specific exercise rehabilitation program. Surgery should be considered when conservative measures have failed and after appropriate investigation. Further studies in histopathology, biomechanics, and prevention will assist in determining future specific management strategies.

REFERENCES

1. Fricker PA, Lovell G. How do you treat chronic groin pain? In: MacAuley T, Best T, eds. *Evidence-Based Sports Medicine.* 2nd Ed. London: Blackwell Science;2007, pp. 491–509.
2. Thorborg K. Assessment and management of long-standing groin pain in athletes: A review of the literature. *Forskning i Fysioterapi* (online). 2004;(2.arg),s:1–14. Available at: http://www.ffy.dk/sw3917.asp (Accessed March 5, 2008).
3. Beer E. Periostitis of the symphysis and descending rami of the pubes following suprapubic operations. *Int J Med Surg.* 1924;37:224–225.
4. Burman M, Weinkle IN, Langsam MJ. Adolescent osteochondritis of the symphysis pubis. *J Bone Joint Surg.* 1934;16:649–657.
5. Klinefelter E. Osteitis pubis: Review of the literature and a case report. *Am J Roentgenol.* 1950;63:368–371.
6. Adams RJ, Chandler FA. Osteitis pubis of traumatic etiology. *J Bone Joint Surg.* 1953;3:685–696.
7. Schnute WJ. Osteitis pubis. *Clin Orthop Relat Res.* 1961;20:187–192.
8. Howse AJG. Osteitis pubis in an olympic road-walker. *Proc Royal Soc Med.* 1964;57:88–90.
9. Cochrane GM. Osteitis pubis in athletes. *Br J Sports Med.* 1971;5:233–235.
10. Harris NH, Murray RO. Lesions of the symphysis in athletes. *Br Med J.* 1974;4:211–214.
11. Koch RA, Jackson DW. Pubic symphysitis in runners: A report of two cases. *Am J Sports Med.* 1981;9(1):62–63.
12. Fricker PA, Taunton JE, Amman W. Osteitis pubis in athletes: Infection, inflammation or injury? *Sports Med.* 1991;12:266–279.
13. Shaker AM, Shaheen MAE, O'Neil PJ. Traumatic aseptic osteitis pubis. *Ann Saudi Med.* 1991;11:205–208.
14. Tuite MJ, DeSmet AA. MRI of selected sports injuries: Muscle tears, groin pain, and osteochondritis dissecans. *Semin Ultrasound CT MR.* 1994;15(5):318–340.
15. Hölmich P. Adductor-related groin pain in athletes. *Sports Med Athrosc Rev.* 1997;5:285–291.
16. Hölmich P. Long-standing groin pain in sportspeople falls into three primary patterns, a "clinical entity" approach: A prospective study of 207 patients. *Br J Sports Med.* 2007;41(4):247–252.
17. Verrall GM, Slavotinek JP, Fon GT. Incidence of pubic bone marrow oedema in Australian rules football players: Relation to groin pain. *Br J Sports Med.* 2001;35(1):28–33.
18. Ekberg O, Sjöberg S, Westlin N. Sports-related groin pain: Evaluation with MR imaging. *Eur Radiol.* 1996;6(1):52–55.
19. Gamble JG, Simmons SC, Freedman M. The symphysis pubis. *Clin Orthop Relat Res.* 1986;(203):261–272.
20. Sutro CJ. The pubic bones and their symphysis. *Arch Surg.* 1936;32:823–841.
21. Putschar W. The structure of the human symphysis pubis with special consideration of parturition and its sequelae. *Am J Phys Anthrop.* 1976;45:589–594.
22. Goncalves da Rocha RC, Chopard RP. Nutrition pathways to the symphysis pubis. *J Anat.* 2004;204(Pt 3):209–215.
23. Robinson P, Salehi F, Grainger A, et al. Cadaveric and MRI study of the musculotendinous contributions to the capsule of the symphysis pubis. *Am J Roentgenol.* 2007;188(5):W440–W445.

24. Zoga A, Morrison W, Kavanagh E, et al. MRI of athletic pubalgia: The rectus abdominis/adductor aponeurotic plate. *RSNA Conf.* 2007. Available at: http://rsna2007.rsna.org/rsna2007/v2007/conference/event_display.cfm?am_id = 2&em_id = 5016115 (Accessed February 21, 2008).
25. Gibbon WW. Groin pain in athletes—letter. *Lancet.* 1999;353:1444–1445.
26. Tuite DJ, Finegan PJ, Saliaris AP, et al. Anatomy of the proximal musculotendinous junction of the adductor longus muscle. *Knee Surg Sports Traumatol Arthrosc.* 1998;6(2):134–137.
27. Maffey L, Emery C. What are the risk factors for groin strain injury in sport? A systematic review of the literature. *Sports Med.* 2007;37(10):881–894.
28. Hölmich P, Uhrskou P, Ulnits L, et al. Effectiveness of active physical training as treatment for long-standing adductor-related groin pain in athletes: Randomised trial. *Lancet.* 1999;353:439–443.
29. Verrall GM, Hamilton IA, Slavotinek JP, et al. Hip joint range of motion reduction in sports-related chronic groin injury diagnosed as pubic bone stress injury. *J Sci Med Sport.* 2005;8(1):77–84.
30. Verrall GM, Slavotinek JP, Barnes PG, et al. Hip joint range of motion restriction precedes athletic chronic groin injury. *J Sci Med Sport.* 2007;10(6):463–466.
31. Dalstra M, Huiskes R. Load transfer across the pelvic bone. *J Biomech.* 1995;28(6):715–724.
32. Wang M, Dumas GA. Mechanical behaviour of the symphysis pubis. *Can Soc Biomech Proc.* 1994;308–309.
33. Brophy RH, Backus SI, Pansy BS, et al. Lower extremity muscle activation and alignment during the soccer instep and side-foot kicks. *J Orthop Sports Phys Ther.* 2007;37(5):260–268.
34. Kadi F, Buskqvist L, Sjoholm O, et al. Strength, muscular endurance and EMG characteristics of thigh adductors. *Isokinetics Exerc Sci.* 2006;14:235–239.
35. Baczkowski K, Marks P, Silberstein M, et al. A new look into kicking a football: An investigation of muscle activity using MRI. *Australas Radiol.* 2006;50(4):324–329.
36. Lovell G, Galloway H, Hopkins W, et al. Osteitis pubis and assessment of bone marrow edema at the pubic symphysis with MRI in an elite junior male soccer squad. *Clin J Sport Med.* 2006;16(2):117–122.
37. Albers SL, Spritzer CE, Garrett WE, et al. MR findings in athletes with pubalgia. *Skeletal Radiol.* 2001;30:270–271.
38. Kiuru MJ, Niva M, Reponen A, et al. Bone stress injuries in asymptomatic elite recruits: A clinical and magnetic resonance imaging study. *Am J Sports Med.* 2005;33(2):272–276.
39. O'Connell MJ, Powell T, McCaffrey NM, et al. Symphyseal cleft injection in the diagnosis and treatment of osteitis pubis in athletes. *Am J Roentgenol.* 2002;179:955–959.
40. Brennan D, O'Connell MJ, Ryan M, et al. Secondary cleft sign as a marker of injury in athletes with groin pain: MR image appearance and interpretation. *Radiology.* 2005;235(1):162–167.
41. Cunningham PM, Brennan D, O'Connell M, et al. Patterns of bone and soft-tissue injury at the symphysis pubis in soccer players: Observations at MRI. *Am J Roentgenol.* 2007;188(3):W291–W296.
42. Paajanen H, Hermunen H, Karonen J. Pubic magnetic resonance imaging findings in athletes during heavy training. *Am J Sports Med.* 2008;36(1):117–121.
43. Kunduracioglu B, Yilmaz C, Yorubulut M, et al. Magnetic resonance findings of osteitis pubis. *J Magn Reson Imaging.* 2007;25(3):535–539.
44. Anderson J, Read JW. *Atlas of Imaging in Sports Medicine.* 2nd Ed. North Ryde, NSW: McGraw-Hill; 2008, pp. 328–333.
45. Coventry MB, Mitchell WC. Osteitis pubis: Observations based on a study of 45 patients. *J Am Med Assoc.* 1961;178:898–905.
46. Grace JN, Sim FH, Shives TC, et al. Wedge resection of the symphysis pubis for the treatment of osteitis pubis. *J Bone Joint Surg (Am).* 1989;71:358–364.
47. Williams PR, Thomas DP, Downes EM. Osteitis pubis and instability of the pubic symphysis: When nonoperative measures fail. *Am J Sports Med.* 2000;28:50–55.
48. Radic R, Annear P. Use of pubic symphysis curettage for treatment-resistant osteitis pubis in athletes. *Am J Sports Med.* 2008;36(1):122–128.
49. Steinbach HL, Petrakis NL, Gilfillan RS, et al. The pathogenesis of osteitis pubis. *J Urol.* 1955;24:840–846.
50. Verrall GM, Oakeshott RD, Henry LW, et al. Bone biopsy of the parasymphyseal region of athletes with osteitis pubis diagnosed by MRI demonstrates new woven bone formation. *Aust J Sci Med Sport.* 2003;6(Suppl 4):95.
51. Benjamin M, McGonagle D. Histopathologic changes at "synovio-entheseal complexes" suggesting a novel mechanism for synovitis in osteoarthritis and spondylarthritis. *Arthritis Rheum.* 2007;56(11):3601–3609.
52. Zimmerman G. Groin pain in athletes. *Aust Fam Physician.* 1988;17(12):1046–1052.
53. Derman WE. A clinical approach to chronic groin pain in the adult athlete. *Int Sportmed J.* 2000;1(1):1–12.
54. Ekberg O, Persson NH, Abrahamsson PA, et al. Longstanding groin pain in athletes: A multidisciplinary approach. *Sports Med.* 1988;6(1):56–61.
55. Lovell G. The diagnosis of chronic groin pain in athletes: A review of 189 cases. *Aust J Sci Med Sport.* 1995;27:76–79.
56. Bradshaw C. The diagnosis of long-standing groin pain—a prospective clinical cohort study. *AFL Symposium,* Melbourne; 2007.
57. Rodriguez C, Miguel A, Lima H, et al. Osteitis pubis syndrome in the professional soccer athlete: A Case Report. *J Athl Train.* 2001;36(4):437–440.
58. Hölmich P, Hölmich LR, Bjerg AM. Clinical examination of athletes with groin pain: An intraobserver and interobserver reliability study. *Br J Sports Med.* 2004;38:446–451.
59. Mozes M, Papa MZ, Zweig A, et al. Iliopsoas injury in soccer players. *Br J Sports Med.* 1985;19:168–170.
60. Verrall GM, Slavotinek JP, Barnes PG, et al. Description of pain provocation tests used for the diagnosis of sports-related chronic groin pain: Relationship of tests to defined clinical (pain and tenderness) and MRI (pubic bone marrow oedema) criteria. *Scand J Med Sci Sports.* 2005;15:36–42.
61. Van Meeteren J, Mens JMA, Stam HJ. Reliability of strength measurement of the hip with a hand-held dynamometer in healthy women. *Eur J Phys Med Rehab.* 1997;7:17–20.
62. Mens J, Inklaar H, Koes BW, et al. A new view on adduction-related groin pain. *Clin J Sport Med.* 2006;16(1):15–19.
63. Kendall FP, McCreary EK. *Muscles, Testing and Function.* 3rd Ed. Baltimore, MD: Williams & Wilkins, Waverly Press; 1983, pp. 176–177.
64. Mandelbaum B, Mora S. Osteitis pubis. *Oper Tech Sports Med.* 2005;13:62–67.
65. Ross JJ, Hu LT. Septic arthritis of the pubic symphysis: Review of 100 cases. *Medicine (Baltimore).* 2003;82(5):340–345.
66. Cross TM, Smart RC, Thomson JE. Exposure to diagnostic ionizing radiation in sports medicine: Assessing and monitoring the risk. *Clin J Sport Med.* 2003;13(3):164–170.
67. Besjakov J, von Scheele C, Ekberg O, et al. Grading scale of radiographic findings in the pubic bone and symphysis in athletes. *Acta Radiologica.* 2003;44:79–83.
68. Chamberlain EW. The symphysis pubis in the roentgen examination of the sacro-iliac joint. *Am J Roentgenol.* 1930;24(6):621–625.
69. Le Jeune JJ, Rochcongar P, Vazelle F, et al. Pubic pain syndrome in sportsmen: Comparison of radiographic and scintigraphic findings. *Eur J Nucl Med.* 1984;9(6):250–253.
70. Omar IM, Kavanagh EC, Koulouris G, et al. Athletic pubalgia and the "sports hernia": Optimal MR imaging of the pubic symphysis region and pictorial review of MR technique and findings. Available at: http://www.bone.tju.edu/download/pubalgia.pdf. (Accessed March 5, 2008).
71. Verrall GM, Slavotinek JP, Fon GT, et al. Outcome of conservative management of athletic chronic groin injury diagnosed as pubic bone stress injury. *Am J Sports Med.* 2007;35(3):467–474.
72. Hölmich P. Exercise rehabilitation for chronic groin pain in athletes. *Int Sportmed J.* 2000;1(1):1–5.
73. Hogan AA. Rehabilitation model for pubic symphysis injuries. In: *Australian Conference of Science and Medicine in Sport (abstracts).* Adelaide: Sports Medicine Australia; 1998, p. 143.
74. Hogan A, Lovell G. Pubic stress tests and rehabilitation of Osteitis Pubis: Key reassessment criteria. In: Reilly T, et al., eds. *Science and Football IV.* London: Routledge. Proceedings Sports Medicine Annual Conference (SA Branch); 2002, pp. 207–211.
75. Wollin M, Lovell G. Osteitis pubis in four young football players: A case series demonstrating successful rehabilitation. *Phys Ther Sport.* 2006;7(3):153–160.
76. Cowan S, Schache AG, Brukner P, et al. Delayed onset of transversus abdominis in long-standing groin pain. *Med Sci Sports Exerc.* 2004;36(12):2040–2045.
77. Hemingway AE, Herrington L, Blower AL. Changes in muscle strength and pain in response to surgical repair of posterior abdominal wall disruption followed by rehabilitation. *Br J Sports Med.* 2003;37:54–58.
78. McKim KR, Taunton JE. The effectiveness of compression shorts in the treatment of athletes with osteitis pubis. *NZ J Sports Med.* 2001;29:70–73.
79. Ekstrand J, Ringborg S. Surgery versus conservative treatment in soccer players with chronic groin pain: A prospective randomised study in soccer players. *Eur J Sports Traumatol Rel Res.* 2001;23:141–145.
80. Gelber J, Byron RJ. Treatment of osteitis pubis with corticotrophin and cortisone. *Arch Surg.* 1954;543–548.
81. Holt MA, Keene JS, Graf BK, et al. Treatment of osteitis pubis in athletes: Results of corticosteroid injections. *Am J Sports Med.* 1995;23(5):601–606.
82. Schilders E, Bismil Q, Robinson P, et al. Adductor-related groin pain in competitive athletes: Role of adductor enthesis, magnetic resonance imaging, and entheseal pubic cleft injections. *J Bone Joint Surg (Am).* 2007;89(10):2173–2178.
83. Topol GA, Reeves KD, Hassanein KM. Efficacy of dextrose prolotherapy in elite male kicking-sport athletes with chronic groin pain. *Arch Phys Med Rehabil.* 2005;86:697–702.
84. Maksymowych WP, Aaron SL, Russell AS. Treatment of refractory symphysitis pubis with intravenous pamidronate. *J Rheumatol.* 2001;28(12):2754–2757.
85. Maksymowych WP. Bisphosphonates for arthritis—a confusing rationale. *J Rheumatol.* 2003;30:430–434.
86. Stewart GW, Brunet ME, Manning MR, et al. Treatment of stress fractures in athletes with intravenous pamidronate. *Clin J Sports Med.* 2005;15:92–94.
87. Watkin NA, Gallegos CR, Moisey CU, et al. Osteitis pubis—a case of successful treatment with anticoagulants. *Acta Orthop Scand.* 1995;65 (6):569–570.
88. Depledge J, McNair PJ, Keal-Smith C, et al. Management of symphysis pubis dysfunction during pregnancy using exercise and pelvic support belts. *Phys Ther.* 2005;85:1290–1300.
89. Martens MA, Hansen L, Mulier JC. Adductor tendinitis and musculus rectus abdominis tendopathy. *Am J Sports Med.* 1987;15(4):353–356.
90. Akermark C, Johansson C. Tenotomy of the adductor longus tendon in the treatment of chronic groin pain in athletes. *Am J Sports Med.* 1992;20(6):640–643.
91. Mulhall KJ, McKenna J, Walsh A, et al. Osteitis pubis in professional soccer players: A report of outcome with symphyseal curettage in cases refractory to conservative management. *Clin J Sports Med.* 2002;12:179–181.
92. Paajanen H, Heikkinen J, Hermunen H, et al. Successful treatment of osteitis pubis by using totally extraperitoneal endoscopic technique. *Int J Sports Med.* 2005;26:303–306.
93. Moore RS Jr, Stover MD, Matta JM. Late posterior instability of the pelvis after resection of the symphysis pubis for the treatment of osteitis pubis: A report of two cases. *J Bone Joint Surg (Am).* 1998;80(7):1043–1048.
94. National Health and Medical Research Council. A guide to the development, implementation and evaluation of clinical practice guidelines. Commonwealth of Australia, Canberra, 1999. Available at: http://www.nhmrc.gov.au/publications/synopses/cp30syn.htm (Accessed March 5, 2008).

CHAPTER

23

Carlos A. Guanche

Sports Hernias

INTRODUCTION

Groin injuries in athletes are being recognized with increasing frequency. Estimates suggest that 5% of all sports injuries occur in the groin. Such injuries are more common in sports that require repetitive twisting and turning movements, such as soccer, hockey, and American football.[1] Injuries to the adductor longus, iliopsoas, and rectus femoris muscles are the most common causes of groin pain in athletes and these are typically muscle strains that resolve with nonoperative measures. Other causes of groin pain include ilioinguinal neuralgia, osteitis pubis, genitourinary sources (prostatitis, epididymitis, urethritis, hydrocele, etc.), bursitis, hip labral injuries, and sports hernias. A poorly understood aspect is the overlap between intra-articular hip pathologies and the associated incidence of groin soft tissue injuries in and about the pelvis.

In general terms, a sports hernia can best be described as incompetence of the abdominal wall musculature in the absence of a clinically detectable hernia bulge. The prevalence of such hernias found at surgical exploration in athletes with chronic groin pain is reported to be as high as 80%.[2,3] However, since up to 50% of these athletes have an occult hernia in the contralateral groin, the presence of a hernia does not necessarily correlate with symptoms.[4]

The common groin injuries can be classified into three major groups: (a) classic hernias, (b) occult groin injuries, and (c) other diagnostic entities (Fig. 23.1). An occult groin injury is defined as a painful, symptomatic injury isolated to the groin or pelvis region in which no clinically obvious signs are present upon exam. This is in contradistinction to the typical inguinal hernia, associated with objective clinical signs. The list of other diagnostic injuries encompasses many of the other chapters in this textbook.

ANATOMY

The pathoanatomy of athletic pubalgia and sports hernia is complex. The potential zone of injury includes the medial extent of the inguinal canal with the transversalis fascia posteriorly, the tendinous rectus abdominis and conjoined tendon anteriorly, and the bony pubic symphysis medially. The adductor tendons and their attachment along the anterior pelvis define the distal extent.[4,5] The various nerves of the inguinal region are commonly involved, and may explain the typical cutaneous pain distribution to the scrotum (as a result of ilioinguinal nerve irritation), ipsilateral and contralateral inguinal area (genitofemoral nerve), and medial thigh (obturator nerve).[3]

Some have classified a "sportsmen's hernia" as an incipient hernia based on the findings of a posterior bulge found in 80% of the operations. This is considered analogous to a classic inguinal hernia, where the absence of striated muscle at the posterior inguinal wall and the passage of the spermatic cord predispose the abdominal wall to a potential site of weakness.[6] Some have defined this hernia as an actual tear in the transversalis fascia in the posterior inguinal wall.[1] The tear is located between the internal inguinal ring and the pubic tubercle, and is typically 3 to 5 cm in length. Others have also identified the area of pathology as the posterior inguinal wall.[7]

Other concepts have centered about the structures about the internal inguinal ring and progressive weakness of the posterior wall. In one study, endoscopic visualization defined a defect in the posterior wall in Hesselbach triangle with forming a true hernia.[8] In general, the concept of "sportsmen's hernia" includes a spectrum of injuries, principally involving the conjoined tendon, inguinal ligament, transversalis fascia, internal oblique muscle, and the external oblique aponeurosis.[9] The general concept is a weakness in the posterior wall between the internal ring and the pubic tubercle without a clinically detectable bulge.

Another broader concept is that of pain generators, leading to the diagnosis and treatment of the entity.[10] In this scheme, there are four general contributors to the groin pain including the adductor or rectus abdominus musculotendinous junctions, osteitis pubis, disruption of the inguinal canal and nerve entrapment (ilioinguinal, genitofemoral and/or obturator).

Another variation with respect to pathoetiology is "Gilmore's groin." This is an entity that falls under the athletic pubalgia category and is described as comprising a torn external oblique aponeurosis, tearing of the conjoined tendon, and avulsion from the pubic tubercle as well as a dehiscence between the conjoined tendon and inguinal ligament.[5] Further confusing the issue, Martens described the concept of associated abdominal muscle and adductor injuries.[11] Subsequently, Meyers introduced athletic pubalgia, upon which the current classification schemes are based.[12]

In summary, it appears that there is a constellation of pathologic findings that have been described to explain the generators of pain about the groin. The variety of described entities points to a general lack of understanding of the inciting

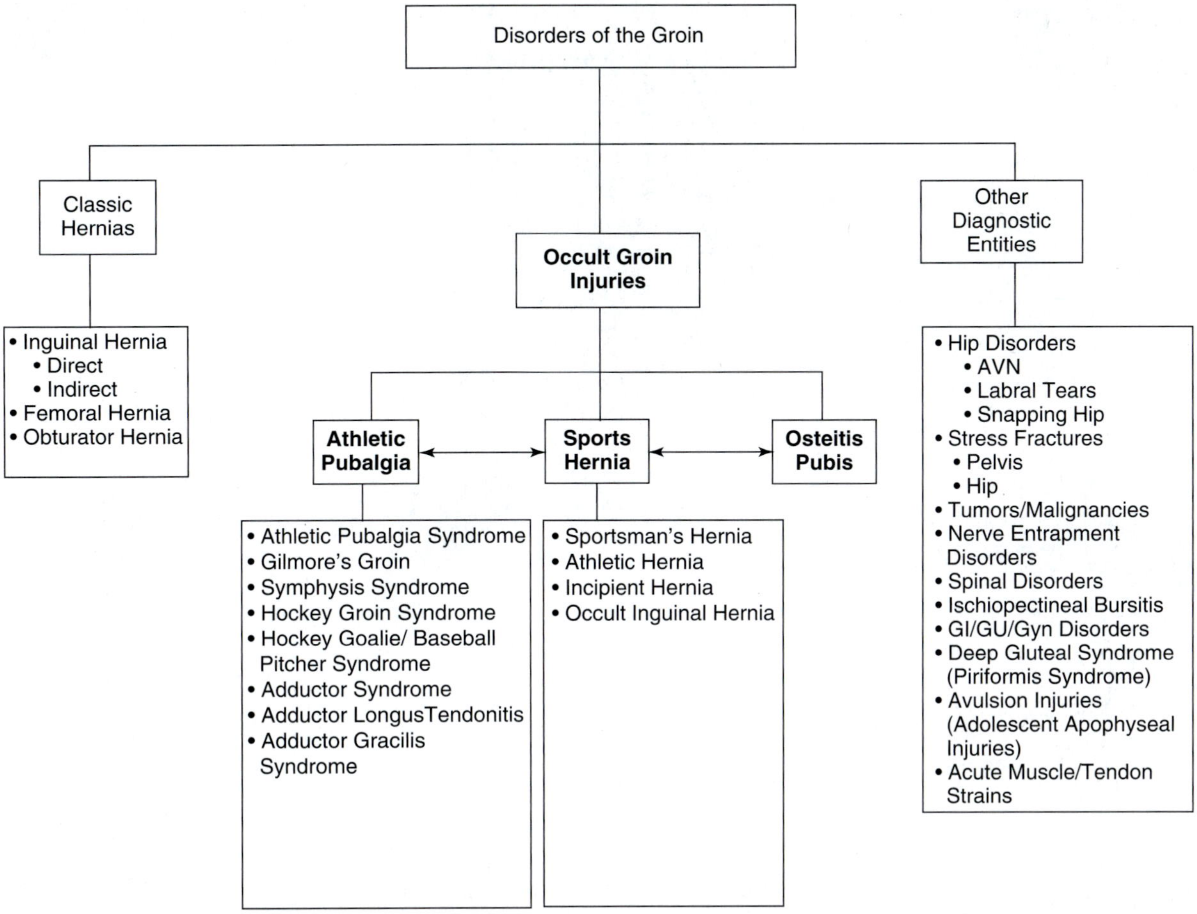

Figure 23.1. Disorders of the groin. (From Pedowitz RA, Johnson DJ. *Practical Orthopaedic Sports Medicine & Arthroscopy*. Philadelphia, PA: Lippincott Williams & Wilkins; 2006, with permission.)

factor(s) and the primary problem causing the symptomatology. With further prospective studies, the possibility of a unifying theory to this aspect of athletic injuries may be delineated.

MECHANISM OF INJURY

Although differing opinions exist, one study has cited the primary site of pathology in athletic pubalgia to be the rectus insertion on the pubis.[12] This syndrome has been described primarily in high-level athletes and almost exclusively in males.[13] The typical mechanism of injury involves repetitive hyperextension of the trunk in association with hyperabduction of the thigh pivoting on the anterior pelvis and pubic symphysis (Fig. 23.2). Kicking and rapid directional changes while running or skating are activities that especially contribute to this mechanism. Although the exact source of pain is unclear, it may be the result of periostitis at either the rectus abdominus insertion or adductor longus origin on the pelvis.[13] As discussed, while there may be attenuation of the abdominal floor musculature in this location, a true hernia is seldom present.

It has been suggested that shearing forces are generated across the pubic symphysis during adductor contraction and these forces stress the posterior inguinal wall. Repetitive stress, or sudden severe force, can therefore lead to separation of the internal oblique and/or the transversalis fascia from the inguinal ligament. This mechanism also accounts for the possible coexistent findings of osteitis pubis and adductor tendonitis in this patient population. In addition, limited hip rotation (developmental or posttraumatic in origin) may play a role in the development of the soft tissue injuries as well as the development of osteitis pubis.[14]

CLINICAL PRESENTATION

HISTORY

Groin pain in athletes is a problem occurring with a frequency of 5% to 28% and includes a wide differential diagnosis.[1,3] It has been studied extensively among European soccer players, Swedish ice hockey players, and Australian Rules football players. While it may occur in recreational athletes, the treatment for this group is much less predictable for unknown reasons.[15] These syndromes occur almost exclusively in males. Women who appear to have a clinical history consistent with athletic pubalgia should be carefully scrutinized and routine laparoscopy should be considered as a result of the high incidence of endometriosis[13] (Table 23.1).

The most common etiologies are musculotendinous injuries (especially of adductor origin), osteitis pubis, and hip joint arthritis.[13,16] Visceral causes include varicocele, hydrocele, prostatitis,

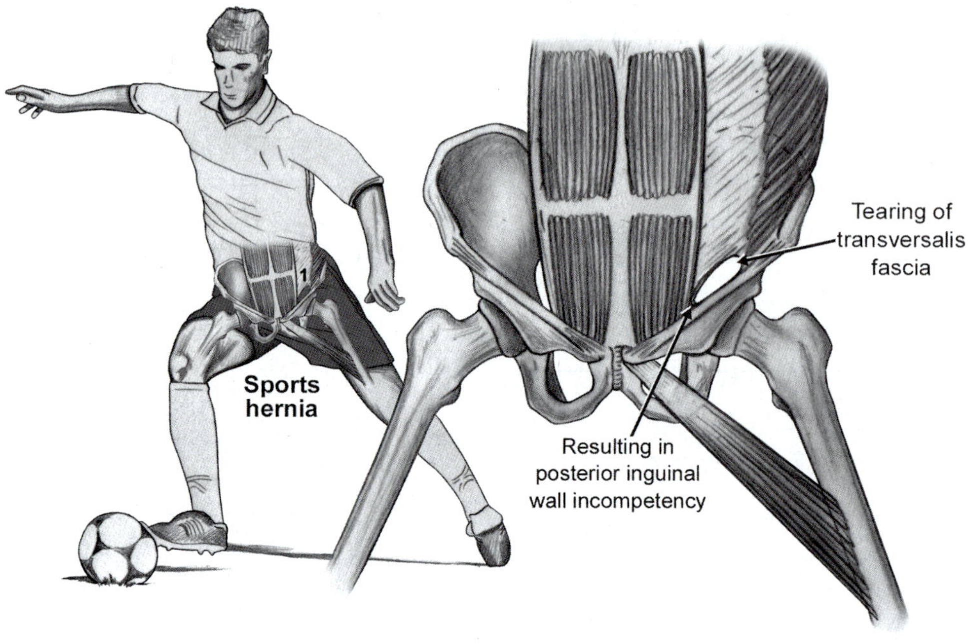

Figure 23.2. Proposed mechanism of injury in *sports hernia.* Primarily involves injury to the transversalis fascia, resulting in eventual incompetency of posterior inguinal wall. (From Pedowitz RA, Johnson DJ. *Practical Orthopaedic Sports Medicine & Arthroscopy.* Philadelphia, PA: Lippincott Williams & Wilkins; 2006, with permission.)

TABLE 23.1 **Summary of Patient Populations from Surgical Series of Sports Hernia Repairs**

Author (Reference)	*Year*	*Number of Patients*	*Patient Population*
Polglase[34]	1991	64	62 men, 2 women; all athletes
Malycha and Lovell[19]	1992	50	Actively involved in sport
Hackney[35]	1993	15	Competitive sports or strenuous activity in the military
Williams and Foster[5]	1995	6	Four soccer players, one rugby player, one cricket player
Simonet and Saylor[29]	1995	10	Elite- or professional-level hockey players
Ingoldby[30]	1997	28	18 professional, 9 amateur athletes
Gilmore[7]	1998	>1200	Soccer players (140 international)
Meyers et al.[13]	2000	175	169 athletes (36% college, 28% pro, 15% amateur, 10% recreational, 6% semi-pro, 5% high school)
Brannigan et al.[31]	2000	85	75% amateur athletes
Srinivasan and Schuricht[32]	2001	15	15 professional athletes

epididymitis, and gastrointestinal disorders. Ilioinguinal neuralgia and nerve entrapment/obturator neuropathy must also be considered, although the pain along specific nerve distributions should make these diagnoses more obvious.[3,6,17] In the diagnosis of groin pain in athletes, one must be aware of the potential for multiple etiologies. One analysis documented that 19 of 21 athletes evaluated for chronic groin pain (>3 months duration) had two or more separate abnormalities contributing to their symptoms.[18]

Athletes with sports hernias usually present with unilateral groin pain, although some will present with bilateral symptoms. The onset of pain is usually insidious, although some will report a sudden onset of symptoms. Initially, symptoms are present with competition or training. With time, symptoms occur during other activities, usually at lower thresholds, such as getting out of bed.[7] By definition, no clinically detectable hernia will be present during examination. The need for a thorough physical exam by an experienced examiner with an understanding of the anatomy cannot be overemphasized.

PHYSICAL EXAMINATION

The incidence of undiagnosed hernias in these patients after all orthopedic and visceral causes have been eliminated has been estimated to be as high as 85%.[4,5,7,19,20] The presence of an inguinal hernia can be difficult to detect on physical exam, even by those experienced in the examination of the inguinal canal. While a quick diagnosis requires a high index of suspicion and a reliable physical exam, the potential for multifactorial causation may require further testing.

When examining those athletes with a possible sports hernia it is important to assess for the presence of a classic inguinal hernia. The examination for this entity is very consistent and reproducible, and in one study it was shown that the majority of tests for pain, strength, and flexibility of the adductor, iliopsoas, and abdominal muscles are reproducible.[21] Specific examination for an inguinal hernia involves placing the patient in the supine position, with examination of the unaffected side performed first to establish a baseline. The tip of the fifth digit is inserted through the scrotum into the external inguinal ring to a depth of approximately 2 to 3 cm. In the sports hernia, there may be slight enlargement of the inguinal ring along with tenderness of the posterior wall of the canal. Sometimes, a subtle defect can be appreciated in the transversalis fascia as it makes up the posterior wall. A cough impulse may also be evident.

Physical examination is extremely useful in ruling out other potential sources of chronic pain such as tress fractures, acetabular labral tears, muscle strains, osteitis pubis, and avulsion injury. The patient with a stress fracture usually has pain with axial loading of the extremity or with standing and/or hopping on the affected leg. Adductor tenderness is very common with athletic pubalgia and this should be elicited, if present. However, focal tenderness over this area is suggestive of adductor muscle injury. Similarly, pain with palpation over the rectus femoris and pain with resisted hip flexion and knee extension suggests a rectus femoris strain. The maximal pain is elicited at the pubic origin with the leg in abduction.[13] In sports hernias, provocative maneuvers such as sit-ups, resisted hip adduction, and Valsalva will often reproduce the symptoms in the affected area. Diffuse tenderness over the pubic tubercle and the peripubic region is common. An examination of the hip with specific attention to internal rotation should also be performed to assess for coexistent hip pathologies. Pain and clicking with passive hip range of motion is suggestive of an acetabular labral tear.

IMAGING

Magnetic resonance, high-speed ultrasound, and bone scan (used to rule out osteitis pubis) have all been used to detect sports hernias.[10,22] High-speed ultrasound can detect posterior wall deficiencies of the inguinal canal and was shown in one series to provide a noninvasive diagnosis.[10] Several authors have published the merits of herniography. It has been shown to be useful in the detection of nonpalpable hernias.[8,9,18,20,23–25] One study showed an 84% incidence of hernias in symptomatic groins and a 49% incidence on the asymptomatic side.[4]

Despite the emphasis on higher technology imaging modalities, it is important to obtain standard radiographs of the pelvis, including the hip joints. Thoughtful analysis of the joint surfaces should be undertaken. In addition, radiographic changes of osteitis pubis including widening, cysts, and hypertrophy of the symphysis pubis should also be documented. Additionally, changes consistent with femoroacetabular impingement should be sought out in order to ensure that this is not a contributing factor in the athlete's problem.[14]

With the wide availability of MRI and its ability to delineate the anatomy in a noninvasive means, many physicians will order these studies. The studies, in most cases, are an attempt to rule out other sources of pathology. Most often, these include adductor muscle strain, acetabular labral tears, stress fractures, iliopsoas bursitis, osteitis pubis, and osteonecrosis of the femoral head. A recent MRI study of athletes with surgically confirmed athletic pubalgia reported that the authors were able to identify several common findings.[13] These included increased signal within one or both pubic bones, attenuation or asymmetry of the abdominal wall musculofascial layers, and increased signal within one or more of the groin muscles. The most useful aspect of MRI appears to be the determination of whether or not to address both sides of the groin.[13] It should be noted, however, that the absence of these findings on MRI does not exclude the diagnosis of athletic pubalgia.

The use of ultrasound, as with other areas, is dependent on the experience of the examiner and the degree of resolution of the device. In one study, a group of Australian Rules football players were assessed with dynamic ultrasound.[10] These studies were able to detect inguinal canal posterior wall insufficiency in young males with no clinically detected hernias.

The use of herniography is advocated in some circumstances. The procedure is performed by injecting contrast material into the peritoneal cavity followed by fluoroscopy to visualize the path of the material. Any extraperitoneal extravasation is consistent with an occult hernia.[26] One of the problems with these studies is a fairly high rate of complications, up to 5% in some studies. The studies can be relatively high yield, however, with one study reporting a true positive rate of 90.5% and a true negative rate of 100% for 43 herniograms.[26] Herniograms should be carefully considered and should be reserved for ambiguous presentations or other carefully selected cases where a clinical decision is expected based on the result of the study.

TREATMENT

Published reports of surgical series have demonstrated a wide variety of anatomic abnormalities, although disruption of the conjoined tendon and/or weakness of the inguinal floor are the most common findings (Table 23.2). This variability underscores the difficulty in forming a true consensus regarding the appropriate therapy in this patient population.

CONSERVATIVE (NONSURGICAL) APPROACH

Complete rest and anti-inflammatory medications may relieve pain but the effect is usually only temporary and symptoms commonly recur with return to the previous level of activities. Injections may provide temporary relief but are rarely curative and should not be done repeatedly. Physical therapy has been shown to be effective for many patients and is aimed at resolving muscular imbalances of hip and pelvic stabilizers.[27] A rehabilitation protocol for athletes suffering from lower abdominal/adductor-related groin pain has been described, and this will be presented in some detail.[28] The protocol serves as a general guideline to attempt return to high-level sporting activities. In addition, it can serve as an important prehabilitation routine for the patient to understand the concepts of recovery following surgical intervention.

Phase I (massage and stretching) Weeks 1 to 2

The first phase includes daily deep tissue massage of the muscles attaching about the posterior, superior, and lateral pelvis (gluteus maximus, minimus and medius, tensor fascia lata, latissimus and lumbodorsal fascia, erector spinae, and other paraspinal

TABLE 23.2 Summary of Operative Findings and Approaches from Surgical Series of Sports Hernia Repairs

Author (Reference)	*Year*	*Surgical Approach*	*Operative Findings*
Polglase[7]	1991	Early: Conjoined tendon repair (Bassini); Later: plication of transversalis fascia with reinforcement of posterior wall	Most common: Deficient posterior wall of the inguinal canal
Malycha and Lovell[19]	1992	Two-layer repair of posterior inguinal wall	80%: Bulge in posterior inguinal wall 14%: No abnormality 2%: Indirect hernia
Hackney[5]	1993	Plication of transversalis fascia with conjoined tendon repair	Weakening of the transversalis fascia with separation of the conjoined tendon
Williams and Foster[5]	1995	Modified herniorrhaphy with repair of external oblique	Small tear in external oblique aponeurosis at neurovascular bundle
Simonet and Saylor[29]	1995	3 conjoined tendon repairs; 7 mesh patch repairs of inguinal floor	Partial or complete tears in internal inguinal ring, injury to the internal oblique musculature
Ingoldby[30]	1997	11 open mesh patch repairs; 3 open conjoined tendon repairs; 14 laparoscopic transperitoneal repairs	Not reported
Gilmore[7]	1998	Six-layered suture repair followed by intensive rehabilitation	Torn external oblique aponeurosis Torn conjoined tendon Conjoined tendon torn from pubic tubercle; dehiscence between conjoined tendon and inguinal ligament No hernia present
Meyers et al.[13]	2000	Open pelvic floor repairs with rectus abdominus reattachment 36 adductor releases also performed	57%: "Loose feeling inguinal floor" 48%: Defects of external oblique aponeurosis 17%: "thin" insertion of rectus abdominus 6%: Tear or injury of rectus abdominus insertion 3 Hernias 12/36 Edema or scarring of adductor
Brannigan et al.[31]	2000	Plication of transversalis fascia and conjoined tendon repair	Aponeurosis of external oblique is frayed Conjoined tendon separated from inguinal ligament Transversalis fascia weakened
Srinivasan and Schuricht[32]	2001	Laparoscopic extraperitoneal	Indirect inguinal hernias in all patients

musculature about the sacroiliac joint, external abdominal obliques, and hamstrings). The focus is applied to especially tender "trigger points" about the iliosacral area. Avoidance of massage or manipulation of the anterior abdominal, adductor, or inguinal musculature is important at this point, with each session lasting 20 to 30 min. This technique requires a therapist familiar with traditional deep tissue and myofascial techniques and should continue daily for 1 week. No sports participation or strengthening occurs during the first week.

The patient is instructed in stretching the hip adductors, hamstrings, hip flexors, hip rotators, and lower back (emphasizing lateral bending and extension of the lower back). Independent gentle stretching several times a day is preferable. An attempt is made to warm the muscles before stretching whenever possible. Athletes may perform light aerobic exercise if not painful (e.g., water walking, stationary bike, treadmill, or other as tolerated). It is important to abstain from running or sports participation.

Phase II (strengthening) Weeks 3 and 4

Module I

A concerted phase of isometric strengthening is begun with static adduction (against ball placed between feet when lying supine), each adduction lasting 30 s and repeated ten times. Abdominal sit-ups both in straight and oblique directions; five sets of ten repetitions are begun concurrently. Another routine is combined abdominal sit-up and hip flexion, starting from a supine position and with a soccer ball placed between the knees ("folding knife"); five sets of ten repetitions. Balance training on a wobble board for 5 min/day is begun. The progression leads to one-foot exercises on a sliding board, with parallel feet as well as with 90° angle between feet; five sets of 1 min continuous work with each leg.

Module II

Progressing with the routine, leg abduction and adduction exercises lying on the contralateral side are instituted with five sets of ten repetitions each. Also begun are low back extension exercises, prone over the end of a table; five sets of ten repetitions. Next are one-leg resisted (theraband or light pulley weight) standing abduction/adduction routines; five sets of ten repetitions each leg. Abdominal sit-ups in straight and oblique directions; five sets of ten repetitions are begun as tolerated.

As the fitness level progresses, one-leg coordination exercise flexing and extending knee and swinging arms in same rhythm (e.g., cross-country skiing on one leg), with five sets of ten repetitions with each leg are instituted. Balance training on a wobble board for 5 min is also continued, with the addition of skating movements on a sliding board for five continuous minutes.

Phase III (functional) Week 5

Running is begun after week four. Shuttle runs, crossovers (cariocas), sidesteps, and other controlled lateral and rotational drills are incorporated into the routine, as tolerance increases. Daily stretching and strengthening are continued and massage only as needed.

Phase IV (return to sport) Week 6

Gradual resumption of sports-specific activities (kicking, passing, shooting, throwing, skating, jumping, etc.) as tolerated can be started in this phase. Team practice and return to competition is allowed once any residual pain has resolved.

SURGICAL APPROACHES

Open surgical exploration of these patients has uniformly shown anatomic derangement as well as inguinal hernias (Table 23.2). As noted earlier, authors have reported a high incidence of multiple abnormalities. One report of 64 athletes, most of which were Australian rules football players, found anatomic defects of the inguinal canal in all patients.[7] Operative findings included a deranged posterior wall of the inguinal canal in 85%, splitting of the conjoined tendon in 26%, and previously occult indirect inguinal hernias in 8%.

Gilmore described a pentad of surgical findings: a torn external oblique aponeurosis, a torn conjoined tendon, conjoined tendon torn from the pubic tubercle, dehiscence between the torn conjoined tendon and the inguinal ligament, and no hernia present.[7] He performed a six-layer suture repair of the inguinal floor. The procedure is performed through a 6 cm incision and includes restoration of the normal anatomy by reconstitution of the posterior inguinal wall, repair of the rectus abdominis and external oblique and reattachment of the conjoined tendon to the pubic tubercle.[7] In his report of 915 cases, 887 (97%) were successful.

The PAIN (Performing Athletes with Abdominal or Inguinal Neuromuscular Pain) study group, summarized its experience combining open inguinal repair in conjunction with adductor tendon release in those athletes who demonstrated concurrent adductor symptoms.[14] The need for a procedure to strengthen the anterior pelvic floor was emphasized, however. Other authors have used the conjoined tendon repair as the basis for inguinal floor abnormalities, sometimes adding modifications such as transversalis fascia plication.[4,19,29–31] Another variation involves a simple suture repair of the external oblique aponeurosis without inguinal canal exploration.[5]

Several authors began their series with repair of sports hernias using a standard open suture repair of the conjoined tendon, but later altered their operative approach to the performance of prosthetic mesh reconstruction.[29,30] As a matter of course, laparoscopic transabdominal hernia repairs with mesh augmentation were eventually described and performed.[30] These appear to be gaining favor as a result of their limited surgical trauma and potentially earlier return to activity.

One approach is a preperitoneal laparoscopic hernia repair with a mesh applied to the area of deficiency. This approach offers improved visualization of the pubis, internal rings, transversalis fascia, Cooper's ligaments, and musculotendinous insertions onto the pubis. The exposure allows mesh reinforcement of the entire myopectineal orifice, allowing structural reinforcement of the region. Documented operative findings have revealed the presence of indirect inguinal hernias in all symptomatic groins of 15 professional athletes.[2,32]

Another issue that is commonly encountered is that of treatment on the asymptomatic side. In one review, Meyers et al.[13] found that 5 out of 86 patients returned for contralateral symptoms. Those surgeons performing the laparoscopic repairs have the option of applying the mesh reinforcement to both inguinal regions. Some perform bilateral mesh reinforcement, citing the need for a balanced repair.[32] There are no studies to support the prophylactic treatment of this entity on the contralateral side, although the laparoscopic approach certainly lends itself to this concept with a minimum of added surgical time and exposure.

RESULTS (TABLE 23.3)

Athletes often desire (or require) a quick return to activity, especially during the competitive season. Often, the postoperative course is long and the rehabilitation necessary for recovery is intense. Such long anticipated recovery times influence an athlete's decision regarding definitive treatment for their groin pain, especially if the groin pain is not completely debilitating. In many situations, the athlete feels compelled to complete their season and delay undergoing surgery until the end of the campaign.

Standard open hernia repair, involving conjoined tendon repair or multilayer suture repair of the inguinal floor, may force

TABLE 23.3 Summary of Return to Activity and follow-up from Surgical Series of Sports Hernia Repairs

Author (Reference)	*Year*	*Return to Activity*	*Long-term Follow-up*
Polglase[7]	1991	Not reported	40/63 returned to sport without further treatment; 20/63 partially satisfied; 3/63 dissatisfied
Malycha and Lovell[19]	1992	Light training begun at 3–4 weeks; Active sport at 6–8 weeks	6 month follow-up: 93% returned to preinjury level (75% good, 23% improved)
Hackney[5]	1993	Stretching/non-weight-bearing exercise at 3 weeks Running at 4–5 weeks Daily training at 6 weeks	18-month to 5-year follow-up: More than 80% return to full activity
Williams and Foster[5]	1995	All returned to full active participation in 6 weeks	No change at 6 weeks
Simonet and Saylor[29]	1995	Not reported	All returned to prior level of play; All reported improvement in symptoms
Ingoldby[30]	1997	Open repair: 9/14 training at 4 weeks Laparoscopic repair: 13/14 training at 4 weeks	Open: One recurrent hernia at 22 months Laparoscopic: One patient with recurrent groin pain at 5 months
Gilmore[7]	1998	Week 1: Walk Week 2: Jog straight Week 3: Run straight Week 4: Sprint, start kicking, may play	97% successful
Meyers et al.[13]	2000	88% at or above preinjury level at 3 months 96% at or above preinjury level at 6 months	89% successful at 6 month follow-up
Brannigan et al.[31]	2000	96% return to competition at 15 weeks	Three long-term failures 96% good results
Srinivasan and Schuricht[32]	2001	87% full return to activity within 4 weeks 100% full return to activity within 6 weeks	Range 6–80 months Median 46 months 100% full return to activity without recurrent symptoms

an athlete out of training for as long as 15 weeks.[5,7,19,30,31] The longest reported return to activity has been as long as 6 months.[13] The least invasive open procedure (suture repair of the external oblique), precludes full activity return for 6 weeks.[5]

Laparoscopic hernia repair offers some athletes a faster return to sports.[2,30,32] One study has reported athletes training immediately with 87% returning to full activity within 4 weeks and all returning to full activity within six weeks.[33] Ingoldby[30] reported 13 of 14 athletes training at 4 weeks.

The long-term outcomes following surgery for sports hernia are difficult to quantify. This is especially true since athletes continue to perform at a very high level of activity, stressing the surgical repair. Long-term follow-up is not reported in most series, although one study has follow-up as long as 5 years and another reports results at 22 months.[5,30] There has been some discrepancy with regard to maintenance of the results. One study reports that 93% of patients returned to preinjury levels (75% good, 23% improved) at 6 months.[19] Another reports only 80% return to activity with an 18 month to 5 year follow-up.[5] One study analyzes an early and a late group. The early group had a mean 78-month follow-up with 94.6% reported to be "successful" or "moderately successful."[13] Finally, one study reports "long-term" follow-up and documents a 100% return to activity with no adverse sequelae or recurrence of symptoms at an average of 12.1 months of follow-up.[31] The difficulty in discerning outcomes includes the variability in the treatments employed, the postoperative treatments, and the specific sports in which the patients participate. With larger series of specific procedures in more homogenous participation populations, consensus for treatment may be developed.

CONCLUSIONS

Groin pain in athletes requires an aggressive multidisciplinary approach to diagnosis and treatment. Clinical analysis and surgical exploration has shown multifactorial causation of chronic groin pain in this population. It is especially important to be thorough in the analysis of all of the anatomical factors involved including muscular, bony, and neural elements. In addition, the incidence of underlying (and perhaps primary) hip pathology has not been well delineated in the literature. An examination of the low back, pelvis, and hip joint in this complex patient population is critical to ensure that an underlying hip rotational deficiency will not lead to failure of an otherwise successful hernia repair. The diagnosis of sports hernia should be made once all other factors are excluded, especially in women.

In a properly diagnosed patient, hernia repair eliminates symptoms and allows return to competitive levels of activity. While length of recovery varies between series, laparoscopic repair appears to allow the quickest return to sport. Most of these laparoscopic approaches have allowed athletes to return to full, unrestricted athletic activity in 4 weeks or less. While the available series show that both alternatives provide good results at follow-up, the overall trend has been toward laparoscopic intervention. Whether the type of repair (open or endoscopic) impacts the long-term outcomes of these patients remains to be seen with further follow-up.

REFERENCES

1. Kemp S, Batt ME. The sports hernia: A common cause of groin pain. *Phys Sports Med.* 1998;26(1):36–44.
2. Azurin DJ, Go LS, Schuricht A, et al. Endoscopic preperitoneal herniorrhaphy in professional athletes with groin pain. *J Laparoendosc Adv Surg Tech.* 1997;7(1):7–12.
3. Akita K, Niga S, Yamato Y, et al. Anatomic basis of chronic groin pain with special reference to sports hernia. *Surgical Rad Anat.* 1999;21(1):1–5.
4. Smedberg SG, Broome AE, Gullmo A, et al. Herniography in athletes with groin pain. *Am J Surg.* 1985;149(3):378–382.
5. Williams P, Foster ME. Gilmore's groin—or is it? *Br J Sports Med.* 1995;29(3):206–208.
6. Syme G, Wilson J, Mackenzie K, et al. Groin pain in athletes–comment. *Lancet.* 1999;353(9162):1444–1445.
7. Gilmore J. Groin pain in the soccer athlete: Fact, fiction and treatment. *Clin Sports Med.* 1998;17(4):787–793.
8. Ekberg O, Abrahamson PA, Kesek P. Inguinal hernia in urological patients: The value of herniography. *J Urol.* 1988;139(6):1253–1255.
9. Jones RL, Wingate JP. Herniography in the investigation of groin pain in adults. *Clin Radiol.* 1998;53(11):805–808.
10. Orchard JW, Read JW, Neophyton J, et al. Groin pain associated with ultrasound finding of inguinal canal posterior wall deficiency in Australian rules footballers. *Br J Sports Med.* 1998;32(2):134–139.
11. Tucker AM. Common soccer injuries: Diagnosis, treatment and rehabilitation. *Sports Med.* 1997;23(1):21–32.
12. Meyers WE, Ricciardi R, Busconi BD, et al. Athletic pubalgia and groin pain. In: Garrett WE, Speer KP, Kirkendall DT, eds. *Orthpaedic Sports Medicine.* Philadelphia, PA: Lippincott Williams & Wilkins; 2000, pp. 223–230.
13. Meyers WC, Foley DP, Garrett WE, et al. Management of severe lower abdominal or inguinal pain in high performance athletes. PAIN (Performing Athletes with abdominal or inguinal Neuromuscular pain study group). *Am J of Sports Med.* 2000;28(1):2–8.
14. Gomes JL, de Castro JV, Becker R. Decreased hip range of motion and noncontact injuries of the anterior cruciate ligament. *Arthroscopy.* 2008;24(9):1034–1037.
15. Joesting DR. Diagnosis and treatment of sportsman's hernia. *Curr Sports Med Rep.* 2002;1:121–124.
16. Taylor DC, Meyers WC, Lohnes J, et al. Abdominal musculature abnormalities as a cause of groin pain in athletes: Inguinal hernias and pubalgia. *Am J Sports Med.* 1991;19(3): 239–242.
17. Bradshaw C, McCrory P, Bell S, et al. Obturator nerve entrapment: A cause of groin pain in athletes. *Am J Sports Med.* 1997;25(3):402–408.
18. Ekberg O, Blomquist P, Fritzdorf J. Herniography in patients with clinically suggested recurrence of inguinal hernia. *Acta Radiol.* 1984;25:225–229.
19. Malycha P, Lovell G. Inguinal surgery in athletes with chronic groin pain: The sportsman's hernia. *Aust NZ J Surg.* 1992;62(2):123–125.
20. Estes NC, Childs EW, Cox G, et al. Role of herniography in the diagnosis of occult hernias. *Am J Surg.* 1991;162(6):608–610.
21. Holmich P, Holmich L, Berg A. Clinical examination of athletes with groin pain: An intraobserver and interobserver reliability study. *Br J Sports Med.* 2004;4:38–41.
22. Ekberg O, Sjoberg S, Westlin N. Sports related groin pain: Evaluation with MR imaging. *Eur Radiol.* 1996;6(1):52–55.
23. Smedberg SG, Broome AE, Elmer O, et al. Herniography in the diagnosis of obscure groin pain. *Acta Chir Scand.* 1985;151(8):663–667.
24. Yilmazlar T, Kizil A, Zorluoglu A, et al. The value of herniography in football players with obscure groin pain. *Acta Chir Belg.* 1996;96(3):115–118.
25. Cohen RH, Turkenberg JL, van Dalen A. Herniography in 79 patients with unexplained pain in the groin: A retrospective study. *Eur J Radiol.* 1990;11(3):184–187.
26. Gwanmesia II, Walsh S, Bury R, et al. Unexplained groin pain: Safety and reliability of herniography for the diagnosis of occult hernia. *Postgrad Med J.* 2001;77:250–251.
27. Holmich P, Uhrskou P, Kanstrup IL, et al. Effectiveness of active physical training as treatment for long-standing adductor related groin pain in athletes. *Lancet.* 1999;353(9151): 439–443.
28. Larson CM, Lohnes JH. Surgical management of athletic pubalgia. *Op Techs Sports Med.* 2002;10:228–232.
29. Simonet WT, Saylor LS III. Abdominal wall muscle tears in hockey players. *Int J Sports Med.* 1995;16(2):126–128.
30. Ingoldby CJH. Laparoscopic and conventional repair of groin disruption in sportsmen. *Br J Surg.* 1997;84:213–215.
31. Brannigan AE, Kerin MJ, McEntee GP. Gilmore's groin repair in athletes. *J Orthop Sports Phys Ther.* 2000;30(6);329–332.
32. Srinivasan A, Schuricht A. Long-term results of laparoscopic preperitoneal hernia repair in professional athletes. *J Laparoendosc Adv Surg Tech.* 2002;12(2):99–104.
33. Susmalian S, Ezri T, Elis M, et al. Corepair of "sportsmen's hernia" in soccer players as treatment of chronic inguinal pain. *Med Sci Monit.* 2004;10:CR52–CR54.
34. Polglase AL, Frydman GM, Framer KC. Inguinal surgery for debilitation chronic groin pain in athletes. *Med J Aust.* 1991;155:674–677.
35. Hackney RG. The sports hernia: a cause of chronic groin pain. *Br J Sports Med.* 1993;27: 58–62.

CHAPTER

24

Michael B. Banffy
Andrew J. Schoenfeld
C. Chambliss Harrod
Mitchel B. Harris

Low Back Pain in Athletes

INTRODUCTION

The lumbar spine and its associated ligaments and muscles are integral in the coordination and power generation of virtually all activities within sports. Injuries to the low back, and associated "low back pain," are a frequent cause of an athlete's lost playing time. The lifetime prevalence of low back pain in the general population is approximately 85%[1] and athletes involved in activities requiring repetitive hyperextension (football, gymnastics, rowing, wrestling, weight lifting, etc.) are at an even greater risk of injury. In addition to specific etiologies, athletes are also victims of the same insidious low back pain that affects the rest of the population. Through the analysis of the anatomy, etiologies, clinical presentation, differential diagnosis, and treatment for low back pain, this chapter will act as a guide for the sports medicine clinician in the analysis of this condition in athletes.

ANATOMY

The bony anatomy of the vertebrae is defined in terms of anterior and posterior elements. The anterior aspect of the vertebrae consists of the body. Posteriorly, there are the pedicles, laminae, superior and inferior facets, transverse processes, and the spinous process. The pars interarticularis exists between the superior and inferior articular processes. The vertebral body has both superior and inferior endplates, which are separated from the adjacent vertebral bodies by the intervertebral disc.

It is generally stated that the intervertebral discs together form approximately 25% of the length of the vertebral column.[2] The intervertebral discs consist of two distinct components. The annulus fibrosus is the outer segment composed of fibrocartilage arranged in concentric rings and consists mainly of type I collagen. The nucleus pulposus is the central portion and is composed of mucoid material consisting of type II collagen and proteoglycans.[3] The principal proteoglycan within the disc is aggrecan, which, because of its high anionic charge, draws water into the disc space and maintains disc height even under high compressive loads. Changes in the composition and content of disc proteoglycans lead to desiccation, a normal part of the aging process. Water content within the nucleus pulposus also diminishes throughout life, with a 22% reduction in water weight appreciated over the first eight decades.[3]

The periphery of the annulus is innervated with afferent pain fibers whereas the inner two thirds and the nucleus pulposus are not.[4] Pain fibers in the disc are derived from the two nerve roots cephalad to the corresponding level. In the lumber spine, the intervertebral discs have a trapezoidal shape, with more height anteriorly than posteriorly. This configuration gives the lumbar spine its characteristic lordosis.

Articulations between the inferior and superior facets of adjacent vertebrae form the functional spinal unit along with the intervertebral disc. In the lumbar spine, the facets of the superior articular processes face posteromedially while the facets of the inferior articular process face anterolaterally. The facets form a diarthrodial joint surrounded by a thin capsular ligament and a synovial membrane. As the facet joint unites the two adjacent vertebrae, this also forms the posterolateral boundaries of the intervertebral foramen through which it traverses the nerve roots.

Several ligaments and muscles also form part of the functional vertebral column and can be a source of low back pain in the form of a strain or sprain. From anterior to posterior, the ligaments include the anterior longitudinal ligament (ALL), the posterior longitudinal ligament (PLL), the ligamentum flavum, and the supraspinous and infraspinous ligaments. The ALL is a broad thick band connecting the anterior aspects of the vertebral bodies while the PLL resembles a series of hourglass formations with thin lateral expansions over the intervertebral discs. Because of this thin arrangement of fibers in the PLL, most disc protrusions are posterolateral.

The paraspinal musculature can also be a frequent source of back pain and should be thought of as two groups of longitudinal muscles. The erector spinae muscle group (iliocostalis, longissimus, and spinalis) and the transversospinalis (semispinalis, multifidus, and rotatores) are involved in coordination, posture, and gait as well as in power generation associated with various sporting activities (e.g., the golfer's swing).

Knowledge of the anatomy of the lumbar spine is critical in the assessment, diagnosis, and treatment of the athlete with low back pain. Furthermore, an understanding of the static anatomy is a prerequisite for an understanding of the dynamic interaction of the anatomical components of the low back. Spinal motion in the lumbar spine occurs in flexion and extension as well as in axial rotation and lateral bending movements. Stress on the supraspinous, as well as other spinal ligaments, stimulates the multifidus muscle to stiffen, thereby limiting instability.[5] Repetition and extremes of motion, along with compressive loads, can cause failure of the anatomic relationships, resulting in low back pain.

CLINICAL PRESENTATION

In the athlete who presents with back pain, it is imperative to obtain a detailed history and physical examination. Besides the history surrounding the patient's low back pain, it is important to inquire into the specific sports that the athlete plays, competitive level within the sport, position within the sport, and number of hours played. All these factors not only assist in determining the etiology of the pain but also help in directing the treatment algorithm and appropriately setting the level of expectations.

Like the history, the physical exam should not focus solely on examination of the low back. The physical exam must be comprehensive as there are many sources of low back pain, both within the axial skeleton and referred to the spine. Conversely, spinal pathology will often present with pain remote from its origin. For example, the classical presentation of a herniated disc is with "searing leg pain." Included in the spinal examination is the assessment of the overall alignment of the spine, with a determination for the presence of hyperlordosis, kyphosis, or scoliosis. Palpation of the paraspinal musculature, as well as bony prominences, is necessary to assess for step-off or areas of focal tenderness. All patients should receive a thorough neurological exam including motor and sensory testing, reflex assessment, and provocative maneuvers (e.g., Lasègue sign, straight leg raise, and slump test). One must document any abnormal sensory complaints or findings, including parathesias, radicular symptoms, or upper motor neuron findings. If there is a history of bowel or bladder dysfunction, it is mandatory that a rectal exam be performed as cauda equina syndrome is a true spinal emergency.

Diagnostic imaging is very useful for the workup of low back pain in the athlete. Numerous studies are available including plain films, computed tomography (CT) scans, discography, magnetic resonance imaging (MRI), single photon emission CT (SPECT), and bone scans. In the following sections, the usefulness of each study will be examined with regard to the pursuant diagnoses.

DIFFERENTIAL DIAGNOSIS

The following disorders are commonly the source of low back pain in the athlete. Not all of the following will be discussed in this chapter but should be excluded in the workup as many disorders may refer pain to the low back.

1. Muscle strain/Sprain
2. Vertebral disc disease
   a. Disc herniation
   b. Degenerative disc disease
3. Spondylolysis/Spondylolisthesis
4. Ring apophyseal injury
5. Sacral stress fractures
6. Acute traumatic lumbar vertebral fracture
7. Discitis/Osteomyelitis
8. Neoplasm
9. Intrapelvic disorders

INTERVERTEBRAL DISC DISEASE IN ATHLETES

INTERVERTEBRAL DISC HERNIATION

Intervertebral disc herniation is a general term that refers to several different acquired pathological morphologies of the intervertebral disc.[6] Thus, it is necessary to clarify this terminology. A disc *bulge* is generally defined as a symmetrical extension of the disc beyond the boundaries of the superior and inferior endplates.[7] A *protrusion* is also an extension of a portion of the disc beyond the interspace, however asymmetric. An *extrusion* represents an extreme extension of the disc beyond the boundary of the endplates with the base narrower than the diameter of the extruded material.[7] Extruded discs remain in contiguity with the disc space. A *sequestration* refers to a piece of disc that is completely separated from the original intervertebral disc and is considered sequestered as it resides beyond the confines of the PLL.[7]

All forms of disc herniation are thought to occur subsequent to an initial injury to the annulus fibrous. Once there is an annular injury, which often occurs simultaneous to the acute disc herniation, the nuclear material is forced from its central disc location through the thick lamellar rings of the annulus toward the periphery of the intervertebral disc.[7] The nucleus pulposus is then either retained by the annulus (extrusion or herniation) or extruded through the annulus and the PLL into the epidural space (sequestration),[7] creating stenosis within the canal or impingement on a nerve root.

The location of the disc herniation is also important and is related to the anatomy of the ALL and the PLL. Because the PLL is weaker than the ALL and only occupies the central portion of the posterior vertebral column, the most common herniation site is posterolateral. With a posterolateral disc herniation, the nerve root affected will be the traversing nerve root as opposed to the exiting nerve root. For example, a L4/L5 disc protrusion will compress the traversing L5 nerve root. There are also far lateral herniations, which affect the exiting nerve root. A far lateral L4/L5 disc herniation will compromise the L4 nerve root. These, however, account for only 6% to 10% of all lumbar disc herniations. The central/posterior herniation is least common and, when occurring in the lumbar segments, can lead to an S1 radiculopathy. This type of herniation is commonly confused with a severely degenerative bulging disc.

Degenerative disease and acute trauma can both lead to damage of the annulus fibrosus and subsequent disc herniation. The specific epidemiology of intervertebral disc herniation within the athletic population is not known. It has been postulated that repetitive movements within a sport may lead to an increased rate of disc degeneration and acute trauma may be more likely within sports as well. For example, offensive football linemen have extremely large compressive loads (>8,600 N) within the intervertebral disc during blocking maneuvers.[8] Small studies have been conducted looking at Olympic athletes with complaints of low back pain and found greater loss of disc height, and higher prevalence of disc bulges, compared with controls.[9]

The patient with a disc herniation may only present with low back pain that is thought to be from the actual injury to the annular fibers. More commonly, however, patients will experience radicular symptoms. Intervertebral disc herniations are most common at the L4/L5 and L5/S1 levels and radicular symptoms are associated with the corresponding affected nerve root. Lasègue sign (pain elicited with flexion of the hip when the knee is extended, but not when the knee is flexed) and the straight leg raising exam are the most specific physical exam findings for intervertebral disc herniation because they consistently reproduce radicular pain as the affected nerve is stretched across the herniated disc. The slump test, where a straight leg raise is performed while the patient flexes the cervical, thoracic, and lumbar spine, has recently been described as a more sensitive test because it adds cephalad gliding of the spinal cord while the straight leg raise stresses only caudal nerve roots.[10] Some researchers advocate using the slump test as a sensitive physical exam tool in patients with symptoms suggestive of a lumbar disc herniation. These authors also advocate using the straight leg raise, which may be more beneficial in identifying patients requiring surgery.[10]

When first evaluating a possible disc herniation, diagnostic imaging should include anteroposterior and lateral plain films.[7] These films can be utilized to assess intervertebral disc height and vertebral column alignment and to identify any structural abnormalities or transitional vertebral relationships. An MRI should also be obtained to evaluate neural compression and to define intervertebral disc anatomy. T2-weighted MRI images have a myelographic effect, which will elucidate areas of stenosis (Fig. 24.1A,B). If a surgical intervention is indicated, flexion–extension radiographs may be obtained to rule out subtle instability prior to discectomy. It has been estimated that with conservative (nonoperative) management in young patients, approximately 90% of the symptoms associated with disc herniations resolve within three months.[11] Treatment should begin with a period of rest for several days. Nonsteroidal anti-inflammatory medications can be used to decrease nerve root irritation in addition to low dose narcotics and the application of local ice. Once the pain has been initially managed and activity becomes more tolerable, the patient should undergo a supervised comprehensive exercise based on physical therapy program. This rehabilitation protocol should focus on core strengthening and flexibility as well as sport-specific exercises to avoid future injury. If the symptoms do not improve, the patient may benefit from a nerve root injection, which may relieve radicular symptoms and allow the patient to undergo further therapy.[12,13]

If the symptoms are persistent over a period of 6 weeks, despite therapy, or if the symptoms are significantly limiting to the point where therapy cannot be initiated, a lumbar discectomy could be considered. Microdiscectomy of the lumbar disc is now the procedure of choice and has replaced laminectomy/discectomy.[7,11] The procedure can be performed with a microscope or with loupe magnification and headlamp. The principal advantages of the operative microscope over loupe magnification are improved lighting and the capacity for an assistant to be more fully integrated into the procedure.

Dissection is performed down to the lamina and ligamentum flavum. The ligamentum is excised leaving the lamina, facet, and capsule intact. Very often, a small amount of lamina or facet excision is required to visualize the lateral aspect of the traversing nerve root in order to safely retract it. The amount of bone resected does not adversely affect the stability of the spine. The affected nerve root is then identified and retracted. The disc is visualized and the exposed disc material is resected. It should be noted that recurrence of disc herniation after surgery is reported at 3% to 12% and remains independent of surgical technique.[7,11,14]

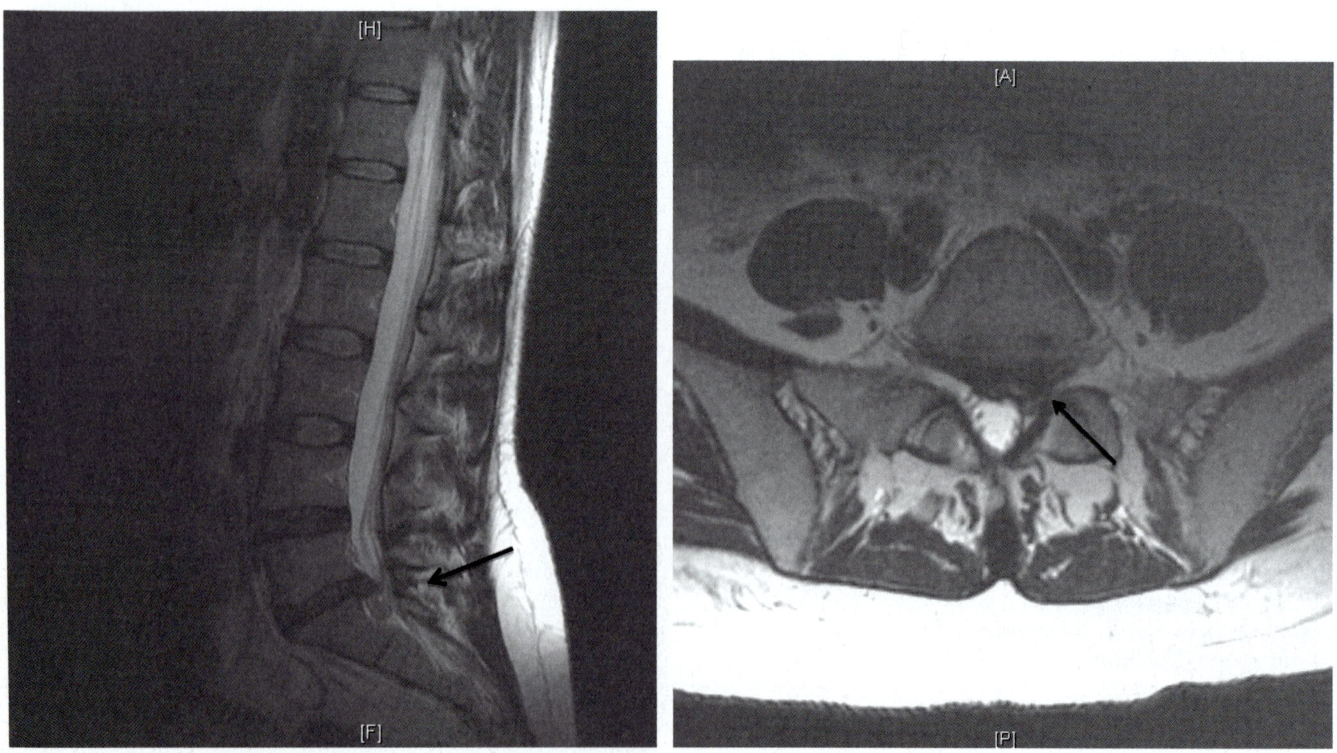

Figure 24.1. Sagittal **(A)** and axial **(B)** images from an MRI in a 40-year-old tri-athlete with left radicular leg pain. MRI demonstrated a left-sided L5–S1 herniated disc (*black arrows*).

Postoperatively, patients should participate in physical therapy involving core strengthening as well as sport specific exercises,[7] although unrestricted activity protocols have also demonstrated success.[15] Return to play depends on the symptoms that remain after the discectomy. If the players are pain free, they may return to play within 3 to 6 months. A retrospective study involving Olympic athletes treated with microdiscectomy had an average return-to-play time of 5.2 months.[16] Other studies involving active young patients and competitive athletes have shown excellent results in regard to pain control and return to high level activity after discectomy.[17,18]

DEGENERATIVE INTERVERTEBRAL DISC DISEASE

Although intervertebral disc herniation provides a precise mechanism for pain generation with impingement of neural structures, the pathophysiology of degenerative disc disease is less clear. Degenerative disease of the intervertebral disc is described as disc space narrowing secondary to circumferential and small radial tears that slowly lead to a loss of disc integrity. Changes in disc nutrition and end plate morphology also contribute to the process, which results in a decreased capacity of the disc to withstand loads.[3] The facet joints are forced to sustain more stress as the disc fails, leading to degeneration of these joints and results in foraminal, as well as central, spinal stenosis.[19] This process ultimately leads to several sources of pain generation.

As stated previously, secondary to the "wear and tear" of sports, degenerative disease of the intervertebral disc is common among athletes. Golfing, bowling, rowing, weight lifting, pitching, gymnastics, football, and skiing all put tremendous amounts of shear and compressive force on the intervertebral discs.[8,20–24] Several studies have correlated low back pain among competitive athletes with degenerative changes on radiographic studies.[24–27] Other studies have shown that sports participation alone is not a risk factor for degenerative disc disease, and may be protective.[28] At the present time, it remains unclear whether participation in athletic activities increases the risk for the development of disc degeneration. Increasing evidence points toward a genetic component to the process and this may prove to be the most important factor.[29]

Patients presenting with degenerative disc disease in the lumbar spine generally describe their pain as located in the low back with or without radiation. Symptoms are typically worse with flexion and are improved with extension of the lumbar spine. Imaging modalities include plain radiographs to assess for the loss of disc height, osteophytes, and facet degeneration. MRI can assess disc desiccation, particularly on T2-weighted images, as well as the latter stages of degenerative disease leading to stenosis (Fig. 24.2).

As with other causes of low back pain, conservative management is the mainstay of treatment. Initial pain control should be managed with nonsteroidal anti-inflammatory medications. Physical therapy should be employed to begin core strengthening as well as plyometrics. It is important to address tight extraspinal musculature, particularly hamstrings and hip flexors. Sport-specific exercises can be introduced when pain levels have decreased and muscle strength and endurance have begun to normalize.[18]

If symptoms persist for greater than four to six months, there is a radiographic documentation of degenerative intervertebral disc disease, and localized tenderness corresponding to the radiographic level, surgical options could be considered.

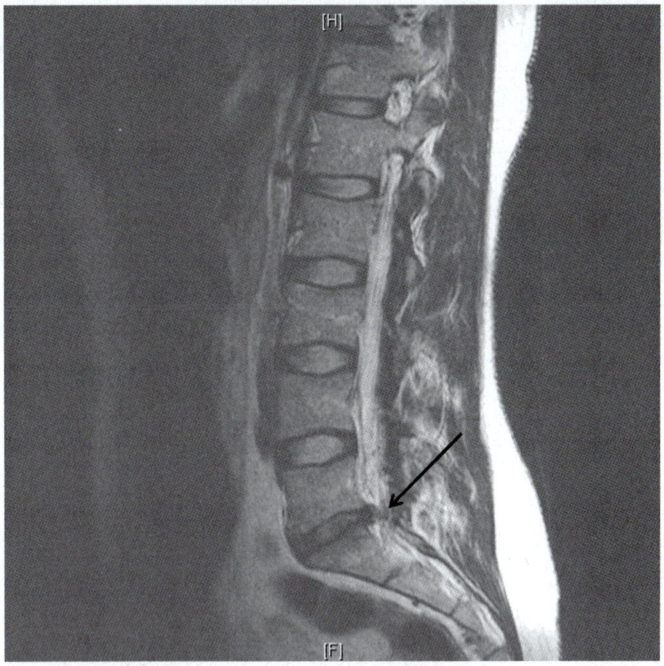

Figure 24.2. Sagittal image from an MRI in a 43-year-old woman with back and leg pain. MRI demonstrated degenerative disc disease at L5–S1 (*black arrow*). This patient was subsequently treated with a transforaminal lumbar interbody fusion (TLIF) at L5–S1 (Fig. 24.3).

However, because surgical treatment generally involves various forms of spinal arthrodesis, this should be taken into consideration as it may require a prolonged period of restriction from sports and does not carry a consistently beneficial outcome. Fusion techniques include posterolateral, interbody (anterior, posterior, or transforaminal), or circumferential fusion.[30] The techniques may be performed with or without instrumentation. Because of higher rates of fusion, and the ability to excise the disc and eliminate a potential pain generator, interbody fusions have gained popularity in recent years (Fig. 24.3).[30–32]

Postoperatively, return to play should not resume until there is a radiographic evidence of a solid fusion. It is also imperative that the patient has adequate postoperative physical therapy to gain strength and flexibility. Because of the potentially long delay to return to sports, a fusion may not be the ideal choice for the professional athletes who require a return to sport for their livelihood. However, in those who are unable to derive satisfactory pain relief from conservative measures, good to excellent results have been reported in 80% to 100% of cases.[33–36]

One concern with fusion techniques is the progression of degenerative disease to adjacent segments. Longitudinal studies have demonstrated the progression of degeneration in adjacent segments after fusion.[37] It is, however, unknown if adjacent segment degeneration results from the fusion or is simply a part of the natural disease process. To potentially address this issue, total disc replacements (TDR) were developed. As a motion-preserving device, many proponents of TDR maintain that adjacent segment degeneration will be reduced. However, to date, such claims remain unsubstantiated in the orthopaedic literature, and long-term data is not available for these devices. As a result, the recommendation for TDR is currently difficult to make, except on an individual case basis, and it would not generally appear suitable for the competitive athlete.

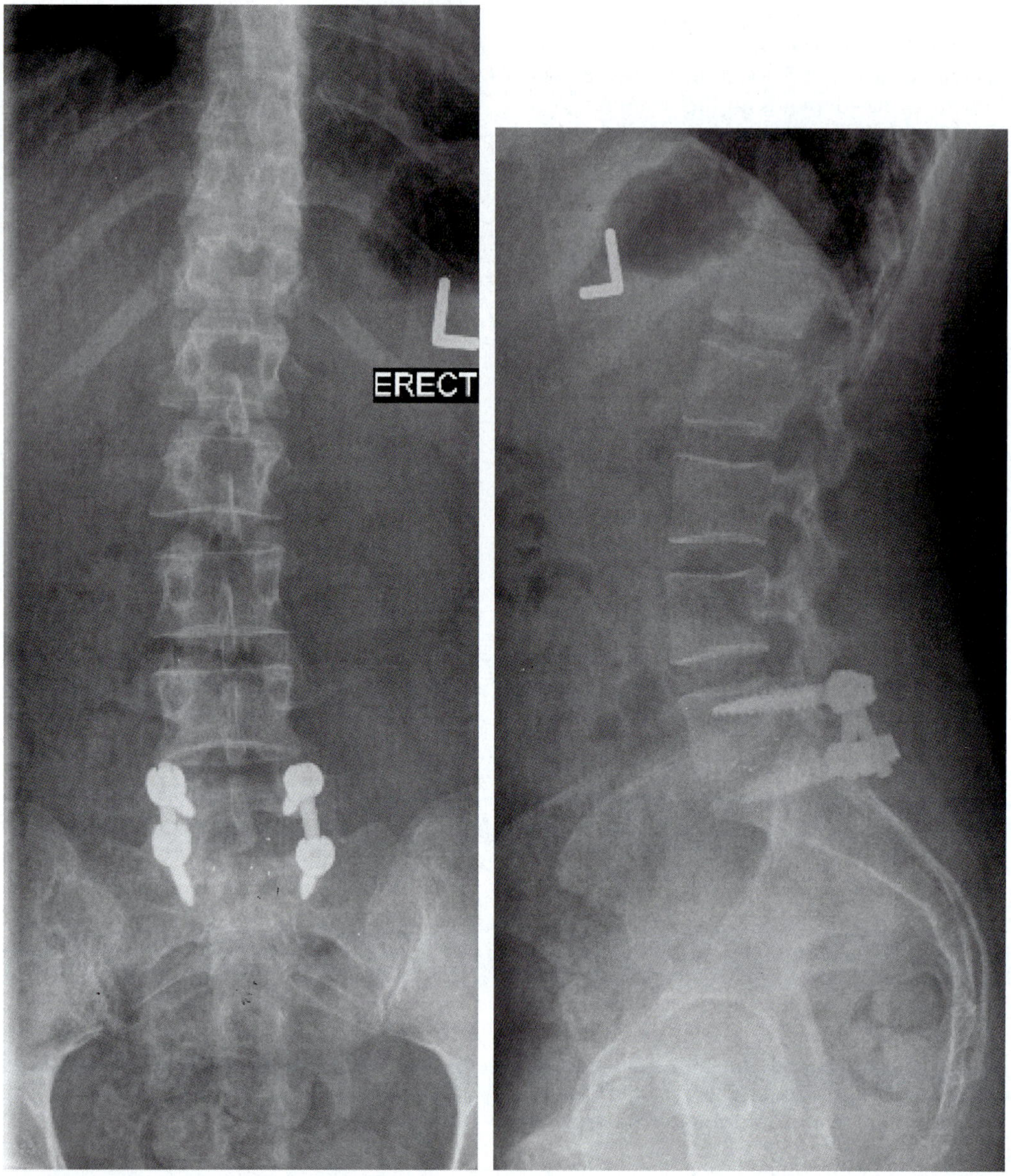

Figure 24.3. Postoperative **(A)** anteroposterior (AP) and **(B)** lateral images from the same patient depicted in Figure 24.2. The patient's symptoms were ultimately treated with a transforaminal lumbar interbody fusion (TLIF) at L5–S1.

SPONDYLOLYSIS/SPONDYLOLISTHESIS

Spondylolysis refers to a bony defect within the pars interarticularis; most commonly found in the lumbar vertebrae. This defect creates a discontinuity between the anterior and posterior elements of the vertebrae. This anatomical condition can lead to pain and instability as well as subluxation of one vertebra on another. When the subluxation occurs, the condition is referred to as spondylolisthesis. The condition of a posterior subluxation of one vertebra relative to its subjacent neighbor is termed retrolisthesis. Spondylolysis can be a developmental defect or an acquired deformity (e.g., secondary to trauma). Athletes who perform repetitive hyperextension of the spine during sport can acquire spondylolysis secondary to stress fracture from the repetitive trauma. Gymnasts, football linemen, and rowers frequently undergo these repetitive actions, causing repetitive loading, and the differential for back pain in these individuals must include this defect.

In the adult population, the incidence of spondylolysis is estimated to be approximately 6%.[38] Males are two times more likely to have a pars defect than females. It is thought that athletes have the same prevalence of spondylolysis as the general population, unless the athlete partakes in one of the high-risk sports mentioned above. It has also been found that adolescent athletes have a higher prevalence of spondylolysis than adult athletes.[39] The most commonly affected spinal segments include the L5 (85% to 95%) and L4 (5% to 15%) vertebral levels.[40] As in the general population, not all spondylolytic defects may be symptomatic in the athlete.

Spondylolisthesis represents a progression from a nondisplaced spondylolytic defect and can be a significant source of pain and instability. The classification system commonly used to differentiate the etiology of spondylolisthesis is the Wiltse–Newman classification (Table 24.1).[41] In the young, active patient population, isthmic spondylolisthesis is the most commonly encountered form.

The Myerding classification is commonly utilized to grade the severity of the subluxation as well as to direct treatment.[5] This grading system is based on the amount of anterior displacement of one vertebra on another. A grade I slip is defined as 0% to 25% of anterior displacement, Grade II is 25% to 50%, grade III is 50% to 75%, and grade IV is >75%. A complete dislocation/slip (grade V) is rare and is termed spondyloptosis.

In a patient with spondylolysis/spondylolisthesis, the most common complaint is low back pain. The initial evaluation should include a comprehensive history and physical examination, including sport specific history and neurological evaluation. The sport-specific history must include the patient's position, level of competition, conditioning, and frequency of training and competitive activity. All of these attributes will contribute to the diagnosis as well as potential treatment/rehabilitation. The pain is typically described as a dull ache and accompanying radiculopathy is uncommon. The patient may complain of pain in the buttock; however, this is more likely secondary to the resultant hamstring tightness. If radiculopathy is truly present, it generally localizes to the exiting nerve root of the level involved. Physical examination will elicit pain with extension of the lumbar spine and there may be an increased lordosis of the lumbar spine. Palpation of the spine may demonstrate point tenderness or a palpable step-off in the case of a high-grade spondylolisthesis. Neurologic examination is typically normal, but radicular symptoms may manifest as pain, weakness, or paresthesias.

Initial radiographic studies should include anteroposterior and lateral lumbar radiographs. If a spondylolysis is suspected but not identified on the initial orthogonal views, oblique views will allow the best appreciation of a defect within the pars, frequently referred to as the broken neck of the "Scottie Dog." Further radiographs can be obtained if an abnormality is demonstrated. Standing full-length films allow appreciation of the sagittal balance, slip angle, and pelvic parameters such as pelvic incidence. These additional parameters will assist in the prognosis for slip progression. Flexion/extension views of the lumbar spine can assist in assessing stability at the affected vertebral level. If the initial radiographs are negative in a patient with persistent pain and suspicion for spondylolysis, further studies can be obtained. These include bone scan, SPECT, CT, and MRI.

A bone scan is an excellent study to obtain when a stress fracture or an impending stress fracture is suspected. Because a bone scan shows areas of increase bone turnover/metabolic activity, it can detect acute fractures and those that are in the process of healing.[42] However, there is lack of specificity with a bone scan as defects that have been present for a long duration of time may not be visualized.

Utilizing gamma cameras and 3D reconstructions, SPECT studies can distinguish an acute lesion from one that is chronic and can help determine if a defect has the capacity to heal.[43,44] SPECT scans are currently the test of choice to detect an occult pars defect because of increased sensitivity compared to other techniques.[45] MRI can be useful if neurological symptoms are present and is also good at predicting an impending pars fracture.[46]

When a lesion is evident but poorly depicted by conventional plain radiographs, it is useful to obtain a CT scan. CT scan provides the best bony details that are not evident on plain radiographs. Furthermore, CT scans can be used to follow lesions to assess bone healing. Spondylolytic lesions, on CT axial images, have been described as resembling degenerative facet joints at the level of the pedicle.[47] Clearly, when assessing the athlete with a suspected spondylolytic lesion, radiographic studies must be obtained in a stepwise and systematic manner depending on the particular history, complaints, and ability of basic studies to differentiate a lesion before a more sophisticated study is obtained.

Once a spondylolytic lesion is found, treatment options vary. An athlete's level of competition, need for early return to sports, neurologic symptoms, and risk of slip progression must all be taken into account. Risk of progression is greater in younger female patients, in those with high-grade slips, and with an increased slip angle or a domed/inclined sacrum.

Once a spondylolytic lesion is determined to be acute, rest and decreased activity level are recommended to promote osseous healing. Some recommend a 12-week hiatus from normal participation in sports, but most authors agree that athletes can return to play once symptom free. A physical therapy rehabilitation program is also initiated, which can include aerobic conditioning, hamstring stretching, and core stabilization/strengthening. Sport specific physical therapy regimens can also be included, which may focus on the kinesthesiological aspects of specific sports and avoidance of certain maneuvers. Conservative treatment has demonstrated good to excellent outcomes in 90% of cases.[12]

In the skeletally immature/adolescent athlete, a thoracolumbosacral orthosis or soft corset may also be used to partially immobilize the spine and prevent hyperlordosis or slip progression. There are, however, few studies that support the effectiveness of such treatment. Some investigators advocate the use of bracing for 6 to 12 weeks, with cessation of use once the patient is pain free and/or there is a radiographic evidence of healing. Bracing in adults is typically reserved for highly symptomatic patients.

It must be noted that with conservative treatment, in the case of spondylolisthesis, there is a risk of slip progression. One study found an approximate 10% risk of progression in

TABLE 24.1	Wiltse–Newman Classification of Spondylolisthesis
Type I—Dysplastic	Congenital facet abnormalities; no pars interarticularis defect
Type II—Isthmic	Defect in the pars interarticularis, allowing anterior subluxation of L5 on S1 a. Lytic—secondary to stress fracture of the pars b. Acute traumatic fracture of the pars
Type III—Degenerative type	Degeneration of long term, leading to instability and subsequent remodeling of articular processes
Type IV—Traumatic	Fracture in area other than the pars
Type V—Pathologic	Secondary to bone disease

a retrospective analysis of 86 adolescent competitive athletes.[48] None of these patients were symptomatic, and some had a decrease in the amount of slip with observational care alone.

When conservative methods fail, operative intervention can be considered. The gold standard of surgical intervention is posterolateral fusion of the affected segments. In the case of spondylolysis alone, direct repair of the pars has been described with a variety of different techniques. Surgical indications for fusion include grade III or higher slip at presentation, progressive slip despite conservative management, neurologic deficit related to the lesion, or failure of a comprehensive conservative treatment course after 6 months.

Posterolateral arthrodesis has been reported to be successful in approximately 90% of cases.[49,50] The fusion is typically performed with posterior instrumentation; however, this is not a requirement and may be unnecessary. In the case of spondylolisthesis, decompression is rarely necessary unless objective neurological signs are present. Classically, unless causing neurological compromise, the affected segments are fused in situ. Two level fusions may be necessary if a higher-grade slip is present (higher than grade II).

In recent years, interbody fusion has become increasingly popular.[51] In this technique, through a variety of different approaches (e.g., posterior lumbar interbody fusion and transforaminal lumbar interbody fusion (TLIF)), adjacent vertebral bodies are fused, resulting in a more stable construct with increased fusion rates. An interbody fusion accompanied by posterior instrumentation may be the optimal choice of treatment in individuals with high-grade slips, especially when an attempt is made to reduce the degree or angle of the slip.

When spondylolysis is present without evidence of spondylolisthesis, direct repair of the pars may be entertained. This technique is becoming more common, with a variety of methods described in the literature.[52–54] Lag screw placement, wiring, pedicle screw-rod constructs, and pedicle screw-laminar hook-rod constructs have all been utilized with success. The technique involves removal of all fibrous tissue, decortication, bone grafting, and fixation utilizing one of the methods mentioned above. Several studies have reported good to excellent results with these techniques.[53,54] This technique is particularly favored when the defect is above the L5 level whereby the alternative treatment, a fusion, would consist of a "floating fusion" adjacent to free segments. Further research, however, is necessary to compare long-term outcomes of arthrodesis to the direct pars repair techniques.

The athlete with back pain demonstrated to have a spondylolysis and/or spondylolisthesis must be treated on a case specific basis. The patient's level of activity, position within sport, "need/desire to return to sport," and severity of injury must all be taken into account. As stated previously, following conservative management, the adult athletes may return to sport once they are asymptomatic. Skeletally immature athletes should generally refrain from athletic participation until they have demonstrated healing of the spondylolytic lesion. Finally, in those cases where surgical intervention is necessary, recommendations regarding return to sport are highly variable. Many feel that, following single level lumbar arthrodesis, a patient could return to noncontact athletics after 6 months. However, it is controversial if patients should ever return to contact sports following posterior fusion, and this decision ultimately rests with the treating surgeon and the athlete.[55–57]

REFERENCES

1. Trainor TJ, Wiesel SW. Epidemiology of back pain in the athlete. *Clin Sports Med.* 2002;21:93–103.
2. Hollinshead HW. *Anatomy for Surgeons: Volume 3. The Back and Limbs.* New York: Hoeber & Harper; 1958.
3. Rao RD, Bagaria V. Pathophysiology of degenerative disk disease and related symptoms. In: Spivak JM, Connolly PJ, eds. *Orthopaedic Knowledge Update: Spine 3.* Rosemont, IL: American Academy of Orthopaedic Surgeons; 2006, pp. 35–41.
4. Bogduk N. The innervation of the lumbar spine. *Spine.* 1983;8:286–293.
5. Solomonow M, Zhou B-H EE, Harris M, et al. The ligamento-muscular stabilizing system of the spine. *Spine.* 1998;23:2552–2562.
6. Jensen M, Brant-Zawadzki M, Obuchowski N, et al. Magnetic resonance imaging of the lumbar spine in people without back pain. *N Engl J Med.* 1994;331:69–73.
7. Bono CM, Wisneski R, Garfin SR. Lumbar disc herniations. In: Herkowitz HN, Garfin SR, Eismont FJ, et al., eds. *The Spine.* 5th Ed. Philadephia, PA: W.B. Saunders; 2006, pp. 967–991.
8. Gatt CJ, Hosea TM, Palumbo RC, et al. Impact loading of the lumbar spine during football blocking. *Am J Sports Med.* 1997;25:317–321.
9. Ong A, Anderson J, Roche J. A pilot study of the prevalence of lumbar disc degeneration in elite athletes with lower back pain at the Sydney 2000 Olympic Games. *Br J Sports Med.* 2003;37:263–266.
10. Majlesi J, Togay H, Unalan H, et al. The sensitivity and specificity of the slump and straight leg raising tests in patients with lumbar disc herniation. *J Clin Rheumatol.* 2008;14:87–91.
11. Bendo JA, Awad JN. Lumbar disk herniation. In: Spivak JM, Connolly PJ, eds. *Orthopaedic Knowledge Update: Spine 3.* Rosemont, IL: American Academy of Orthopaedic Surgeons; 2006, pp. 289–297.
12. Wang JC, Lin E, Brodke DS, et al. Epidural injections for the treatment of symptomatic lumbar herniated discs. *J Spinal Disord.* 2002;15:269–272.
13. Weber H. Lumbar disc herniation: A controlled, prospective study with ten years of observations. *Spine.* 1983;8:131–140.
14. Jonsson B, Stromqvist B. Clinical characteristics of recurrent sciatica after lumbar discectomy. *Spine.* 1996;21:500–505.
15. Carragee EJ, Han MY, Yang B, et al. Activity restrictions after posterior lumbar discectomy: A prospective study of outcomes in 152 cases with no postoperative restrictions. *Spine.* 1999;24:2346–2351.
16. Watkins RG, Williams LA, Watkins RG. Microscopic lumbar discectomy results for 60 cases in professional and Olympic athletes. *Spine.* 2003;3:100–105.
17. Wang J, Shapiro M, Hatch J, et al. The outcome of lumbar discectomy in elite athletes. *Spine.* 1999;24:570–573.
18. Cooke PM, Lutz GE. Internal disc disruption and axial back pain in the athlete. *Phys Med Rehabil Clin N Am.* 2000;11:837–865.
19. Kirkaldy-Willis WH, Frafan HF. Instability of the lumbar spine. *Clin Orthop.* 1982;165: 110–123.
20. Hosea TM, Boland AL. Rowing injuries. *Postgrad Adv Sports Med.* 1989;III:1–17.
21. Elliott B, Khangure M. Disk degeneration and fast bowling in cricket: An intervention study. *Med Sci Sports Exerc.* 2002;34:1714–1718.
22. Cholewicki J, McGill SM, Norman RW. Lumbar spine loads during the lifting of extremely heavy weights. *Med Sci Sports Exerc.* 1991;23:1179–1186.
23. Cappozzo A, Felici F, Figura F, et al. Lumbar spine loading during half squat exercises. *Med Sci Sports Exerc.* 1985;17:613–620.
24. Videman T, Sarna S, Battle MC, et al. The long term effects of physical loading and exercise lifestyles on back-related symptoms, disability, and spinal pathology among men. *Spine.* 1995;20:699–709.
25. Ogon M, Riedl-Huter C, Sterzinger W, et al. Radiologic abnormalities and low back pain in elite skiers. *Clin Orthop.* 2001;390:151–162.
26. Lundin O, Hellstrom M, Nilsson I, et al. Back pain and radiological changes in the thoraco-lumbar spine of athletes: A long-term follow-up. *Scand J Med Sci Sports.* 2001;11:103–109.
27. Sward L, Helistrom M, Jacobsson B, et al. Disc degeneration and associated abnormalities of the spine in elite gymnasts: A magnetic resonance imaging study. *Spine.* 191;16:437–443.
28. Dickerman RD, Zigler JE. Discogenic back pain. In: Spivak JM, Connolly PJ, eds. *Orthopaedic Knowledge Update: Spine 3.* Rosemont, IL: American Academy of Orthopaedic Surgeons; 2006, pp. 319–329.
29. Hartvigsen J, Christensen K, Frederiksen H, et al. Genetic and environmental contributions to back pain in old age: A study of 2108 Danish twins aged 70 and older. *Spine.* 2004;29:897–901.
30. DiPaola CP, Molinari RW. Posterior lumbar interbody fusion. *J Am Acad Orthop Surg.* 2008;16:130–139.
31. DeBerard MS, Colledge AL, Masters KS, et al. Outcomes of posterolateral versus BAK titanium cage interbody lumbar fusion in injured workers: A retrospective cohort study. *J South Orthop Assoc.* 2002;11:157–166.
32. Hackenberg L, Halm H, Bullmann V, et al. Transforaminal lumbar interbody fusion: A safe technique with satisfactory three to five year results. *Eur Spine K.* 2005;14:551–558.
33. Lee CK, Vessa P, Lee KJ. Chronic disabling low back pain syndrome caused by internal disc derangements: The results of disc excision and posterior lumbar interbody fusion. *Spine.* 1995;20:356–361.
34. Kuslich SD, Ulstrom CL, Griffith SL, et al. The Bagby and Kuslich method of lumbar interbody fusion: History, techniques, and 2 year follow-up results of a United States prospective, multicenter trial. *Spine.* 1998;23:1267–1279.

35. Pearson AM, Blood EA, Frymoyer JW, et al. SPORT lumbar intervertebral disk herniation and back pain: Does treatment, location, or morphology matter? *Spine.* 2008;33(4):428–435.
36. Brantigan JW, Steffee AD, Lewis ML, et al. Lumbar interbody fusion using the Brantigan I/F cage for posterior lumbar interbody fusion and the variable pedicle screw placement system: Two year results from a Food and Drug Administration investigational device exemption clinical trial. *Spine.* 2000;25:1437–1446.
37. Cheh G, Bridwell KH, Lenke LG, et al. Adjacent segment disease following lumbar/thoracolumbar fusion with pedicle screw instrumentation: A minimum 5-year follow-up. *Spine.* 2007;32:2253–2257.
38. Beutler WJ, Fredrickson BE, Murtland A, et al. The natural history of spondylolysis and spondylolisthesis: 45 year follow-up evaluation. *Spine.* 2003;10:1027–1035.
39. Micheli LJ. Back pain in young athletes: Significant differences from adults in causes and patterns. *Arch Pediatr Adolesc Med.* 1995;149:15.
40. Standaert CJ. Spondylolysis. *Phys Med Rehabil Clin N Am.* 2000;11:785–803.
41. Wiltse LL, Newman PH, Macnab I. Classification of spondylolysis and spondylolisthesis. *Clin Orthop.* 1976;117:23–29.
42. Jackson DW, Wiltse LL, Dingeman RD, et al. Stress reactions involving the pars interarticularis in young athletes. *Am J Sports Med.* 1981;9:304–312.
43. Bellah RD, Summerville DA, et al. Low back pain in adolescent athletes: Detection of stress injury to the pars interarticularis with SPECT. *Radiology.* 1991;180:509–512.
44. Kanstrup IL. Bone scintigraphy in sports medicine: A review. *Scand J Med Sci Sports.* 1997;7:322–330.
45. Standaert CJ, Herring SA. Expert opinion and controversies in sports and musculoskeletal medicine: The diagnosis and treatment of spondylolysis in adolescent athletes. *Arch Phys Med Rehab.* 2007;88:537–540.
46. Yamane T, Yoshida T, Mimatsu K. et al. Early diagnosis of lumbar spondylolysis by MRI. *J Bone Joint Surg Br.* 1993;75:764–768.
47. Bono CM. Low back pain in athletes. *J Bone Joint Surg Am.* 2004;86:382–396.
48. Muschik M, Hahnel H, Robinson PN, et al. Competitive sports and the progression of spondylolisthesis. *J Ped Orthop.* 1996;16:364–369.
49. Wiltse LL. Jackson treatment of spondylolysis and spondylolisthesis in children. *Clin Orthop.* 1976;117:92–110.
50. Seitsalso S, Osterman K, Hyvarinen H, et al. Severe spondylolisthesis in children and adolescents. A long term review of fusion in situ. *J Bone Joint Surg Br.* 1990;72:259–265.
51. La Rosa G, Conti A, Cacciola F, et al. Pedicle screw fixation for isthmic spondylolisthesis: Does posterior lumbar interbody fusion improve outcome over posterolateral fusion? *J Neurosurg.* 2003;99(Suppl. 2):143–150.
52. Debnath UK, Freeman BJ, Gregory P, et al. Clinical outcome and return to sport after the surgical treatment of spondylolysis in young athletes. *J Bone Joint Surg Br.* 2003;85: 244–249.
53. Nozawa S, Shimizu K, Miyamoto K, et al. Repair of pars interarticularis defect by segmental wire fixation in young athletes with spondylolysis. *Am J Sports Med.* 2003;31:359–364.
54. Gillet P, Petit M. Direct repair of spondylolysis without spondylolisthesis, using a rod screw construct and bone grafting of the pars defect. *Spine.* 1999;24:1252–1256.
55. Dewing CB, Provencher MT, Riffenburgh RH, et al. The outcomes of lumbar microdiscectomy in a young, active population: Correlation by herniation type and level. *Spine.* 2008;33:33–38.
56. Myerding HW. Spondylolisthesis. *Surg Gynecol Obstet.* 1932;54:371–377.
57. Miller SF, Congeni J, Swanson K. Long-term functional and anatomical follow-up of early detected spondylolysis in young athletes. *Am J Sports Med.* 2004;32:928–933.

CHAPTER

25

Jeffrey R. Vargo
Erik J. Wolpert

Rehabilitation of the Postarthroscopic Hip

INTRODUCTION

Rehabilitation of the hip joint is better achieved through considerable knowledge of the joint's mechanics, ligamentous structures, and muscular function. As these topics have been detailed in prior chapters, it will not be repeated at this time. This chapter will focus on rehabilitation of the hip in regard to the innovative arthroscopic interventions described. The following chapter will review the purpose and goals of physical therapy intervention in the postoperative patient. We will discuss the adverse effects of labrum and joint injuries, the contraindications and considerations during the therapeutic process, and the patient presentation following arthroscopy. Lastly, the chapter will present the rehabilitative protocols designed for the postarthroscopic hip.

PURPOSE OF PHYSICAL THERAPY

The emphasis of physical therapy is to intervene on structures in the hip girdle that can be affected by therapeutic exercises, manual procedures, and physical agents. A physical therapist equipped with the understanding of hip arthroscopy and proper protocols can insure a positive outcome and speed the recovery process toward optimal function. The rehabilitation process is essential for proper recovery and can prevent issues in arthrokinematic and muscular dysfunctions that may interfere with a return to desired activity level.

For effective physical therapy intervention, it is imperative for the clinician to identify the clinical and functional problems that each individual presents. This ability facilitates sound treatment rationale to achieve the desired clinical goals (Table 25.1) which will lead to functional outcomes. Once problems and goals are clearly defined, an individualized and effective treatment plan can be implemented. Figure 25.1 demonstrates the clinical reasoning process to achieve effective treatment planning.

ADVERSE EFFECTS OF LABRAL AND JOINT INJURIES AND SURGICAL INTERVENTION ON THE HIP

It is important to comprehend the inherent issues that accompany intracapsular injuries to the hip. Injury and subsequent arthroscopic surgery to the hip manifest multiple clinical and functional problems. Each must be considered and addressed in order to eliminate potential lingering deficits that may limit function. Table 25.2 describes the most common deficits observed from injury and arthroscopic surgery.

Intracapsular injuries characteristically present problems with range of motion (ROM), gait abnormalities, localized pain, and compensatory pain. Arthroscopic intervention will remove the physical and anatomical sources of these problems. However, restoration of these issues is left to therapeutic intervention.

Surgery presents a set of clinical challenges as well. Despite being arthroscopic, the hip will present itself with moderate to severe swelling, muscle inhibition due to joint and incisional pain, weight-bearing sensitivity, and significant cardiovascular deconditioning. When properly identified, resolution of injury-related and postarthroscopic issues may be significantly facilitated through appropriate manual therapies, physical agents, and therapeutic exercise.

PRESENTATION TO REHABILITATION AFTER ARTHROSCOPIC PROCEDURES

The arthroscopic hip patient will typically begin physical therapy between 1 and 4 weeks after surgery. Depending on the specific procedure, the patient will be present with crutches and instructions for either toe touch weight bearing (TTWB) or nonweight bearing (NWB) on the affected lower extremity. Compression hose is typically utilized to prevent lower extremity swelling and reduce risk of embolism. The patient will often need assistance moving the lower extremity on and off the examination table in the early phase following surgery, as severe swelling and moderate pain levels cause muscular inhibition.

Once the patient is on the table, closer examination of the involved region will show evidence of healing arthroscopic incisions with adhesive strips maintaining approximation. These strips will fall off when the incisions are healed. Severe swelling is present at the hip and often spills over into the pelvis and thigh. Additionally, despite compression hose, there will be moderate swelling in the knee and lower leg. Active ROM (AROM) is severely limited due to the pain and swelling inhibition.

TABLE 25.1 Goals of Physical Therapy/Hip Rehabilitation

- Clinical
  1. Eliminate inflammation of periarticular tissues
  2. Retard muscle atrophy and normalize neuromuscular recruitment patterns
  3. Normalize joint accessory motion
  4. Normalize joint AROM in all directions
  5. Normalize strength of the hip
- Functional
  1. Normalize gait: Eliminate compensations leading to asymmetry and microtraumas to other joints (S-I and L/S). Improve efficiency in bipedal locomotion
  2. Improve hip contribution to normal body and lifting mechanics efficiency
  3. Return to recreational activity

During the initial evaluation, the physical therapist will document the available AROM and passive ROM (PROM). While assessing ROM, the physical therapist will find moderate to severe limitations depending upon the pain level and the procedure the patient has undergone. The swelling mentioned previously will disguise muscle atrophy. However, inhibited or slowed muscle recruitment patterns in the hip, quadriceps, and hamstring muscles are noteworthy. After completing the thorough assessment of ROM, acute neuromuscular deficits, and noting functional deficits, the physical therapist may begin the individualized plan within the protocol guidelines.

TREATMENT INTERVENTION

Treatment of the hip after arthroscopic intervention may begin after the evaluation and assessment by the physical therapist.

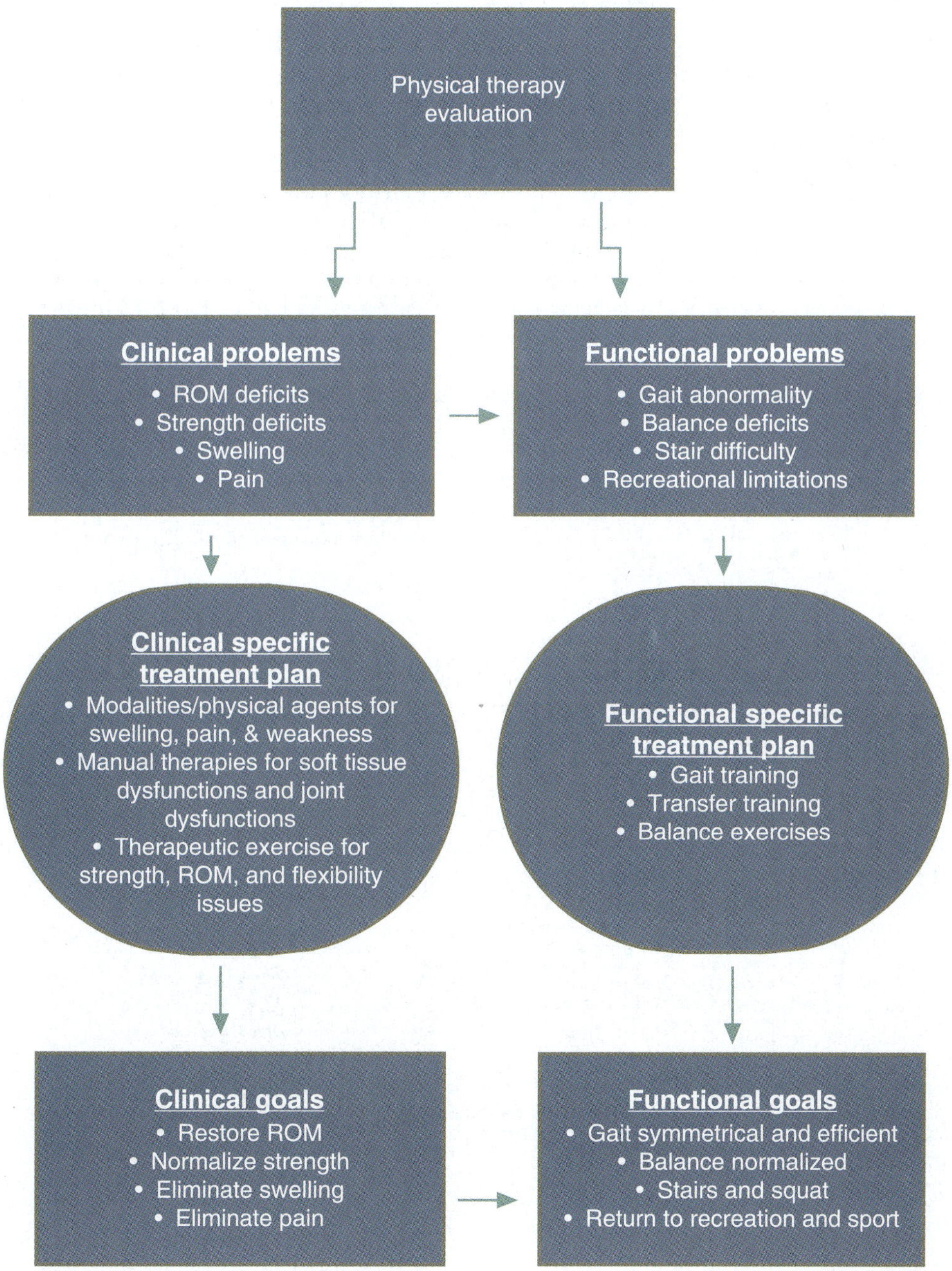

Figure 25.1. Clinical rationale for treatment planning.

TABLE 25.2 Adverse Effects of Intracapsular Injury and Surgery

- Injury
  1. ROM restrictions
  2. Gait abnormalities
     a. Ipsilateral trunk lean
     b. Decreased trailing limb posture due to extension limitation or sensitivity
  3. Acute and chronic hip flexor pain/strain
  4. Lumbar and S-I pain due to compensation
- Surgery
  1. Swelling of periarticular tissues and entire lower extremity
  2. Muscle inhibition/weakness
  3. Healing incision sites
  4. Weight-bearing sensitivity
  5. Cardiovascular deconditioning

TABLE 25.3 Treatment Contraindications and Precautions Following Hip Arthroscopy

- Internal rotation with the hip flexed to 90° is discouraged in the early phases.
- Impact activity should not begin until 6 weeks post-op on hip arthroscopy or debridement or femoral neck debridement.
- Impact activity should not begin until 12 weeks post-op in labral repairs.
- Femoral neck debridement should be NWB or TTWB for 2–4 weeks after surgery, and should not be full weight bearing (FWB) until Week 6.
- Avoid forward straight leg raises until 4 weeks.
- Do not push the arthritic hip to gain ROM.

There are a wide variety of physical agents and modalities available to a physical therapist to aid in the healing process, alleviating pain and swelling, and improving muscle recruitment and function. Manual therapy intervention is also important in reducing swelling, restoring ROM, and re-educating neuromusculoskeletal movement patterns for function and gait. We encourage an approach that incorporates both physical agents and manual therapy along with the exercise protocol provided, in order to achieve optimal outcomes and return to function for the patient.

Physical agents and manual therapy may be applied liberally throughout the rehabilitation protocol. Precautions should be taken when considering mobilization and ROM procedures in order to protect structures that have been repaired and areas of weakened bone. A list of general treatment contraindications and precautions is provided in Table 25.3.

The remainder of this chapter will focus on exercise protocols that have been designed for the patient who has had arthroscopic surgery on the hip. The protocols provided in Table 25.4 encompass exercises prescribed from the day of surgery through return to function and sport. The protocols include exercise schedules for the three most typical hip arthroscopy procedures: labral debridement, labral repair, and femoral neck debridement. Again, attention at all times should be directed toward precautions and contraindications, as well as activity and weight-bearing limitations in order to prevent exacerbation of symptoms or reinjury of the hip.

The protocols for rehabilitation of the hip after arthroscopy focus on normalizing joint accessory motion, stretching the periarticular structures, and strengthening the hip movers and stabilizers. The end result of these exercises and interventions should be consistent with the functional goals previously listed in Figure 25.1. The pictures provided in Figures 25.2–25.16 demonstrate many of the key exercises of the hip protocols.

TABLE 25.4 Exercise Protocols

Time	*Hip Arthroscopy*	*Labral Repair*	*Femoral Neck Debridement*
Same day	Isometric exercise • Gluteal AROM • Ankle pumps	Isometric exercise • Gluteal sets AROM • Ankle pumps	Isometric exercise • Gluteal sets AROM • Ankle pumps
Week 1	Isometric exercise • Gluteal, quadriceps, hamstrings, adductors, abductors sets Active assistive ROM • All planes on table, ball slides for flexion Open chain • Standing flexion, abduction, adduction, and extension Closed chain • Bridging, standing weight shifts, balance (as tolerated) Weight bearing: as tolerated (WBAT)	Isometric exercise • Gluteal, quadriceps, hamstrings, adductors, abductors sets Active assistive ROM • All planes on table, ball slides for flexion Open chain • Standing flexion, abduction, adduction, and extension Weight bearing: NWB	Isometric exercise • Gluteal, quadriceps, hamstrings, adductors, abductors sets Active assistive ROM • All planes on table, ball slides for flexion Open chain • Standing flexion, abduction, adduction, and extension Weight bearing: NWB

(Continued)

TABLE 25.4 Continued

Time	*Hip Arthroscopy*	*Labral Repair*	*Femoral Neck Debridement*
Weeks 2–4	Open chain AROM without restrictions Progressive resistive exercises (PREs) • Resisted above knee flexion, abduction, adduction, and extension • Theraband or pulley Closed chain Single limb bridge Advanced balance Cardiovascular • Bicycle • Pool Joint mobilization may be initiated Weight bearing: FWB wean from assistive devices and normalize gait	Open chain AROM with restrictions PREs • Resisted above knee flexion, abduction, adduction, and extension • Theraband or pulley Cardiovascular • Pool as tolerated Weight bearing: NWB Joint mobilization may be initiated	Open chain AROM with restrictions • Bike-assisted ROM PREs • Resisted above knee flexion, abduction, adduction, and extension • Theraband or pulley Cardiovascular • Pool Weight bearing: NWB until 4th week then WBAT with crutches Joint mobilization may be initiated
Weeks 5 and 6	Flexibility • Stretching to full range Open chain • PREs of hip without restriction in all planes of motion • Quadriceps and hamstrings • Start straight leg raises Closed chain without limits • Ball squats • Single limb balance • Step downs and up Cardiovascular • Bike • Stairmaster or elliptical	Flexibility • Gentle stretching Open chain • PREs of hip in all planes of motion • Quadriceps and hamstrings • Start straight leg raises Closed chain • Bridging bilateral • Weight shift • Balance Cardiovascular • Bike (recumbent preferred) Weight bearing: WBAT, weaning from assistive devices. • Avoid pivot or twisting on hip	Flexibility • Gentle stretching Open chain • PREs of hip in all planes of motion • Quadriceps and hamstrings • Start straight leg raises Closed chain • Bridging bilateral • Weight shift • Balance Cardiovascular • Bike (recumbent preferred) • Stairmaster or elliptical Weight bearing: FWB wean from assistive devices and normalize gait • Avoid pivot or twisting of hip
Weeks 7 and 8	Function-specific exercises Sport-specific training and increasing impact activity	Flexibility • Stretching to full range Open chain • PREs of hip and knee without restriction Closed chain without limits • Unilateral bridging • Ball squats • Single limb balance • Step downs and up Cardiovascular • Bike • Stairmaster or elliptical Weight bearing: Controlled pivot and twist	Flexibility • Stretching to full range Open chain • PREs of hip and knee without restriction Closed chain without limits • Unilateral bridging • Ball squats • Single limb balance • Step downs and up Cardiovascular • Bike • Stairmaster or elliptical Weight bearing: Controlled pivot and twist
Weeks 9 and 10	Return to sport	Function-specific exercises Sport-specific training and increasing impact activity	Function-specific exercises Sport-specific training and increasing impact activity
Week 12		Return to sport	Return to sport

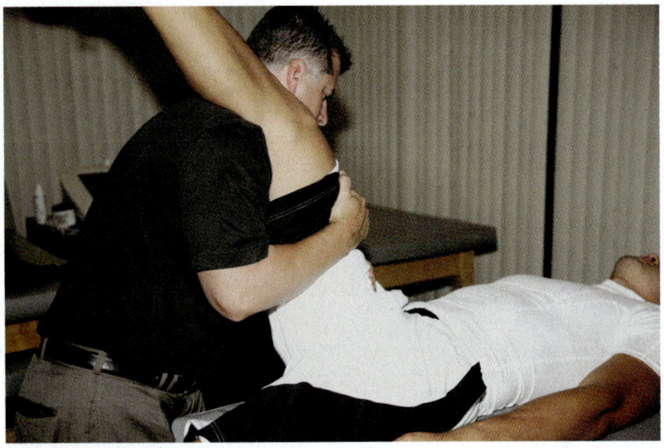

Figure 25.2. Hip inferior glide mobilization.

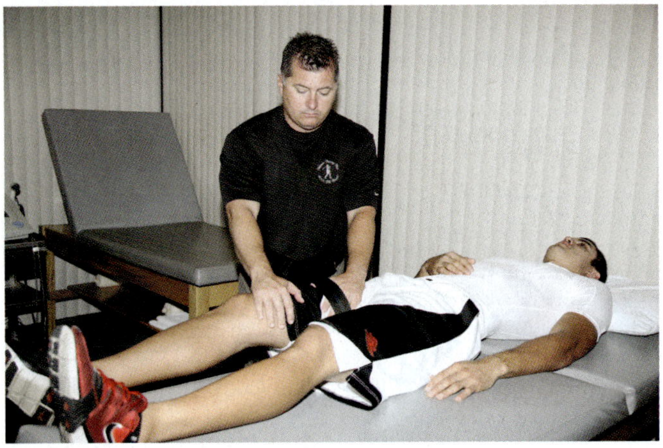

Figure 25.3. Hip lateral glide mobilization.

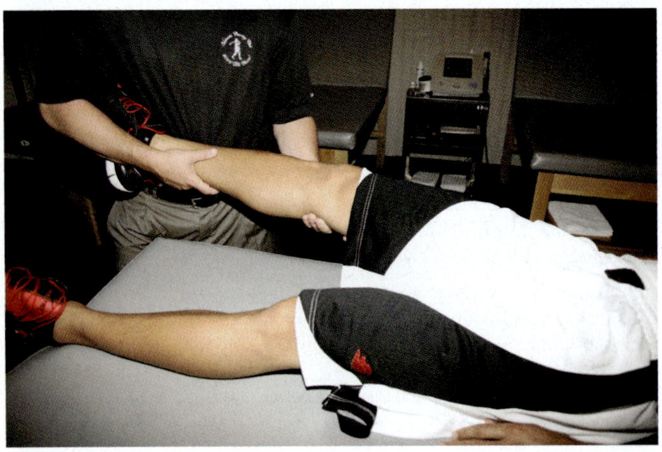

Figure 25.4. Hip distraction mobilization.

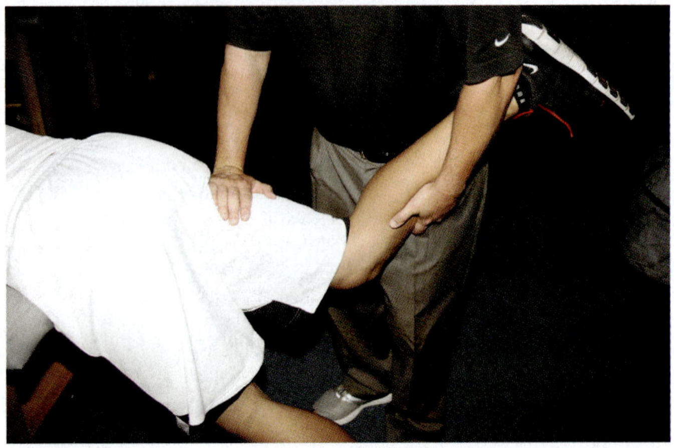

Figure 25.5. Hip posterior–anterior mobilization.

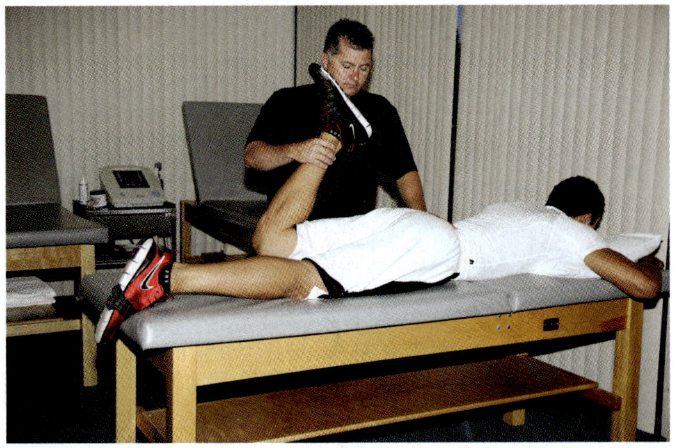

Figure 25.6. Prone knee bent to stretch hip flexors and quadriceps.

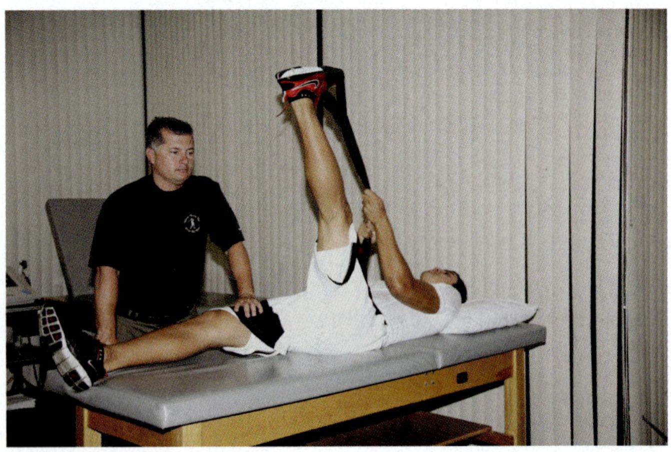

Figure 25.7. Hamstring stretch and opposite side hip flexor stretch.

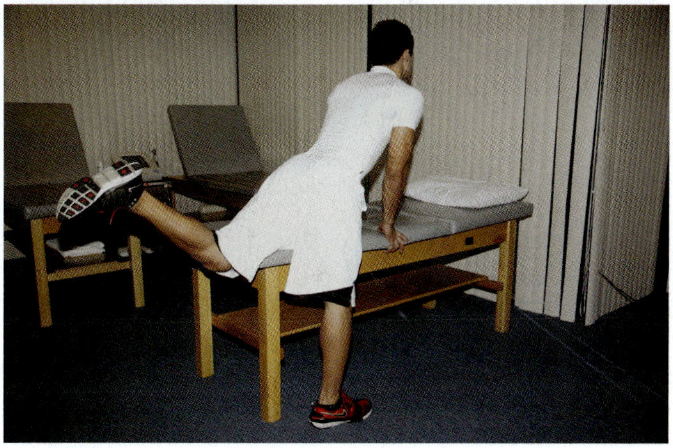

Figure 25.8. Standing hip flexor stretch.

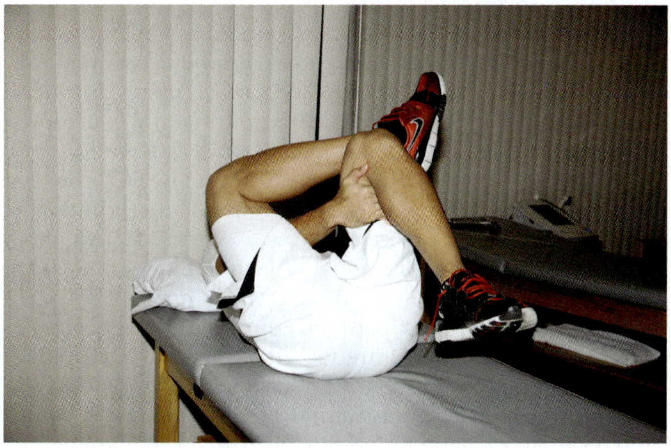

Figure 25.9. Gluteal stretch.

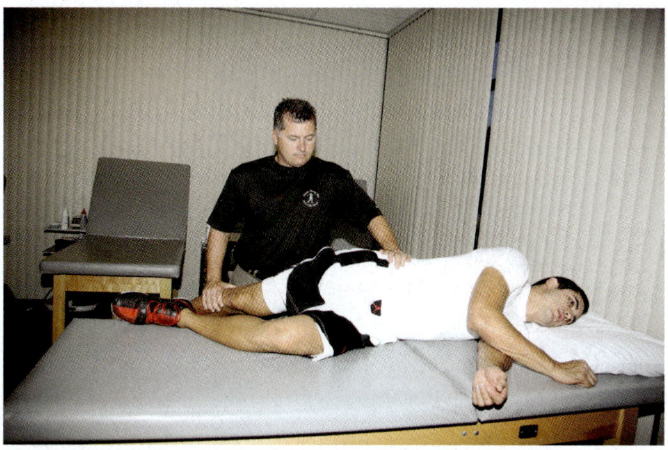

Figure 25.10. Tensor fascia latae/abductor stretch.

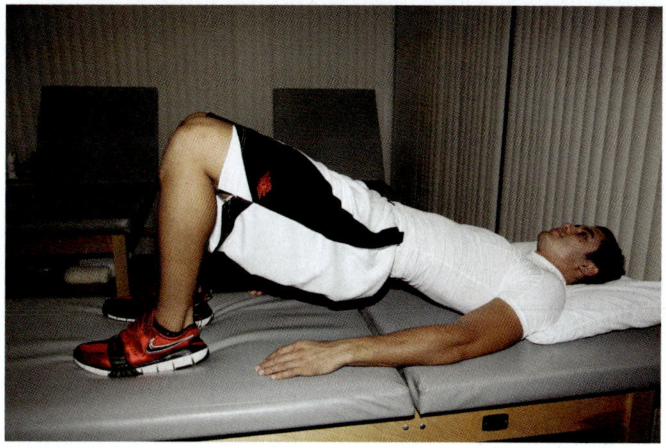

Figure 25.11. Bilateral bridging.

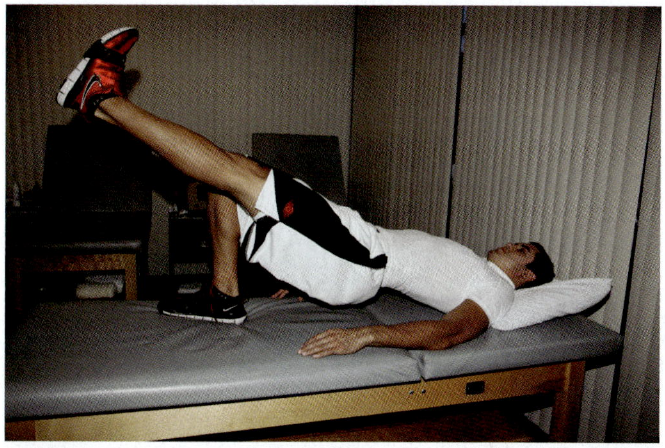

Figure 25.12. Unilateral bridging.

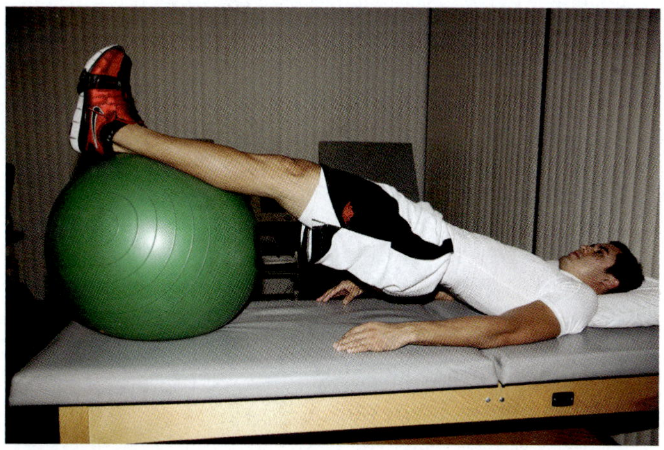

Figure 25.13. Bridging over ball.

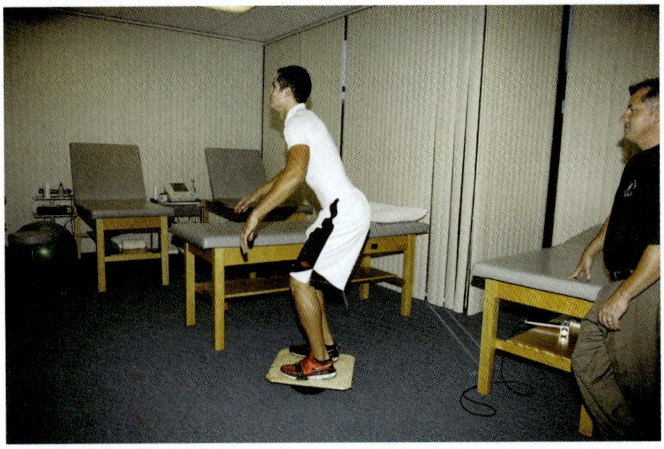

Figure 25.14. Bilateral balance on balance board.

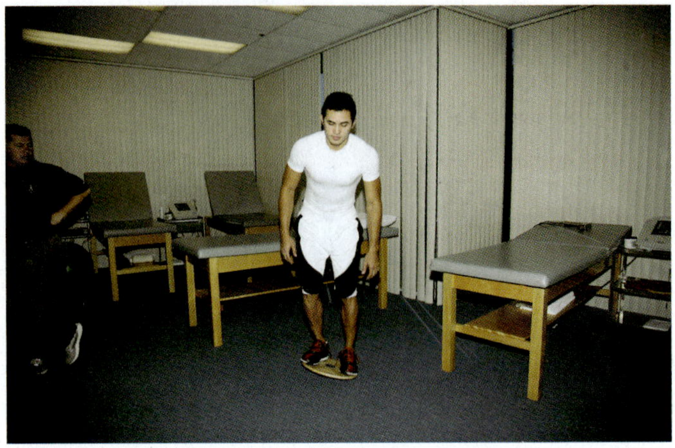

Figure 25.16. Bilateral balance on balance disc.

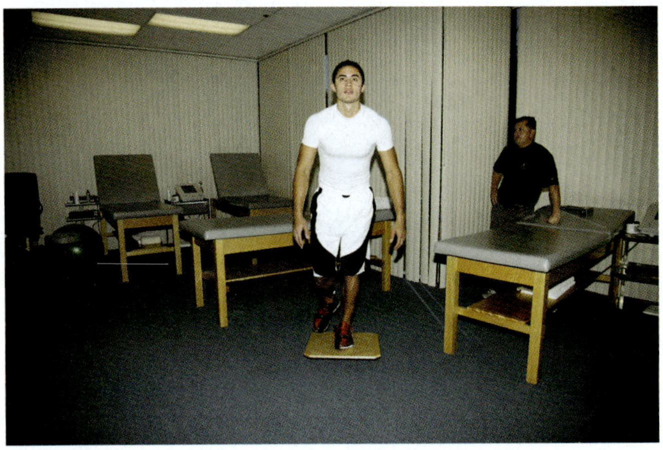

Figure 25.15. Single leg balance on balance board.

Figures 25.2–25.5 provide photographic examples of mobilizing the hip joint in multiple planes in order to prevent capsular contracture and reduce postoperative pain. Hip mobilization may be introduced as early as 2 weeks if performed cautiously. Figures 25.6–25.10 demonstrate stretching techniques of the hip musculature. Restoring muscles to normal flexibility improves the length–tension relationship that is necessary for efficient muscle contraction and strengthening. Furthermore, it allows for normal hip motion in gait and facilitates more dynamic movement needed for higher level activity, recreation, and sport. Lastly, Figures 25.11–25.16 provide examples of hip and pelvis strengthening statically and dynamically. Bridging is an important exercise in restoring pelvic stability, gluteal strength, and trunk strength. Progression of this exercise includes one leg bridging and dynamic bridging on an exercise ball. Balance can be retrained on multiple sorts of balance boards or dynamic surfaces in order to improve dynamic strength and pelvic stability. Progressions include balance on one leg and multiplanar surfaces.

Index

Page numbers followed by an "f" indicate figures; those followed by a "t" denote tables.